Physiology

FIFTH EDITION

Linda S. Costanzo, PhD

Professor of Physiology and Biophysics
Virginia Commonwealth University School of Medicine
Richmond, Virginia

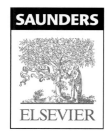

SAUNDERS

ELSEVIER

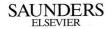

SAUNDERS
ELSEVIER

1600 John F. Kennedy Blvd.
Ste. 1800
Philadelphia, PA 19103-2899

PHYSIOLOGY
Copyright © 2014 by Saunders, an imprint of Elsevier Inc.

ISBN: 978-1-4557-0847-5

Notices

Previous editions copyrighted 2010, 2006, 2002, 1998

ISBN: 978-1-4557-0847-5

Senior Content Strategist: Elyse O'Grady
Content Development Specialist: Andrea Vosburgh
Publishing Services Manager: Patricia Tannian
Senior Project Manager: John Casey
Design Manager: Louis Forgione
Illustrator: Matt Chansky

Printed in China

Last digit is the print number: 9 8 7 6 5 4 3 2 1

Working together
to grow libraries in
developing countries

www.elsevier.com • www.bookaid.org

To
Heinz Valtin and **Arthur C. Guyton,**
who have written so well for students of physiology

Richard, Dan, Rebecca, Sheila, Elise, and **Max,**
who make everything worthwhile

Preface

Physiology is the foundation of medical practice. A firm grasp of its principles is essential for the medical student and the practicing physician. This book is intended for students of medicine and related disciplines who are engaged in the study of physiology. It can be used either as a companion to lectures and syllabi in discipline-based curricula or as a primary source in integrated or problem-based curricula. For advanced students, the book can serve as a reference in pathophysiology courses and in clinical clerkships.

In the fifth edition of this book, as in the previous editions, the important concepts in physiology are covered at the organ system and cellular levels. Chapters 1 and 2 present the underlying principles of cellular physiology and the autonomic nervous system. Chapters 3 through 10 present the major organ systems: neurophysiology and cardiovascular, respiratory, renal, acid-base, gastrointestinal, endocrine, and reproductive physiology. The relationships between organ systems are emphasized to underscore the integrative mechanisms for homeostasis.

This edition includes the following features designed to facilitate the study of physiology:

◆ **Text** that is easy to read and concise: Clear headings orient the student to the organization and hierarchy of the material. Complex physiologic information is presented systematically, logically, and step-wise. When a process occurs in a specific sequence, the steps are numbered in the text and often correlate with numbers shown in a figure. Bullets are used to separate and highlight the features of a process. Rhetorical questions are posed throughout the text to anticipate the questions that students may be asking; by first contemplating and then answering these questions, students learn to explain difficult concepts and rationalize unexpected or paradoxical findings. References at the end of each chapter direct the student to monographs, texts, review articles, and classic papers that offer further detail or historical perspective. Chapter summaries provide a brief overview.

◆ **Tables and illustrations** that can be used in concert with the text or, because they are designed to stand alone, as a review: The tables summarize, organize, and make comparisons. Examples are (1) a table that compares the gastrointestinal hormones with respect to hormone family, site of and stimuli for secretion, and hormone actions; (2) a table that compares the pathophysiologic features of disorders of Ca^{2+} homeostasis; and (3) a table that compares the features of the action potential in different cardiac tissues. The illustrations are clearly labeled, often with main headings, and include simple diagrams, complex diagrams with numbered steps, and flow charts.

◆ **Equations and sample problems** that are integrated into the text: All terms and units in equations are defined, and each equation is restated in words to place it in a physiologic context. Sample problems are followed by complete numerical solutions and explanations that guide the student through the proper steps in reasoning; by following the steps provided, students acquire the skills and confidence to solve similar or related problems.

◆ **Clinical physiology** presented in boxes: Each box features a fictitious patient with a classic disorder. The clinical findings and proposed treatment are explained in terms of underlying physiologic principles. An integrative approach to the patient is used to emphasize the relationships between organ systems. For example, the case of type I diabetes mellitus involves a disorder not only of the endocrine system but also of the renal, acid-base, respiratory, and cardiovascular systems.

◆ **Practice questions** in "Challenge Yourself" sections at the end of each chapter: Practice questions, which are designed for short answers (a word, a phrase, or a numerical solution), challenge the student to apply principles and concepts in problem solving rather than to recall isolated facts. The questions are posed in varying formats and are given in random order. They will be most helpful when used as a tool after studying each chapter and without referring to the text. In that way, the student can confirm his or her understanding of the material and can determine areas of weakness. Answers are provided at the end of the book.

◆ **Abbreviations and normal values** presented in appendices. As students refer to and use these common abbreviations and values throughout the book, they will find that they become second nature.

This book embodies three beliefs that I hold about teaching: (1) even complex information can be transmitted clearly if the presentation is systematic, logical, and presented step-wise; (2) the presentation can be just as effective in print as in person; and (3) beginning medical students wish for nonreference teaching materials that are accurate and didactically strong but without the details that primarily concern experts. In essence, a book can "teach" if the teacher's voice is present, if the material is carefully selected to include essential information, and if great care is paid to logic and sequence. This text offers a down-to-earth and professional presentation written *to* students and *for* students.

I hope that the readers of this book enjoy their study of physiology. Those who learn its principles well will be rewarded throughout their professional careers!

Linda S. Costanzo

Acknowledgments

I gratefully acknowledge the contributions of Elyse O'Grady, Andrea Vosburgh, and John Casey at Elsevier in preparing the fifth edition of *Physiology*. The artist, Matthew Chansky, revised existing figures and created new figures—all of which beautifully complement the text.

Colleagues at Virginia Commonwealth University have faithfully answered my questions, especially Drs. Clive Baumgarten, Diomedes Logothetis, Roland Pittman, and Raphael Witorsch. Sincere thanks also go to the medical students worldwide who have generously written to me about their experiences with earlier editions of the book.

My husband, Richard, our children, Dan and Rebecca, our daughter-in-law, Sheila, and our grandchildren, Elise and Max, have provided enthusiastic support and unqualified love, which give the book its spirit.

Contents

Cellular Physiology

Understanding the functions of the organ systems requires profound knowledge of basic cellular mechanisms. Although each organ system differs in its overall function, all are undergirded by a common set of physiologic principles.

The following basic principles of physiology are introduced in this chapter: body fluids, with particular emphasis on the differences in composition of intracellular fluid and extracellular fluid; creation of these concentration differences by transport processes in cell membranes; the origin of the electrical potential difference across cell membranes, particularly in excitable cells such as nerve and muscle; generation of action potentials and their propagation in excitable cells; transmission of information between cells across synapses and the role of neurotransmitters; and the mechanisms that couple the action potentials to contraction in muscle cells.

These principles of cellular physiology constitute a set of recurring and interlocking themes. Once these principles are understood, they can be applied and integrated into the function of each organ system.

VOLUME AND COMPOSITION OF BODY FLUIDS

Distribution of Water in the Body Fluid Compartments

In the human body, water constitutes a high proportion of body weight. The total amount of fluid or water is called **total body water,** which accounts for 50% to 70% of body weight. For example, a 70-kilogram (kg) man whose total body water is 65% of his body weight has 45.5 kg or 45.5 liters (L) of water (1 kg water ≈ 1 L water). In general, total body water correlates inversely with body fat. Thus, total body water is a higher percentage of body weight when body fat is low and a lower percentage when body fat is high. Because females have a higher percentage of adipose tissue than males, they tend to have less body water. The distribution of water among body fluid compartments is described briefly in this chapter and in greater detail in Chapter 6.

Total body water is distributed between two major body fluid compartments: intracellular fluid (ICF) and extracellular fluid (ECF) (Fig. 1-1). The **ICF** is contained within the cells and is two thirds of total body water; the **ECF** is outside the cells and is one third of total body water. ICF and ECF are separated by the cell membranes.

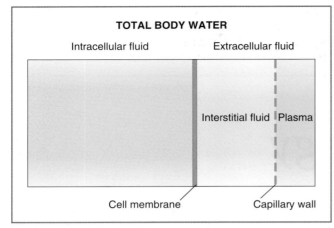

TOTAL BODY WATER

Intracellular fluid   Extracellular fluid

Interstitial fluid | Plasma

Cell membrane   Capillary wall

Figure 1–1   Body fluid compartments.

ECF is further divided into two compartments: plasma and interstitial fluid. **Plasma** is the fluid circulating in the blood vessels and is the smaller of the two ECF subcompartments. **Interstitial fluid** is the fluid that actually bathes the cells and is the larger of the two subcompartments. Plasma and interstitial fluid are separated by the capillary wall. Interstitial fluid is an **ultrafiltrate** of plasma, formed by filtration processes across the capillary wall. Because the capillary wall is virtually impermeable to large molecules such as plasma proteins, interstitial fluid contains little, if any, protein.

The method for estimating the volume of the body fluid compartments is presented in Chapter 6.

Composition of Body Fluid Compartments

The composition of the body fluids is not uniform. ICF and ECF have vastly different concentrations of various solutes. There are also certain predictable differences in solute concentrations between plasma and interstitial fluid that occur as a result of the exclusion of protein from interstitial fluid.

Units for Measuring Solute Concentrations

Typically, **amounts** of solute are expressed in moles, equivalents, or osmoles. Likewise, **concentrations** of solutes are expressed in moles per liter (mol/L), equivalents per liter (Eq/L), or osmoles per liter (Osm/L). In biologic solutions, concentrations of solutes are usually quite low and are expressed in *milli*moles per liter (mmol/L), *milli*equivalents per liter (mEq/L), or *milli*osmoles per liter (mOsm/L).

One **mole** is 6×10^{23} molecules of a substance. One **millimole** is 1/1000 or 10^{-3} moles. A glucose concentration of 1 mmol/L has 1×10^{-3} moles of glucose in 1 L of solution.

An **equivalent** is used to describe the amount of charged (ionized) solute and is the number of moles of

the solute multiplied by its valence. For example, one mole of potassium chloride (KCl) in solution dissociates into one equivalent of potassium (K^+) and one equivalent of chloride (Cl^-). Likewise, one mole of calcium chloride ($CaCl_2$) in solution dissociates into *two* equivalents of calcium (Ca^{2+}) and *two* equivalents of chloride (Cl^-); accordingly, a Ca^{2+} concentration of 1 mmol/L corresponds to 2 mEq/L.

One **osmole** is the number of particles into which a solute dissociates in solution. **Osmolarity** is the concentration of particles in solution expressed as osmoles per liter. If a solute does not dissociate in solution (e.g., glucose), then its osmolarity is equal to its molarity. If a solute dissociates into more than one particle in solution (e.g., NaCl), then its osmolarity equals the molarity multiplied by the number of particles in solution. For example, a solution containing 1 mmol/L NaCl is 2 mOsm/L because NaCl dissociates into two particles.

pH is a logarithmic term that is used to express hydrogen (H^+) concentration. Because the H^+ concentration of body fluids is very low (e.g., 40×10^{-9} Eq/L in arterial blood), it is more conveniently expressed as a logarithmic term, pH. The negative sign means that pH decreases as the concentration of H^+ increases, and pH increases as the concentration of H^+ decreases. Thus,

$$pH = -\log_{10}[H^+]$$

SAMPLE PROBLEM. Two men, Subject A and Subject B, have disorders that cause excessive acid production in the body. The laboratory reports the acidity of Subject A's blood in terms of [H^+] and the acidity of Subject B's blood in terms of pH. Subject A has an arterial [H^+] of 65×10^{-9} Eq/L, and Subject B has an arterial pH of 7.3. *Which subject has the higher concentration of H^+ in his blood?*

SOLUTION. To compare the acidity of the blood of each subject, convert the [H^+] for Subject A to pH as follows:

$$pH = -\log_{10}[H^+]$$
$$= -\log_{10}(65 \times 10^{-9} \text{ Eq/L})$$
$$= -\log_{10}(6.5 \times 10^{-8} \text{ Eq/L})$$
$$\log_{10} 6.5 = 0.81$$
$$\log_{10} 10^{-8} = -8.0$$
$$\log_{10} 6.5 \times 10^{-8} = 0.81 + (-8.0) = -7.19$$
$$pH = -(-7.19) = 7.19$$

Thus, Subject A has a blood pH of 7.19 computed from the [H^+], and Subject B has a reported blood pH of 7.3. Subject A has a lower blood pH, reflecting a higher [H^+] and a more acidic condition.

Electroneutrality of Body Fluid Compartments

Each body fluid compartment must obey the **principle of macroscopic electroneutrality**; that is, each compartment must have the same concentration, in mEq/L, of positive charges (**cations**) as of negative charges (**anions**). There can be no more cations than anions, or vice versa. Even when there is a potential difference across the cell membrane, charge balance still is maintained in the bulk (macroscopic) solutions. Because potential differences are created by the separation of just a few charges adjacent to the membrane, this small separation of charges is not enough to measurably change bulk concentrations.

Composition of Intracellular Fluid and Extracellular Fluid

The compositions of ICF and ECF are strikingly different, as shown in Table 1-1. The major cation in **ECF** is sodium (Na^+), and the balancing anions are chloride (Cl^-) and bicarbonate (HCO_3^-). The major cations in **ICF** are potassium (K^+) and magnesium (Mg^{2+}), and the balancing anions are proteins and organic phosphates. Other notable differences in composition involve Ca^{2+} and pH. Typically, ICF has a very low concentration of ionized Ca^{2+} ($\approx 10^{-7}$ mol/L), whereas the Ca^{2+} concentration in ECF is higher by approximately four orders of magnitude. ICF is more acidic (has a lower pH) than ECF. Thus, substances found in high concentration in ECF are found in low concentration in ICF, and vice versa.

Remarkably, given all of the concentration differences for individual solutes, the total solute concentration (**osmolarity**) is the same in ICF and ECF. This equality is achieved because water flows freely across cell membranes. Any transient differences in osmolarity that occur between ICF and ECF are quickly dissipated by water movement into or out of cells to reestablish the equality.

Creation of Concentration Differences across Cell Membranes

The differences in solute concentration across cell membranes are created and maintained by energy-consuming transport mechanisms in the cell membranes.

The best known of these transport mechanisms is the Na^+-K^+ ATPase (Na^+-K^+ pump), which transports Na^+ from ICF to ECF and simultaneously transports K^+ from ECF to ICF. Both Na^+ and K^+ are transported against their respective electrochemical gradients; therefore, an energy source, adenosine triphosphate (ATP), is required. The Na^+-K^+ ATPase is responsible for creating the large concentration gradients for Na^+ and K^+ that exist across cell membranes (i.e., the low intracellular Na^+ concentration and the high intracellular K^+ concentration).

Similarly, the intracellular Ca^{2+} concentration is maintained at a level much lower than the extracellular Ca^{2+} concentration. This concentration difference is established, in part, by a cell membrane Ca^{2+} ATPase that pumps Ca^{2+} against its electrochemical gradient. Like the Na^+-K^+ ATPase, the Ca^{2+} ATPase uses ATP as a direct energy source.

In addition to the transporters that use ATP directly, other transporters establish concentration differences across the cell membrane by utilizing the transmembrane Na^+ concentration gradient (established by the Na^+-K^+ ATPase) as an energy source. These transporters create concentration gradients for glucose, amino acids, Ca^{2+}, and H^+ without the direct utilization of ATP.

Clearly, cell membranes have the machinery to establish large concentration gradients. However, if cell membranes were freely permeable to all solutes, these gradients would quickly dissipate. Thus, it is critically important that cell membranes are *not* freely permeable to all substances but, rather, have selective permeabilities that maintain the concentration gradients established by energy-consuming transport processes.

Directly or indirectly, the differences in composition between ICF and ECF underlie every important physiologic function, as the following examples illustrate: (1) The resting membrane potential of nerve and muscle critically depends on the difference in concentration of K^+ across the cell membrane; (2) The upstroke of the action potential of these same excitable cells depends on the differences in Na^+ concentration across the cell membrane; (3) Excitation-contraction coupling in muscle cells depends on the differences in Ca^{2+} concentration across the cell membrane and the membrane

Table 1–1 Approximate Compositions of Extracellular and Intracellular Fluids

Substance and Units	Extracellular Fluid	Intracellular Fluid*
Na^+ (mEq/L)	140	14
K^+ (mEq/L)	4	120
Ca^{2+}, ionized (mEq/L)	2.5[†]	1×10^{-4}
Cl^- (mEq/L)	105	10
HCO_3^- (mEq/L)	24	10
pH[‡]	7.4	7.1
Osmolarity (mOsm/L)	290	290

*The major anions of intracellular fluid are proteins and organic phosphates.

[†]The corresponding total $[Ca^{2+}]$ in extracellular fluid is 5 mEq/L or 10 mg/dL.

[‡]pH is $-\log_{10}$ of the $[H^+]$; pH 7.4 corresponds to $[H^+]$ of 40×10^{-9} Eq/L.

of the sarcoplasmic reticulum; and (4) Absorption of essential nutrients depends on the transmembrane Na^+ concentration gradient (e.g., glucose absorption in the small intestine or glucose reabsorption in the renal proximal tubule).

Concentration Differences between Plasma and Interstitial Fluids

As previously discussed, ECF consists of two subcompartments: interstitial fluid and plasma. The most significant difference in composition between these two compartments is the presence of proteins (e.g., albumin) in the plasma compartment. Plasma proteins do not readily cross capillary walls because of their large molecular size and, therefore, are excluded from interstitial fluid.

The exclusion of proteins from interstitial fluid has secondary consequences. The plasma proteins are negatively charged, and this negative charge causes a redistribution of small, permeant cations and anions across the capillary wall, called a **Gibbs-Donnan equilibrium.** The redistribution can be explained as follows: The plasma compartment contains the impermeant, negatively charged proteins. Because of the requirement for electroneutrality, the plasma compartment must have a slightly lower concentration of small anions (e.g., Cl^-) and a slightly higher concentration of small cations (e.g., Na^+ and K^+) than that of interstitial fluid. The small concentration difference for permeant ions is expressed in the **Gibbs-Donnan ratio,** which gives the plasma concentration relative to the interstitial fluid concentration for anions and interstitial fluid relative to plasma for cations. For example, the Cl^- concentration in plasma is slightly less than the Cl^- concentration in interstitial fluid (due to the effect of the impermeant plasma proteins); the Gibbs-Donnan ratio for Cl^- is 0.95, meaning that $[Cl^-]_{plasma}/[Cl^-]_{interstitial\ fluid}$ equals 0.95. For Na^+, the Gibbs-Donnan ratio is also 0.95, but Na^+, being positively charged, is oriented the opposite way, and $[Na^+]_{interstitial\ fluid}/[Na^+]_{plasma}$ equals 0.95. Generally, these minor differences in concentration for small cations and anions are ignored.

CHARACTERISTICS OF CELL MEMBRANES

Cell membranes are composed primarily of lipids and proteins. The lipid component consists of phospholipids, cholesterol, and glycolipids and is responsible for the high permeability of cell membranes to lipid-soluble substances such as carbon dioxide, oxygen, fatty acids, and steroid hormones. The lipid component of cell membranes is also responsible for the low permeability of cell membranes to water-soluble substances such as

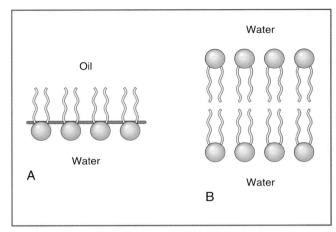

Figure 1–2 **Orientation of phospholipid molecules at oil and water interfaces.** Depicted are the orientation of phospholipid at an oil-water interface **(A)** and the orientation of phospholipid in a bilayer, as occurs in the cell membrane **(B)**.

ions, glucose, and amino acids. The protein component of the membrane consists of transporters, enzymes, hormone receptors, cell-surface antigens, and ion and water channels.

Phospholipid Component of Cell Membranes

Phospholipids consist of a phosphorylated glycerol backbone ("head") and two fatty acid "tails" (Fig. 1-2). The glycerol backbone is **hydrophilic** (water soluble), and the fatty acid tails are **hydrophobic** (water insoluble). Thus, phospholipid molecules have both hydrophilic and hydrophobic properties and are called **amphipathic.** At an oil-water interface (see Fig. 1-2A), molecules of phospholipids form a monolayer and orient themselves so that the glycerol backbone dissolves in the water phase and the fatty acid tails dissolve in the oil phase. In cell membranes (see Fig. 1-2B), phospholipids orient so that the lipid-soluble fatty acid tails face each other and the water-soluble glycerol heads point away from each other, dissolving in the aqueous solutions of the ICF or ECF. This orientation creates a **lipid bilayer.**

Protein Component of Cell Membranes

Proteins in cell membranes may be either integral or peripheral, depending on whether they span the membrane or whether they are present on only one side. The distribution of proteins in a phospholipid bilayer is illustrated in the **fluid mosaic model,** shown in Figure 1-3.

♦ **Integral membrane proteins** are embedded in, and anchored to, the cell membrane by **hydrophobic**

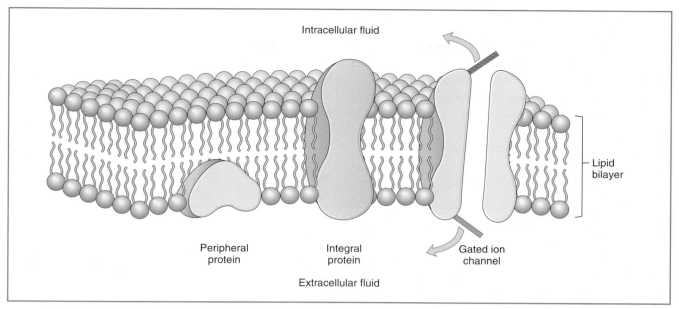

Figure 1–3 **Fluid mosaic model for cell membranes.**

interactions. To remove an integral protein from the cell membrane, its attachments to the lipid bilayer must be disrupted (e.g., by detergents). Some integral proteins are **transmembrane proteins,** meaning they span the lipid bilayer one or more times; thus, transmembrane proteins are in contact with both ECF and ICF. Examples of transmembrane integral proteins are ligand-binding receptors (e.g., for hormones or neurotransmitters), transport proteins (e.g., Na$^+$-K$^+$ ATPase), pores, ion channels, cell adhesion molecules, and GTP-binding proteins (G proteins). Other integral proteins are embedded in the membrane but do not span it.

♦ **Peripheral membrane proteins** are *not* embedded in the membrane and are *not* covalently bound to cell membrane components. They are loosely attached to either the intracellular or extracellular side of the cell membrane by **electrostatic interactions** (e.g., with integral proteins) and can be removed with mild treatments that disrupt ionic or hydrogen bonds. One example of a peripheral membrane protein is **ankyrin,** which "anchors" the cytoskeleton of red blood cells to an integral membrane transport protein, the Cl$^-$-HCO$_3^-$ exchanger (also called band 3 protein).

TRANSPORT ACROSS CELL MEMBRANES

Several types of mechanisms are responsible for transport of substances across cell membranes (Table 1-2).

Substances may be transported down an electrochemical gradient (downhill) or against an electrochemical gradient (uphill). **Downhill** transport occurs by diffusion, either simple or facilitated, and requires no input of metabolic energy. **Uphill** transport occurs by active transport, which may be primary or secondary. Primary and secondary active transport processes are distinguished by their energy source. Primary active transport requires a *direct* input of metabolic energy; secondary active transport utilizes an *indirect* input of metabolic energy.

Further distinctions among transport mechanisms are based on whether the process involves a protein carrier. Simple diffusion is the only form of transport that is *not* carrier mediated. Facilitated diffusion, primary active transport, and secondary active transport all involve integral membrane proteins and are called **carrier-mediated transport.** All forms of carrier-mediated transport share the following three features: saturation, stereospecificity, and competition.

♦ **Saturation.** Saturability is based on the concept that carrier proteins have a limited number of binding sites for the solute. Figure 1-4 shows the relationship between the rate of carrier-mediated transport and solute concentration. At low solute concentrations, many binding sites are available and the rate of transport increases steeply as the concentration increases. However, at high solute concentrations, the available binding sites become scarce and the rate of transport levels off. Finally, when all of the binding sites are occupied, saturation is achieved at a point called the **transport maximum,** or **T$_m$**. The

Table 1-2 Summary of Membrane Transport

Type of Transport	Active or Passive	Carrier-Mediated	Uses Metabolic Energy	Dependent on Na⁺ Gradient
Simple diffusion	Passive; downhill	No	No	No
Facilitated diffusion	Passive; downhill	Yes	No	No
Primary active transport	Active; uphill	Yes	Yes; direct	No
Cotransport	Secondary active*	Yes	Yes; indirect	Yes (solutes move in same direction as Na⁺ across cell membrane)
Countertransport	Secondary active*	Yes	Yes; indirect	Yes (solutes move in opposite direction as Na⁺ across cell membrane)

*Na⁺ is transported downhill and one or more solutes are transported uphill.

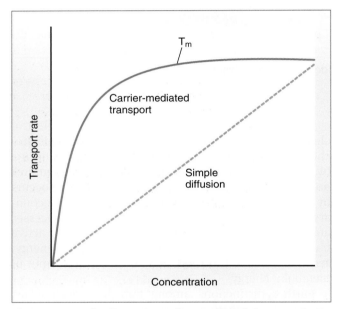

Figure 1-4 Kinetics of carrier-mediated transport. T_m, Transport maximum.

kinetics of carrier-mediated transport are similar to Michaelis-Menten enzyme kinetics—both involve proteins with a limited number of binding sites. (The T_m is analogous to the V_{max} of enzyme kinetics.) T_m-limited glucose transport in the proximal tubule of the kidney is an example of saturable transport.

♦ **Stereospecificity.** The binding sites for solute on the transport proteins are stereospecific. For example, the transporter for glucose in the renal proximal tubule recognizes and transports the natural isomer D-glucose, but it does not recognize or transport the unnatural isomer L-glucose. In contrast, simple diffusion does not distinguish between the two glucose isomers because no protein carrier is involved.

♦ **Competition.** Although the binding sites for transported solutes are quite specific, they may recognize, bind, and even transport chemically related solutes. For example, the transporter for glucose is specific for D-glucose, but it also recognizes and transports a closely related sugar, D-galactose. Therefore, the presence of D-galactose inhibits the transport of D-glucose by occupying some of the binding sites and making them unavailable for glucose.

Simple Diffusion

Diffusion of Nonelectrolytes

Simple diffusion occurs as a result of the random thermal motion of molecules, as shown in Figure 1-5. Two solutions, A and B, are separated by a membrane that is permeable to the solute. The solute concentration in A is initially twice that of B. The solute molecules are in constant motion, with equal probability that a given molecule will cross the membrane to the other solution. However, because there are twice as many solute molecules in Solution A as in Solution B, there will be greater movement of molecules from A to B than from B to A. In other words, there will be **net diffusion** of the solute from A to B, which will continue until the solute concentrations of the two solutions become equal (although the random movement of molecules will go on forever).

Net diffusion of the solute is called **flux,** or **flow (J),** and depends on the following variables: size of the concentration gradient, partition coefficient, diffusion coefficient, thickness of the membrane, and surface area available for diffusion.

CONCENTRATION GRADIENT ($C_A - C_B$)

The concentration gradient across the membrane is the driving force for net diffusion. The larger the difference in solute concentration between Solution A and

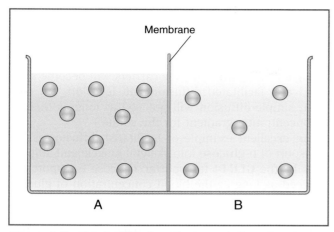

Figure 1–5 Simple diffusion. The two solutions, **A** and **B**, are separated by a membrane, which is permeable to the solute (*circles*). Solution A initially contains a higher concentration of the solute than does Solution B.

Solution B, the greater the driving force and the greater the net diffusion. It also follows that, if the concentrations in the two solutions are equal, there is no driving force and no net diffusion.

PARTITION COEFFICIENT (K)

The partition coefficient, by definition, describes the solubility of a solute in oil relative to its solubility in water. The greater the relative solubility in oil, the higher the partition coefficient and the more easily the solute can dissolve in the cell membrane's lipid bilayer. Nonpolar solutes tend to be soluble in oil and have high values for partition coefficient, whereas polar solutes tend to be insoluble in oil and have low values for partition coefficient. The partition coefficient can be measured by adding the solute to a mixture of olive oil and water and then measuring its concentration in the oil phase relative to its concentration in the water phase. Thus,

$$K = \frac{\text{Concentration in olive oil}}{\text{Concentration in water}}$$

DIFFUSION COEFFICIENT (D)

The diffusion coefficient depends on such characteristics as size of the solute molecule and the viscosity of the medium. It is defined by the Stokes-Einstein equation (see later). The diffusion coefficient correlates *inversely* with the molecular radius of the solute and the viscosity of the medium. Thus, small solutes in nonviscous solutions have the largest diffusion coefficients and diffuse most readily; large solutes in viscous solutions have the smallest diffusion coefficients and diffuse least readily. Thus,

$$D = \frac{KT}{6\pi r\eta}$$

where

D = Diffusion coefficient
K = Boltzmann's constant
T = Absolute temperature (K)
r = Molecular radius
η = Viscosity of the medium

THICKNESS OF THE MEMBRANE (ΔX)

The thicker the cell membrane, the greater the distance the solute must diffuse and the lower the rate of diffusion.

SURFACE AREA (A)

The greater the surface area of membrane available, the higher the rate of diffusion. For example, lipid-soluble gases such as oxygen and carbon dioxide have particularly high rates of diffusion across cell membranes. These high rates can be attributed to the large surface area for diffusion provided by the lipid component of the membrane.

To simplify the description of diffusion, several of the previously cited characteristics can be combined into a single term called **permeability** (**P**). Permeability includes the partition coefficient, the diffusion coefficient, and the membrane thickness. Thus,

$$P = \frac{KD}{\Delta x}$$

By combining several variables into permeability, the rate of net diffusion is simplified to the following expression:

$$J = PA(C_A - C_B)$$

where

J = Net rate of diffusion (mmol/sec)
P = Permeability (cm/sec)
A = Surface area for diffusion (cm^2)
C_A = Concentration in Solution A (mmol/L)
C_B = Concentration in Solution B (mmol/L)

Diffusion of Electrolytes

Thus far, the discussion concerning diffusion has assumed that the solute is a nonelectrolyte (i.e., it is uncharged). However, if the diffusing solute is an **ion** or an **electrolyte,** there are two additional consequences of the presence of charge on the solute.

First, if there is a potential difference across the membrane, that potential difference will alter the net rate of diffusion of a charged solute. (A potential difference does not alter the rate of diffusion of a nonelectrolyte.) For example, the diffusion of K$^+$ ions will be

SAMPLE PROBLEM. Solution A and Solution B are separated by a membrane whose permeability to urea is 2×10^{-5} cm/sec and whose surface area is 1 cm². The concentration of urea in A is 10 mg/mL, and the concentration of urea in B is 1 mg/mL. The partition coefficient for urea is 10^{-3}, as measured in an oil-water mixture. *What are the initial rate and direction of net diffusion of urea?*

SOLUTION. Note that the partition coefficient is extraneous information because the value for permeability, which already includes the partition coefficient, is given. Net flux can be calculated by substituting the following values in the equation for net diffusion: Assume that 1 mL of water = 1 cm³. Thus,

$$J = PA(C_A - C_B)$$

where

$J = 2 \times 10^{-5}$ cm/sec $\times 1$ cm² $\times (10$ mg/mL $- 1$ mg/mL$)$

$J = 2 \times 10^{-5}$ cm/sec $\times 1$ cm² $\times (10$ mg/cm³ $- 1$ mg/cm³$)$

$\quad = 1.8 \times 10^{-4}$ mg/sec

The *magnitude* of net flux has been calculated as 1.8×10^{-4} mg/sec. The *direction* of net flux can be determined intuitively because net flux will occur from the area of high concentration (Solution A) to the area of low concentration (Solution B). Net diffusion will continue until the urea concentrations of the two solutions become equal, at which point the driving force will be zero.

slowed if K^+ is diffusing into an area of positive charge, and it will be accelerated if K^+ is diffusing into an area of negative charge. This effect of potential difference can either add to or negate the effects of differences in concentrations, depending on the orientation of the potential difference and the charge on the diffusing ion. If the concentration gradient and the charge effect are oriented in the same direction across the membrane, they will combine; if they are oriented in opposite directions, they may cancel each other out.

Second, when a charged solute diffuses down a concentration gradient, that diffusion can *itself* generate a potential difference across a membrane called a **diffusion potential.** The concept of diffusion potential will be discussed more fully in a following section.

Facilitated Diffusion

Like simple diffusion, facilitated diffusion occurs down an electrochemical potential gradient; thus, it requires no input of metabolic energy. Unlike simple diffusion, however, facilitated diffusion uses a membrane carrier and exhibits all the characteristics of carrier-mediated transport: saturation, stereospecificity, and competition. At low solute concentration, facilitated diffusion typically proceeds faster than simple diffusion (i.e., is facilitated) because of the function of the carrier. However, at higher concentrations, the carriers will become saturated and facilitated diffusion will level off. (In contrast, simple diffusion will proceed as long as there is a concentration gradient for the solute.)

An excellent example of facilitated diffusion is the transport of **D-glucose** into skeletal muscle and adipose cells by the **GLUT4** transporter. Glucose transport can proceed as long as the blood concentration of glucose is higher than the intracellular concentration of glucose and as long as the carriers are not saturated. Other monosaccharides such as D-galactose, 3-O-methyl glucose, and phlorizin competitively inhibit the transport of glucose because they bind to transport sites on the carrier. The competitive solute may itself be transported (e.g., D-galactose), or it may simply occupy the binding sites and prevent the attachment of glucose (e.g., phlorizin). As noted previously, the nonphysiologic stereoisomer, L-glucose, is not recognized by the carrier for facilitated diffusion and, therefore, is not bound or transported.

Primary Active Transport

In active transport, one or more solutes are moved against an electrochemical potential gradient (uphill). In other words, solute is moved from an area of low concentration (or low electrochemical potential) to an area of high concentration (or high electrochemical potential). Because movement of a solute *uphill* is work, metabolic energy in the form of ATP must be provided. In the process, ATP is hydrolyzed to adenosine diphosphate (ADP) and inorganic phosphate (P_i), releasing energy from the terminal high-energy phosphate bond of ATP. When the terminal phosphate is released, it is transferred to the transport protein, initiating a cycle of phosphorylation and dephosphorylation. When the ATP energy source is directly coupled to the transport process, it is called *primary* active transport. Three examples of primary active transport in physiologic systems are the Na^+-K^+ ATPase present in all cell membranes, the Ca^{2+} ATPase present in sarcoplasmic and endoplasmic reticulum, and the H^+-K^+ ATPase present in gastric parietal cells.

Na⁺-K⁺ ATPase (Na⁺-K⁺ Pump)

Na^+-K^+ ATPase is present in the membranes of all cells. It pumps Na^+ from ICF to ECF and K^+ from ECF to ICF (Fig. 1-6). Each ion moves against its respective electrochemical gradient. The stoichiometry can vary but, typically, for every three Na^+ ions pumped out of the cell, two K^+ ions are pumped into the cell. This stoichiometry of three Na^+ ions per two K^+ ions means that,

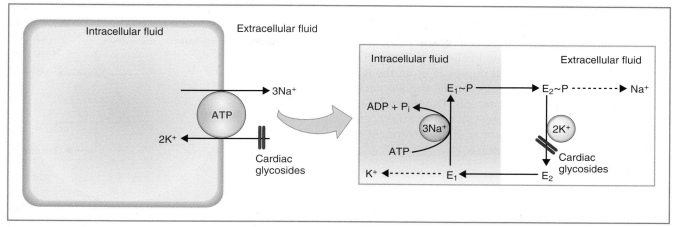

Figure 1–6   Na⁺-K⁺ pump of cell membranes. ADP, Adenosine diphosphate; ATP, adenosine triphosphate; E, Na⁺-K⁺ ATPase; E ~ P, phosphorylated Na⁺-K⁺ ATPase; P_i, inorganic phosphate.

for each cycle of the Na⁺-K⁺ ATPase, more positive charge is pumped out of the cell than is pumped into the cell. Thus, the process is termed **electrogenic** because it creates a charge separation and a potential difference. The Na⁺-K⁺ ATPase is responsible for maintaining concentration gradients for both Na⁺ and K⁺ across cell membranes, keeping the intracellular Na⁺ concentration low and the intracellular K⁺ concentration high.

The Na⁺-K⁺ ATPase consists of α and β subunits. The α subunit contains the ATPase activity, as well as the binding sites for the transported ions, Na⁺ and K⁺. The Na⁺-K⁺ ATPase switches between two major conformational states, E_1 and E_2. In the **E_1 state,** the binding sites for Na⁺ and K⁺ face the intracellular fluid and the enzyme has a high affinity for Na⁺. In the **E_2 state,** the binding sites for Na⁺ and K⁺ face the extracellular fluid and the enzyme has a high affinity for K⁺. The enzyme's ion-transporting function (i.e., pumping Na⁺ out of the cell and K⁺ into the cell) is based on cycling between the E_1 and E_2 states and is powered by ATP hydrolysis.

The **transport cycle** is illustrated in Figure 1-6. The cycle begins with the enzyme in the E_1 state, bound to ATP. In the E_1 state, the ion-binding sites face the intracellular fluid, and the enzyme has a high affinity for Na⁺; three Na⁺ ions bind, ATP is hydrolyzed, and the terminal phosphate of ATP is transferred to the enzyme, producing a high-energy state, $E_1 \sim P$. Now, a major conformational change occurs, and the enzyme switches from $E_1 \sim P$ to $E_2 \sim P$. In the E_2 state, the ion-binding sites face the extracellular fluid, the affinity for Na⁺ is low, and the affinity for K⁺ is high. The three Na⁺ ions are released from the enzyme to extracellular fluid, two K⁺ ions are bound, and inorganic phosphate is released from E_2. The enzyme now binds intracellular ATP, and another major conformational change occurs that returns the enzyme to the E_1 state; the two K⁺ ions

are released to intracellular fluid, and the enzyme is ready for another cycle.

Cardiac glycosides (e.g., **ouabain** and **digitalis**) are a class of drugs that inhibits Na⁺-K⁺ ATPase. Treatment with this class of drugs causes certain predictable changes in intracellular ionic concentration: The intracellular Na⁺ concentration will increase, and the intracellular K⁺ concentration will decrease. Cardiac glycosides inhibit the Na⁺-K⁺ATPase by binding to the $E_2 \sim P$ form near the K⁺-binding site on the extracellular side, thereby preventing the conversion of $E_2 \sim P$ back to E_1. By disrupting the cycle of phosphorylation-dephosphorylation, these drugs disrupt the entire enzyme cycle and its transport functions.

Ca²⁺ ATPase (Ca²⁺ Pump)

Most **cell (plasma) membranes** contain a Ca²⁺ ATPase, or plasma-membrane Ca²⁺ ATPase (**PMCA**), whose function is to extrude Ca²⁺ from the cell against an electrochemical gradient; one Ca²⁺ ion is extruded for each ATP hydrolyzed. PMCA is responsible, in part, for maintaining the very low intracellular Ca²⁺ concentration. In addition, the **sarcoplasmic reticulum** of muscle cells and the **endoplasmic reticulum** of other cells contain variants of Ca²⁺ ATPase that pump two Ca²⁺ ions (for each ATP hydrolyzed) from intracellular fluid into the interior of the sarcoplasmic or endoplasmic reticulum (i.e., Ca²⁺ sequestration). These variants are called sarcoplasmic and endoplasmic reticulum Ca²⁺ ATPase (**SERCA**). Ca²⁺ ATPase functions similarly to Na⁺-K⁺ ATPase, with E_1 and E_2 states that have, respectively, high and low affinities for Ca²⁺. For PMCA, the E_1 state binds Ca²⁺ on the intracellular side, a conformational change to the E_2 state occurs, and the E_2 state releases Ca²⁺ to extracellular fluid. For SERCA, the E_1 state binds Ca²⁺ on the intracellular side and the E_2 state releases Ca²⁺ to the lumen of the sarcoplasmic or endoplasmic reticulum.

H^+-K^+ ATPase (H^+-K^+ Pump)

H^+-K^+ ATPase is found in the parietal cells of the gastric mucosa and in the α-intercalated cells of the renal collecting duct. In the stomach, it pumps H^+ from the ICF of the parietal cells into the lumen of the stomach, where it acidifies the gastric contents. **Omeprazole,** an inhibitor of gastric H^+-K^+ ATPase, can be used therapeutically to reduce the secretion of H^+ in the treatment of some types of peptic ulcer disease.

Secondary Active Transport

Secondary active transport processes are those in which the transport of two or more solutes is coupled. One of the solutes, usually Na^+, moves down its electrochemical gradient (downhill), and the other solute moves against its electrochemical gradient (uphill). The downhill movement of Na^+ provides energy for the uphill movement of the other solute. Thus, metabolic energy, as ATP, is not used directly, but it is supplied indirectly in the Na^+ concentration gradient across the cell membrane. (The Na^+-K^+ ATPase, utilizing ATP, creates and maintains this Na^+ gradient.) The name *secondary* active transport, therefore, refers to the *indirect* utilization of ATP as an energy source.

Inhibition of the Na^+-K^+ ATPase (e.g., by treatment with ouabain) diminishes the transport of Na^+ from ICF to ECF, causing the intracellular Na^+ concentration to increase and thereby decreasing the size of the transmembrane Na^+ gradient. Thus, indirectly, all secondary active transport processes are diminished by inhibitors of the Na^+-K^+ ATPase because their energy source, the Na^+ gradient, is diminished.

There are two types of secondary active transport, distinguishable by the direction of movement of the uphill solute. If the uphill solute moves in the same direction as Na^+, it is called **cotransport, or symport.** If the uphill solute moves in the opposite direction of Na^+, it is called **countertransport, antiport,** or **exchange.**

Cotransport

Cotransport (symport) is a form of secondary active transport in which all solutes are transported in the **same direction** across the cell membrane. Na^+ moves *into* the cell on the carrier down its electrochemical gradient; the solutes, cotransported with Na^+, also move *into* the cell. Cotransport is involved in several critical physiologic processes, particularly in the absorbing epithelia of the small intestine and the renal tubule. For example, **Na^+-glucose cotransport** (SGLT) and **Na^+-amino acid cotransport** are present in the luminal membranes of the epithelial cells of both small intestine and renal proximal tubule. Another example of cotransport involving the renal tubule is

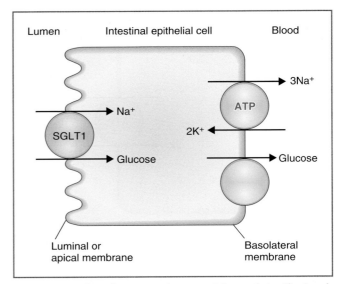

Figure 1–7 **Na^+-glucose cotransport in an intestinal epithelial cell.** ATP, Adenosine triphosphate; SGLT1, Na^+-glucose transport protein 1.

Na^+-K^+-$2Cl^-$ cotransport, which is present in the luminal membrane of epithelial cells of the thick ascending limb. In each example, the Na^+ gradient established by the Na^+-K^+ ATPase is used to transport solutes such as glucose, amino acids, K^+, or Cl^- against electrochemical gradients.

Figure 1-7 illustrates the principles of cotransport using the example of Na^+-glucose cotransport (**SGLT1,** or Na-glucose transport protein 1) in intestinal epithelial cells. The cotransporter is present in the luminal membrane of these cells and can be visualized as having two specific recognition sites, one for Na^+ ions and the other for glucose. When both Na^+ and glucose are present in the lumen of the small intestine, they bind to the transporter. In this configuration, the cotransport protein rotates and releases both Na^+ and glucose to the interior of the cell. (Subsequently, both solutes are transported out of the cell across the basolateral membrane—Na^+ by the Na^+-K^+ ATPase and glucose by facilitated diffusion.) If either Na^+ or glucose is missing from the intestinal lumen, the cotransporter cannot rotate. Thus, both solutes are required, and neither can be transported in the absence of the other (Box 1-1).

Finally, the role of the intestinal Na^+-glucose cotransport process can be understood in the context of overall intestinal absorption of carbohydrates. Dietary carbohydrates are digested by gastrointestinal enzymes to an absorbable form, the monosaccharides. One of these monosaccharides is glucose, which is absorbed across the intestinal epithelial cells by a combination of Na^+-glucose cotransport in the luminal membrane and facilitated diffusion of glucose in the basolateral membrane. Na^+-glucose cotransport is the active step,

---

BOX 1–1   Clinical Physiology: Glucosuria Due to Diabetes Mellitus

DESCRIPTION OF CASE. At his annual physical examination, a 14-year-old boy reports symptoms of frequent urination and severe thirst. A dipstick test of his urine shows elevated levels of glucose. The physician orders a glucose tolerance test, which indicates that the boy has type I diabetes mellitus. He is treated with insulin by injection, and his dipstick test is subsequently normal.

EXPLANATION OF CASE. Although type I diabetes mellitus is a complex disease, this discussion is limited to the symptom of frequent urination and the finding of glucosuria (glucose in the urine). Glucose is normally handled by the kidney in the following manner: Glucose in the blood is filtered across the glomerular capillaries. The epithelial cells, which line the renal proximal tubule, then reabsorb all of the filtered glucose so that no glucose is excreted in the urine. Thus, a normal dipstick test would show no glucose in the urine. If the epithelial cells in the proximal tubule do not reabsorb all of the filtered glucose back into the blood, the glucose that escapes reabsorption is excreted. The cellular mechanism for this glucose reabsorption is the Na^+-glucose cotransporter in the luminal membrane of the proximal tubule cells. Because this is a carrier-mediated transporter, there are a finite number of binding sites for glucose. Once these binding sites

are fully occupied, saturation of transport occurs (transport maximum).

In this patient with type I diabetes mellitus, the hormone insulin is not produced in sufficient amounts by the pancreatic β cells. Insulin is required for normal uptake of glucose into liver, muscle, and other cells. Without insulin, the blood glucose concentration increases because glucose is not taken up by the cells. When the blood glucose concentration increases to high levels, more glucose is filtered by the renal glomeruli and the amount of glucose filtered exceeds the capacity of the Na^+-glucose cotransporter. The glucose that cannot be reabsorbed because of saturation of this transporter is then "spilled" in the urine.

TREATMENT. Treatment of the patient with type I diabetes mellitus consists of administering exogenous insulin by injection. Whether secreted normally from the pancreatic β cells or administered by injection, insulin lowers the blood glucose concentration by promoting glucose uptake into cells. When this patient received insulin, his blood glucose concentration was reduced; thus, the amount of glucose filtered was reduced, and the Na^+-glucose cotransporters were no longer saturated. All of the filtered glucose could be reabsorbed, and therefore, no glucose was excreted, or "spilled," in the urine.

---

allowing glucose to be absorbed into the blood against an electrochemical gradient.

Countertransport

Countertransport (antiport or exchange) is a form of secondary active transport in which solutes move in *opposite directions* across the cell membrane. Na^+ moves *into* the cell on the carrier down its electrochemical gradient; the solutes that are countertransported or exchanged for Na^+ move *out of* the cell. Countertransport is illustrated by Ca^{2+}-Na^+ exchange (Fig. 1-8) and by Na^+-H^+ exchange. As with cotransport, each process uses the Na^+ gradient established by the Na^+-K^+ ATPase as an energy source; Na^+ moves downhill and Ca^{2+} or H^+ moves uphill.

Ca^{2+}-Na^+ exchange is one of the transport mechanisms, along with the Ca^{2+} ATPase, that helps maintain the intracellular Ca^{2+} concentration at very low levels ($\approx 10^{-7}$ molar). To accomplish Ca^{2+}-Na^+ exchange, active transport must be involved because Ca^{2+} moves out of the cell against its electrochemical gradient. Figure 1-8 illustrates the concept of Ca^{2+}-Na^+ exchange in a muscle cell membrane. The exchange protein has recognition sites for both Ca^{2+} and Na^+. The protein must bind Ca^{2+} on the intracellular side of the membrane and,

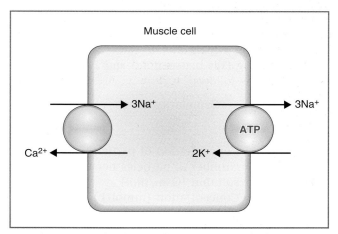

Figure 1–8 Ca^{2+}-Na^+ **countertransport (exchange) in a muscle cell.** ATP, Adenosine triphosphate.

simultaneously, bind Na^+ on the extracellular side. In this configuration, the exchange protein rotates and delivers Ca^{2+} to the exterior of the cell and Na^+ to the interior of the cell.

The stoichiometry of Ca^{2+}-Na^+ exchange varies between different cell types and may even vary for a single cell type under different conditions. Usually, however, three Na^+ ions enter the cell for each Ca^{2+} ion extruded from the cell. With this stoichiometry of three Na^+ ions per one Ca^{2+} ion, three positive charges move into the cell in exchange for two positive charges leaving the cell, making the Ca^{2+}-Na^+ exchanger **electrogenic.**

Osmosis

Osmosis is the flow of water across a semipermeable membrane because of differences in solute concentration. Concentration differences of impermeant solutes establish osmotic pressure differences, and this osmotic pressure difference causes water to flow by osmosis. Osmosis of water is *not* diffusion of water: Osmosis occurs because of a pressure difference, whereas diffusion occurs because of a concentration (or activity) difference of water.

Osmolarity

The osmolarity of a solution is its concentration of osmotically active particles, expressed as osmoles per liter or milliosmoles per liter. To calculate osmolarity, it is necessary to know the concentration of solute and whether the solute dissociates in solution. For example, glucose does not dissociate in solution; theoretically, NaCl dissociates into two particles and $CaCl_2$ dissociates into three particles. The symbol "g" gives the number of particles in solution and also takes into account whether there is complete or only partial dissociation. Thus, if NaCl is completely dissociated into two particles, g equals 2.0; if NaCl dissociates only partially, then g falls between 1.0 and 2.0. Osmolarity is calculated as follows:

$$\text{Osmolarity} = g\ C$$

where

$$\text{Osmolarity} = \text{Concentration of particles (mOsm/L)}$$
$$g = \text{Number of particles per mole in solution (Osm/mol)}$$
$$C = \text{Concentration (mmol/L)}$$

If two solutions have the same calculated osmolarity, they are called **isosmotic.** If two solutions have different calculated osmolarities, the solution with the higher osmolarity is called **hyperosmotic** and the solution with the lower osmolarity is called **hyposmotic.**

Osmolality

Osmolality is similar to osmolarity, except that it is the concentration of osmotically active particles, expressed as osmoles (or milliosmoles) *per kg of water*. Because 1 kg of water is approximately equivalent to 1 L of

---

SAMPLE PROBLEM. Solution A is 2 mmol/L urea, and Solution B is 1 mmol/L NaCl. Assume that $g_{NaCl} = 1.85$. *Are the two solutions isosmotic?*

SOLUTION. Calculate the osmolarities of both solutions to compare them. Solution A contains urea, which does not dissociate in solution. Solution B contains NaCl, which dissociates partially in solution but not completely (i.e., $g < 2.0$). Thus,

$$\text{Osmolarity}_A = 1\ \text{Osm/mol} \times 2\ \text{mmol/L}$$
$$= 2\ \text{mOsm/L}$$
$$\text{Osmolarity}_B = 1.85\ \text{Osm/mol} \times 1\ \text{mmol/L}$$
$$= 1.85\ \text{mOsm/L}$$

The two solutions do not have the same calculated osmolarity; therefore, they are *not isosmotic.* Solution A has a higher osmolarity than Solution B and is hyperosmotic; Solution B is hyposmotic.

---

water, osmolarity and osmolality will have essentially the same numerical value.

Osmotic Pressure

Osmosis is the flow of water across a semipermeable membrane due to a difference in solute concentration. The difference in solute concentration creates an osmotic pressure difference across the membrane and that pressure difference is the driving force for osmotic water flow.

Figure 1-9 illustrates the concept of osmosis. Two aqueous solutions, open to the atmosphere, are shown in Figure 1-9*A*. The membrane separating the solutions is permeable to water but is impermeable to the solute. Initially, solute is present only in Solution 1. The solute in Solution 1 produces an osmotic pressure and causes, by the interaction of solute with pores in the membrane, a reduction in hydrostatic pressure of Solution 1. The resulting hydrostatic pressure difference across the membrane then causes water to flow from Solution 2 into Solution 1. With time, water flow causes the volume of Solution 1 to increase and the volume of Solution 2 to decrease.

Figure 1-9*B* shows a similar pair of solutions; however, the preparation has been modified so that water flow into Solution 1 is prevented by applying pressure to a piston. *The pressure required to stop the flow of water is the osmotic pressure of Solution 1.*

The osmotic pressure (π) of Solution 1 depends on two factors: the concentration of osmotically active particles and whether the solute remains in Solution 1 (i.e., whether the solute can cross the membrane or not). Osmotic pressure is calculated by the **van't Hoff equation** (as follows), which converts the concentration of particles to a pressure, taking into account whether the solute is retained in the original solution.

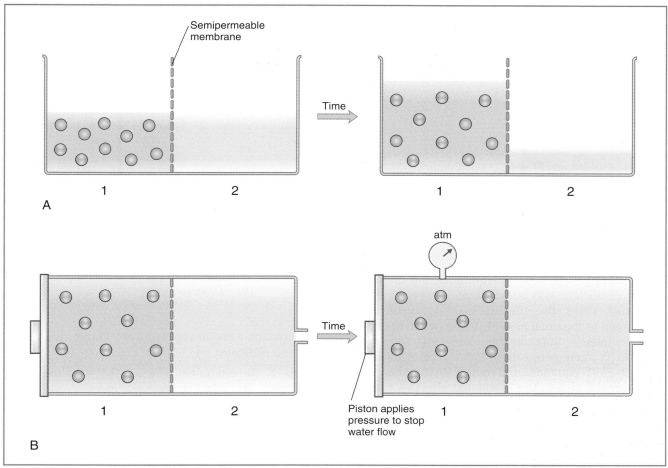

Figure 1–9 **Osmosis across a semipermeable membrane. A,** Solute (*circles*) is present on one side of a semipermeable membrane; with time, the osmotic pressure created by the solute causes water to flow from Solution 2 to Solution 1. The resulting volume changes are shown. **B,** The solutions are closed to the atmosphere, and a piston is applied to stop the flow of water into Solution 1. The pressure needed to stop the flow of water is the effective osmotic pressure of Solution 1. Atm, Atmosphere.

Thus,

$$\pi = g\,C\,\sigma\,R\,T$$

where

   π = Osmotic pressure (atm or mm Hg)
   g = Number of particles per mole in solution (Osm/mol)
   C = Concentration (mmol/L)
   σ = Reflection coefficient (varies from 0 to 1)
   R = Gas constant (0.082 L – atm/mol – K)
   T = Absolute temperature (K)

The **reflection coefficient** (σ) is a dimensionless number ranging between 0 and 1 that describes the ease with which a solute crosses a membrane. Reflection coefficients can be described for the following three conditions (Fig. 1-10):

♦ **σ = 1.0** (see Fig. 1-10*A*). If the membrane is impermeable to the solute, σ is 1.0, and the solute will be retained in the original solution and exert its full osmotic effect. In this case, the effective osmotic pressure will be maximal and will cause maximal water flow. For example, **serum albumin** and **intracellular proteins** are solutes where σ = 1.

♦ **σ = 0** (see Fig. 1-10*C*). If the membrane is freely permeable to the solute, σ is 0, and the solute will diffuse across the membrane down its concentration gradient until the solute concentrations of the two solutions are equal. In other words, the solute behaves as if it were water. In this case, there will be *no* effective osmotic pressure difference across the membrane and, therefore, no driving force for osmotic water flow. Refer again to the van't Hoff equation and notice that, when σ = 0, the calculated effective osmotic pressure becomes zero. **Urea** is an example of a solute where σ = 0 (or nearly 0).

♦ **σ = a value between 0 and 1** (see Fig. 1-10*B*). Most solutes are neither impermeant (σ = 1) nor freely

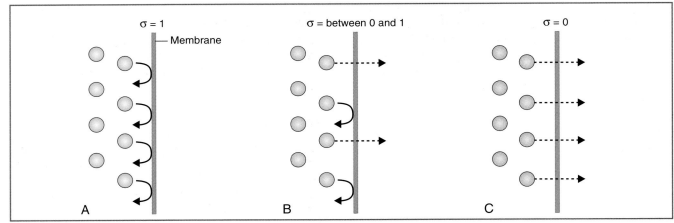

Figure 1-10 Reflection coefficient (σ).

permeant (σ = 0) across membranes, but the reflection coefficient falls somewhere between 0 and 1. In such cases, the effective osmotic pressure lies between its maximal possible value (when the solute is completely impermeable) and zero (when the solute is freely permeable). Refer once again to the van't Hoff equation and notice that, when σ is between 0 and 1, the calculated effective osmotic pressure will be less than its maximal possible value, but greater than zero.

When two solutions separated by a semipermeable membrane have the same effective osmotic pressure, they are **isotonic;** that is, no water will flow between them because there is no effective osmotic pressure difference across the membrane. When two solutions have different effective osmotic pressures, the solution with the lower effective osmotic pressure is **hypotonic** and the solution with the higher effective osmotic pressure is **hypertonic.** *Water will flow from the hypotonic solution into the hypertonic solution.*

SAMPLE PROBLEM. A solution of 1 mol/L NaCl is separated from a solution of 2 mol/L urea by a semipermeable membrane. Assume that NaCl is completely dissociated, that σ_{NaCl} = 0.3, and σ_{urea} = 0.05. *Are the two solutions isosmotic and/or isotonic? Is there net water flow, and what is its direction?*

SOLUTION. STEP 1. To determine whether the solutions are isosmotic, simply calculate the osmolarity of each solution (g×C) and compare the two values. It was stated that NaCl is completely dissociated (i.e., separated into two particles); thus, for NaCl, g = 2.0. Urea does not dissociate in solution; thus, for urea, g = 1.0.

$$\text{NaCl: Osmolarity} = g\,C$$
$$= 2.0 \times 1\,\text{mol/L}$$
$$= 2\,\text{Osm/L}$$

$$\text{Urea: Osmolarity} = g\,C$$
$$= 1.0 \times 2\,\text{mol/L}$$
$$= 2\,\text{Osm/L}$$

Each solution has an osmolarity of 2 Osm/L—they are indeed isosmotic.

Step 2. To determine whether the solutions are isotonic, the effective osmotic pressure of each solution must be determined. Assume that at 37°C (310 K), RT = 25.45 L-atm/mol. Thus,

$$\text{NaCl: } \pi = g\,C\,\sigma\,RT$$
$$= 2 \times 1\,\text{mol/L} \times 0.3 \times RT$$
$$= 0.6\,RT$$
$$= 15.3\,\text{atm}$$

$$\text{Urea: } \pi = g\,C\,\sigma\,RT$$
$$= 1 \times 2\,\text{mol/L} \times 0.05 \times RT$$
$$= 0.1\,RT$$
$$= 2.5\,\text{atm}$$

Although the two solutions have the same calculated osmolarities and are isosmotic (Step 1), they have different effective osmotic pressures and they are not isotonic (Step 2). This difference occurs because the reflection coefficient for NaCl is much higher than the reflection coefficient for urea and, thus, NaCl creates the greater *effective* osmotic pressure. Water will flow from the urea solution into the NaCl solution, from the hypotonic solution to the hypertonic solution.

DIFFUSION POTENTIALS AND EQUILIBRIUM POTENTIALS

Ion Channels

Ion channels are integral, membrane-spanning proteins that, when open, permit the passage of certain ions. Thus, ion channels are **selective** and allow ions with specific characteristics to move through them. This selectivity is based on both the size of the channel and the charges lining it. For example, channels lined with negative charges typically permit the passage of cations but exclude anions; channels lined with positive charges permit the passage of anions but exclude cations. Channels also discriminate on the basis of size. For example, a cation-selective channel lined with negative charges might permit the passage of Na^+ but exclude K^+; another cation-selective channel (e.g., nicotinic receptor on the motor end plate) might have less selectivity and permit the passage of several different small cations.

Ion channels are controlled by **gates,** and, depending on the position of the gates, the channels may be open or closed. When a channel is open, the ions for which it is selective can flow through it by passive diffusion, down the existing electrochemical gradient. When the channel is closed, the ions cannot flow through it, no matter what the size of the electrochemical gradient. The **conductance** of a channel depends on the probability that it is open. The higher the probability that the channel is open, the higher is its conductance or permeability.

The gates on ion channels are controlled by three types of **sensors.** One type of gate has sensors that respond to changes in membrane potential (i.e., voltage-gated channels); a second type of gate responds to changes in signaling molecules (i.e., second-messenger-gated channels); and a third type of gate responds to changes in ligands such as hormones or neurotransmitters (i.e., ligand-gated channels).

- ♦ **Voltage-gated channels** have gates that are controlled by changes in membrane potential. For example, the **activation gate on the nerve Na^+ channel** is *opened* by depolarization of the nerve cell membrane; opening of this channel is responsible for the upstroke of the action potential. Interestingly, another gate on the Na^+ channel, an **inactivation gate,** is *closed* by depolarization. Because the activation gate responds more rapidly to depolarization than the inactivation gate, the Na^+ channel first opens and then closes. This difference in response times of the two gates accounts for the shape and time course of the action potential.

- ♦ **Second messenger-gated channels** have gates that are controlled by changes in levels of intracellular signaling molecules such as cyclic adenosine monophosphate (cyclic AMP) or inositol 1,4,5-triphosphate (IP_3). Thus, the sensors for these gates are on the intracellular side of the ion channel. For example, the gates on Na^+ channels in cardiac sinoatrial node are opened by increased intracellular cyclic AMP.

- ♦ **Ligand-gated channels** have gates that are controlled by hormones and neurotransmitters. The sensors for these gates are located on the extracellular side of the ion channel. For example, the **nicotinic receptor** on the **motor end plate** is actually an ion channel that opens when acetylcholine (ACh) binds to it; when open, it is permeable to Na^+ and K^+ ions.

Diffusion Potentials

A diffusion potential is the potential difference generated across a membrane when a charged solute (an ion) diffuses down its concentration gradient. Therefore, a **diffusion potential is caused by diffusion of ions.** It follows, then, that a diffusion potential can be generated *only* if the membrane is permeable to that ion. Furthermore, if the membrane is not permeable to the ion, no diffusion potential will be generated no matter how large a concentration gradient is present.

The **magnitude** of a diffusion potential, measured in millivolts (mV), depends on the size of the concentration gradient, where the concentration gradient is the driving force. The **sign** of the diffusion potential depends on the charge of the diffusing ion. Finally, as noted, diffusion potentials are created by the movement of only a few ions, and they do not cause changes in the concentration of ions in bulk solution.

Equilibrium Potentials

The concept of equilibrium potential is simply an extension of the concept of diffusion potential. If there is a concentration difference for an ion across a membrane and the membrane is permeable to that ion, a potential difference (the diffusion potential) is created. Eventually, net diffusion of the ion slows and then stops because of that potential difference. In other words, if a cation diffuses down its concentration gradient, it carries a positive charge across the membrane, which will retard and eventually stop further diffusion of the cation. If an anion diffuses down its concentration gradient, it carries a negative charge, which will retard and then stop further diffusion of the anion. The **equilibrium potential** is the diffusion potential that exactly balances or opposes the tendency for diffusion down the concentration difference. At **electrochemical equilibrium,** the chemical and electrical driving forces acting on an ion are equal and opposite, and no further net diffusion occurs.

The following examples of a diffusing cation and a diffusing anion illustrate the concepts of equilibrium potential and electrochemical equilibrium:

Example of Na⁺ Equilibrium Potential

Figure 1-11 shows two solutions separated by a theoretical membrane that is permeable to Na^+ but not to Cl^-. The NaCl concentration is higher in Solution 1 than

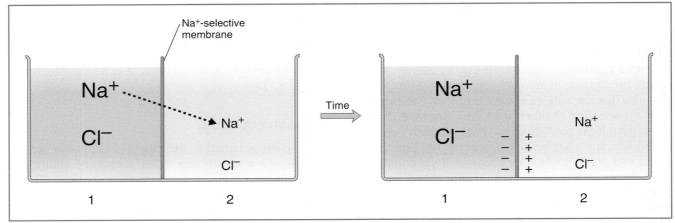

Figure 1–11 Generation of an Na⁺ diffusion potential.

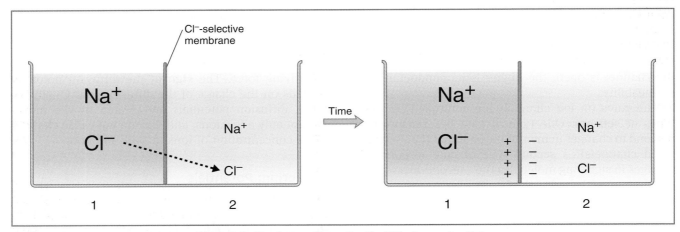

Figure 1–12 Generation of a Cl⁻ diffusion potential.

in Solution 2. The permeant ion, Na⁺, will diffuse down its concentration gradient from Solution 1 to Solution 2, but the impermeant ion, Cl⁻, will not accompany it. As a result of the net movement of positive charge to Solution 2, an **Na⁺ diffusion potential** develops and Solution 2 becomes positive with respect to Solution 1. The positivity in Solution 2 opposes further diffusion of Na⁺, and eventually it is large enough to prevent further net diffusion. The potential difference that exactly balances the tendency of Na⁺ to diffuse down its concentration gradient is the **Na⁺ equilibrium potential.** When the chemical and electrical driving forces on Na⁺ are equal and opposite, Na⁺ is said to be at **electrochemical equilibrium.** This diffusion of a *few* Na⁺ ions, sufficient to create the diffusion potential, does not produce any change in Na⁺ concentration in the bulk solutions.

Example of Cl⁻ Equilibrium Potential

Figure 1-12 shows the same pair of solutions as in Figure 1-11; however, in Figure 1-12, the theoretical

membrane is permeable to Cl⁻ rather than to Na⁺. Cl⁻ will diffuse from Solution 1 to Solution 2 down its concentration gradient, but Na⁺ will not accompany it. A diffusion potential will be established, and Solution 2 will become negative relative to Solution 1. The potential difference that exactly balances the tendency of Cl⁻ to diffuse down its concentration gradient is the **Cl⁻ equilibrium potential.** When the chemical and electrical driving forces on Cl⁻ are equal and opposite, then Cl⁻ is at **electrochemical equilibrium.** Again, diffusion of these few Cl⁻ ions will not change the Cl⁻ concentration in the bulk solutions.

Nernst Equation

The Nernst equation is used to calculate the equilibrium potential for an ion at a given concentration difference across a membrane, assuming that the membrane is permeable to that ion. By definition, the equilibrium potential is calculated for *one ion at a time.* Thus,

$$E_X = \frac{-2.3RT}{zF} \log_{10} \frac{[C_i]}{[C_e]}$$

where

E_X = Equilibrium potential (mV) for a given ion, X

$\dfrac{2.3RT}{F}$ = Constant (60 mV at 37°C)

z = Charge on the ion (+1 for Na^+; +2 for Ca^{2+}; −1 for Cl^-)

C_i = Intracellular concentration of X (mmol/L)

C_e = Extracellular concentration of X (mmol/L)

In words, the Nernst equation converts a concentration difference for an ion into a voltage. This conversion is accomplished by the various constants: R is the gas constant, T is the absolute temperature, and F is Faraday's constant; multiplying by 2.3 converts natural logarithm to $\log_{10}$.

By convention, *membrane potential is expressed as intracellular potential relative to extracellular potential.* Hence, a transmembrane potential difference of −70 mV means 70 mV, cell interior negative.

Typical values for equilibrium potential for common ions, calculated as previously described and assuming typical concentration gradients across cell membranes, are as follows:

$$E_{Na^+} = +65 \text{ mV}$$

$$E_{Ca^{2+}} = +120 \text{ mV}$$

$$E_{K^+} = -85 \text{ mV}$$

$$E_{Cl^-} = -90 \text{ mV}$$

It is useful to keep these values in mind when considering the concepts of resting membrane potential and action potentials.

SAMPLE PROBLEM. *If the intracellular $[Ca^{2+}]$ is 10^{-7} mol/L and the extracellular $[Ca^{2+}]$ is 2×10^{-3} mol/L, at what potential difference across the cell membrane will Ca^{2+} be at electrochemical equilibrium? Assume that 2.3RT/F = 60 mV at body temperature (37°C).*

SOLUTION. Another way of posing the question is to ask what the membrane potential will be, given this concentration gradient across the membrane, if Ca^{2+} is the only permeant ion. Remember, Ca^{2+} is divalent, so z = +2. Thus,

$$\begin{aligned} E_{Ca^{2+}} &= \frac{-60 \text{ mV}}{z} \log_{10} \frac{C_i}{C_e} \\ &= \frac{-60 \text{ mV}}{+2} \log_{10} \frac{10^{-7} \text{ mol/L}}{2 \times 10^{-3} \text{ mol/L}} \\ &= -30 \text{ mV} \log_{10} 5 \times 10^{-5} \\ &= -30 \text{ mV} (-4.3) \\ &= +129 \text{ mV} \end{aligned}$$

Because this is a log function, it is not necessary to remember which concentration goes in the numerator. Simply complete the calculation either way to arrive at 129 mV, and then determine the correct sign with an intuitive approach. The intuitive approach depends on the knowledge that, because the $[Ca^{2+}]$ is much higher in ECF than in ICF, Ca^{2+} will tend to diffuse down this concentration gradient from ECF into ICF, making the inside of the cell positive. Thus, Ca^{2+} will be at electrochemical equilibrium when the membrane potential is +129 mV (cell interior positive).

Be aware that the equilibrium potential has been calculated at a given concentration gradient for Ca^{2+} ions. With a different concentration gradient, the calculated equilibrium potential would be different.

Driving Force

When dealing with uncharged solutes, the driving force for net diffusion is simply the concentration difference of the solute across the cell membrane. However, when dealing with charged solutes (i.e., ions), the driving force for net diffusion must consider both concentration difference and electrical potential difference across the cell membrane.

The **driving force** on a given ion is the difference between the actual, measured membrane potential (E_m) and the ion's calculated equilibrium potential (E_X). In other words, it is the difference between E_m and what that ion would "like" the membrane potential to be (its equilibrium potential, as calculated by the Nernst equation). The driving force on a given ion, X, is therefore calculated as:

$$\text{Net driving force (mV)} = E_m - E_X$$

where

Driving force = Driving force (mV)

E_m = Actual membrane potential (mV)

E_X = Equilibrium potential for X (mV)

When the driving force is negative (i.e., E_m is more negative than the ion's equilibrium potential), that ion X will enter the cell if it is a cation and will leave the cell if it is an anion. In other words, ion X "thinks" the membrane potential is too negative and tries to bring the membrane potential toward its equilibrium potential by diffusing in the appropriate direction across the cell membrane. Conversely, if the driving force is positive (E_m is more positive than the ion's equilibrium potential), then ion X will leave the cell if it is a cation and will enter the cell if it is an anion; in this case, ion X "thinks" the membrane potential is too positive and tries to bring the membrane potential toward its equilibrium potential by diffusing in the appropriate direction across the cell membrane. Finally, if E_m is equal to the ion's equilibrium potential, then the driving force on the ion is zero, and the ion is, by definition, at electrochemical equilibrium.

Ionic Current

Ionic current (I_X), or current flow, occurs when there is movement of an ion across the cell membrane. Ions will move across the cell membrane through ion channels when two conditions are met: (1) there is a driving force on the ion and (2) the membrane has a conductance to that ion (i.e., its ion channels are open). Thus,

$$I_X = G_X(E_m - E_X)$$

Where

$$I_X = \text{ionic current (mAmps)}$$
$$G_X = \text{ionic conductance (1/ohms),}$$
$$\text{where conductance is the}$$
$$\text{reciprocal of resistance}$$
$$E_m - E_X = \text{driving force on ion X (mV)}$$

You will notice that the equation for ionic current is simply a rearrangement of Ohm's law, where $V = IR$ or $I = V/R$ (where V is the same thing as E). Because conductance (G) is the reciprocal of resistance (R), $I = G \times V$.

The **direction of ionic current** is determined by the direction of the driving force, as described in the previous section. The **magnitude of ionic current** is determined by the size of the driving force and the conductance. For a given conductance, the greater the driving force, the greater the current flow. For a given driving force, the greater the conductance, the greater the current flow. Lastly, if either the driving force or the conductance of an ion is zero, there can be no diffusion of that ion across the cell membrane and no current flow.

RESTING MEMBRANE POTENTIAL

The resting membrane potential is the potential difference that exists across the membrane of excitable cells such as nerve and muscle in the period between action potentials (i.e., at rest). As stated previously, in expressing the membrane potential, it is conventional to refer the intracellular potential to the extracellular potential.

The resting membrane potential is established by diffusion potentials, which result from the concentration differences for various ions across the cell membrane. (Recall that these concentration differences have been established by primary and secondary active transport mechanisms.) *Each permeant ion*

attempts to drive the membrane potential toward its own equilibrium potential. Ions with the highest permeabilities or conductances at rest will make the greatest contributions to the resting membrane potential, and those with the lowest permeabilities will make little or no contribution.

The resting membrane potential of excitable cells falls in the range of **−70 to −80 mV.** These values can best be explained by the concept of relative permeabilities of the cell membrane. Thus, the resting membrane potential is *close to* the equilibrium potentials for K^+ and Cl^- because the permeability to these ions at rest is high. The resting membrane potential is *far from* the equilibrium potentials for Na^+ and Ca^{2+} because the permeability to these ions at rest is low.

One way of evaluating the contribution each ion makes to the membrane potential is by using the **chord conductance equation,** which weights the equilibrium potential for each ion (calculated by the Nernst equation) by its relative conductance. Ions with the highest conductance drive the membrane potential toward their equilibrium potentials, whereas those with low conductance have little influence on the membrane potential. (An alternative approach to the same question applies the **Goldman equation,** which considers the contribution of each ion by its relative permeability rather than by its conductance.) The chord conductance equation is written as follows:

$$E_m = \frac{g_{K^+}}{g_T}E_{K^+} + \frac{g_{Na^+}}{g_T}E_{Na^+} + \frac{g_{Cl^-}}{g_T}E_{Cl^-} + \frac{g_{Ca^{2+}}}{g_T}E_{Ca^{2+}}$$

where

$$E_m = \text{Membrane potential (mV)}$$
$$g_{K^+} \text{ etc.} = K^+ \text{ conductance etc. (mho, reciprocal of}$$
$$\text{resistance)}$$
$$g_T = \text{Total conductance (mho)}$$
$$E_{K^+} \text{ etc.} = K^+ \text{ equilibrium potential etc. (mV)}$$

At rest, the membranes of excitable cells are far more permeable to K^+ and Cl^- than to Na^+ and Ca^{2+}. These differences in permeability account for the resting membrane potential.

What role, if any, does the Na^+-K^+ATPase play in creating the resting membrane potential? The answer has two parts. First, there is a small *direct* electrogenic contribution of the Na^+-K^+ ATPase, which is based on the stoichiometry of three Na^+ ions pumped out of the cell for every two K^+ ions pumped into the cell. Second, the more important *indirect* contribution is in maintaining the concentration gradient for K^+ across the cell membrane, which then is responsible for the K^+ diffusion potential that drives the membrane potential toward the K^+ equilibrium potential. Thus, the Na^+-K^+ ATPase is necessary to create and maintain the K^+ concentration gradient, which establishes the resting membrane potential. (A similar argument can be made for the role of the Na$^+$-K$^+$ ATPase in the upstroke of the action potential, where it maintains the ionic gradient for Na$^+$ across the cell membrane.)

ACTION POTENTIALS

The action potential is a phenomenon of excitable cells such as nerve and muscle and consists of a rapid depolarization (upstroke) followed by repolarization of the membrane potential. Action potentials are the basic mechanism for transmission of information in the nervous system and in all types of muscle.

Terminology

The following terminology will be used for discussion of the action potential, the refractory periods, and the propagation of action potentials:

♦ **Depolarization** is the process of making the membrane potential *less negative*. As noted, the usual resting membrane potential of excitable cells is oriented with the cell interior negative. Depolarization makes the interior of the cell less negative, or it may even cause the cell interior to become positive. A change in membrane potential should not be described as "increasing" or "decreasing" because those terms are ambiguous. (For example, when the membrane potential depolarizes, or becomes less negative, has the membrane potential increased or decreased?)

♦ **Hyperpolarization** is the process of making the membrane potential *more negative*. As with depolarization, the terms "increasing" or "decreasing" should not be used to describe a change that makes the membrane potential more negative.

♦ **Inward current** is the flow of positive charge into the cell. Thus, inward currents *depolarize* the membrane potential. An example of an inward current is the flow of Na$^+$ into the cell during the upstroke of the action potential.

♦ **Outward current** is the flow of positive charge out of the cell. Outward currents *hyperpolarize* the membrane potential. An example of an outward current is the flow of K$^+$ out of the cell during the repolarization phase of the action potential.

♦ **Threshold potential** is the membrane potential at which occurrence of the action potential is inevitable. Because the threshold potential is less negative than the resting membrane potential, an inward current is required to depolarize the membrane potential to threshold. At threshold potential, net inward current (e.g., inward Na$^+$ current) becomes larger than net outward current (e.g., outward K$^+$ current), and the resulting depolarization becomes self-sustaining, giving rise to the upstroke of the action potential. If net inward current is less than net outward current, the membrane will not be depolarized to threshold and no action potential will occur (see all-or-none response).

♦ **Overshoot** is that portion of the action potential where the membrane potential is positive (cell interior positive).

♦ **Undershoot,** or **hyperpolarizing afterpotential,** is that portion of the action potential, following repolarization, where the membrane potential is actually more negative than it is at rest.

♦ **Refractory period** is a period during which another normal action potential cannot be elicited in an excitable cell. Refractory periods can be absolute or relative.

Characteristics of Action Potentials

Action potentials have three basic characteristics: stereotypical size and shape, propagation, and all-or-none response.

♦ **Stereotypical size and shape.** Each *normal* action potential for a given cell type looks identical, depolarizes to the same potential, and repolarizes back to the same resting potential.

♦ **Propagation.** An action potential at one site causes depolarization at adjacent sites, bringing those adjacent sites to threshold. Propagation of action potentials from one site to the next is *nondecremental.*

♦ **All-or-none response.** An action potential either occurs or does not occur. If an excitable cell is depolarized to threshold in a *normal* manner, then the occurrence of an action potential is inevitable. On the other hand, if the membrane is not depolarized to threshold, no action potential can occur. Indeed, if the stimulus is applied during the refractory period, then either no action potential occurs, or the action potential will occur but not have the stereotypical size and shape.

Ionic Basis of the Action Potential

The action potential is a fast depolarization (the upstroke), followed by repolarization back to the resting membrane potential. Figure 1-13 illustrates the events of the action potential in nerve and skeletal muscle, which occur in the following steps:

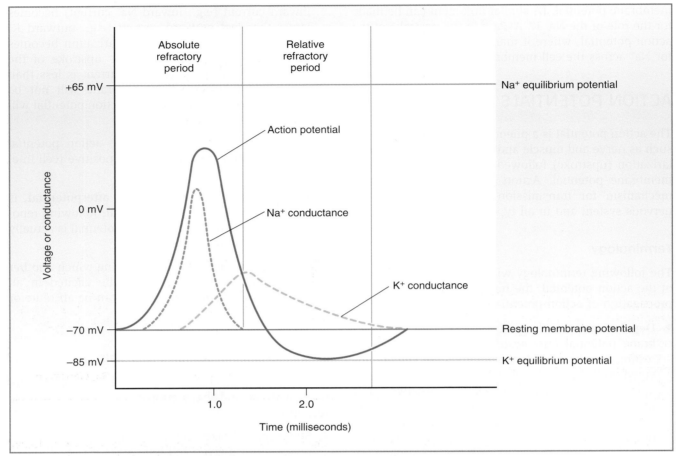

Figure 1–13 **Time course of voltage and conductance changes during the action potential of nerve.**

1. **Resting membrane potential.** At rest, the membrane potential is approximately −70 mV (cell interior negative). The **K⁺ conductance or permeability is high** and K⁺ channels are almost fully open, allowing K⁺ ions to diffuse out of the cell down the existing concentration gradient. This diffusion creates a K⁺ diffusion potential, which drives the membrane potential toward the K⁺ equilibrium potential. The conductance to Cl⁻ (not shown) also is high, and, at rest, Cl⁻ also is near electrochemical equilibrium. At rest, the **Na⁺ conductance is low,** and, thus, the resting membrane potential is far from the Na⁺ equilibrium potential.

2. **Upstroke of the action potential.** An inward current, usually the result of current spread from action potentials at neighboring sites, causes depolarization of the nerve cell membrane to threshold, which occurs at approximately −60 mV. This initial depolarization causes rapid opening of the **activation gates** of the Na⁺ channel, and the Na⁺ conductance promptly increases and becomes even higher than the K⁺ conductance (Fig. 1-14). The increase in Na⁺ conductance results in an

inward Na⁺ current; the membrane potential is further depolarized toward, but does not quite reach, the Na⁺ equilibrium potential of +65 mV. **Tetrodotoxin** (a toxin from the Japanese puffer fish) and the local anesthetic **lidocaine** block these voltage-sensitive Na⁺ channels and prevent the occurrence of nerve action potentials.

3. **Repolarization of the action potential.** The upstroke is terminated, and the membrane potential repolarizes to the resting level as a result of two events. First, the inactivation gates on the Na⁺ channels respond to depolarization by closing, but their response is slower than the opening of the activation gates. Thus, after a delay, the **inactivation gates** close the Na⁺ channels, terminating the upstroke. Second, depolarization opens K⁺ channels and increases K⁺ conductance to a value even higher than occurs at rest. The combined effect of closing of the Na⁺ channels and greater opening of the K⁺ channels makes the K⁺ conductance much higher than the Na⁺ conductance. Thus, an **outward K⁺ current** results, and the membrane is repolarized. **Tetraethylammonium (TEA)** blocks these

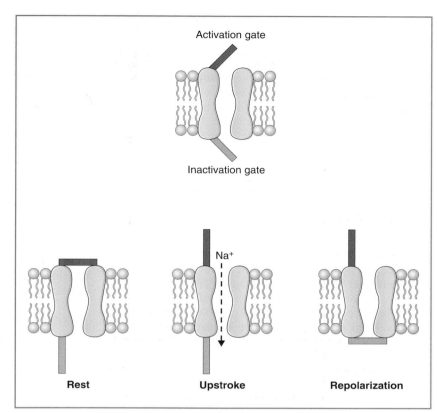

Figure 1–14 Functions of activation and inactivation gates on the nerve Na⁺ channel. At rest, the activation gate is closed and the inactivation gate is open. During the upstroke of the action potential, both gates are open and Na⁺ flows into the cell down its electrochemical potential gradient. During repolarization, the activation gate remains open but the inactivation gate is closed.

voltage-gated K⁺ channels, the outward K⁺ current, and repolarization.

4. **Hyperpolarizing afterpotential (undershoot).** For a brief period following repolarization, the K⁺ conductance is higher than at rest and the membrane potential is driven even closer to the K⁺ equilibrium potential (hyperpolarizing afterpotential). Eventually, the K⁺ conductance returns to the resting level, and the membrane potential depolarizes slightly, back to the resting membrane potential. The membrane is now ready, if stimulated, to generate another action potential.

The Nerve Na⁺ Channel

A voltage-gated Na⁺ channel is responsible for the upstroke of the action potential in nerve and skeletal muscle. This channel is an integral membrane protein, consisting of a large α subunit and two β subunits. The α subunit has four domains, each of which has six transmembrane α-helices. The repeats of transmembrane α-helices surround a central pore, through which Na⁺ ions can flow (if the channel's gates are open). A conceptual model of the Na⁺ channel demonstrating the function of the activation and inactivation gates is shown in Figure 1-14. The basic assumption of this model is that in order for Na⁺ to move through the

channel, *both gates on the channel must be open.* Recall how these gates respond to depolarization: The activation gate opens quickly, and the inactivation gate closes after a time delay.

1. At **rest,** the activation gate is closed. Although the inactivation gate is open (because the membrane potential is hyperpolarized), Na⁺ cannot move through the channel.

2. During the **upstroke of the action potential,** depolarization to threshold causes the activation gate to open quickly. The inactivation gate is still open because it responds to depolarization more slowly than the activation gate. Thus, both gates are open briefly, and Na⁺ can flow through the channel into the cell, causing further depolarization (the upstroke).

3. At the **peak of the action potential,** the slow inactivation gate finally responds and closes, and the channel itself is closed. Repolarization begins. When the membrane potential has repolarized back to its resting level, the activation gate will be closed and the inactivation gate will be open, both in their original positions.

Refractory Periods

During the refractory periods, excitable cells are *incapable* of producing normal action potentials (see Fig. 1-13).

BOX 1–2   Clinical Physiology: Hyperkalemia with Muscle Weakness

DESCRIPTION OF CASE. A 48-year-old woman with insulin-dependent diabetes mellitus reports to her physician that she is experiencing severe muscle weakness. She is being treated for hypertension with propranolol, a β-adrenergic blocking agent. Her physician immediately orders blood studies, which reveal a serum [K⁺] of 6.5 mEq/L (normal, 4.5 mEq/L) and elevated BUN (blood urea nitrogen). The physician tapers off the dosage of propranolol, with eventual discontinuation of the drug. He adjusts her insulin dosage. Within a few days, the patient's serum [K⁺] has decreased to 4.7 mEq/L, and she reports that her muscle strength has returned to normal.

EXPLANATION OF CASE. This diabetic patient has severe hyperkalemia caused by several factors: (1) Because her insulin dosage is insufficient, the lack of adequate insulin has caused a shift of K⁺ out of cells into blood (insulin promotes K⁺ uptake into cells). (2) Propranolol, the β-blocking agent used to treat the woman's hypertension, also shifts K⁺ out of cells into blood. (3) Elevated BUN suggests that the woman is developing renal failure; her failing kidneys are unable to excrete the extra K⁺ that is accumulating in her blood. These mechanisms involve concepts related to renal physiology and endocrine physiology.

It is important to understand that this woman has a severely elevated blood [K⁺] (hyperkalemia) and that her muscle weakness results from this hyperkalemia. The basis for this weakness can be explained as follows: The resting membrane potential of muscle cells is determined by the concentration gradient for K⁺ across the cell membrane (Nernst equation). At rest, the cell membrane is very permeable to K⁺, and K⁺ diffuses out of the cell down its concentration gradient, creating a K⁺ diffusion potential. This K⁺ diffusion potential is responsible for the resting membrane potential, which is cell interior negative. The larger the K⁺ concentration gradient, the greater the negativity in the cell. When the blood [K⁺] is elevated, the concentration gradient across the cell membrane is less than normal; resting membrane potential will therefore be less negative (i.e., depolarized).

It might be expected that this depolarization would make it easier to generate action potentials in the muscle because the resting membrane potential would be closer to threshold. A more important effect of depolarization, however, is that it closes the inactivation gates on Na⁺ channels. When these inactivation gates are closed, no action potentials can be generated, even if the activation gates are open. Without action potentials in the muscle, there can be no contraction.

TREATMENT. Treatment of this patient is based on shifting K⁺ back into the cells by increasing the woman's insulin dosages and by discontinuing propranolol. By reducing the woman's blood [K⁺] to normal levels, the resting membrane potential of her skeletal muscle cells will return to normal, the inactivation gates on the Na⁺ channels will be open at the resting membrane potential (as they should be), and normal action potentials can occur.

The refractory period includes an absolute refractory period and a relative refractory period (Box 1-2).

Absolute Refractory Period

The absolute refractory period overlaps with almost the entire duration of the action potential. During this period, no matter how great the stimulus, another action potential cannot be elicited. The basis for the absolute refractory period is closure of the inactivation gates of the Na⁺ channel in response to depolarization. These inactivation gates are in the closed position until the cell is repolarized back to the resting membrane potential (see Fig. 1-14).

Relative Refractory Period

The relative refractory period begins at the end of the absolute refractory period and overlaps primarily with the period of the hyperpolarizing afterpotential. During this period, an action potential can be elicited, but only if a greater than usual depolarizing (inward) current is applied. The basis for the relative refractory period is the higher K⁺ conductance than is present at rest. Because the membrane potential is closer to the K⁺ equilibrium potential, more inward current is needed to bring the membrane to threshold for the next action potential to be initiated.

Accommodation

When a nerve or muscle cell is depolarized slowly or is held at a depolarized level, the usual threshold potential may pass without an action potential having been fired. This process, called accommodation, occurs because depolarization closes inactivation gates on the Na⁺ channels. If depolarization occurs slowly enough, the Na⁺ channels close and remain closed. The upstroke of the action potential cannot occur because there are not enough Na⁺ channels available to carry inward current. An example of accommodation is seen in persons who have an elevated serum K⁺ concentration, or **hyperkalemia.** At rest, nerve and muscle cell

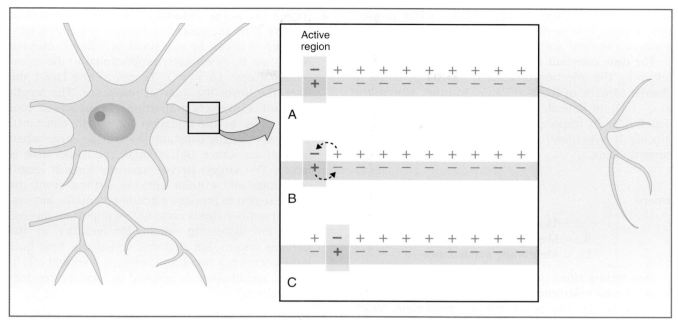

Figure 1–15 **Spread of depolarization down a nerve fiber by local currents. A,** The initial segment of the axon has fired an action potential, and the potential difference across the cell membrane has reversed to become inside positive. The adjacent area is inactive and remains at the resting membrane potential, inside negative. **B,** At the active site, positive charges inside the nerve flow to the adjacent inactive area. **C,** Local current flow causes the adjacent area to be depolarized to threshold and to fire action potentials; the original active region has repolarized back to the resting membrane potential.

membranes are very permeable to K^+; an increase in extracellular K^+ concentration causes depolarization of the resting membrane (as dictated by the Nernst equation). This depolarization brings the cell membrane closer to threshold and would seem to make it more likely to fire an action potential. However, the cell is actually *less* likely to fire an action potential because this sustained depolarization closes the inactivation gates on the Na^+ channels.

Propagation of Action Potentials

Propagation of action potentials down a nerve or muscle fiber occurs by the spread of **local currents** from active regions to adjacent inactive regions. Figure 1-15 shows a nerve cell body with its dendritic tree and an axon. At rest, the entire nerve axon is at the resting membrane potential, with the cell interior negative. Action potentials are initiated in the initial segment of the axon, nearest the nerve cell body. They propagate down the axon by spread of local currents, as illustrated in the figure.

In Figure 1-15*A* the initial segment of the nerve axon is depolarized to threshold and fires an action potential (the active region). As the result of an inward Na^+ current, at the peak of the action potential, the polarity of the membrane potential is reversed and

the cell interior becomes positive. The adjacent region of the axon remains inactive, with its cell interior negative.

Figure 1-15*B* illustrates the spread of local current from the depolarized active region to the adjacent inactive region. At the active site, positive charges inside the cell flow toward negative charges at the adjacent inactive site. This current flow causes the adjacent region to depolarize to threshold.

In Figure 1-15*C* the adjacent region of the nerve axon, having been depolarized to threshold, now fires an action potential. The polarity of its membrane potential is reversed, and the cell interior becomes positive. At this time, the *original* active region has been repolarized back to the resting membrane potential and restored to its inside-negative polarity. The process continues, transmitting the action potential sequentially down the axon.

Conduction Velocity

The speed at which action potentials are conducted along a nerve or muscle fiber is the conduction velocity. This property is of great physiologic importance because it determines the speed at which information can be transmitted in the nervous system. To understand conduction velocity in excitable tissues, two major concepts must be explained: the time constant and the length constant. These concepts, called **cable properties,** explain how nerves and muscles act as cables to conduct electrical activity.

The **time constant** (τ) is the amount of time it takes following the injection of current for the potential to change to 63% of its final value. In other words, the time constant indicates how quickly a cell membrane depolarizes in response to an inward current or how quickly it hyperpolarizes in response to an outward current. Thus,

$$\tau = R_m C_m$$

where

τ = Time constant
R_m = Membrane resistance
C_m = Membrane capacitance

Two factors affect the time constant. The first factor is **membrane resistance (R_m)**. When R_m is high, current does not readily flow across the cell membrane, which makes it difficult to change the membrane potential, thus increasing the time constant. The second factor, **membrane capacitance (C_m)**, is the ability of the cell membrane to store charge. When C_m is high, the time constant is increased because injected current first must discharge the membrane capacitor before it can depolarize the membrane. Thus, the time constant is greatest (i.e., takes longest) when R_m and C_m are high.

The **length constant** (λ) is the distance from the site of current injection where the potential has fallen by 63% of its original value. The length constant indicates how far a depolarizing current will spread along a nerve. In other words, the longer the length constant, the farther the current spreads down the nerve fiber. Thus,

$$\lambda \propto \sqrt{R_m / R_i}$$

where

λ = Length constant
R_m = Membrane resistance
R_i = Internal resistance

Again, R_m represents membrane resistance. Internal resistance, R_i, is inversely related to the ease of current flow in the cytoplasm of the nerve fiber. Therefore, the length constant will be greatest (i.e., current will travel the farthest) when the diameter of the nerve is large, when membrane resistance is high, and when internal resistance is low. In other words, current flows along the path of least resistance.

Changes in Conduction Velocity

There are two mechanisms that *increase* conduction velocity along a nerve: increasing the size of the nerve fiber and myelinating the nerve fiber. These mechanisms can best be understood in terms of the cable properties of time constant and length constant.

♦ **Increasing nerve diameter.** Increasing the size of a nerve fiber increases conduction velocity, a relationship that can be explained as follows: Internal resistance, R_i, is inversely proportional to the cross-sectional area ($A = \pi r^2$). Therefore, the larger the fiber, the lower the internal resistance. The length constant is inversely proportional to the square root of R_i (refer to the equation for length constant). Thus, the length constant (λ) will be large when internal resistance (R_i) is small (i.e., fiber size is large). The largest nerves have the longest length constants, and current spreads farthest from the active region to propagate action potentials. Increasing nerve fiber size is certainly an important mechanism for increasing conduction velocity in the nervous system, but anatomic constraints limit how large nerves can become. Therefore, a second mechanism, myelination, is invoked to increase conduction velocity.

♦ **Myelination.** Myelin is a lipid insulator of nerve axons that increases membrane resistance and decreases membrane capacitance. The **increased membrane resistance** forces current to flow along the path of least resistance of the axon interior rather than across the high resistance path of the axonal membrane. The **decreased membrane capacitance** produces a decrease in time constant; thus, at breaks in the myelin sheath (see following), the axonal membrane depolarizes faster in response to inward current. Together, the effects of increased membrane resistance and decreased membrane capacitance result in **increased conduction velocity** (Box 1-3).

If the entire nerve were coated with the lipid myelin sheath, however, no action potentials could occur because there would be no low resistance breaks in the membrane across which depolarizing current could flow. Therefore, it is important to note that at intervals of 1 to 2 mm, there are breaks in the myelin sheath, at the **nodes of Ranvier.** At the nodes, membrane resistance is low, current can flow across the membrane, and action potentials can occur. Thus, conduction of action potentials is faster in myelinated nerves than in unmyelinated nerves because action potentials "jump" long distances from one node to the next, a process called **saltatory conduction.**

SYNAPTIC AND NEUROMUSCULAR TRANSMISSION

A **synapse** is a site where information is transmitted from one cell to another. The information can be transmitted either electrically (electrical synapse) or via a chemical transmitter (chemical synapse).

BOX 1–3   Clinical Physiology: Multiple Sclerosis

DESCRIPTION OF CASE. A 32-year-old woman had her first episode of blurred vision 5 years ago. She had trouble reading the newspaper and the fine print on labels. Her vision returned to normal on its own, but 10 months later, the blurred vision recurred, this time with other symptoms including double vision, and a "pins and needles" feeling and severe weakness in her legs. She was too weak to walk even a single flight of stairs. She was referred to a neurologist, who ordered a series of tests. Magnetic resonance testing (MRI) of the brain showed lesions typical of multiple sclerosis. Visual evoked potentials had a prolonged latency that was consistent with decreased nerve conduction velocity. Since the diagnosis, she has had two relapses and she is currently being treated with interferon beta.

EXPLANATION OF CASE. Action potentials are propagated along nerve fibers by spread of local currents as follows: When an action potential occurs, the inward current of the upstroke of the action potential depolarizes the membrane at that site and reverses the polarity (i.e., that site briefly becomes inside positive). The depolarization then spreads to adjacent sites along the nerve fiber by local current flow. Importantly, if these local currents depolarize an adjacent region to threshold, it will fire an action potential (i.e., the action potential will be propagated). The speed of propagation of the action potential is called conduction velocity. The further local currents can spread without decay (expressed as the length constant), the faster the conduction velocity. There are two main factors that increase length constant and, therefore, increase conduction velocity in nerves: increased nerve diameter and myelination.

Myelin is an insulator of axons that increases membrane resistance and decreases membrane capacitance. By increasing membrane resistance, current is forced to flow down the axon interior and less current is lost across the cell membrane (increasing length constant); because more current flows down the axon, conduction velocity is increased. By decreasing membrane capacitance, local currents depolarize the membrane more rapidly, which also increases conduction velocity. In order for action potentials to be conducted in myelinated nerves, there must be periodic breaks in the myelin sheath (at the nodes of Ranvier), where there is a concentration of Na^+ and K^+ channels. Thus, at the nodes, the ionic currents necessary for the action potential can flow across the membrane (e.g., the inward Na^+ current necessary for the upstroke of the action potential). Between nodes, membrane resistance is very high and current is forced to flow rapidly down the nerve axon to the next node, where the next action potential can be generated. Thus, the action potential appears to "jump" from one node of Ranvier to the next. This is called saltatory conduction.

Multiple sclerosis is the most common demyelinating disease of the central nervous system. Loss of the myelin sheath around nerves causes a decrease in membrane resistance, which means that current "leaks out" across the membrane during conduction of local currents. For this reason, local currents decay more rapidly as they flow down the axon (decreased length constant) and, because of this decay, may be insufficient to generate an action potential when they reach the next node of Ranvier.

Types of Synapses

Electrical Synapses

Electrical synapses allow current to flow from one excitable cell to the next via low resistance pathways between the cells called **gap junctions.** Gap junctions are found in cardiac muscle and in some types of smooth muscle and account for the very fast conduction in these tissues. For example, rapid cell-to-cell conduction occurs in cardiac ventricular muscle, in the uterus, and in the bladder, allowing cells in these tissues to be activated simultaneously and ensuring that contraction occurs in a coordinated manner.

Chemical Synapses

In chemical synapses, there is a gap between the presynaptic cell membrane and the postsynaptic cell membrane, known as the **synaptic cleft.** Information is transmitted across the synaptic cleft via a neurotransmitter, a substance that is released from the presynaptic terminal and binds to receptors on the postsynaptic terminal.

The following sequence of events occurs at chemical synapses: An action potential in the presynaptic cell causes Ca^{2+} channels to open. An influx of Ca^{2+} into the presynaptic terminal causes the neurotransmitter, which is stored in synaptic vesicles, to be released by exocytosis. The neurotransmitter diffuses across the synaptic cleft, binds to receptors on the postsynaptic membrane, and produces a change in membrane potential on the postsynaptic cell.

The change in membrane potential on the postsynaptic cell membrane can be either excitatory or inhibitory, depending on the nature of the neurotransmitter released from the presynaptic nerve terminal. If the neurotransmitter is excitatory, it causes depolarization

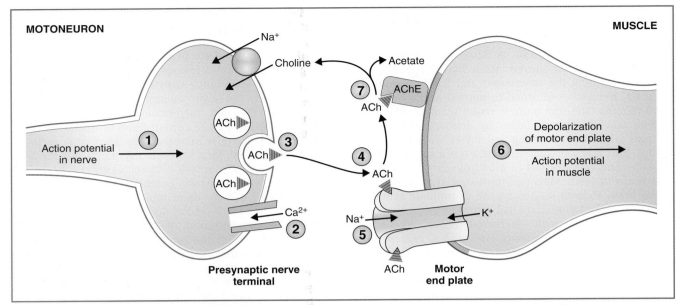

MOTONEURON

Na+

Choline

Acetate

7

AChE

ACh

ACh

1

Action potential
in nerve

ACh

ACh

3

4

ACh

Ca2+

2

Na+

5

K+

ACh

MUSCLE

6

Depolarization
of motor end plate

Action potential
in muscle

**Presynaptic nerve
terminal**

**Motor
end plate**

Figure 1–16 Sequence of events in neuromuscular transmission. *1,* Action potential travels down the motoneuron to the presynaptic terminal. *2,* Depolarization of the presynaptic terminal opens Ca^{2+} channels, and Ca^{2+} flows into the terminal. *3,* Acetylcholine (ACh) is extruded into the synapse by exocytosis. *4,* ACh binds to its receptor on the motor end plate. *5,* Channels for Na^+ and K^+ are opened in the motor end plate. *6,* Depolarization of the motor end plate causes action potentials to be generated in the adjacent muscle tissue. *7,* ACh is degraded to choline and acetate by acetylcholinesterase (AChE); choline is taken back into the presynaptic terminal on an Na^+-choline cotransporter.

of the postsynaptic cell; if the neurotransmitter is inhibitory, it causes hyperpolarization of the postsynaptic cell.

In contrast to electrical synapses, neurotransmission across chemical synapses is **unidirectional** (from presynaptic cell to postsynaptic cell). The **synaptic delay** is the time required for the multiple steps in chemical neurotransmission to occur.

Neuromuscular Junction—Example of a Chemical Synapse

Motor Units

Motoneurons are the nerves that innervate muscle fibers. A **motor unit** comprises a single motoneuron and the muscle fibers it innervates. Motor units vary considerably in size: A single motoneuron may activate a few muscle fibers or thousands of muscle fibers. Predictably, small motor units are involved in fine motor activities (e.g., facial expressions), and large motor units are involved in gross muscular activities (e.g., quadriceps muscles used in running).

Sequence of Events at the Neuromuscular Junction

The synapse between a motoneuron and a muscle fiber is called the **neuromuscular junction** (Fig. 1-16). An action potential in the motoneuron produces an action potential in the muscle fibers it innervates by the

following sequence of events: The numbered steps correlate with the circled numbers in Figure 1-16.

1. Action potentials are propagated down the motoneuron, as described previously. Local currents depolarize each adjacent region to threshold. Finally, the presynaptic terminal is depolarized, and this depolarization causes voltage-gated **Ca^{2+} channels** in the presynaptic membrane to open.

2. When these Ca^{2+} channels open, the Ca^{2+} permeability of the presynaptic terminal increases, and Ca^{2+} flows into the terminal down its electrochemical gradient.

3. Ca^{2+} uptake into the terminal causes release of the neurotransmitter **acetylcholine (ACh),** which has been previously synthesized and stored in synaptic vesicles. To release ACh, the synaptic vesicles fuse with the plasma membrane and empty their contents into the synaptic cleft by exocytosis.

   ACh is formed from acetyl coenzyme A (acetyl CoA) and choline by the action of the enzyme **choline acetyltransferase** (Fig. 1-17). ACh is stored in vesicles with ATP and proteoglycan for subsequent release. On stimulation, the entire content of a synaptic vesicle is released into the synaptic cleft. The smallest possible amount of ACh that can be released is the content of one synaptic vesicle (one quantum), and for this reason, the release of ACh is said to be **quantal.**

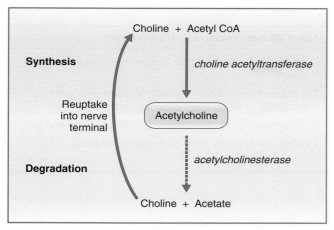

Figure 1–17 **Synthesis and degradation of acetylcholine.**

4. ACh diffuses across the synaptic cleft to the post-synaptic membrane. This specialized region of the muscle fiber is called the **motor end plate,** which contains **nicotinic receptors** for ACh. ACh binds to the α subunits of the nicotinic receptor and causes a conformational change. It is important to note that the nicotinic receptor for ACh is an example of a ligand-gated ion channel: It *also* is an Na^+ and K^+ channel. When the conformational change occurs, the central core of the channel opens, and the permeability of the motor end plate to both Na^+ and K^+ increases.

5. When these channels open, both Na^+ and K^+ flow down their respective electrochemical gradients, Na^+ moving into the end plate and K^+ moving out, each ion attempting to drive the motor end plate potential to its equilibrium potential. Indeed, if there were no other ion channels in the motor end plate, the end plate would depolarize to a value about halfway between the equilibrium potentials for Na^+ and K^+, or approximately 0 mV. (In this case, zero is not a "magic number"—it simply happens to be the value about halfway between the two equilibrium potentials.) In practice, however, because other ion channels that influence membrane potential are present in the end plate, the motor end plate only depolarizes to about −50 mV, which is the **end plate potential** (**EPP**). The EPP is not an action potential but is simply a local depolarization of the specialized motor end plate.

The content of a single synaptic vesicle produces the smallest possible change in membrane potential of the motor end plate, the **miniature end plate potential** (**MEPP**). MEPPs summate to produce the full-fledged EPP. The spontaneous appearance of MEPPs proves the quantal nature of ACh release at the neuromuscular junction.

Each MEPP, which represents the content of one synaptic vesicle, depolarizes the motor end plate by about 0.4 mV. An EPP is a multiple of these 0.4 mV units of depolarization. *How many such quanta are required to depolarize the motor end plate to the EPP?* Because the motor end plate must be depolarized from its resting potential of −90 mV to the threshold potential of −50 mV, it must, therefore, depolarize by 40 mV. Depolarization by 40 mV requires 100 quanta (because each quantum or vesicle depolarizes the motor end plate by 0.4 mV).

6. Depolarization of the motor end plate (the EPP) then spreads by local currents to adjacent muscle fibers, which are depolarized to threshold and fire action potentials. Although the motor end plate itself cannot fire action potentials, it depolarizes sufficiently to initiate the process in the neighboring "regular" muscle cells. Action potentials are propagated down the muscle fiber by a continuation of this process.

7. The EPP at the motor end plate is terminated when ACh is degraded to choline and acetate by **acetyl-cholinesterase** (**AChE**) on the motor end plate. Approximately 50% of the choline is returned to the presynaptic terminal by **Na^+-choline cotransport,** to be used again in the synthesis of new ACh.

Agents That Alter Neuromuscular Function

Several agents interfere with normal activity at the neuromuscular junction, and their mechanisms of action can be readily understood by considering the steps involved in neuromuscular transmission (Table 1-3; see Fig. 1-16).

♦ **Botulinus toxin** blocks the release of ACh from presynaptic terminals, causing total blockade of neuromuscular transmission, paralysis of skeletal muscle, and, eventually, death from respiratory failure.

♦ **Curare** competes with ACh for the nicotinic receptors on the motor end plate, decreasing the size of the EPP. When administered in maximal doses, curare causes paralysis and death. D-**Tubocurarine,** a form of curare, is used therapeutically to cause relaxation of skeletal muscle during anesthesia. A related substance, **α-bungarotoxin,** binds irreversibly to ACh receptors. Binding of radioactive α-bungarotoxin has provided an experimental tool for measuring the density of ACh receptors on the motor end plate.

♦ **AChE inhibitors** (anticholinesterases) such as **neostigmine** prevent degradation of ACh in the synaptic cleft, and they prolong and enhance the action of ACh at the motor end plate. AChE inhibitors can be used in the treatment of **myasthenia gravis,** a

Table 1-3 Agents Affecting Neuromuscular Transmission

Example	Action	Effect on Neuromuscular Transmission
Botulinus toxin	Blocks ACh release from presynaptic terminals	Total blockade, paralysis of respiratory muscles, and death
Curare	Competes with ACh for receptors on motor end plate	Decreases size of EPP; in maximal doses produces paralysis of respiratory muscles and death
Neostigmine	AChE inhibitor (anticholinesterase)	Prolongs and enhances action of ACh at motor end plate
Hemicholinium	Blocks reuptake of choline into presynaptic terminal	Depletes ACh stores from presynaptic terminal

ACh, Acetylcholine; AChE, acetylcholinesterase; EPP, end plate potential.

BOX 1–4   Clinical Physiology: Myasthenia Gravis

DESCRIPTION OF CASE. An 18-year-old college woman comes to the student health service complaining of progressive weakness. She reports that occasionally her eyelids "droop" and that she tires easily, even when completing ordinary daily tasks such as brushing her hair. She has fallen several times while climbing a flight of stairs. These symptoms improve with rest. The physician orders blood studies, which reveal elevated levels of antibodies to ACh receptors. Nerve stimulation studies show decreased responsiveness of skeletal muscle on repeated stimulation of motoneurons. The woman is diagnosed with myasthenia gravis and is treated with the drug pyridostigmine. After treatment, she reports a return of muscle strength.

EXPLANATION OF CASE. This young woman has classic myasthenia gravis. In the autoimmune form of the disease, antibodies are produced to ACh receptors on the motor end plates of skeletal muscle. Her symptoms of severe muscle weakness (eye muscles; arms and legs) are explainable by the presence of antibodies that block ACh receptors. Although ACh is released in normal amounts from the terminals of

motoneurons, binding of ACh to its receptors on the motor end plates is impaired. Because ACh cannot bind, depolarization of the motor end plate (end plate potential, EPP) will not occur and normal action potentials cannot be generated in the skeletal muscle. Muscle weakness and fatigability ensue.

TREATMENT. Treatment of the patient with myasthenia gravis depends on a clear understanding of the physiology of the neuromuscular junction. Because this patient's condition improved with the administration of pyridostigmine (a long-acting acetylcholinesterase [AChE] inhibitor), the success of the treatment confirmed the diagnosis of myasthenia gravis. AChE on the motor end plate normally degrades ACh (i.e., AChE terminates the action of ACh). By inhibiting the ACh-degradative enzyme with pyridostigmine, ACh levels in the neuromuscular junction are maintained at a high level, prolonging the time available for ACh to activate its receptors on the motor end plate. Thus, a more normal EPP in the muscle fiber can be produced even though many of the ACh receptors are blocked by antibodies.

---

disease characterized by skeletal muscle weakness and fatigability, in which ACh receptors are blocked by antibodies (Box 1-4).

♦ **Hemicholinium** blocks choline reuptake into presynaptic terminals, thus depleting choline stores from the motoneuron terminal and decreasing the synthesis of ACh.

Types of Synaptic Arrangements

There are several types of relationships between the input to a synapse (the presynaptic element) and the output (the postsynaptic element): one-to-one, one-to-many, or many-to-one.

♦ **One-to-one synapses.** The one-to-one synapse is illustrated by the **neuromuscular junction** (see Fig. 1-16). A single action potential in the presynaptic cell, the motoneuron, causes a single action potential in the postsynaptic cell, the muscle fiber.

♦ **One-to-many synapses.** The one-to-many synapse is uncommon, but it is found, for example, at the synapses of motoneurons on Renshaw cells of the spinal cord. An action potential in the presynaptic cell, the motoneuron, causes a burst of action potentials in the postsynaptic cells. This arrangement causes amplification of activity.

♦ **Many-to-one synapses.** The many-to-one synapse is a very common arrangement in the nervous system.

In these synapses, an action potential in the presynaptic cell is insufficient to produce an action potential in the postsynaptic cell. Instead, many presynaptic cells converge on the postsynaptic cell, these inputs summate, and the sum of the inputs determines whether the postsynaptic cell will fire an action potential.

Synaptic Input—Excitatory and Inhibitory Postsynaptic Potentials

The many-to-one synaptic arrangement is a common configuration in which many presynaptic cells converge on a single postsynaptic cell, with the inputs being either **excitatory** or **inhibitory.** The postsynaptic cell integrates all the converging information, and if the sum of the inputs is sufficient to bring the postsynaptic cell to threshold, it will then fire an action potential.

Excitatory Postsynaptic Potentials

Excitatory postsynaptic potentials (EPSPs) are synaptic inputs that **depolarize** the postsynaptic cell, bringing the membrane potential closer to threshold and closer to firing an action potential. EPSPs are produced by **opening Na$^+$ and K$^+$ channels,** similar to the nicotinic ACh receptor. The membrane potential is driven to a value approximately halfway between the equilibrium potentials for Na$^+$ and K$^+$, or 0 mV, which is a depolarized state. Excitatory neurotransmitters include ACh, norepinephrine, epinephrine, dopamine, glutamate, and serotonin.

Inhibitory Postsynaptic Potentials

Inhibitory postsynaptic potentials (IPSPs) are synaptic inputs that **hyperpolarize** the postsynaptic cell, taking the membrane potential away from threshold and farther from firing an action potential. IPSPs are produced by **opening Cl$^-$ channels.** The membrane potential is driven toward the Cl$^-$ equilibrium potential (approximately –90 mV), which is a hyperpolarized state. Inhibitory neurotransmitters are γ-aminobutyric acid (GABA) and glycine.

Integration of Synaptic Information

The presynaptic information that arrives at the synapse may be integrated in one of two ways, spatially or temporally.

Spatial Summation

Spatial summation occurs when two or more presynaptic inputs arrive at a postsynaptic cell simultaneously. If both inputs are excitatory, they will combine to produce greater depolarization than either input would produce separately. If one input is excitatory and the other is inhibitory, they will cancel each other out.

Spatial summation may occur, even if the inputs are far apart on the nerve cell body, because EPSPs and IPSPs are conducted so rapidly over the cell membrane.

Temporal Summation

Temporal summation occurs when two presynaptic inputs arrive at the postsynaptic cell in rapid succession. Because the inputs overlap in time, they summate.

Other Phenomena That Alter Synaptic Activity

Facilitation, augmentation, and **post-tetanic potentiation** are phenomena that may occur at synapses. In each instance, repeated stimulation causes the response of the postsynaptic cell to be greater than expected. The common underlying mechanism is believed to be an increased release of neurotransmitter into the synapse, possibly caused by accumulation of Ca^{2+} in the presynaptic terminal. **Long-term potentiation** occurs in storage of memories and involves both increased release of neurotransmitter from presynaptic terminals and increased sensitivity of postsynaptic membranes to the transmitter.

Synaptic fatigue may occur where repeated stimulation produces a smaller than expected response in the postsynaptic cell, possibly resulting from the depletion of neurotransmitter stores from the presynaptic terminal.

Neurotransmitters

The transmission of information at chemical synapses involves the release of a neurotransmitter from a presynaptic cell, diffusion across the synaptic cleft, and binding of the neurotransmitter to specific receptors on the postsynaptic membrane to produce a change in membrane potential.

The following criteria are used to formally designate a substance as a neurotransmitter: The substance must be synthesized in the presynaptic cell; the substance must be released by the presynaptic cell on stimulation; and, if the substance is applied exogenously to the postsynaptic membrane at physiologic concentration, the response of the postsynaptic cell must mimic the in vivo response.

Neurotransmitter substances can be grouped into the following categories: acetylcholine, biogenic amines, amino acids, and neuropeptides (Table 1-4).

Acetylcholine

The role of acetylcholine (ACh) as a neurotransmitter is vitally important for several reasons. ACh is the *only* neurotransmitter that is utilized at the neuromuscular junction. It is the neurotransmitter released from *all* preganglionic and most postganglionic neurons in the parasympathetic nervous system and from *all*

Table 1-4 Classification of Neurotransmitter Substances

Choline Esters	Biogenic Amines	Amino Acids	Neuropeptides
Acetylcholine (ACh)	Dopamine	γ-Aminobutyric acid	Adrenocorticotropin (ACTH)
	Epinephrine	(GABA)	Cholecystokinin
	Histamine	Glutamate	Dynorphin
	Norepinephrine	Glycine	Endorphins
	Serotonin		Enkephalins
			Glucose-dependent insulinotropic peptide (GIP)
			Glucagon
			Neurotensin
			Oxytocin
			Secretin
			Substance P
			Thyrotropin-releasing hormone (TRH)
			Vasopressin
			Vasoactive intestinal peptide (VIP)

preganglionic neurons in the sympathetic nervous system. It is also the neurotransmitter that is released from presynaptic neurons of the adrenal medulla.

Figure 1-17 illustrates the synthetic and degradative pathways for ACh. In the presynaptic terminal, choline and acetyl CoA combine to form ACh, catalyzed by choline acetyltransferase. When ACh is released from the presynaptic nerve terminal, it diffuses to the post-synaptic membrane, where it binds to and activates nicotinic ACh receptors. AChE is present on the post-synaptic membrane, where it degrades ACh to choline and acetate. This degradation terminates the action of ACh at the postsynaptic membrane. Approximately one half of the choline that is released from the degradation of ACh is taken back into the presynaptic terminal to be reutilized for synthesis of new ACh.

Norepinephrine, Epinephrine, and Dopamine

Norepinephrine, epinephrine, and dopamine are members of the same family of biogenic amines: They share a common precursor, tyrosine, and a common biosynthetic pathway (Fig. 1-18). Tyrosine is converted to L-dopa by tyrosine hydroxylase, and L-dopa is converted to **dopamine** by dopa decarboxylase. If dopamine β-hydroxylase is present in small dense-core vesicles of the nerve terminal, dopamine is converted to **norepinephrine.** If phenylethanolamine-N-methyl transferase (PNMT) is present (with S-adenosylmethionine as the methyl donor), then norepinephrine is methylated to form **epinephrine.**

The specific neurotransmitter secreted depends on which portion, or portions, of the enzymatic pathway are present in a particular type of nerve or gland. Thus, **dopaminergic neurons** secrete dopamine because the presynaptic nerve terminal contains tyrosine hydroxylase and dopa decarboxylase, but not the other enzymes. **Adrenergic neurons** secrete norepinephrine because they contain dopamine β-hydroxylase, in addition to

tyrosine hydroxylase and dopa decarboxylase, but not PNMT. The **adrenal medulla** contains the complete enzymatic pathway; therefore, it secretes primarily epinephrine.

The degradation of dopamine, norepinephrine, and epinephrine to inactive substances occurs via two enzymes: catechol-O-methyltransferase (COMT) and monoamine oxidase (MAO). **COMT,** a methylating enzyme, is *not found in nerve terminals,* but it is distributed widely in other tissues including the liver. **MAO** is located in presynaptic nerve terminals and catalyzes oxidative deamination. If a neurotransmitter is to be degraded by MAO, there must be reuptake of the neurotransmitter from the synapse.

Each of the biogenic amines can be degraded by MAO alone, by COMT alone, or by both MAO and COMT (in any order). Thus, there are three possible degradative products from each neurotransmitter, and typically these products are excreted in the urine (see Fig. 1-18). The major metabolite of norepinephrine is **normetanephrine.** The major metabolite of epinephrine is **metanephrine.** Both norepinephrine and epinephrine are degraded to **3-methoxy-4-hydroxymandelic acid (VMA).**

Serotonin

Serotonin, another biogenic amine, is produced from tryptophan in serotonergic neurons in the brain and in the gastrointestinal tract (Fig. 1-19). Following its release from presynaptic neurons, serotonin may be returned intact to the nerve terminal, or it may be degraded in the presynaptic terminal by MAO to 5-hydroxyindoleacetic acid. Additionally, serotonin serves as the precursor to melatonin in the pineal gland.

Histamine

Histamine, a biogenic amine, is synthesized from histidine, catalyzed by histidine decarboxylase. It is present

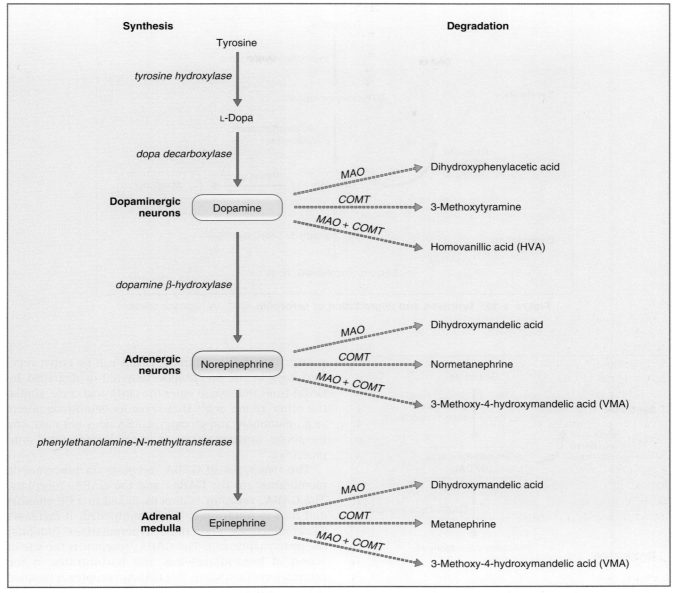

Figure 1–18 **Synthesis and degradation of dopamine, norepinephrine, and epinephrine.** COMT, Catechol-*O*-methyltransferase; MAO, monoamine oxidase.

in neurons of the hypothalamus, as well as in nonneural tissue such as **mast cells** of the gastrointestinal tract.

Glutamate

Glutamate, an amino acid, is the major **excitatory** neurotransmitter in the central nervous system. It plays a significant role in the spinal cord and cerebellum. There are four subtypes of glutamate receptors. Three of the subtypes are **ionotropic receptors,** or ligand-gated ion channels including the **NMDA** (*N*-methyl-D-aspartate) receptor that is widely distributed throughout the central nervous system. A fourth subtype comprises

metabotropic receptors, which are coupled via heterotrimeric guanosine triphosphate (GTP)–binding proteins (G proteins) to ion channels.

Glycine

Glycine, an amino acid, is an **inhibitory** neurotransmitter that is found in the spinal cord and brain stem. Its mechanism of action is to **increase Cl⁻ conductance** of the postsynaptic cell membrane. By increasing Cl⁻ conductance, the membrane potential is driven closer to the Cl⁻ equilibrium potential. Thus, the postsynaptic cell membrane is hyperpolarized or inhibited.

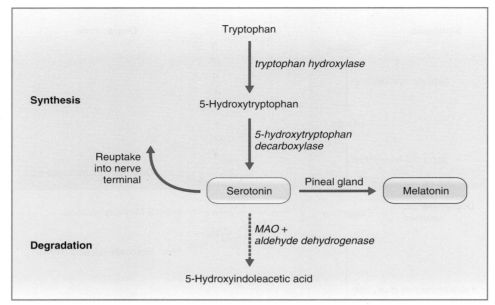

Figure 1–19 Synthesis and degradation of serotonin. MAO, Monoamine oxidase.

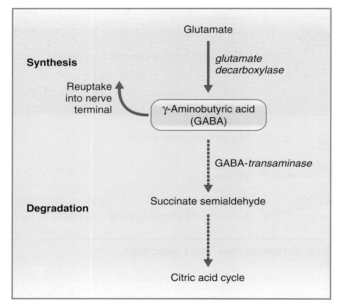

Figure 1–20 Synthesis and degradation of γ-aminobutyric acid (GABA).

γ-Aminobutyric Acid (GABA)

γ-Aminobutyric acid (GABA) is an amino acid and an **inhibitory** neurotransmitter that is distributed widely in the central nervous system in GABAergic neurons. GABA is synthesized from glutamic acid, catalyzed by glutamic acid decarboxylase, an enzyme that is unique to GABAergic neurons (Fig. 1-20). Following its release from presynaptic nerves and its action at the postsynaptic cell membrane, GABA can be either recycled back to the presynaptic terminal or degraded by GABA transaminase to enter the citric acid cycle. Unlike the other amino acids that serve as neurotransmitters (e.g., glutamate and glycine), GABA does not have any metabolic functions (i.e., it is not incorporated into proteins).

The two types of GABA receptors on postsynaptic membranes are the $GABA_A$ and the $GABA_B$ receptors. The **$GABA_A$ receptor** is directly linked to a Cl^- channel and thus is **ionotropic.** When stimulated, it increases Cl^- conductance and, thus, hyperpolarizes (inhibits) the postsynaptic cell. The $GABA_A$ receptor is the site of action of **benzodiazepines** and **barbiturates** in the central nervous system. The **$GABA_B$ receptor** is coupled via a G protein to a K^+ channel and thus is **metabotropic.** When stimulated, it increases K^+ conductance and hyperpolarizes the postsynaptic cell.

Huntington disease is associated with GABA deficiency. The disease is characterized by hyperkinetic choreiform movements related to a deficiency of GABA in the projections from the striatum to the globus pallidus. The characteristic uncontrolled movements are, in part, attributed to lack of GABA-dependent inhibition of neural pathways.

Nitric Oxide

Nitric oxide (NO) is a short-acting inhibitory neurotransmitter in the gastrointestinal tract and the central nervous system. In presynaptic nerve terminals, the enzyme **NO synthase** converts arginine to citrulline and NO. Then, NO, a permeant gas, simply diffuses from the presynaptic terminal to its target cell (instead of the usual packaging of neurotransmitter in synaptic vesicles and release by exocytosis). In addition to serving as a neurotransmitter, NO also functions in signal transduction of guanylyl cyclase in a variety of tissues including vascular smooth muscle (see Chapter 4).

Neuropeptides

There is a long and growing list of neuropeptides that function as neuromodulators, neurohormones, and neurotransmitters (see Table 1-4 for a partial list).

♦ **Neuromodulators** are substances that act on the presynaptic cell to alter the amount of neurotransmitter released in response to stimulation. Alternatively, a neuromodulator may be cosecreted with a neurotransmitter and alter the response of the postsynaptic cell to the neurotransmitter.

♦ **Neurohormones,** like other hormones, are released from secretory cells (in these cases, neurons) into the blood to act at a distant site.

♦ In several instances, **neuropeptides** are copackaged and cosecreted from presynaptic vesicles along with the classical neurotransmitters. For example, vasoactive intestinal peptide (VIP) is stored and secreted with ACh, particularly in neurons of the gastrointestinal tract. Somatostatin, enkephalin, and neurotensin are secreted with norepinephrine. Substance P is secreted with serotonin.

In contrast to classical neurotransmitters, which are synthesized in presynaptic nerve terminals, neuropeptides are synthesized in the nerve cell body. As occurs in all protein synthesis, the cell's DNA is transcribed into specific messenger RNA, which is translated into polypeptides on the ribosomes. Typically, a preliminary polypeptide containing a signal peptide sequence is synthesized first. The signal peptide is removed in the endoplasmic reticulum, and the final peptide is delivered to secretory vesicles. The secretory vesicles are then moved rapidly down the nerve by **axonal transport** to the presynaptic terminal, where they become the synaptic vesicles.

Purines

Adenosine triphosphate (ATP) and adenosine function as neuromodulators in the autonomic and central nervous systems. For example, **ATP** is synthesized in the sympathetic neurons that innervate vascular smooth muscle. It is costored and cosecreted with the "regular" neurotransmitter of these neurons, norepinephrine. When stimulated, the neuron releases both ATP and norepinephrine and both transmitters cause contraction of the smooth muscle; in fact, the ATP-induced contraction precedes the norepinephrine-induced contraction.

SKELETAL MUSCLE

Contraction of skeletal muscle is under voluntary control. Each skeletal muscle cell is innervated by a branch of a motoneuron. Action potentials are propagated along the motoneurons, leading to release of ACh at the neuromuscular junction, depolarization of the motor end plate, and initiation of action potentials in the muscle fiber.

What events, then, elicit contraction of the muscle fiber? These events, occurring between the action potential in the muscle fiber and contraction of the muscle fiber, are called **excitation-contraction coupling.** The mechanisms of excitation-contraction coupling in skeletal muscle and smooth muscle are discussed in this chapter, and the mechanisms of excitation-contraction coupling in cardiac muscle are discussed in Chapter 4.

Muscle Filaments

Each muscle fiber behaves as a single unit, is multinucleate, and contains myofibrils. The myofibrils are surrounded by sarcoplasmic reticulum and are invaginated by transverse tubules (T tubules). Each myofibril contains interdigitating thick and thin filaments, which are arranged longitudinally and cross-sectionally in sarcomeres (Fig. 1-21). The repeating units of sarcomeres account for the unique banding pattern seen in striated muscle (which includes both skeletal and cardiac muscle).

Thick Filaments

The thick filaments comprise a large molecular weight protein called **myosin,** which has six polypeptide chains including one pair of **heavy chains** and two pairs of **light chains** (see Figure 1-21A). Most of the heavy-chain myosin has an α-helical structure, in which the two chains coil around each other to form the "**tail**" of the myosin molecule. The four light chains and the N terminus of each heavy chain form two globular "**heads**" on the myosin molecule. These globular heads have an actin-binding site, which is necessary for cross-bridge formation, and a site that binds and hydrolyzes ATP (myosin ATPase).

Thin Filaments

The thin filaments are composed of three proteins: actin, tropomyosin, and troponin (see Fig. 1-21B).

Actin is a globular protein and, in this globular form, is called G-actin. In the thin filaments, G-actin is polymerized into two strands that are twisted into an α-helical structure to form filamentous actin, called F-actin. Actin has myosin-binding sites. When the muscle is at rest, the myosin-binding sites are covered by tropomyosin so that actin and myosin cannot interact.

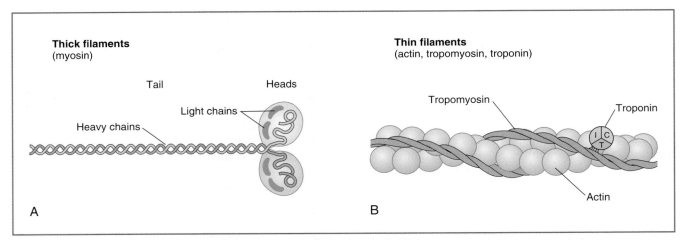

Figure 1–21 **Structure of thick (A) and thin (B) filaments of skeletal muscle.** Troponin is a complex of three proteins: I, troponin I; T, troponin T; and C, troponin C.

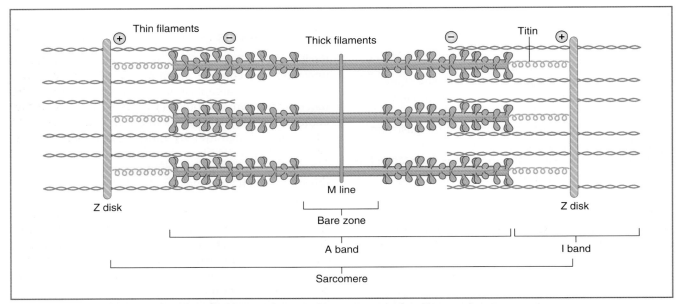

Figure 1–22 **Arrangement of thick and thin filaments of skeletal muscle in sarcomeres.**

Tropomyosin is a filamentous protein that runs along the groove of each twisted actin filament. At rest, its function is to block the myosin-binding sites on actin. If contraction is to occur, tropomyosin must be moved out of the way so that actin and myosin can interact.

Troponin is a complex of three globular proteins (troponin T, troponin I, and troponin C) located at regular intervals along the tropomyosin filaments. **Troponin T** (T for tropomyosin) attaches the troponin complex to tropomyosin. **Troponin I** (I for inhibition), along with tropomyosin, inhibits the interaction of actin and myosin by covering the myosin-binding site on actin. **Troponin C** (C for Ca^{2+}) is a Ca^{2+}-binding protein that plays a central role in the initiation of contraction. When the intracellular Ca^{2+} concentration increases, Ca^{2+} binds to troponin C, producing a conformational change in the troponin complex. This conformational change moves tropomyosin out of the way, permitting the binding of actin to the myosin heads.

Arrangement of Thick and Thin Filaments in Sarcomeres

The **sarcomere** is the basic contractile unit, and it is delineated by the Z disks. Each sarcomere contains a full A band in the center and one half of two I bands on either side of the A band (Fig. 1-22).

The **A bands** are located in the center of the sarcomere and contain the thick (myosin) filaments, which appear dark when viewed under polarized light. Thick and thin filaments may overlap in the A band; these

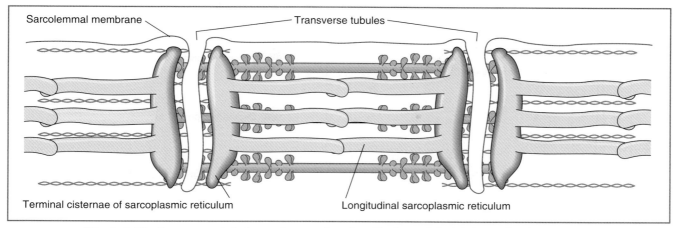

Sarcolemmal membrane

Transverse tubules

Terminal cisternae of sarcoplasmic reticulum

Longitudinal sarcoplasmic reticulum

Figure 1–23 **Transverse tubules and sarcoplasmic reticulum of skeletal muscle.** The transverse tubules are continuous with the sarcolemmal membrane and invaginate deep into the muscle fiber, making contact with terminal cisternae of the sarcoplasmic reticulum.

areas of overlap are potential sites of cross-bridge formation.

The **I bands** are located on either side of the A band and appear light when viewed under polarized light. They contain the thin (actin) filaments, intermediate filamentous proteins, and Z disks. They have no thick filaments.

The **Z disks** are darkly staining structures that run down the middle of each I band, delineating the ends of each sarcomere.

The **bare zone** is located in the center of each sarcomere. There are no thin filaments in the bare zone; thus, there can be no overlap of thick and thin filaments or cross-bridge formation in this region.

The **M line** bisects the bare zone and contains darkly staining proteins that link the central portions of the thick filaments together.

Cytoskeletal Proteins

Cytoskeletal proteins establish the architecture of the myofibrils, ensuring that the thick and thin filaments are aligned correctly and at proper distances with respect to each other.

Transverse cytoskeletal proteins link thick and thin filaments, forming a "scaffold" for the myofibrils and linking sarcomeres of adjacent myofibrils. A system of intermediate filaments holds the myofibrils together, side by side. The entire myofibrillar array is anchored to the cell membrane by an actin-binding protein called **dystrophin.** (In patients with muscular dystrophy, dystrophin is defective or absent.)

Longitudinal cytoskeletal proteins include two large proteins called titin and nebulin. **Titin,** which is associated with thick filaments, is a large molecular weight protein that extends from the M lines to the Z disks. Part of the titin molecule passes through the thick filament; the rest of the molecule, which is elastic or springlike, is anchored to the Z disk. As the length of the sarcomere changes, so does the elastic portion of the titin molecule. Titin also helps center the thick filaments in the sarcomere. **Nebulin** is associated with thin filaments. A single nebulin molecule extends from one end of the thin filament to the other. Nebulin serves as a "molecular ruler," setting the length of thin filaments during their assembly. **α-Actinin** anchors the thin filaments to the Z disk.

Transverse Tubules and the Sarcoplasmic Reticulum

The **transverse (T) tubules** are an extensive network of muscle cell membrane (sarcolemmal membrane) that invaginates deep into the muscle fiber. The T tubules are responsible for carrying depolarization from action potentials at the muscle cell surface to the interior of the fiber. The T tubules make contact with the terminal cisternae of the sarcoplasmic reticulum and contain a voltage-sensitive protein called the **dihydropyridine receptor,** named for the drug that inhibits it (Fig. 1-23).

The **sarcoplasmic reticulum** is an internal tubular structure, which is the site of storage and release of Ca^{2+} for excitation-contraction coupling. As previously noted, the terminal cisternae of the sarcoplasmic reticulum make contact with the T tubules in a triad arrangement. The sarcoplasmic reticulum contains a Ca^{2+}-release channel called the **ryanodine receptor** (named for the plant alkaloid that opens this release channel). The significance of the physical relationship between the T tubules (and their dihydropyridine receptor) and the sarcoplasmic reticulum (and its ryanodine receptor) is described in the section on excitation-contraction coupling.

Ca^{2+} is accumulated in the sarcoplasmic reticulum by the action of **Ca^{2+} ATPase (SERCA)** in the

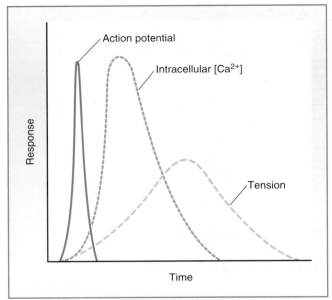

Figure 1–24 Temporal sequence of events in excitation-contraction coupling in skeletal muscle. The muscle action potential precedes a rise in intracellular [Ca²⁺], which precedes contraction.

sarcoplasmic reticulum membrane. The Ca²⁺ ATPase pumps Ca²⁺ from the ICF of the muscle fiber into the interior of the sarcoplasmic reticulum, keeping the intracellular Ca²⁺ concentration low when the muscle fiber is at rest. Within the sarcoplasmic reticulum, Ca²⁺ is bound to **calsequestrin**, a low-affinity, high-capacity Ca²⁺-binding protein. Calsequestrin, by binding Ca²⁺, helps to maintain a low free Ca²⁺ concentration inside the sarcoplasmic reticulum, thereby reducing the work of the Ca²⁺ ATPase pump. Thus, a large quantity of Ca²⁺ can be stored inside the sarcoplasmic reticulum in *bound* form, while the intrasarcoplasmic reticulum *free* Ca²⁺ concentration remains extremely low.

Excitation-Contraction Coupling in Skeletal Muscle

The mechanism that translates the muscle action potential into the production of tension is excitation-contraction coupling. Figure 1-24 shows the temporal relationships between an action potential in the skeletal muscle fiber, the subsequent increase in intracellular free Ca²⁺ concentration (which is released from the sarcoplasmic reticulum), and contraction of the muscle fiber. These temporal relationships are critical in that the action potential always *precedes* the rise in intracellular Ca²⁺ concentration, which always *precedes* contraction.

The steps involved in excitation-contraction coupling are described as follows and illustrated in Figure 1-25. (Step 6 is illustrated in Fig. 1-26):

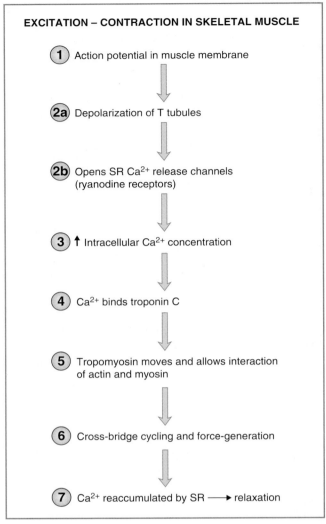

Figure 1–25 Steps in excitation-contraction in skeletal muscle. SR, Sarcoplasmic reticulum; T tubules, transverse tubules. See text for explanation of the circled numbers.

1. **Action potentials** in the muscle cell membrane are propagated to the **T tubules** by the spread of local currents. Thus, the T tubules are continuous with the sarcolemmal membrane and carry the depolarization from the surface to the interior of the muscle fiber.

2a. and b. **Depolarization of the T tubules** causes a critical conformational change in their voltage-sensitive **dihydropyridine receptors.** This conformational change opens Ca²⁺-release channels (**ryanodine receptors**) on the nearby sarcoplasmic reticulum. (As an aside, although the T tubules' dihydropyridine receptors are L-type voltage-gated Ca²⁺ channels, Ca²⁺ influx into the cell through these channels is *not* required for excitation-contraction coupling in skeletal muscle.)

Position of Actin and Myosin During Cross-bridge Cycling	Events	ATP/ADP
A	Rigor	No nucleotides bound
B	ATP binds to cleft on myosin head Conformational change in myosin Decreased affinity of myosin for actin Myosin released	ATP bound
C	Cleft closes around ATP Conformational change Myosin head displaced toward ⊕ end of actin ATP hydrolysis	ATP ⟶ ADP + P$_i$ ADP + P$_i$ bound
D	Myosin head binds new site on actin Power stroke = force	ADP bound
E	ADP released Rigor	No nucleotides bound

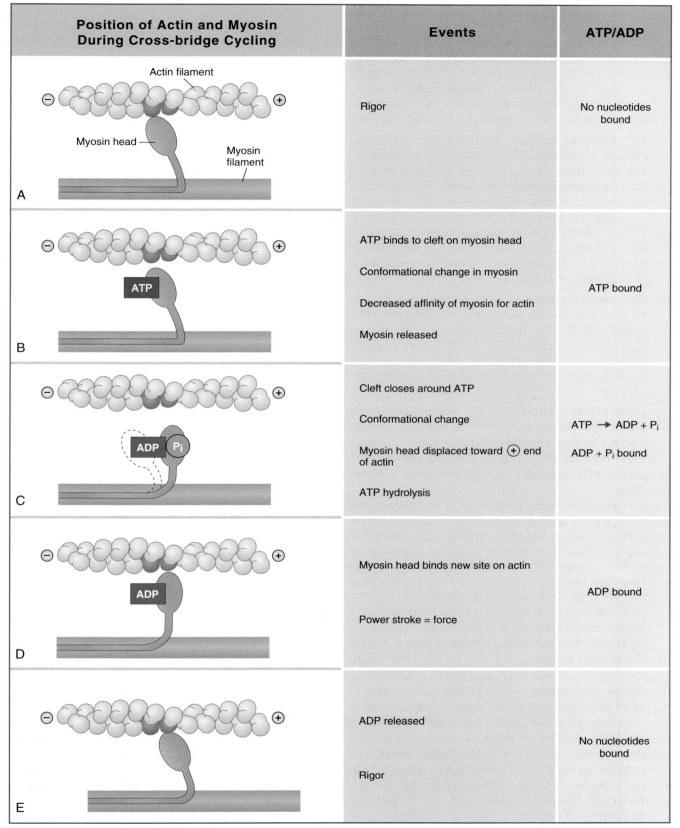

Figure 1–26 Cross-bridge cycle in skeletal muscle. Mechanism by which myosin "walks" toward the plus end of the actin filament. **A–E**, See the discussion in the text. ADP, Adenosine diphosphate; ATP, adenosine triphosphate; P$_i$, inorganic phosphate.

3. When these Ca^{2+}-release channels open, Ca^{2+} is released from its storage site in the sarcoplasmic reticulum into the ICF of the muscle fiber, resulting in an **increase in intracellular Ca^{2+} concentration.** At rest, the intracellular free Ca^{2+} concentration is less than 10^{-7} M. After its release from the sarcoplasmic reticulum, intracellular free Ca^{2+} concentration increases to levels between 10^{-7} M and 10^{-6} M.

4. **Ca^{2+} binds to troponin C** on the thin filaments, causing a conformational change in the troponin complex. Troponin C can bind as many as four Ca^{2+} ions per molecule of protein. Because this binding is cooperative, each molecule of bound Ca^{2+} increases the affinity of troponin C for the next Ca^{2+}. Thus, even a small increase in Ca^{2+} concentration increases the likelihood that all of the binding sites will be occupied to produce the necessary conformational change in the troponin complex.

5. The **conformational change in troponin** causes tropomyosin (which was previously blocking the interaction of actin and myosin) to be moved out of the way so that cross-bridge cycling can begin. When tropomyosin is moved away, the myosin-binding sites on actin, previously covered, are exposed.

6. **Cross-bridge cycling.** With Ca^{2+} bound to troponin C and tropomyosin moved out of the way, myosin heads can now bind to actin and form so-called **cross-bridges.** Formation of cross-bridges is associated with hydrolysis of ATP and generation of force.

    The sequence of events in the cross-bridge cycle is shown in Figure 1-26. *A,* At the beginning of the cycle, no ATP is bound to myosin, and myosin is tightly attached to actin in a "rigor" position. In rapidly contracting muscle, this state is brief. However, in the absence of ATP, this state is permanent (i.e., rigor mortis). *B,* The binding of ATP to a cleft on the back of the myosin head produces a conformational change in myosin that decreases its affinity for actin; thus, myosin is released from the original actin-binding site. *C,* The cleft closes around the bound ATP molecule, producing a further conformational change that causes myosin to be displaced toward the plus end of actin. ATP is hydrolyzed to ADP and P_i, which remain attached to myosin. *D,* Myosin binds to a new site on actin (toward the plus end), constituting the force-generating, or power, stroke. Each cross-bridge cycle "walks" the myosin head 10 nanometers (10^{-8} meters) along the actin filament. *E,* ADP is released, and myosin is returned to its original state with no nucleotides bound (*A*). Cross-bridge cycling continues, with myosin "walking" toward the plus end of the actin filament, as long as Ca^{2+} is bound to troponin C.

7. **Relaxation** occurs when Ca^{2+} is reaccumulated in the sarcoplasmic reticulum by the Ca^{2+} ATPase of the sarcoplasmic reticulum membrane (**SERCA**). When the intracellular Ca^{2+} concentration decreases to less than 10^{-7} M, there is insufficient Ca^{2+} for binding to troponin C. When Ca^{2+} is released from troponin C, tropomyosin returns to its resting position, where it blocks the myosin-binding site on actin. As long as the intracellular Ca^{2+} is low, cross-bridge cycling cannot occur and the muscle will relax.

The cross-bridge cycle produces force (tension) at the level of the contractile elements. In order for this force to be transmitted to the muscle surface, the series elastic elements (e.g., titin) must first be stretched out. As a result, there is a delay in transmission of force from the cross-bridges to the muscle surface (see Fig. 1-24). Once cross-bridge cycling has concluded, there is also a delay in the fall of muscle tension; the series elastic elements remain stretched out and thus force transmission to the muscle surface continues after intracellular Ca^{2+} has fallen and cross-bridge cycling has ceased.

Mechanism of Tetanus

A single action potential results in the release of a fixed amount of Ca^{2+} from the sarcoplasmic reticulum, which produces a single twitch. The twitch is terminated (relaxation occurs) when the sarcoplasmic reticulum reaccumulates this Ca^{2+}. However, if the muscle is stimulated repeatedly, there is insufficient time for the sarcoplasmic reticulum to reaccumulate Ca^{2+}, and the intracellular Ca^{2+} concentration never returns to the low levels that exist during relaxation. Instead, the level of intracellular Ca^{2+} concentration remains high, resulting in continued binding of Ca^{2+} to troponin C and continued cross-bridge cycling. In this state, there is a sustained contraction called **tetanus,** rather than just a single twitch.

Length-Tension Relationship

The length-tension relationship in muscle refers to the effect of muscle fiber length on the amount of tension the fiber can develop (Fig. 1-27). The amount of tension is determined for a muscle undergoing an **isometric contraction,** in which the muscle is allowed to develop tension at a preset length (called **preload**) but is not allowed to shorten. (Imagine trying to lift a 500-lb barbell. The tension developed would be great, but no shortening or movement of muscle would occur!) The following measurements of tension can be made as a function of preset length (or preload):

♦ **Passive tension** is the tension developed by simply stretching a muscle to different lengths. (Think of

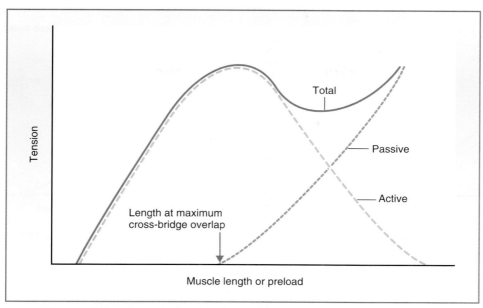

Figure 1–27 Length-tension relationship in skeletal muscle. Maximal active tension occurs at muscle lengths where there is maximal overlap of thick and thin filaments.

the tension produced in a rubber band as it is progressively stretched to longer lengths.)

♦ **Total tension** is the tension developed when a muscle is stimulated to contract at different preloads. It is the sum of the active tension developed by the cross-bridge cycling in the sarcomeres and the passive tension caused by stretching the muscle.

♦ **Active tension** is determined by subtracting the passive tension from the total tension. It represents the active force developed during cross-bridge cycling.

The unusual relationship between active tension and muscle length is the **length-tension relationship** and can be explained by the mechanisms involved in the cross-bridge cycle (see Fig. 1-27). The *active tension developed is proportional to the number of cross-bridges that cycle.* Therefore, the active tension is maximal when there is maximal overlap of thick and thin filaments and maximal possible cross-bridges. When the muscle is stretched to longer lengths, the number of possible cross-bridges is reduced and active tension is reduced. Likewise, when muscle length is decreased, the thin filaments collide with each other in the center of the sarcomere, reducing the number of possible cross-bridges and reducing active tension.

Force-Velocity Relationship

The force-velocity relationship, shown in Figure 1-28, describes the velocity of shortening when the force against which the muscle contracts, the **afterload,** is varied (see Fig. 1-28, *left*). In contrast to the length-tension relationship, the force-velocity relationship is determined by allowing the muscle to shorten. The force, rather than the length, is fixed, and therefore, it is called an **isotonic contraction.** The velocity of shortening reflects the **speed of cross-bridge cycling.** As is intuitively obvious, the velocity of shortening will be maximal (V_{max}) when the afterload on the muscle is zero. As the afterload on the muscle increases, the velocity will be decreased because crossbridges can cycle less rapidly against the higher resistance. As the afterload increases to even higher levels, the velocity of shortening is reduced to zero. (Imagine how quickly you can lift a feather as opposed to a ton of bricks!)

The effect of afterload on the velocity of shortening can be further demonstrated by setting the muscle to a preset length (preload) and then measuring the velocity of shortening at various levels of afterload (see Fig. 1-28, *right*). A "family" of curves is generated, each one representing a different fixed preload. The curves always intersect at V_{max}, the point where afterload is zero and where velocity of shortening is maximal.

SMOOTH MUSCLE

Smooth muscle lacks striations, which distinguishes it from skeletal and cardiac muscle. The striations found in skeletal and cardiac muscle are created by the banding patterns of thick and thin filaments in the sarcomeres. In smooth muscle, there are no striations because the thick and thin filaments, while present, are not organized in sarcomeres.

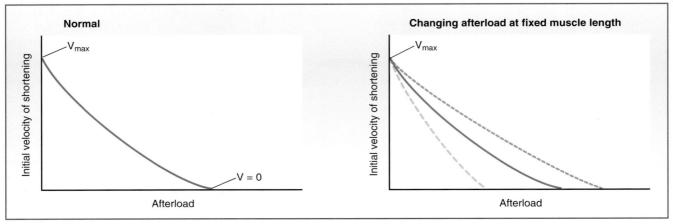

Figure 1-28 Initial velocity of shortening as a function of afterload in skeletal muscle.

Smooth muscle is found in the walls of hollow organs such as the gastrointestinal tract, the bladder, and the uterus, as well as in the vasculature, the ureters, the bronchioles, and the muscles of the eye. The functions of smooth muscle are twofold: to produce motility (e.g., to propel chyme along the gastrointestinal tract or to propel urine along the ureter) and to maintain tension (e.g., smooth muscle in the walls of blood vessels).

Types of Smooth Muscle

Smooth muscles are classified as multiunit or unitary, depending on whether the cells are electrically coupled. Unitary smooth muscle has gap junctions between cells, which allow for the fast spread of electrical activity throughout the organ, followed by a coordinated contraction. Multiunit smooth muscle has little or no coupling between cells. A third type, a combination of unitary and multiunit smooth muscle, is found in vascular smooth muscle.

Unitary Smooth Muscle

Unitary (single unit) smooth muscle is present in the gastrointestinal tract, bladder, uterus, and ureter. The smooth muscle in these organs contracts in a coordinated fashion because the cells are linked by **gap junctions.** Gap junctions are low-resistance pathways for current flow, which permit electrical coupling between cells. For example, action potentials occur simultaneously in the smooth muscle cells of the bladder so that contraction (and emptying) of the entire organ can occur at once.

Unitary smooth muscle is also characterized by spontaneous pacemaker activity, or **slow waves.** The frequency of slow waves sets a characteristic pattern of action potentials within an organ, which then determines the frequency of contractions.

Multiunit Smooth Muscle

Multiunit smooth muscle is present in the iris, in the ciliary muscles of the lens, and in the vas deferens. Each muscle fiber behaves as a separate motor unit (similar to skeletal muscle), and there is little or no coupling between cells. Multiunit smooth muscle cells are densely innervated by postganglionic fibers of the parasympathetic and sympathetic nervous systems, and it is these innervations that regulate function.

Excitation-Contraction Coupling in Smooth Muscle

The mechanism of excitation-contraction coupling in smooth muscle differs from that of skeletal muscle. Recall that in skeletal muscle binding of actin and myosin is permitted when Ca^{2+} binds troponin C. In smooth muscle, however, there is no troponin. Rather, the interaction of actin and myosin is controlled by the binding of Ca^{2+} to another protein, **calmodulin.** In turn, Ca^{2+}-calmodulin regulates myosin-light-chain kinase, which regulates cross-bridge cycling.

Steps in Excitation-Contraction Coupling in Smooth Muscle

The steps involved in excitation-contraction coupling in smooth muscle are illustrated in Figure 1-29 and occur as follows:

1. **Depolarization of smooth muscle** opens voltage-gated Ca^{2+} channels in the sarcolemmal membrane. With these Ca^{2+} channels open, Ca^{2+} flows into the cell down its electrochemical gradient. This influx of Ca^{2+} from the ECF causes an **increase in intracellular Ca^{2+} concentration.** In contrast to skeletal muscle, where action potentials are required to produce contraction, in smooth muscle, subthreshold depolarization (which does not lead to an action

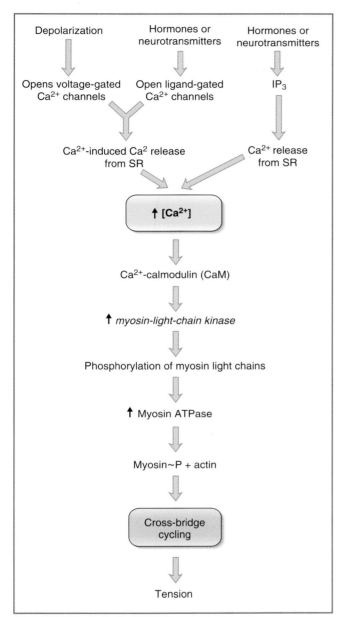

Figure 1–29 **The sequence of molecular events in contraction of smooth muscle.** ADP, Adenosine diphosphate; ATP, adenosine triphosphate; Myosin~P, phosphorylated myosin; P_i, inorganic phosphate. CaM, calmodulin; ATPase, adenosine triphosphatase; IP_3, inositol 1,4,5 triphosphate; SR, sarcoplasmic reticulum.

potential) can open these voltage-gated Ca^{2+} channels and cause an increase in intracellular Ca^{2+} concentration. *If* the depolarization of the smooth muscle membrane reaches threshold, then **action potentials** *can occur,* causing even greater depolarization and even greater opening of voltage-gated Ca^{2+} channels.

Ca^{2+} that enters the smooth muscle cells through voltage-gated Ca^{2+} channels releases additional Ca^{2+} from the SR (called **Ca^{2+}-induced Ca^{2+} release**).

Thus, the rise in intracellular Ca^{2+} is partly due to Ca^{2+} entry across the sarcolemmal membrane and partly due to Ca^{2+} release from intracellular SR stores.

2. Two additional mechanisms may contribute to the increase in intracellular Ca^{2+} concentration: ligand-gated Ca^{2+} channels and inositol 1,4,5-triphosphate (IP_3)–gated Ca^{2+} release channels. **Ligand-gated Ca^{2+} channels** in the sarcolemmal membrane may be opened by various hormones and neurotransmitters, permitting the entry of *additional* Ca^{2+} from the ECF. **IP_3-gated Ca^{2+} release channels** in the membrane of the sarcoplasmic reticulum may be opened by hormones and neurotransmitters. Either of these mechanisms may augment the rise in intracellular Ca^{2+} concentration caused by depolarization.

3. The rise in intracellular Ca^{2+} concentration causes Ca^{2+} to bind to **calmodulin.** Like troponin C in skeletal muscle, calmodulin binds four ions of Ca^{2+} in a cooperative fashion. The Ca^{2+}-calmodulin complex binds to and activates **myosin-light-chain kinase.**

4. When activated, myosin-light-chain kinase **phosphorylates myosin light chain.** When myosin light chain is phosphorylated, the conformation of the myosin head is altered, greatly increasing its ATPase activity. (In contrast, skeletal muscle myosin ATPase activity is always high.) The increase in myosin ATPase activity allows myosin to bind actin, thus initiating cross-bridge cycling and production of tension. The amount of tension is proportional to the intracellular Ca^{2+} concentration.

5. Ca^{2+}-calmodulin, in addition to the effects on myosin described earlier, also has effects on two thin filament proteins, **calponin** and **caldesmon.** At low levels of intracellular Ca^{2+}, calponin and caldesmon bind actin, inhibiting myosin ATPase and preventing the interaction of actin and myosin. When the intracellular Ca^{2+} increases, the Ca^{2+}-calmodulin complex leads to phosphorylation of calponin and caldesmon, releasing their inhibition of myosin ATPase and facilitating the formation of cross-bridges between actin and myosin.

6. **Relaxation** of smooth muscle occurs when the intracellular Ca^{2+} concentration falls below the level needed to form Ca^{2+}-calmodulin complexes. A fall in intracellular Ca^{2+} concentration can occur by a variety of mechanisms including hyperpolarization (which closes voltage-gated Ca^{2+} channels); direct inhibition of Ca^{2+} channels by ligands such as cyclic AMP and cyclic GMP; inhibition of IP_3 production and decreased release of Ca^{2+} from sarcoplasmic reticulum; and increased Ca^{2+} ATPase activity in sarcoplasmic reticulum. Additionally, relaxation of

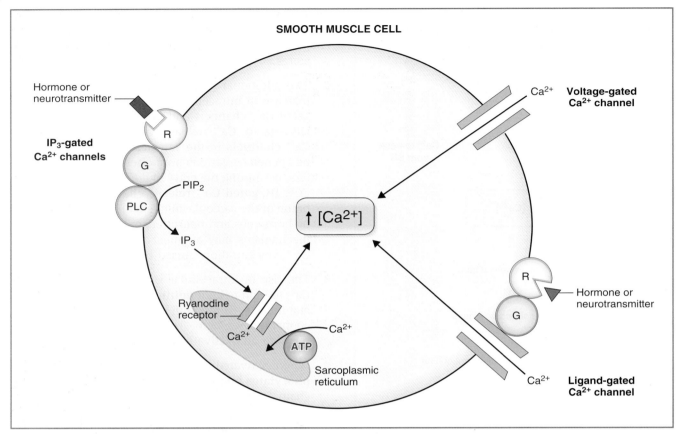

Figure 1–30 **Mechanisms for increasing intracellular [Ca²⁺] in smooth muscle.** ATP, Adenosine triphosphate; G, GTP-binding protein (G protein); IP₃, inositol 1,4,5-triphosphate; PIP₂, phosphatidylinositol 4,5-diphosphate; PLC, phospholipase C; R, receptor for hormone or neurotransmitter.

smooth muscle can involve activation of myosin-light-chain phosphatase, which dephosphorylates myosin light chain, leading to inhibition of myosin ATPase.

Mechanisms That Increase Intracellular Ca²⁺ Concentration in Smooth Muscle

Depolarization of smooth muscle opens sarcolemmal voltage-gated Ca²⁺ channels and Ca²⁺ enters the cell from ECF. As already noted, this is only *one* source of Ca²⁺ for contraction. Ca²⁺ also can enter the cell through ligand-gated channels in the sarcolemmal membrane, or it can be released from the sarcoplasmic reticulum by second messenger (IP₃)-gated mechanisms (Fig. 1-30). (In contrast, recall that in skeletal muscle the rise in intracellular Ca²⁺ concentration is caused exclusively by release from the sarcoplasmic reticulum—Ca²⁺ does not enter the cell from the ECF.) The three mechanisms involved in Ca²⁺ entry in smooth muscle are described as follows:

♦ **Voltage-gated Ca²⁺ channels** are sarcolemmal Ca²⁺ channels that open when the cell membrane potential depolarizes. Thus, action potentials in the smooth muscle cell membrane cause voltage-gated Ca²⁺ channels to open, allowing Ca²⁺ to flow into the cell down its electrochemical potential gradient.

♦ **Ligand-gated Ca²⁺ channels** also are present in the sarcolemmal membrane. They are not regulated by changes in membrane potential, but by receptor-mediated events. Various hormones and neurotransmitters interact with specific receptors in the sarcolemmal membrane, which are coupled via a GTP-binding protein (G protein) to the Ca²⁺ channels. When the channel is open, Ca²⁺ flows into the cell down its electrochemical gradient. (See Chapters 2 and 9 for further discussion of G proteins.)

♦ **IP₃-gated Ca²⁺ channels** are present in the sarcoplasmic reticulum membrane. The process begins at the cell membrane, but the source of the Ca²⁺ is the sarcoplasmic reticulum rather than the ECF. Hormones or neurotransmitters interact with specific receptors on the sarcolemmal membrane (e.g., norepinephrine with α₁ receptors). These receptors are coupled, via a G protein, to phospholipase C (PLC). **Phospholipase C** catalyzes the hydrolysis of phosphatidylinositol 4,5-diphosphate (PIP_2) to IP_3 and diacylglycerol (DAG). **IP_3** then diffuses to the sarcoplasmic reticulum, where it opens Ca^{2+} release channels (similar to the mechanism of the ryanodine receptor in skeletal muscle). When these Ca^{2+} channels are open, Ca^{2+} flows from its storage site in the sarcoplasmic reticulum into the ICF. (See Chapter 9 for discussion of IP_3-mediated hormone action.)

Ca^{2+}-Independent Changes in Smooth Muscle Contraction

In addition to the contractile mechanisms in smooth muscle that depend on changes in intracellular Ca^{2+} concentration, the degree of contraction also can be regulated by Ca^{2+}-independent mechanisms. For example, in the presence of a constant level of intracellular Ca^{2+}, if there is activation of myosin-light-chain kinase, more cross-bridges will cycle and more tension will be produced (**Ca^{2+}-sensitization**); conversely, if there is activation of myosin-light-chain phosphatase, fewer cross-bridges will cycle and less tension will be produced (**Ca^{2+}-desensitization**).

SUMMARY

■ Water, a major component of the body, is distributed among two major compartments, ICF and ECF. ECF is further distributed among the plasma and the interstitial fluid. The differences in composition of ICF and ECF are created and maintained by transport proteins in the cell membranes.

■ Transport may be either passive or active. If transport occurs down an electrochemical gradient, it is passive and does not consume energy. If transport occurs against an electrochemical gradient, it is active. The energy for active transport may be primary (using ATP) or secondary (using energy from the Na^+ gradient). Osmosis occurs when an impermeable solute creates an osmotic pressure difference across a membrane, which drives water flow.

■ Ion channels provide routes for charged solutes to move across cell membranes. The conductance of ion channels is controlled by gates, which are regulated by voltage or by ligands. Diffusion of a permeable ion down a concentration gradient creates a diffusion potential, which, at electrochemical equilibrium, is calculated by the Nernst equation. When several ions are permeable, each attempts to drive the membrane toward its equilibrium potential. Ions with the highest permeabilities make the greatest contribution to the resting membrane potential.

■ Action potentials in nerve and muscle consist of rapid depolarization (upstroke), followed by repolarization caused by the opening and closing of ion channels. Action potentials are propagated down nerve and muscle fibers by the spread of local currents, with the speed of conduction depending on the tissue's cable properties. Conduction velocity is increased by increasing fiber size and by myelination.

■ Synapses between cells may be electrical or, more commonly, chemical. The prototype of the chemical synapse is the neuromuscular junction, which uses ACh as a neurotransmitter. ACh is released from presynaptic nerve terminals and diffuses across the synapse to cause depolarization of the motor end plate. Neurotransmitters at other synapses may be either excitatory (causing depolarization) or inhibitory (causing hyperpolarization).

■ In muscle, action potentials precede contraction. The mechanisms that translate the action potential into contraction are called excitation-contraction coupling. In both skeletal and smooth muscle, Ca^{2+} plays a central role in the coupling.

■ In skeletal muscle, the action potential is carried to the cell interior by the T tubules, where depolarization releases Ca^{2+} from terminal cisternae of the nearby sarcoplasmic reticulum. Ca^{2+} then binds to troponin C on the thin filaments, causing a conformational change, which removes the inhibition of myosin-binding sites. When actin and myosin bind, cross-bridge cycling begins, producing tension.

■ In smooth muscle, Ca^{2+} enters the cell during the action potential via voltage-gated Ca^{2+} channels. Ca^{2+} then binds to calmodulin, and the Ca^{2+}-calmodulin complex activates myosin-light-chain kinase, which phosphorylates myosin. Myosin $\sim$ P can bind actin, form cross-bridges, and generate tension. Other sources of intracellular Ca^{2+} in smooth muscle are ligand-gated Ca^{2+} channels in the sarcolemmal membrane and IP_3-gated Ca^{2+} channels in the sarcoplasmic reticulum membrane.

Challenge Yourself

Answer each question with a word, phrase, sentence, or numerical solution. When a list of possible answers is supplied with the question, one, more than one, or none of the choices may be correct. Correct answers are provided at the end of the book.

1 *Solution A contains 100 mM NaCl, Solution B contains 10 mM NaCl, and the membrane separating them is permeable to Cl^- but not Na^+. What is the orientation of the potential difference that will be established across the membrane?*

2 *The osmolarity of a solution of 50 mmol/L $CaCl_2$ is closest to the osmolarity of which of the following: 50 mmol/L NaCl, 100 mmol/L urea, 150 mmol/L NaCl, or 150 mmol/L urea?*

3 *How does the intracellular Na^+ concentration change following inhibition of Na^+-K^+ ATPase?*

4 *Which phase of the nerve action potential is responsible for propagation of the action potential to neighboring sites?*

5 *How many quanta of acetylcholine (ACh) are required to depolarize the motor end plate from −80 mV to −70 mV if a miniature end plate potential (MEPP) is 0.4 mV?*

6 *A man is poisoned with curare. Which of the following agents would worsen his condition: neostigmine, nicotine, botulinus toxin, ACh?*

7 *Put these events in the correct temporal order: end plate potential (EPP), action potential in muscle fiber, ACh release from presynaptic terminal, MEPP, opening ligand-gated ion channels, opening Ca^{2+} channels in presynaptic terminal, binding of ACh to nicotinic receptors, action potential in nerve fiber.*

8 *In skeletal muscle, at muscle lengths less than the length that generates maximum active tension, is active tension greater than, less than, or approximately equal to total tension?*

9 *Which of the following neurotransmitters would be inactivated by peptidases: ACh, Substance P, dopamine, glutamate, GABA, histamine, vasopressin, nitric oxide (NO)?*

10 *Solution A contains 10 mmol/L glucose, and Solution B contains 1 mmol/L glucose. If the glucose concentration in both solutions is doubled, by how much will the flux (flow) of glucose between the two solutions change (e.g., halve, remain unchanged, double, triple, quadruple)?*

11 *Adrenergic neurons synthesize which of the following: norepinephrine, epinephrine, ACh, dopamine, L-dopa, serotonin?*

12 *What effect would each of the following have on conduction velocity: increasing nerve diameter, increasing internal resistance (R_i), increasing membrane resistance (R_m), decreasing membrane capacitance (C_m), increasing length constant, increasing time constant?*

13 *How does hyperkalemia alter resting membrane potential (depolarizes, hyperpolarizes, or has no effect), and why does this cause muscle weakness?*

14 *During which of the following steps in cross-bridge cycling in skeletal muscle is ATP bound to myosin: rigor, conformational change in myosin that reduces its affinity for actin, power stroke?*

15 *Which of the following classes of drugs are contraindicated in a patient with myasthenia gravis: nicotinic receptor antagonist, inhibitor of choline reuptake, acetylcholinesterase (AChE) inhibitor, inhibitor of ACh release?*

16 *Solution A contains 100 mmol/L glucose and Solution B contains 50 mmol/L NaCl. Assume that g_{NaCl} is 2.0, $\sigma_{glucose}$ is 0.5, and σ_{NaCl} is 0.8. If a semipermeable membrane separates the two solutions, what is the direction of water flow across the membrane?*

SELECTED READINGS

Berne RM, Levy MN: Physiology, 5th ed. St Louis, Mosby, 2004, section 1.

Gamble JL: Chemical Anatomy, Physiology and Pathology of Extracellular Fluid. Cambridge, Mass, Harvard University Press, 1958.

Hille B: Ionic Channels of Excitable Membranes. Sunderland, Mass, Sindauer Associates, 1984.

Hodgkin AL, Huxley AF: A quantitative description of membrane current and its application to conduction and excitation in nerve. J Physiol 117:500–544, 1952.

Kandel ER, Schwartz JH: Principles of Neural Science, 4th ed. New York, Elsevier, 2000.

Katz B: Nerve, Muscle, and Synapse. New York, McGraw-Hill, 1966.

Katz B, Miledi R: The release of acetylcholine from nerve endings by graded electrical pulses. Proc Royal Soc London 167:23–38, 1967.

Singer SJ, Nicolson GL: The fluid mosaic model of the structure of cell membranes. Science 175:720–731, 1972.

Autonomic Nervous System

The motor (efferent) nervous system has two components: the somatic and the autonomic. These two systems differ in a number of ways but are chiefly distinguished by the types of effector organs they innervate and the types of functions they control.

The **somatic nervous system** is a **voluntary** motor system under conscious control. Each of its pathways consists of a single motoneuron and the skeletal muscle fibers it innervates. The cell body of the motoneuron is located in the central nervous system (CNS), in either the brain stem or spinal cord, and its axon synapses directly on skeletal muscle, the effector organ. The neurotransmitter acetylcholine (ACh) is released from presynaptic terminals of the motoneurons and activates nicotinic receptors located on the motor end plates of the skeletal muscle. An action potential in the motoneuron causes an action potential in the muscle fiber, which causes the muscle to contract. (For a complete discussion of the somatic nervous system, see Chapter 1.)

The **autonomic nervous system** is an **involuntary** system that controls and modulates the functions primarily of visceral organs. Each pathway in the autonomic nervous system consists of two neurons: a preganglionic neuron and a postganglionic neuron. The cell body of each preganglionic neuron resides in the CNS. The axons of these preganglionic neurons synapse on the cell bodies of postganglionic neurons in one of several autonomic ganglia located outside the CNS. The axons of the postganglionic neurons then travel to the periphery, where they synapse on visceral effector organs such as the heart, bronchioles, vascular smooth muscle, gastrointestinal tract, bladder, and genitalia. All preganglionic neurons of the autonomic nervous system release ACh. Postganglionic neurons release either ACh or norepinephrine, or, in some cases, neuropeptides.

ORGANIZATION AND GENERAL FEATURES OF THE AUTONOMIC NERVOUS SYSTEM

The autonomic nervous system has two major divisions: the sympathetic and the parasympathetic, which often complement each other in the regulation of organ system function. A third division of the autonomic nervous system, the enteric nervous system, is located in plexuses of the gastrointestinal tract. (The enteric nervous system is discussed in Chapter 8.)

The organization of the autonomic nervous system is described in Figure 2-1 and its companion, Table 2-1. The sympathetic and parasympathetic divisions are included and, for comparison, so is the somatic nervous system.

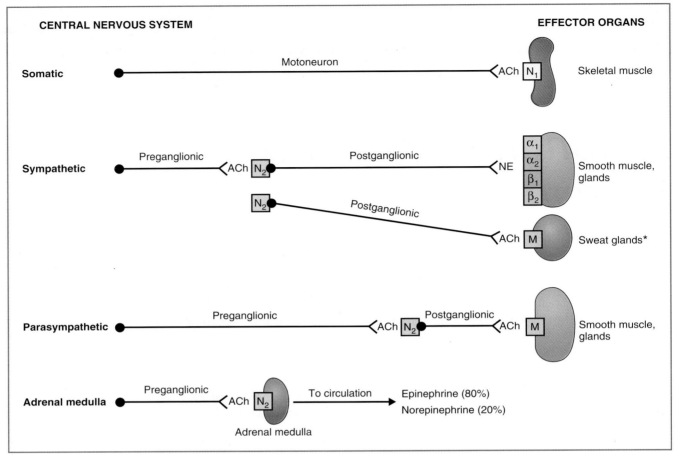

CENTRAL NERVOUS SYSTEM

EFFECTOR ORGANS

Figure 2–1 Organization of the autonomic nervous system. The somatic nervous system is included for comparison. ACh, Acetylcholine; M, muscarinic receptor; N, nicotinic receptor; NE, norepinephrine. *Sweat glands have sympathetic cholinergic innervation.

Terminology

The terms sympathetic and parasympathetic are strictly *anatomic* terms and refer to the *anatomic* origin of the preganglionic neurons in the CNS (see Table 2-1). Preganglionic neurons in the **sympathetic division** originate in the thoracolumbar spinal cord. Preganglionic neurons in the **parasympathetic division** originate in the brain stem and sacral spinal cord.

The terms adrenergic and cholinergic are used to describe neurons of *either* division, according to which neurotransmitter they synthesize and release. **Adrenergic** neurons release **norepinephrine;** receptors for norepinephrine on the effector organs are called **adrenoreceptors.** Adrenoreceptors may be activated by norepinephrine, which is released from adrenergic neurons, or by epinephrine, which is secreted into the circulation by the adrenal medulla. **Cholinergic** neurons release **ACh;** receptors for ACh are called **cholinoreceptors.** (A third term is **nonadrenergic, noncholinergic,** which describes *some* postganglionic parasympathetic neurons of the gastrointestinal tract that release

peptides [e.g., substance P] or other substances [e.g., nitric oxide] as their neurotransmitter rather than ACh.)

To summarize, whether located in the sympathetic division or in the parasympathetic division, all preganglionic neurons release ACh and, therefore, are called cholinergic. Postganglionic neurons may be either adrenergic (they release norepinephrine) or cholinergic (they release ACh). Most postganglionic parasympathetic neurons are cholinergic; postganglionic sympathetic neurons may be either adrenergic or cholinergic.

Neuroeffector Junctions of the Autonomic Nervous System

The junctions between postganglionic autonomic neurons and their effectors (target tissues), the **neuroeffector junctions,** are analogous to the neuromuscular junctions of the somatic nervous system. There are, however, several structural and functional differences with the neuromuscular junction. (1) The neuromuscular junction (discussed in Chapter 1) has a discrete arrangement, whereby the "effector," a skeletal muscle

Table 2–1   Organization of the Autonomic Nervous System

Characteristics	Sympathetic Division	Parasympathetic Division	Somatic Nervous System*
Origin of preganglionic neurons	Spinal cord segments T1–L3 (thoracolumbar)	Nuclei of CN III, VII, IX, and X; spinal cord segments S2–S4 (craniosacral)	—
Location of autonomic ganglia	Paravertebral and prevertebral	In or near effector organs	—
Length of preganglionic axons	Short	Long	—
Length of postganglionic axons	Long	Short	—
Effector organs	Smooth muscle; cardiac muscle; glands	Smooth muscle; cardiac muscle; glands	Skeletal muscle
Neuroeffector junctions	Diffuse, branching; receptors not concentrated in one region	Diffuse, branching; receptors not concentrated in one region	Discrete, organized; ACh receptors localized on motor end plate
Neurotransmitter and receptor type in ganglion	ACh/nicotinic receptor	ACh/nicotinic receptor	—
Neurotransmitter in effector organs	Norepinephrine (except sweat glands)	ACh	Ach
Receptor types in effector organs	α_1, α_2, β_1, β_2	Muscarinic	Nicotinic

ACh, Acetylcholine; CN, cranial nerve.
*Somatic nervous system is included for comparison.

fiber, is innervated by a single motoneuron. In contrast, in the autonomic nervous system, the postganglionic neurons that innervate target tissues form **diffuse, branching** networks. Beads, or **varicosities,** line these branches and are the sites of neurotransmitter synthesis, storage, and release. The varicosities are therefore analogous to the presynaptic nerve terminals of the neuromuscular junction. (2) There is overlap in the branching networks from different postganglionic neurons, such that target tissues may be innervated by many postganglionic neurons. (3) In the autonomic nervous system, postsynaptic receptors are widely distributed on the target tissues, and there is no specialized region of receptors analogous to the motor end plate of skeletal muscle.

Sympathetic Nervous System

The overall function of the sympathetic nervous system is to **mobilize the body for activity.** In the extreme, if a person is exposed to a stressful situation, the sympathetic nervous system is activated with a response known as "fight or flight," which includes increased arterial pressure, increased blood flow to active muscles, increased metabolic rate, increased blood glucose concentration, and increased mental activity and alertness. Although this response, *per se,* is rarely employed, the sympathetic nervous system operates continuously to modulate the functions of many organ systems such as heart, blood vessels, gastrointestinal tract, bronchi, and sweat glands.

Figure 2-2 depicts the organization of the sympathetic nervous system in relation to the spinal cord, the sympathetic ganglia, and the effector organs in the periphery. The preganglionic sympathetic neurons originate in nuclei of the thoracolumbar spinal cord, leave the spinal cord via the ventral motor roots and white rami, and project either to the paravertebral ganglia of the sympathetic chain or to a series of prevertebral ganglia. Thus, one category of preganglionic neuron synapses on postganglionic neurons within the **sympathetic chain.** These synapses may occur in ganglia at the same segmental level of the chain, or the preganglionic fibers may turn in the cranial or caudal direction and innervate ganglia at higher or lower levels in the chain, thereby permitting synapses in multiple ganglia (consistent with the diffuseness of sympathetic functions). The other category of preganglionic neuron passes through the sympathetic chain without synapsing and continues on to synapse in **prevertebral ganglia** (celiac, superior mesenteric, and inferior mesenteric) that supply visceral organs, glands, and the enteric nervous system of the gastrointestinal tract. In the ganglia, the preganglionic neurons synapse on postganglionic neurons, which travel to the periphery and innervate the effector organs.

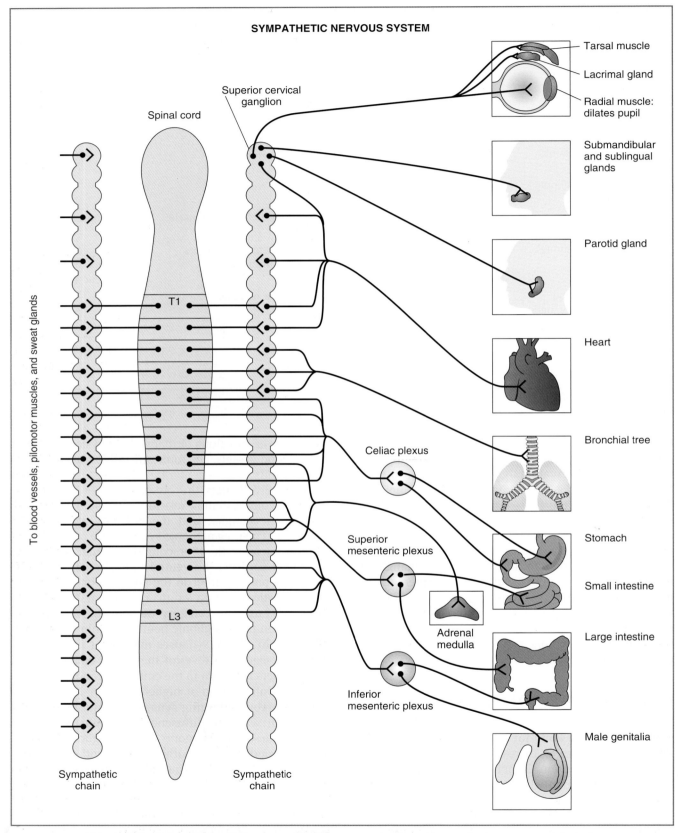

SYMPATHETIC NERVOUS SYSTEM

Figure 2–2 Innervation of the sympathetic nervous system. Preganglionic neurons originate in thoracic and lumbar segments of the spinal cord (T1–L3).

The features of the sympathetic nervous system discussed in the following sections are listed in Table 2-1 and are illustrated in Figure 2-2.

Origin of Preganglionic Neurons

The preganglionic neurons of the sympathetic division arise from nuclei in the thoracic and lumbar spinal cord segments, specifically from the first thoracic segment to the third lumbar segment (T1–L3). Thus, the sympathetic division is referred to as **thoracolumbar.**

Generally, the origin of preganglionic neurons in the spinal cord is anatomically consistent with the projection to the periphery. Thus, the sympathetic pathways to organs in the thorax (e.g., heart) have preganglionic neurons originating in the *upper thoracic* spinal cord. Sympathetic pathways to organs in the pelvis (e.g., colon, genitals) have preganglionic neurons that originate in the *lumbar* spinal cord. Blood vessels, thermoregulatory sweat glands, and pilomotor muscles of the skin have preganglionic neurons that synapse on multiple postganglionic neurons up and down the sympathetic chain, reflecting their broad distribution throughout the body.

Location of Autonomic Ganglia

The ganglia of the sympathetic nervous system are located **near the spinal cord,** either in the paravertebral ganglia (known as the sympathetic chain) or in the prevertebral ganglia. Again, the anatomy is logical. The superior cervical ganglion projects to organs in the head such as the eyes and the salivary glands. The celiac ganglion projects to the stomach and the small intestine. The superior mesenteric ganglion projects to the small and large intestine, and the inferior mesenteric ganglion projects to the lower large intestine, anus, bladder, and genitalia.

The adrenal medulla is simply a specialized sympathetic ganglion whose preganglionic neurons originate in the thoracic spinal cord (T5–T9), pass through the sympathetic chain and the celiac ganglion without synapsing, and travel in the greater splanchnic nerve to the adrenal gland.

Length of Preganglionic and Postganglionic Axons

Because the sympathetic ganglia are located *near* the spinal cord, the preganglionic nerve axons are short and the postganglionic nerve axons are long (so that they can reach the peripheral effector organs).

Neurotransmitters and Types of Receptors

Preganglionic neurons of the sympathetic division are always **cholinergic.** They release ACh, which interacts with nicotinic receptors on the cell bodies of postganglionic neurons. **Postganglionic neurons** of the sympathetic division are adrenergic in all of the effector organs, *except* in the thermoregulatory sweat glands (where they are cholinergic). The effector organs that are innervated by sympathetic adrenergic neurons have one or more of the following types of adrenoreceptors: alpha₁, alpha₂, beta₁, or beta₂ (α_1, α_2, β_1, or β_2). The thermoregulatory sweat glands innervated by sympathetic cholinergic neurons have muscarinic cholinoreceptors.

Sympathetic Adrenergic Varicosities

As described previously, **sympathetic postganglionic adrenergic nerves** release their neurotransmitters from varicosities onto their target tissues (e.g., vascular smooth muscle). The sympathetic adrenergic **varicosities** contain both the classic neurotransmitter (norepinephrine) and nonclassic neurotransmitters (ATP and neuropeptide Y). The classic neurotransmitter, **norepinephrine,** is synthesized from tyrosine in the varicosities (see Fig. 1-18) and stored in *small* **dense-core vesicles,** ready for release; these small dense-core vesicles also contain dopamine β-hydroxylase, which catalyzes the conversion of dopamine to norepinephrine (the final step in the synthetic pathway), and **ATP.** ATP is said to be "colocalized" with norepinephrine. A separate group of *large* **dense-core vesicles** contain **neuropeptide Y.**

When sympathetic postganglionic adrenergic neurons are stimulated, norepinephrine and ATP are released from the small dense-core vesicles. Both norepinephrine and ATP serve as neurotransmitters at the neuroeffector junction, binding to and activating their respective receptors on the target tissue (e.g., vascular smooth muscle). Actually, ATP acts first, binding to purinergic receptors on the target tissue and causing a physiologic effect (e.g., contraction of the vascular smooth muscle). The action of norepinephrine follows ATP; norepinephrine binds to its receptors on the target tissue (e.g., α_1-adrenergic receptors on vascular smooth muscle) and causes a second, more prolonged contraction. Finally, with more intense or higher-frequency stimulation, the large dense-core vesicles release neuropeptide Y, which binds to its receptor on the target tissue, causing a third, slower phase of contraction.

Adrenal Medulla

The adrenal medulla is a specialized ganglion in the sympathetic division of the autonomic nervous system. The cell bodies of its preganglionic neurons are located in the thoracic spinal cord. The axons of these preganglionic neurons travel in the greater splanchnic nerve to the adrenal medulla, where they synapse on **chromaffin cells** and release ACh, which activates nicotinic receptors. When activated, the chromaffin cells of the adrenal medulla secrete catecholamines (epinephrine and norepinephrine) into the general circulation. In contrast with sympathetic postganglionic neurons, which release only norepinephrine, the adrenal medulla secretes mainly **epinephrine** (80%) and a small amount of **norepinephrine** (20%). The reason for this difference is the presence of **phenylethanolamine-N-methyltransferase** (PNMT) in the adrenal medulla, but not in sympathetic postganglionic adrenergic neurons (see Fig. 1-18). PNMT catalyzes the conversion of norepinephrine to epinephrine, a step that, interestingly, requires cortisol from the nearby adrenal *cortex;* cortisol is supplied to the adrenal medulla in venous effluent from the adrenal cortex.

A tumor of the adrenal medulla, or **pheochromocytoma,** may be located on or near the adrenal medulla, or at a distant (ectopic) location in the body (Box 2-1). Unlike the normal adrenal medulla, which secretes mainly epinephrine, a pheochromocytoma secretes mainly **norepinephrine**, which is explained by the fact that the tumor is too far from the adrenal cortex to receive the cortisol that is required by PNMT.

Fight or Flight Response

The body responds to fear, extreme stress, and intense exercise with a massive, coordinated activation of the sympathetic nervous system including the adrenal medulla. This activation, the fight or flight response, ensures that the body can respond appropriately to a stressful situation (e.g., take a difficult exam, run away from a burning house, fight an attacker). The response includes increases in heart rate, cardiac output, and blood pressure; redistribution of blood flow away from skin, kidneys, and splanchnic regions and toward skeletal muscle; increased ventilation, with dilation of the airways; decreased gastrointestinal motility and secretions; and increased blood glucose concentration.

BOX 2–1 Clinical Physiology: Pheochromocytoma

DESCRIPTION OF CASE. A 48-year-old woman visits her physician complaining of what she calls "panic attacks." She reports that she has experienced a racing heart and that she can feel (and even see) her heart pounding in her chest. She also complains of throbbing headaches, cold hands and cold feet, feeling hot, visual disturbances, and nausea and vomiting. In the physician's office, her blood pressure is severely elevated (230/125). She is admitted to the hospital for evaluation of her hypertension.

A 24-hour urine sample reveals elevated levels of metanephrine, normetanephrine, and 3-methoxy-4-hydroxymandelic acid (VMA). After the physician rules out other causes for hypertension, he concludes that she has a tumor of the adrenal medulla, called a pheochromocytoma. A computerized tomographic scan of the abdomen reveals a 3.5-cm mass on her right adrenal medulla. The patient is administered an α_1 antagonist, and surgery is performed. The woman recovers fully; her blood pressure returns to normal, and her other symptoms disappear.

EXPLANATION OF CASE. The woman has a classic pheochromocytoma, a tumor of the chromaffin cells of the adrenal medulla. The tumor secretes excessive amounts of norepinephrine and epinephrine, which produce all of the woman's symptoms and result in elevated levels of catecholamine metabolites in her urine. In contrast to normal adrenal medulla, which secretes mainly epinephrine, pheochromocytomas secrete mainly norepinephrine.

The patient's symptoms can be interpreted by understanding the physiologic effects of catecholamines. Any tissue where adrenoreceptors are present will be activated by the increased levels of epinephrine and norepinephrine, which reach the tissues via the circulation. The woman's most prominent symptoms are cardiovascular: pounding heart, increased heart rate, increased blood pressure, and cold hands and feet. These symptoms can be understood by considering the functions of adrenoreceptors in the heart and blood vessels. The increased amounts of circulating catecholamines activated β_1 receptors in the heart, increasing the heart rate and increasing contractility (pounding of the heart). Activation of α_1 receptors in vascular smooth muscle of the skin produced vasoconstriction, which presented as cold hands and feet. The patient felt hot, however, because this vasoconstriction in the skin impaired the ability to dissipate heat. Her extremely elevated blood pressure was caused by the combination of increased heart rate, increased contractility, and increased constriction (resistance) of the blood vessels. The patient's headache was secondary to her elevated blood pressure.

The woman's other symptoms also can be explained by the activation of adrenoreceptors in other organ systems (i.e., gastrointestinal symptoms of nausea and vomiting and visual disturbances).

TREATMENT. The patient's treatment consisted of locating and excising the tumor, thereby removing the source of excess catecholamines. Alternatively, if the tumor had not been excised, the woman could have been treated pharmacologically with a combination of α_1 antagonists (e.g., phenoxybenzamine or prazosin) and β_1 antagonists (e.g., propranolol) to prevent the actions of the endogenous catecholamines at the receptor level.

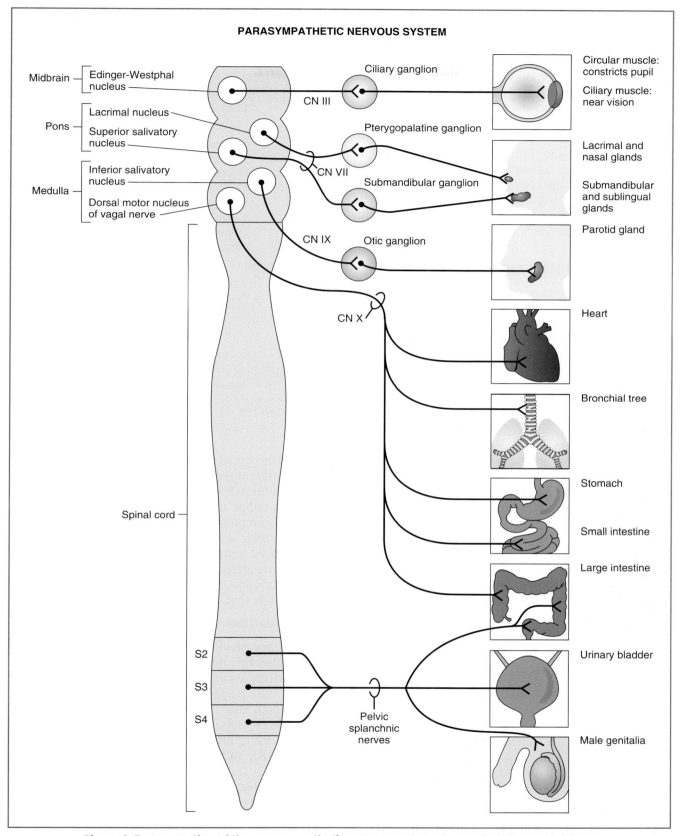

Figure 2–3 **Innervation of the parasympathetic nervous system.** Preganglionic neurons originate in nuclei of the brain stem (midbrain, pons, medulla) and in sacral segments (S2–S4) of the spinal cord. CN, Cranial nerve.

Parasympathetic Nervous System

The overall function of the parasympathetic nervous system is **restorative,** to **conserve energy.** Figure 2-3 depicts the organization of the parasympathetic nervous system in relation to the CNS (brain stem and spinal cord), the parasympathetic ganglia, and the effector organs. Preganglionic neurons of the parasympathetic division have their cell bodies in either the brain stem (midbrain, pons, and medulla) or the sacral spinal cord. Preganglionic axons project to a series of ganglia located near or in the effector organs.

The following features of the parasympathetic nervous system can be noted and compared with the sympathetic nervous system (see Table 2-1 and Fig. 2-3).

Origin of Preganglionic Neurons

Preganglionic neurons of the parasympathetic division arise from nuclei of cranial nerves (CN) III, VII, IX, and X or from sacral spinal cord segments S2–S4; therefore, the parasympathetic division is called **craniosacral.** As in the sympathetic division, the origin of the preganglionic neurons in the CNS is consistent with the projection to effector organs in the periphery. For example, the parasympathetic innervation of eye muscles originates in the Edinger-Westphal nucleus in the midbrain and travels to the periphery in CN III; the parasympathetic innervation of the heart, bronchioles, and gastrointestinal tract originates in nuclei of the medulla and travels to the periphery in CN X (vagus nerve); and the parasympathetic innervation of the genitourinary organs originates in the sacral spinal cord and travels to the periphery in the pelvic nerves.

Location of Autonomic Ganglia

In contrast to the sympathetic ganglia, which are located near the CNS, the ganglia of the parasympathetic nervous system are located **near, on,** or **in the effector organs** (e.g., ciliary, pterygopalatine, submandibular, otic).

Length of Preganglionic and Postganglionic Axons

The relative length of preganglionic and postganglionic axons in the parasympathetic division is the reverse of the relative lengths in the sympathetic division. This difference reflects the location of the ganglia. The parasympathetic ganglia are located near or in the effector organs; therefore, the preganglionic neurons have long axons and the postganglionic neurons have short axons.

Neurotransmitters and Types of Receptors

As in the sympathetic division, all **preganglionic neurons** are **cholinergic** and release ACh, which interacts at nicotinic receptors on the cell bodies of

Table 2-2 Prototypes of Agonists and Antagonists to Autonomic Receptors

Receptor	Agonists	Antagonists
Adrenoreceptors		
α_1	Norepinephrine Phenylephrine	Phenoxybenzamine Prazosin
α_2	Clonidine	Yohimbine
β_1	Norepinephrine Epinephrine Isoproterenol Dobutamine	Propranolol Metoprolol
β_2	Epinephrine Norepinephrine Isoproterenol Albuterol	Propranolol Butoxamine
Cholinoreceptors		
Nicotinic	Ach Nicotine	Curare (blocks neuromuscular N_1 receptors) Hexamethonium (blocks ganglionic N_2 receptors)
Muscarinic	Ach Muscarine	Atropine

ACh, Acetylcholine.

postganglionic neurons. Most **postganglionic neurons** of the parasympathetic division are also **cholinergic.** Receptors for ACh in the effector organs are muscarinic receptors rather than nicotinic receptors. Thus, ACh released from preganglionic neurons of the parasympathetic division activates nicotinic receptors, whereas ACh released from postganglionic neurons of the parasympathetic division activates muscarinic receptors. These receptors and their functions are distinguished by the drugs that activate or inhibit them (Table 2-2).

Parasympathetic Cholinergic Varicosities

As described previously, **parasympathetic postganglionic cholinergic nerves** release their neurotransmitters from varicosities onto their target tissues (e.g., smooth muscle). The parasympathetic cholinergic **varicosities** release both the classic neurotransmitter (ACh) and nonclassic neurotransmitters (e.g., vasoactive intestinal peptide [VIP], nitric oxide [NO]). The classic neurotransmitter, **ACh,** is synthesized in the varicosities from choline and acetyl CoA (see Fig. 1-17) and stored in **small, clear vesicles.** A separate group of **large dense-core vesicles** contains peptides such as **VIP.** Lastly, the varicosities contain nitric oxide synthase and can synthesize **NO** on demand.

When parasympathetic postganglionic cholinergic neurons are stimulated, ACh is released from the

Table 2-3 Effects of the Autonomic Nervous System on Organ System Function

Organ	Sympathetic Action	Receptor	Parasympathetic Action	Receptor
Heart				
SA node, heart rate	↑	β_1	↓	M
AV nodal conduction	↑	β_1	↓	M
Contractility	↑	β_1	↓ (atria only)	M
Vascular Smooth Muscle				
Skin; splanchnic	Constricts	α_1		
Skeletal muscle	Dilates	β_2		
Skeletal muscle	Constricts	α_1		
Endothelium			Releases EDRF	M
Bronchioles	Dilates	β_2	Constricts	M
Gastrointestinal Tract				
Smooth muscle, walls	Relaxes	α_2, β_2	Contracts	M
Smooth muscle, sphincters	Contracts	α_1	Relaxes	M
Saliva secretion	↑	β_1	↑	M
Gastric acid secretion			↑	M
Pancreatic secretion			↑	M
Bladder				
Wall, detrusor muscle	Relaxes	β_2	Contracts	M
Sphincter	Contracts	α_1	Relaxes	M
Male Genitalia	Ejaculation	α	Erection	M
Eye				
Radial muscle, iris	Dilates pupil (mydriasis)	α_1		
Circular sphincter muscle, iris			Constricts pupil (miosis)	M
Ciliary muscle	Dilates (far vision)	β	Contracts (near vision)	M
Skin				
Sweat glands, thermoregulatory	↑	M*		
Sweat glands, stress	↑	α		
Pilomotor muscle (goose bumps)	Contracts	α		
Lacrimal Glands			Secretion	M
Liver	Gluconeogenesis; glycogenolysis	α, β_2		
Adipose Tissue	Lipolysis	β_1		
Kidney	Renin secretion	β_1		

AV, Atrioventricular; EDRF, endothelial-derived relaxing factor; M, muscarinic receptor; SA, sinoatrial.
*Sympathetic cholinergic neurons.

varicosities and binds to muscarinic receptors on the target tissue, which direct its physiologic action. With intense or high-frequency stimulation, the large dense-core vesicles release their peptides (e.g., VIP), which bind to receptors on the target tissues and augment the actions of ACh.

Autonomic Innervation of the Organ Systems

Table 2-3 serves as a reference for information concerning autonomic control of organ system function. This table lists the sympathetic and parasympathetic innervations of the major organ systems and the receptor types that are present in these tissues. Table 2-3 will be most valuable if the information it contains is seen as a set of recurring themes rather than as a random list of actions and receptors.

Reciprocal Functions—Sympathetic and Parasympathetic

Most organs have both sympathetic and parasympathetic innervation. These innervations operate **reciprocally** or **synergistically** to produce coordinated responses. For example, the heart has both sympathetic and parasympathetic innervations that function reciprocally to regulate heart rate, conduction velocity, and the force of contraction (contractility). The smooth muscle walls of the gastrointestinal tract and the bladder have both sympathetic innervation (which produces relaxation) and parasympathetic innervation (which produces contraction). The radial muscles of the iris are responsible for dilation of the pupil (mydriasis) and have sympathetic innervation; the circular muscle of the iris is responsible for constriction of the pupil (miosis) and has parasympathetic innervation. In this example of the eye muscles, different muscles control pupil size, but the *overall* effects of sympathetic and parasympathetic activity are reciprocal. In the male genitalia, sympathetic activity controls ejaculation and parasympathetic activity controls erection, which, together, are responsible for the male sexual response.

The following three examples further illustrate the reciprocity and synergism of the sympathetic and parasympathetic divisions.

SINOATRIAL NODE

The autonomic innervation of the **sinoatrial (SA) node** in the heart is an excellent example of coordinated control of function. The SA node is the normal pacemaker of the heart, and its rate of depolarization sets the overall heart rate. The SA node has both sympathetic and parasympathetic innervations, which function reciprocally to modulate the heart rate. Thus, an increase in sympathetic activity increases heart rate, and an increase in parasympathetic activity decreases heart rate. These reciprocal functions are illustrated as follows: If there is a decrease in blood pressure, vasomotor centers in the brain stem respond to this decrease and produce, simultaneously, an increase in sympathetic activity to the SA node and a decrease in parasympathetic activity. Each of these actions, directed and coordinated by the brain stem vasomotor center, has the effect of increasing heart rate. The sympathetic and parasympathetic actions do not compete with each other but work synergistically to increase the heart rate (which helps restore normal blood pressure).

URINARY BLADDER

The **urinary bladder** is another example of reciprocal innervations by sympathetic and parasympathetic divisions (Fig. 2-4). In adults, **micturition,** or emptying of the bladder, is under voluntary control because the external sphincter is composed of skeletal muscle. However, the micturition reflex itself is controlled by the autonomic nervous system. This reflex occurs when the bladder is sensed as being "full." The detrusor muscle of the bladder wall and the internal bladder sphincter are composed of smooth muscle; each has both sympathetic and parasympathetic innervations. The sympathetic innervation of the detrusor muscle and the internal sphincter originates in the lumbar spinal cord (L1–L3), and the parasympathetic innervation originates in the sacral spinal cord (S2–S4).

When the **bladder is filling** with urine, **sympathetic** control predominates. This sympathetic activity produces relaxation of the detrusor muscle, via β_2 receptors, and contraction of the internal sphincter muscle, via α_1 receptors. The external sphincter is simultaneously closed by trained voluntary action. When the muscle wall is relaxed and the sphincters are closed, the bladder can fill with urine.

When the **bladder is full,** this fullness is sensed by mechanoreceptors in the bladder wall, and afferent neurons transmit this information to the spinal cord and then to the brain stem. The micturition reflex is coordinated by centers in the midbrain, and now **parasympathetic** control predominates. Parasympathetic activity produces contraction of the detrusor muscle (to increase pressure and eject urine) and relaxation of the internal sphincters. Simultaneously, the external sphincter is relaxed by a voluntary action.

Clearly, the sympathetic and parasympathetic actions on the bladder structures are opposite, but coordinated: The sympathetic actions dominate for bladder filling, and the parasympathetic actions dominate for bladder emptying.

PUPIL

The **size of the pupil** is reciprocally controlled by two muscles of the iris: the pupillary dilator (radial) muscle and pupillary constrictor (sphincter) muscle. The **pupillary dilator muscle** is controlled by sympathetic innervation through α_1 receptors. Activation of these α_1 receptors causes *constriction* of the radial muscle, which causes *dilation* of the pupil, or mydriasis. The **pupillary constrictor muscle** is controlled by parasympathetic innervation through muscarinic receptors. Activation of these muscarinic receptors causes *constriction* of the sphincter muscle, which causes *constriction* of the pupil, or miosis.

For example, in the **pupillary light reflex,** light strikes the retina and, through a series of CNS

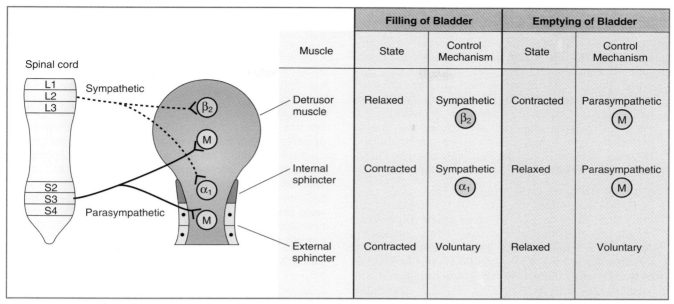

Figure 2-4 Autonomic control of bladder function. During filling of the bladder, sympathetic control predominates, causing relaxation of the detrusor muscle and contraction of the internal sphincter. During micturition, parasympathetic control predominates, causing contraction of the detrusor muscle and relaxation of the internal sphincter. *Dashed lines* represent sympathetic innervation; *solid lines* represent parasympathetic innervation. α_1, Adrenoreceptor in internal sphincter; β_2, adrenoreceptor in detrusor muscle; L1–L3, lumbar segments; M, muscarinic cholinoreceptor in detrusor muscle and internal sphincter; S2–S4, sacral segments.

connections, activates parasympathetic preganglionic nerves in the Edinger-Westphal nucleus; activation of these parasympathetic fibers causes contraction of the sphincter muscle and pupillary constriction. In the **accommodation response,** a blurred retinal image activates parasympathetic preganglionic neurons in the Edinger-Westphal nuclei and leads to contraction of the sphincter muscle and pupillary constriction. At the same time, the ciliary muscle contracts, causing the lens to "round up" and its refractive power to increase.

There are some notable *exceptions* to the generalization of reciprocal innervation. Several organs have *only* **sympathetic innervation:** sweat glands, vascular smooth muscle, pilomotor muscles of the skin, liver, adipose tissue, and kidney.

Coordination of Function within Organs

Coordination of function within the organ systems, as orchestrated by the autonomic nervous system, is another recurring physiologic theme (Box 2-2).

This control is exquisitely clear, for example, when considering the function of the **urinary bladder.** In this organ, there must be a timely coordination between activity of the detrusor muscle in the bladder wall and in the sphincters (see Fig. 2-4). Thus, sympathetic activity dominates when the bladder is filling to produce relaxation of the bladder wall and, simultaneously,

contraction of the internal bladder sphincter. The bladder can fill because the bladder wall is relaxed and the sphincter is closed. During micturition, parasympathetic activity dominates, producing contraction of the bladder wall and, simultaneously, relaxation of the sphincter.

Similar reasoning can be applied to the autonomic control of the **gastrointestinal tract:** Contraction of the wall of the gastrointestinal tract is accompanied by relaxation of the sphincters (parasympathetic), allowing the contents of the gastrointestinal tract to be propelled forward. Relaxation of the wall of the gastrointestinal tract is accompanied by contraction of the sphincters (sympathetic); the combined effect of these actions is to slow or stop movement of the contents.

Types of Receptors

Inspection of Table 2-3 permits some generalizations about types of receptors and their mechanisms of action. These generalizations are as follows: (1) In the parasympathetic division, effector organs have *only* muscarinic receptors. (2) In the sympathetic division, there are multiple receptor types in effector organs including the four adrenoreceptors (α_1, α_2, β_1, β_2), and in tissues with sympathetic cholinergic innervation, there are muscarinic receptors. (3) Among the sympathetic adrenoreceptors, receptor type is related

---

BOX 2–2 Clinical Physiology: Horner Syndrome

DESCRIPTION OF CASE. A 66-year-old man who suffered a stroke on the right side has a drooping right eyelid (ptosis), constriction of his right pupil (miosis), and lack of sweating on the right side of his face (anhidrosis). His physician orders a test with cocaine eye drops. When a solution of 10% cocaine was applied in the left eye, it caused dilation of the pupil (mydriasis). However, when the cocaine solution was applied in the right eye, it failed to cause dilation of that pupil.

EXPLANATION OF CASE. The man has a classic case of Horner syndrome, secondary to his stroke. In this syndrome, there is loss of sympathetic innervation on the affected side of the face. Thus, the loss of sympathetic innervation to smooth muscle elevating the right eyelid caused ptosis on the right side. The loss of sympathetic innervation of the right pupillary dilator

muscle caused constriction of the right pupil. And loss of sympathetic innervation of the sweat glands of the right side of the face caused anhidrosis on the right side.

When cocaine drops were instilled in the left eye (the unaffected side), the cocaine blocked reuptake of norepinephrine into sympathetic nerves innervating the pupillary dilator muscle; with higher norepinephrine levels in those adrenergic synapses, there was constriction of the radial muscle of the iris, leading to prolonged dilation of the pupil. When cocaine drops were instilled in the right eye, because there was less norepinephrine in those synapses, pupillary dilation did not occur.

TREATMENT. The treatment of Horner syndrome is to address the underlying cause.

---

to function. The α receptors and α_1 receptors cause contraction of smooth muscle such as vascular smooth muscle, gastrointestinal and bladder sphincters, pilomotor muscles, and the radial muscle of the iris. The β_1 receptors are involved in metabolic functions such as gluconeogenesis, lipolysis, renin secretion, and in all functions in the heart. The β_2 receptors cause relaxation of smooth muscle in bronchioles, wall of the bladder, and wall of the gastrointestinal tract.

Hypothalamic and Brain Stem Centers

Centers in the hypothalamus and brain stem coordinate the autonomic regulation of organ system functions. Figure 2-5 summarizes the locations of these centers, which are responsible for temperature regulation, thirst, food intake (satiety), micturition, breathing, and cardiovascular (vasomotor) function. For example, the vasomotor center receives information about blood pressure from baroreceptors in the carotid sinus and compares this information to a blood pressure set point. If corrections are necessary, the vasomotor center orchestrates changes in output of both the sympathetic and the parasympathetic innervation of the heart and blood vessels to bring about the necessary change in blood pressure. These higher autonomic centers are discussed throughout this book in the context of each organ system.

AUTONOMIC RECEPTORS

As noted in the preceding discussion, autonomic receptors are present at the neuromuscular junction, on the cell bodies of postganglionic neurons, and in the

effector organs. The type of receptor and its mechanism of action determine the nature of the physiologic response. Furthermore, the physiologic responses are tissue specific and cell type specific.

To illustrate this specificity, compare the effect of activating adrenergic β_1 receptors in the SA node to the effect of activating β_1 receptors in ventricular muscle. Both the SA node and the ventricular muscle are located in the heart, and their adrenergic receptors and mechanisms of action are the same. The resulting physiologic actions, however, are entirely different. The **β_1 receptor in the SA node** is coupled to mechanisms that increase the spontaneous rate of depolarization and increase heart rate; binding of an agonist such as norepinephrine to *this* β_1 receptor increases the heart rate. The **β_1 receptor in ventricular muscle** is coupled to mechanisms that increase intracellular Ca^{2+} concentration and contractility; binding of an agonist such as norepinephrine to *this* β_1 receptor increases contractility, but it has no direct effect on the heart rate.

The type of receptor also predicts which pharmacologic agonists or antagonists will activate it or block it. The effects of such drugs can be readily predicted by understanding the *normal* physiologic responses. For example, drugs that are β_1 agonists are expected to cause increased heart rate and increased contractility, and drugs that are β_1 antagonists are expected to cause decreased heart rate and decreased contractility.

Table 2-4 summarizes the adrenergic and cholinergic receptors, their target tissues, and their mechanisms of action. Table 2-2, its companion, is arranged similarly by receptor type and lists the prototypical drugs that either activate (**agonists**) or block (**antagonists**) the receptors. Together, the two tables should be used as a reference for the following discussion about

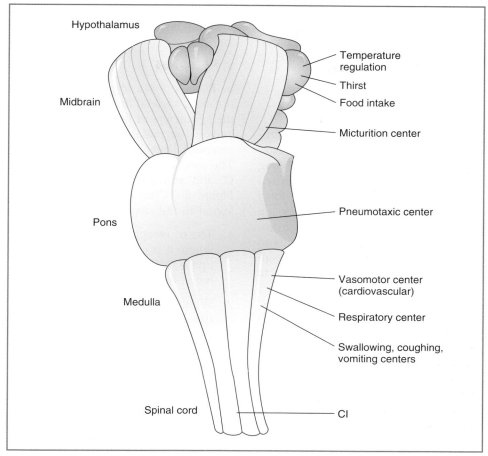

Figure 2–5 **Autonomic centers in the hypothalamus and brain stem.** CI, First cervical spinal cord segment.

Table 2–4 Location and Mechanism of Action of Autonomic Receptors

Receptor	Target Tissue	Mechanism of Action
Adrenoreceptors		
α_1	Vascular smooth muscle, skin, renal, and splanchnic Gastrointestinal tract, sphincters Bladder, sphincter Radial muscle, iris	IP_3, ↑ intracellular $[Ca^{2+}]$
α_2	Gastrointestinal tract, wall Presynaptic adrenergic neurons	Inhibition of adenylyl cyclase, ↓ cAMP
β_1	Heart Salivary glands Adipose tissue Kidney	Stimulation of adenylyl cyclase, ↑ cAMP
β_2	Vascular smooth muscle of skeletal muscle Gastrointestinal tract, wall Bladder, wall Bronchioles	Stimulation of adenylyl cyclase, ↑ cAMP
Cholinoreceptors		
Nicotinic	Skeletal muscle, motor end plate (N_1) Postganglionic neurons, SNS and PNS (N_2) Adrenal medulla (N_2)	Opening Na^+ and K^+ channels → depolarization
Muscarinic	All effector organs, PNS Sweat glands, SNS	IP_3, ↑ intracellular $[Ca^{2+}]$ (M_1, M_3, M_5) ↓ adenylyl cyclase, ↓ cAMP (M_2, M_4)

cAMP, Cyclic adenosine monophosphate; PNS, parasympathetic nervous system; SNS, sympathetic nervous system.

mechanisms of action. These mechanisms involving guanosine triphosphate (GTP)-binding proteins (G proteins), adenylyl cyclase, and inositol 1,4,5-triphosphate (IP_3) also are discussed in Chapter 9 in the context of hormone action.

G Proteins

Autonomic receptors are coupled to GTP-binding proteins (G proteins) and, therefore, are called **G protein–linked receptors.** G protein–linked receptors, including those in the autonomic nervous system, are composed of a single polypeptide chain that winds back and forth across the cell membrane seven times; thus, they are also known as seven-pass transmembrane receptor proteins. The ligand (e.g., ACh, norepinephrine) binds to the extracellular domain of its G protein–linked receptor. The intracellular domain of the receptor binds to (is "linked" to) a G protein.

These G proteins are **heterotrimeric.** In other words, they have three different subunits: α, β, and γ. The α subunit binds either guanosine diphosphate (GDP) or guanosine triphosphate (GTP). When GDP is bound, the α subunit is inactive; when GTP is bound, the α subunit is active. Thus, activity of the G protein resides in its α subunit, and the G protein switches between active and inactive states according to whether it is bound to GDP or GTP. For example, when the G protein releases GDP and binds GTP, it switches from the inactive state to the active state; when GTP is converted back to GDP through intrinsic GTPase activity of the G protein, it switches from the active state to the inactive state.

G proteins couple G protein–linked autonomic receptors to enzymes that execute physiologic actions. These enzymes are adenylyl cyclase and phospholipase C, which, when activated, generate a second messenger (cyclic adenosine monophosphate [cAMP] or IP_3, respectively). The second messenger then amplifies the message and executes the final physiologic action. In some cases (e.g., certain muscarinic receptors), the G protein directly alters the function of an ion channel without the mediation of a second messenger.

Adrenoreceptors

Adrenoreceptors are found in target tissues of the sympathetic nervous system and are activated by the catecholamines norepinephrine and epinephrine. Norepinephrine is released from postganglionic neurons of the sympathetic nervous system. Epinephrine is secreted by the adrenal medulla and reaches the target tissues via the circulation. Adrenoreceptors are divided into two types, α and β, which are further designated as α_1, α_2, β_1, and β_2 receptors. Each of the receptor types has a different mechanism of action (except the β_1 and β_2

receptors, which have the same mechanism of action), resulting in different physiologic effects (see Tables 2-3 and 2-4).

α_1 Receptors

α_1 Receptors are found in vascular smooth muscle of the skin, skeletal muscle, and the splanchnic region, in the sphincters of the gastrointestinal tract and bladder, and in the radial muscle of the iris. Activation of α_1 receptors leads to **contraction** in each of these tissues. The mechanism of action involves a G protein called G_q and **activation of phospholipase C,** illustrated in Figure 2-6. The circled numbers in the figure correspond to the steps discussed as follows:

1. The α_1 receptor is embedded in the cell membrane, where it is coupled, via the G_q protein, to phospholipase C. In the inactive state, the α_q subunit of the heterotrimeric G_q protein is bound to GDP.

2. When an agonist such as norepinephrine binds to the α_1 receptor (Step 1), a conformational change occurs in the α_q subunit of the G_q protein. This conformational change has two effects (Step 2): GDP is released from the α_q subunit and replaced by GTP, and the α_q subunit (with GTP attached) detaches from the rest of the G_q protein.

3. The α_q-GTP complex migrates within the cell membrane and binds to and activates phospholipase C (Step 3). Intrinsic GTPase activity then converts GTP back to GDP, and the α_q subunit returns to the inactive state (not shown).

4. Activated phospholipase C catalyzes the liberation of diacylglycerol and IP_3 from phosphatidylinositol 4,5-diphosphate (Step 4). The **IP_3** that is generated causes the release of **Ca^{2+}** from intracellular stores in the endoplasmic or sarcoplasmic reticulum, resulting in an increase in intracellular Ca^{2+} concentration (Step 5). Together, Ca^{2+} and diacylglycerol activate protein kinase C (Step 6), which phosphorylates proteins. These phosphorylated proteins execute the final physiologic actions (Step 7) such as contraction of smooth muscle.

α_2 Receptors

α_2 Receptors are inhibitory, are located both presynaptically and postsynaptically, and are less common than α_1 receptors. They are found on presynaptic adrenergic and cholinergic nerve terminals and in the gastrointestinal tract. α_2 receptors are found in two forms, autoreceptors and heteroreceptors.

α_2 Receptors present on sympathetic postganglionic nerve terminals are called **autoreceptors.** In this function, activation of α_2 receptors by norepinephrine released from presynaptic nerve terminals inhibits

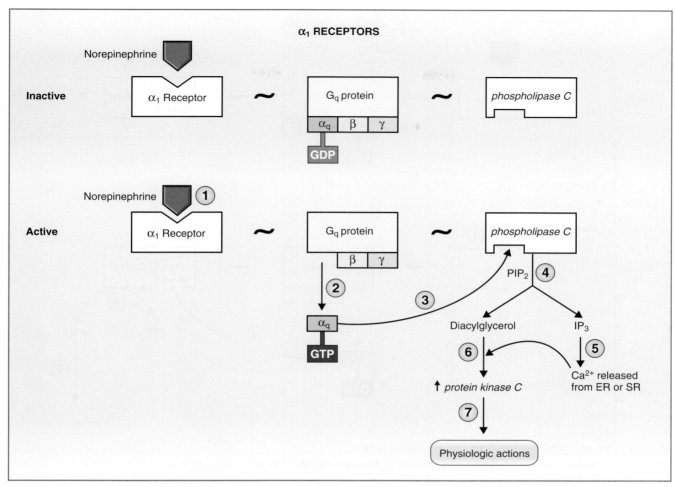

Figure 2–6 **Mechanism of action of** α_1 **adrenoreceptors.** In the inactive state, the α_q subunit of the G_q protein is bound to GDP. In the active state, with norepinephrine bound to the α_1 receptor, the α_q subunit is bound to GTP. α_q, β, and γ are subunits of the G_q protein. The circled numbers correspond to steps discussed in the text. ER, Endoplasmic reticulum; GDP, guanosine diphosphate; G_q, G protein; GTP, guanosine triphosphate; PIP_2, phosphatidylinositol 4,5-diphosphate; SR, sarcoplasmic reticulum.

further release of norepinephrine from the same terminals; this negative feedback conserves norepinephrine in states of high stimulation of the sympathetic nervous system. Interestingly, the adrenal medulla does not have α_2 receptors and, therefore, is not subject to feedback inhibition; consequently, the adrenal medulla can become depleted of catecholamines during periods of prolonged stress.

α_2 Receptors present on parasympathetic postganglionic nerve terminals of the gastrointestinal tract are called **heteroreceptors.** Norepinephrine is released from sympathetic postganglionic fibers that synapse on these parasympathetic postganglionic fibers. When activated by norepinephrine, the α_2 receptors cause inhibition of release of acetylcholine from the parasympathetic postganglionic nerve terminals. In this way, the sympathetic nervous system indirectly inhibits gastrointestinal function (i.e., by inhibiting the parasympathetic activity).

The mechanism of action of these receptors involves the **inhibition of adenylyl cyclase,** described by the following steps:

1. The agonist (e.g., norepinephrine) binds to the α_2 receptor, which is coupled to adenylyl cyclase by an inhibitory G protein, G_i.

2. When norepinephrine is bound, the G_i protein releases GDP and binds GTP, and the α_i subunit dissociates from the G protein complex.

3. The α_i subunit then migrates in the membrane and binds to and **inhibits adenylyl cyclase.** As a result, cAMP levels decrease, producing the final physiologic action.

β_1 Receptors

β_1 Receptors are prominent in the heart. They are present in the SA node, in the atrioventricular (AV)

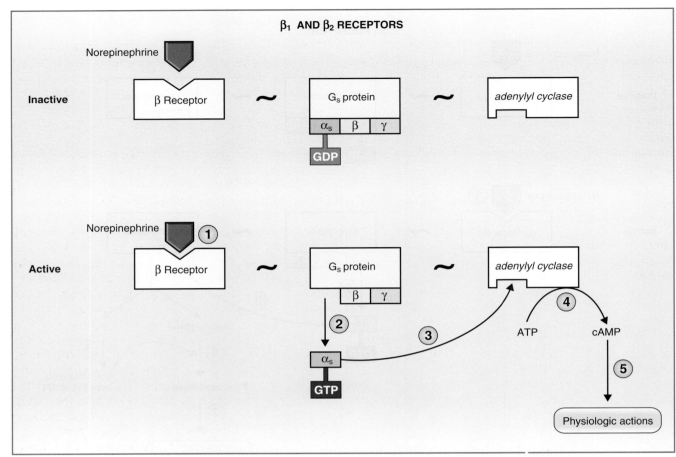

β₁ AND β₂ RECEPTORS

Figure 2–7 **Mechanism of action of β adrenoreceptors.** In the inactive state, the α_s subunit of the G_s protein is bound to GDP. In the active state, with norepinephrine bound to the β receptor, the α_s subunit is bound to GTP. β₁ and β₂ receptors have the same mechanism of action. The circled numbers correspond to steps discussed in the text. ATP, Adenosine triphosphate; cAMP, cyclic adenosine monophosphate; GDP, guanosine diphosphate; GTP, guanosine triphosphate.

node, and in ventricular muscle. Activation of β₁ receptors in these tissues produces increased heart rate in the SA node, increased conduction velocity in the AV node, and increased contractility in ventricular muscle, respectively. β₁ Receptors also are located in the salivary glands, in adipose tissue, and in the kidney (where they promote renin secretion). The mechanism of action of β₁ receptors involves a G_s protein and **activation of adenylyl cyclase.** This action is illustrated in Figure 2-7 and involves the following steps, which correspond to the circled numbers in the figure:

1. Similar to other autonomic receptors, β₁ receptors are embedded in the cell membrane. They are coupled, via a G_s protein, to adenylyl cyclase. In the inactive state, the α_s subunit of the G_s protein is bound to GDP.

2. When an agonist such as norepinephrine binds to the β₁ receptor (Step 1), a conformational change occurs in the α_s subunit. This change has two effects (Step 2): GDP is released from the α_s subunit

and replaced by GTP, and the activated α_s subunit detaches from the G protein complex.

3. The α_s-GTP complex migrates within the cell membrane and binds to and activates adenylyl cyclase (Step 3). GTPase activity converts GTP back to GDP, and the α_s subunit is returned to its inactive state (not shown).

4. Activated adenylyl cyclase catalyzes the conversion of ATP to cAMP, which serves as the second messenger (Step 4). **cAMP**, via steps involving activation of protein kinases, initiates the final physiologic actions (Step 5). As mentioned previously, these physiologic actions are tissue specific and cell type specific. When β₁ receptors are activated in the SA node, heart rate increases; when β₁ receptors are activated in ventricular muscle, contractility increases; when β₁ receptors are activated in the salivary gland, secretion increases; when β₁ receptors are activated in the kidney, renin is secreted.

β_2 Receptors

β_2 Receptors are found in the vascular smooth muscle of skeletal muscle, in the walls of the gastrointestinal tract and bladder, and in the bronchioles. The activation of β_2 receptors in these tissues leads to **relaxation** or dilation. The β_2 receptors have a mechanism of action similar to that of β_1 receptors: activation of a G_s protein, release of the α_s subunit, **stimulation of adenylyl cyclase,** and generation of cAMP (see Fig. 2-7).

Responses of Adrenoreceptors to Norepinephrine and Epinephrine

There are significant differences in the responses of α_1, β_1, and β_2 adrenoreceptors to the catecholamines epinephrine and norepinephrine. These differences are explained as follows, recalling that norepinephrine is the catecholamine released from postganglionic sympathetic adrenergic nerve fibers, while epinephrine is the primary catecholamine released from the adrenal medulla: (1) Norepinephrine and epinephrine have almost the same potency at α_1 **receptors,** with epinephrine being slightly more potent. However, compared with β receptors, α_1 receptors are relatively insensitive to catecholamines. Higher concentrations of catecholamines are necessary to activate α_1 receptors than to activate β receptors. Physiologically, such high concentrations are reached locally when norepinephrine is released from postganglionic sympathetic nerve fibers but not when catecholamines are released from the adrenal medulla. For example, the amount of epinephrine (and norepinephrine) released from the adrenal medulla in the fight or flight response is insufficient to activate α_1 receptors. (2) Norepinephrine and epinephrine are equipotent at β_1 receptors. As noted previously, much lower concentrations of catecholamines will activate β_1 receptors than will activate α_1 receptors. Thus, norepinephrine released from sympathetic nerve fibers or epinephrine released from the adrenal medulla will activate β_1 receptors. (3) β_2 **receptors** are preferentially activated by epinephrine. Thus, epinephrine released from the adrenal medulla is expected to activate β_2 receptors, whereas norepinephrine released from sympathetic nerve endings is not.

Cholinoreceptors

There are two types of cholinoreceptors: nicotinic and muscarinic. Nicotinic receptors are found on the motor end plate, in all autonomic ganglia, and on chromaffin cells of the adrenal medulla. Muscarinic receptors are found in all effector organs of the parasympathetic division and in a few effector organs of the sympathetic division.

Nicotinic Receptors

Nicotinic receptors are found in several important locations: on the motor end plate of skeletal muscle, on all postganglionic neurons of both sympathetic and parasympathetic nervous systems, and on the chromaffin cells of the adrenal medulla. ACh is the natural agonist, which is released from motoneurons and from all preganglionic neurons.

The question arises as to whether the nicotinic receptor on the motor end plate is identical to the nicotinic receptor in the autonomic ganglia. This question can be answered by examining the actions of drugs that serve as agonists or antagonists to the nicotinic receptor. The nicotinic receptors at the two loci are certainly similar: Both are activated by the agonists ACh, nicotine, and carbachol, and both are antagonized by the drug **curare** (see Table 2-2). However, another antagonist to the nicotinic receptor, **hexamethonium,** blocks the nicotinic receptor in the ganglia but not the nicotinic receptor on the motor end plate. Thus, it can be concluded that the receptors at the two loci are similar but not identical, where the nicotinic receptor on the skeletal muscle end plate is designated N_1 and the nicotinic receptor in the autonomic ganglia is designated N_2. This pharmacologic distinction predicts that drugs such as hexamethonium will be ganglionic-blocking agents but not neuromuscular-blocking agents.

A second conclusion can be drawn about **ganglionic-blocking agents** such as hexamethonium. These agents should inhibit nicotinic receptors in *both* sympathetic and parasympathetic ganglia, and thus, they should produce widespread effects on autonomic function. However, to predict the actions of ganglionic-blocking agents on a particular organ system, it is necessary to know whether sympathetic or parasympathetic control is dominant in that organ. For example, **vascular smooth muscle** has *only* sympathetic innervation, which causes vasoconstriction; thus, ganglionic-blocking agents produce relaxation of vascular smooth muscle and vasodilation. (Because of this property, ganglionic-blocking agents can be used to treat hypertension.) On the other hand, **male sexual function** is dramatically impaired by ganglionic-blocking agents because the male sexual response has both sympathetic (ejaculation) and parasympathetic (erection) components.

The **mechanism of action** of nicotinic receptors, whether at the motor end plate or in the ganglia, is based on the fact that this ACh receptor is also an ion channel for Na^+ and K^+. When the nicotinic receptor is activated by ACh, the channel opens and both Na^+ and K^+ flow through the channel, down their respective electrochemical gradients.

Figure 2-8 illustrates the function of the nicotinic receptor/channel in two states: closed and open. The

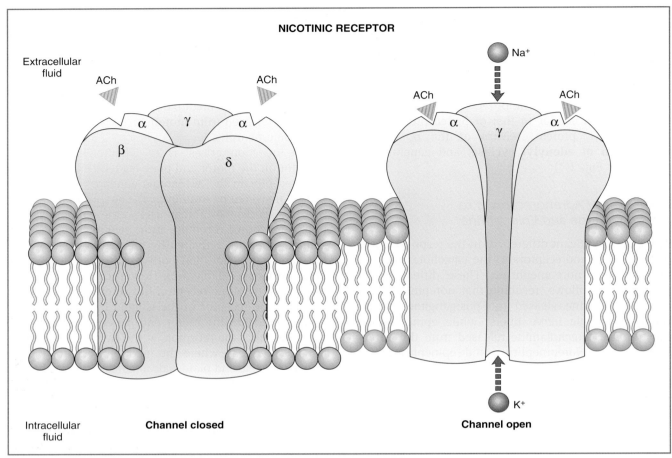

NICOTINIC RECEPTOR

Extracellular fluid

Intracellular fluid

Channel closed

Channel open

Figure 2–8 **Mechanism of action of nicotinic cholinoreceptors.** The nicotinic receptor for acetylcholine (ACh) is an ion channel for Na^+ and K^+. The receptor has five subunits: two α, one β, one δ, and one γ. (Modified from Kandel ER, Schwartz JH: Principles of Neural Science, 4th ed. New York, Elsevier, 2000.)

nicotinic receptor is an integral cell membrane protein consisting of five subunits: two α, one β, one delta (δ), and one gamma (γ). These five subunits form a funnel around the mouth of a central core. When *no ACh is bound,* the mouth of the channel is closed. When *ACh is bound* to each of the two α subunits, a conformational change occurs in all of the subunits, resulting in opening of the central core of the channel. When the core of the channel opens, Na^+ and K^+ flow down their respective electrochemical gradients (Na^+ into the cell, and K^+ out of the cell), with each ion attempting to drive the membrane potential to its equilibrium potential. The resulting membrane potential is midway between the Na^+ and K^+ equilibrium potentials, approximately 0 millivolts, which is a depolarized state.

Muscarinic Receptors

Muscarinic receptors are located in all of the effector organs of the parasympathetic nervous system: in the heart, gastrointestinal tract, bronchioles, bladder, and male sex organs. These receptors also are found in

certain effector organs of the sympathetic nervous system, specifically, in sweat glands.

Some muscarinic receptors (e.g., M_1, M_3, and M_5) have the same **mechanism of action** as the α_1 adrenoreceptors (see Fig. 2-6). In these cases, binding of the agonist (ACh) to the muscarinic receptor causes dissociation of the α subunit of the G protein, activation of **phospholipase C,** and generation of **IP_3** and diacylglycerol. IP_3 releases stored Ca^{2+}, and the increased intracellular Ca^{2+} with diacylglycerol produces the tissue-specific physiologic actions.

Other muscarinic receptors (e.g., M_4) act by inhibiting adenylyl cyclase and decreasing intracellular cAMP levels.

Other muscarinic receptors (M_2) alter physiologic processes via a **direct action of the G protein.** In these cases, no other second messenger is involved. For example, muscarinic receptors in the cardiac **SA node,** when activated by ACh, produce activation of a G_i protein and release of the α_i subunit, which binds *directly* to K^+ channels of the SA node. When the α_i

---

BOX 2–3   Clinical Physiology: Treatment of Motion Sickness with a Muscarinic Receptor Antagonist

DESCRIPTION OF CASE. A woman planning a 10-day cruise asks her physician for medication to prevent motion sickness. The physician prescribes scopolamine, a drug related to atropine, and recommends that she take it for the entire duration of the cruise. While taking the drug, the woman experiences no nausea or vomiting, as hoped. However, she does experience dry mouth, dilation of the pupils (mydriasis), increased heart rate (tachycardia), and difficulty voiding urine.

EXPLANATION OF CASE. Scopolamine, like atropine, blocks cholinergic muscarinic receptors in target tissues. Indeed, it can be used effectively to treat motion sickness, whose etiology involves muscarinic receptors in the vestibular system. The adverse effects that the woman experienced while taking scopolamine can

be explained by understanding the physiology of muscarinic receptors in target tissues.

Activation of muscarinic receptors causes increased salivation, constriction of the pupils, decreased heart rate (bradycardia), and contraction of the bladder wall during voiding (see Table 2-2). Therefore, *inhibition* of the muscarinic receptors with scopolamine would be expected to cause symptoms of decreased salivation (dry mouth), dilation of the pupils (due to the unopposed influence of the sympathetic nervous system on the radial muscles), increased heart rate, and slowed voiding of urine (caused by the loss of contractile tone of the bladder wall).

TREATMENT. Scopolamine is discontinued.

---

subunits bind to K^+ channels, the channels open, slowing the rate of depolarization of the SA node and decreasing the heart rate. In this mechanism, there is no stimulation or inhibition of either adenylyl cyclase or phospholipase C and no involvement of any second messenger; rather, the G_i protein acts directly on the ion channel (Box 2-3).

SUMMARY

■ The autonomic nervous system is composed of two major divisions, the sympathetic and the parasympathetic, which operate in a coordinated fashion to regulate involuntary functions. The sympathetic division is thoracolumbar, referring to its origin in the spinal cord. The parasympathetic division is craniosacral, referring to its origin in the brain stem and sacral spinal cord.

■ Efferent pathways in the autonomic nervous system consist of a preganglionic and a postganglionic neuron, which synapse in autonomic ganglia. The axons of postganglionic neurons then travel to the periphery to innervate the effector organs. The adrenal medulla is a specialized ganglion of the sympathetic division; when stimulated, it secretes catecholamines into the circulation.

■ Often, the sympathetic and parasympathetic innervations of organs or organ systems have reciprocal effects. These effects are coordinated by autonomic centers in the brain stem. For example, autonomic centers in the brain stem control the heart rate by modulating sympathetic and parasympathetic activity to the SA node.

■ Receptors for neurotransmitters in the autonomic nervous system are either adrenergic (adrenoreceptors) or cholinergic (cholinoreceptors). Adrenoreceptors are

activated by the catecholamines norepinephrine and epinephrine. Cholinoreceptors are activated by ACh.

■ Autonomic receptors are coupled to G proteins, which may be stimulatory (G_s) or inhibitory (G_i). The G proteins in turn activate or inhibit enzymes that are responsible for the final physiologic actions.

■ The mechanism of action of the adrenoreceptors can be explained as follows: α_1 Receptors act through activation of phospholipase C and generation of IP_3. β_1 and β_2 receptors act through activation of adenylyl cyclase and generation of cAMP. α_2 Receptors act through inhibition of adenylyl cyclase.

■ The mechanism of action of cholinoreceptors can be explained as follows: Nicotinic receptors act as ion channels for Na^+ and K^+. Many muscarinic receptors have the same mechanism of action as α_1 receptors; some muscarinic receptors act by inhibiting adenylyl cyclase; a few muscarinic receptors involve direct action of a G protein on the physiologic mechanism.

Challenge Yourself

Answer each question with a word, phrase, sentence, or numerical solution. When a list of possible answers is supplied with the question, one, more than one, or none of the choices may be correct. The correct answers are provided at the end of the book.

1 *Which of the following actions is/are mediated by β_2 receptors: increased heart rate, contraction of gastrointestinal sphincters, contraction of vascular smooth muscle, dilation of airways, relaxation of bladder wall?*

2 *A woman who is taking atropine for a gastrointestinal disorder notices that her pupils are dilated. This has occurred because atropine blocks _____ receptors on the _____ muscle of the iris.*

3 *Which of the following is/are characteristic of the parasympathetic nervous system, but not of the sympathetic nervous system: ganglia in or near target tissues, nicotinic receptors on postganglionic neurons, muscarinic receptors on some target tissues, β_1 receptors on some target tissues, cholinergic preganglionic neurons?*

4 *Propranolol causes a decrease in heart rate because it _____ the _____ receptors in the sinoatrial node of the heart.*

5 *Which of the following actions is/are mediated by the adenylyl cyclase mechanism: effect of parasympathetic nervous system to increase gastric acid secretion, effect of epinephrine to increase cardiac contractility, effect of epinephrine to increase heart rate, effect of acetylcholine to decrease heart rate, effect of acetylcholine to constrict airways, constriction of vascular smooth muscle in splanchnic blood vessels?*

6 *What enzyme is responsible for the fact that the adrenal medulla synthesizes more epinephrine than norepinephrine?*

7 *A man had a pheochromocytoma that caused severe elevation of his blood pressure. Prior to surgery to remove the tumor, he received the wrong drug, which caused a further elevation in blood pressure. Name two classes of drugs that may have been given in error to cause this further elevation.*

8 *A man's bladder is full. When he voids (micturition), _____ receptors cause _____ of the detrusor muscle and _____ receptors cause _____ of the internal sphincter.*

9 *In the action of α_1 receptors, what is the correct order of steps: α_q binds to GDP, α_q binds to GTP, generation of IP_3, release of Ca^{2+} from intracellular stores, activation of protein kinase, activation of phospholipase C?*

10 *Which of the following actions are mediated by muscarinic receptors? Slowing of conduction velocity in AV node; gastric acid secretion, mydriasis, contraction of gastrointestinal sphincters, erection, renin secretion, sweating on a hot day.*

SELECTED READINGS

Burnstock G, Hoyle CHV: Autonomic Neuroeffector Mechanisms. Newark, NJ, Harwood Academic Publishers, 1992.

Changeux J-P: The acetylcholine receptor: An "allosteric" membrane protein. Harvey Lect 75:85–254, 1981.

Gilman AG: Guanine nucleotide-binding regulatory proteins and dual control of adenylate cyclase. J Clin Invest 73:1–4, 1984.

Houslay MD, Milligan G: G Proteins as Mediators of Cellular Signalling Processes. New York, John Wiley, 1990.

Lefkowitz RJ, Stadel JM, Caron MG: Adenylate cyclase-coupled beta-adrenergic receptors: Structure and mechanisms of activation and desensitization. Annu Rev Biochem 52:159–186, 1983.

Pick J: The Autonomic Nervous System: Morphological, Comparative, Clinical and Surgical Aspects. Philadelphia, JB Lippincott, 1970.

Neurophysiology

The nervous system is a complex network that allows an organism to communicate with its environment. The network includes sensory components, which detect changes in environmental stimuli, and motor components, which generate movement, contraction of cardiac and smooth muscle, and glandular secretions. Integrative components of the nervous system receive, store, and process sensory information and then orchestrate the appropriate motor responses.

ORGANIZATION OF THE NERVOUS SYSTEM

To understand neurophysiology, it is necessary to appreciate the organization of the nervous system and the gross anatomic arrangement of structures. A comprehensive presentation of neuroanatomy would be the subject of an entire text. Thus, in this chapter, the anatomy will be described briefly, as is appropriate for the physiologic context.

The nervous system is composed of two divisions: the **central nervous system (CNS),** which includes the brain and the spinal cord, and the **peripheral nervous system (PNS),** which includes sensory receptors, sensory nerves, and ganglia outside the CNS. The CNS and PNS communicate extensively with each other.

Further distinction can be made between the sensory and motor divisions of the nervous system. The **sensory or afferent division** brings information *into* the nervous system, usually beginning with events in sensory receptors in the periphery. These receptors include, but are not limited to, visual receptors, auditory receptors, chemoreceptors, and somatosensory (touch) receptors. This afferent information is then transmitted to progressively higher levels of the nervous system, and finally to the cerebral cortex. The **motor or efferent division** carries information *out of* the nervous system to the periphery. This efferent information results in contraction of skeletal muscle, smooth muscle, and cardiac muscle or secretion by endocrine and exocrine glands.

To illustrate and compare the functions of the sensory and motor divisions of the nervous system, consider an example introduced in Chapter 2: regulation of arterial blood pressure. Arterial blood pressure is sensed by baroreceptors located in the walls of the carotid sinus. This information is transmitted, via the glossopharyngeal nerve (cranial nerve IX), to the vasomotor center in the medulla of the brain stem—this is the sensory or afferent limb of blood pressure regulation. In the medulla, the sensed blood

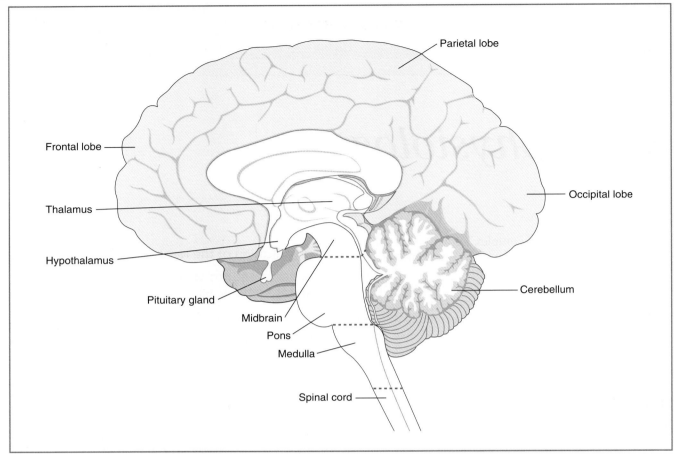

Figure 3–1 Midsagittal section of the brain. Relationships are shown between the lobes of the cerebral cortex, the cerebellum, the thalamus and hypothalamus, the brain stem, and the spinal cord.

pressure is compared with a set point, and the medullary vasomotor center directs changes in sympathetic and parasympathetic outflow to the heart and blood vessels, which produce appropriate adjustments in arterial pressure—this is the motor or efferent limb of blood pressure regulation.

The CNS includes the **brain** and **spinal cord.** The organization of major structures of the CNS is shown in Figures 3-1 and 3-2. Figure 3-1 shows the structures in their correct anatomic positions. These same structures are illustrated schematically in Figure 3-2, which may prove more useful as a reference.

The major divisions of the CNS are the spinal cord; brain stem (medulla, pons, and midbrain); cerebellum; diencephalon (thalamus and hypothalamus); and cerebral hemispheres (cerebral cortex, white matter, basal ganglia, hippocampal formation, and amygdala).

Spinal Cord

The spinal cord is the most caudal portion of the CNS, extending from the base of the skull to the first lumbar vertebra. The spinal cord is segmented, with 31 pairs of spinal nerves that contain both **sensory** (afferent) nerves and **motor** (efferent) nerves. Sensory nerves carry information *to* the spinal cord from the skin, joints, muscles, and visceral organs in the periphery via dorsal root and cranial nerve ganglia. Motor nerves carry information *from* the spinal cord to the periphery and include both somatic motor nerves, which innervate skeletal muscle, and motor nerves of the autonomic nervous system, which innervate cardiac muscle, smooth muscle, glands, and secretory cells (see Chapter 2).

Information also travels up and down within the spinal cord. **Ascending pathways** in the spinal cord carry sensory information from the periphery to higher levels of the CNS. **Descending pathways** in the spinal cord carry motor information from higher levels of the CNS to the motor nerves that innervate the periphery.

Brain Stem

The medulla, pons, and midbrain are collectively called the brain stem. Ten of the 12 cranial nerves (CN III–XII) arise in the brain stem. They carry sensory information

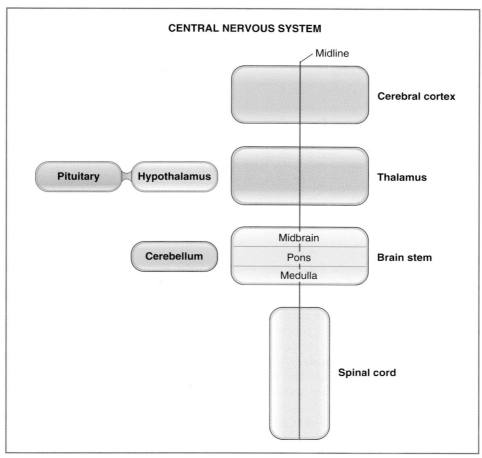

CENTRAL NERVOUS SYSTEM

Midline

Cerebral cortex

Pituitary — Hypothalamus

Thalamus

Midbrain
Pons
Medulla

Cerebellum

Brain stem

Spinal cord

Figure 3-2 **Schematic diagram of the central nervous system.**

to the brain stem and motor information away from it. The components of the brain stem are as follows:

♦ The **medulla** is the rostral extension of the spinal cord. It contains autonomic centers that regulate breathing and blood pressure, as well as the centers that coordinate swallowing, coughing, and vomiting reflexes (see Chapter 2, Fig. 2-5).

♦ The **pons** is rostral to the medulla and, together with centers in the medulla, participates in balance and maintenance of posture and in regulation of breathing. In addition, the pons relays information from the cerebral hemispheres to the cerebellum.

♦ The **midbrain** is rostral to the pons and participates in control of eye movements. It also contains relay nuclei of the auditory and visual systems.

Cerebellum

The cerebellum is a foliated ("leafy") structure that is attached to the brain stem and lies dorsal to the pons and medulla. The functions of the cerebellum are coordination of movement, planning and execution of

movement, maintenance of posture, and coordination of head and eye movements. Thus, the cerebellum, conveniently positioned between the cerebral cortex and the spinal cord, integrates sensory information about position from the spinal cord, motor information from the cerebral cortex, and information about balance from the vestibular organs of the inner ear.

Thalamus and Hypothalamus

Together, the thalamus and hypothalamus form the **diencephalon,** which means "between brain." The term refers to the location of the thalamus and hypothalamus between the cerebral hemispheres and the brain stem.

The **thalamus** processes almost all sensory information *going to* the cerebral cortex and almost all motor information *coming from* the cerebral cortex to the brain stem and spinal cord.

The **hypothalamus** lies ventral to the thalamus and contains centers that regulate body temperature, food intake, and water balance. The hypothalamus is also an endocrine gland that controls the hormone secretions of the pituitary gland. The hypothalamus secretes releasing hormones and release-inhibiting hormones into hypophysial portal blood that cause release (or inhibition of release) of the anterior pituitary hormones. The hypothalamus also contains the cell bodies of neurons of the posterior pituitary gland that secrete antidiuretic hormone (ADH) and oxytocin.

Cerebral Hemispheres

The cerebral hemispheres consist of the cerebral cortex, an underlying white matter, and three deep nuclei (basal ganglia, hippocampus, and amygdala). The functions of the cerebral hemispheres are perception, higher motor functions, cognition, memory, and emotion.

♦ **Cerebral cortex.** The cerebral cortex is the convoluted surface of the cerebral hemispheres and consists of four lobes: **frontal, parietal, temporal,** and **occipital.** These lobes are separated by sulci or grooves. The cerebral cortex receives and processes sensory information and integrates motor functions. These sensory and motor areas of the cortex are further designated as **"primary," "secondary,"** and **"tertiary,"** depending on how directly they deal with sensory or motor processing. The primary areas are the most direct and involve the fewest number of synapses; the tertiary areas require the most complex processing and involve the greatest number of synapses. **Association areas** integrate diverse information for purposeful actions. For example, the limbic association area is involved in motivation, memory, and emotions. The following examples illustrate the nomenclature: (1) The *primary* motor cortex contains the upper motoneurons, which project directly to the spinal cord and activate lower motoneurons that innervate skeletal muscle. (2) The *primary* sensory cortices consist of the primary visual cortex, primary auditory cortex, and primary somatosensory cortex and receive information from sensory receptors in the periphery, with only a few intervening synapses. (3) *Secondary* and *tertiary* sensory and motor areas surround the primary areas and are involved with more complex processing by connecting to association areas.

♦ **Basal ganglia, hippocampus, and amygdala.** There are three deep nuclei of the cerebral hemispheres. The **basal ganglia** consist of the caudate nucleus, the putamen, and the globus pallidus. The basal ganglia receive input from all lobes of the cerebral cortex and have projections, via the thalamus, to the frontal cortex to assist in regulating movement. The **hippocampus** and **amygdala** are part of the limbic system. The hippocampus is involved in memory; the amygdala is involved with the emotions and communicates with the autonomic nervous system

via the hypothalamus (e.g., effect of the emotions on heart rate, pupil size, and hypothalamic hormone secretion).

GENERAL FEATURES OF SENSORY AND MOTOR SYSTEMS

Before proceeding to specific discussions about the major sensory and motor systems, some common organizational features will be considered. Although the details of each system will vary, these features can be appreciated as a set of recurring themes throughout neurophysiology.

Synaptic Relays

The simplest synapses are one-to-one connections consisting of a presynaptic element (e.g., motoneuron) and a postsynaptic element (e.g., skeletal muscle fiber). In the nervous system, however, many synapses are more complicated and use synapses in **relay nuclei** to integrate converging information. Relay nuclei are found throughout the CNS, but they are especially prominent in the thalamus.

Relay nuclei contain several different types of neurons including local **interneurons** and **projection neurons.** The projection neurons extend long axons out of the nuclei to synapse in other relay nuclei or in the cerebral cortex. Almost all information going to and coming from the cerebral cortex is processed in thalamic relay nuclei.

Topographic Organization

One of the striking features of sensory and motor systems is that information is encoded in **neural maps.** For example, in the somatosensory system, a **somatotopic map** is formed by an array of neurons that receive information *from* and send information *to* specific locations on the body. The topographic coding is preserved at each level of the nervous system, even as high as the cerebral cortex. Thus, in the somatosensory system, the topographic information is represented as a sensory homunculus in the cerebral cortex (see Fig. 3-11). In the visual system, the topographic representation is called **retinotopic,** in the auditory system it is called **tonotopic,** and so forth.

Decussations

Almost all sensory and motor pathways are bilaterally symmetric, and information crosses from one side (ipsilateral) to the other (contralateral) side of the brain or spinal cord. Thus, sensory activity on one side of the

Table 3-1 Classification of Nerve Fibers

Classification	Type of Nerve Fiber	Example	Relative Diameter	Relative Conduction Velocity	Myelination
Sensory and Motor	A alpha (Aα)	α Motoneurons	Largest	Fastest	Yes
	A beta (Aβ)	Touch, pressure	Medium	Medium	Yes
	A gamma (Aγ)	γ Motoneurons to muscle spindles (intrafusal fibers)	Medium	Medium	Yes
	A delta (Aδ)	Touch, pressure, temperature, fast pain	Small	Medium	Yes
	B	Preganglionic autonomic nerves	Small	Medium	Yes
	C	Slow pain; postganglionic autonomic nerves; olfaction	Smallest	Slowest	No
Sensory Only	Ia	Muscle spindle afferents	Largest	Fastest	Yes
	Ib	Golgi tendon organ afferents	Largest	Fastest	Yes
	II	Secondary afferents of muscle spindles; touch, pressure	Medium	Medium	Yes
	III	Touch, pressure, fast pain, temperature	Small	Medium	Yes
	IV	Pain, temperature; olfaction	Smallest	Slowest	No

body is relayed to the contralateral cerebral hemisphere; likewise, motor activity on one side of the body is controlled by the contralateral cerebral hemisphere.

All pathways do not cross at the same level of the CNS, however. Some pathways cross in the spinal cord (e.g., pain), and many cross in the brain stem. These crossings are called **decussations.** Areas of the brain that contain only decussating axons are called **commissures;** for example, the corpus callosum is the commissure connecting the two cerebral hemispheres.

Some systems are mixed, having both crossed and uncrossed pathways. For example, in the visual system, half of the axons from each retina cross to the contralateral side and half remain ipsilateral. Visual fibers that cross do so in the **optic chiasm.**

Types of Nerve Fibers

Nerve fibers are classified according to their conduction velocity, which depends on the size of the fibers and the presence or absence of myelination. The effects of fiber diameter and myelination on conduction velocity are explained in Chapter 1. Briefly, the larger the fiber, the higher the conduction velocity. Conduction velocity also is increased by the presence of a myelin sheath around the nerve fiber. Thus, large myelinated nerve fibers have the fastest conduction velocities, and small unmyelinated nerve fibers have the slowest conduction velocities.

Two classification systems, which are based on differences in conduction velocity, are used. The first system, described by Erlanger and Gasser, applies to *both* sensory (afferent) and motor (efferent) nerve fibers and uses a lettered nomenclature of A, B, and C. The second system, described by Lloyd and Hunt, applies *only* to sensory nerve fibers and uses a Roman numeral nomenclature of I, II, III, and IV. Table 3-1 provides a summary of nerve fiber types within each classification, examples of each type, information about fiber diameter and conduction velocity, and whether the fibers are myelinated or unmyelinated.

SENSORY SYSTEMS

Sensory Pathways

Sensory systems receive information from the environment via specialized receptors in the periphery and transmit this information through a series of neurons and synaptic relays to the CNS. The following steps are involved in transmitting sensory information (Fig. 3-3):

1. **Sensory receptors.** Sensory receptors are activated by stimuli in the environment. The nature of the receptors varies from one sensory modality to the next. In the visual, taste, and auditory systems, the receptors are specialized epithelial cells. In the somatosensory and olfactory systems, the receptors are first-order, or primary afferent, neurons. Regardless of these differences, the basic function of the receptors is the same: to convert a stimulus (e.g., sound waves, electromagnetic waves, or pressure)

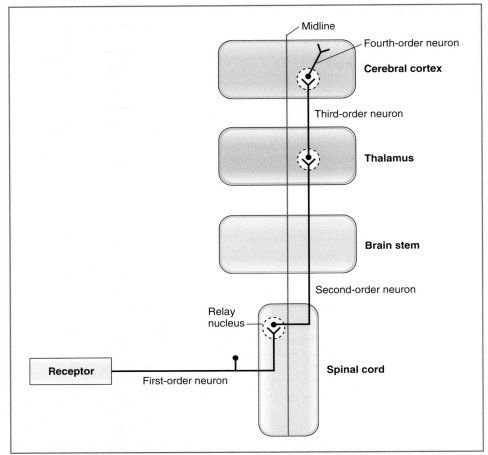

Figure 3–3 Schematic diagram of sensory pathways in the nervous system. Information is transmitted, via a series of neurons, from receptors in the periphery to the cerebral cortex. Synapses are made in relay nuclei between first- and second-order neurons, between second- and third-order neurons, and between third- and fourth-order neurons. Second-order neurons cross the midline either in the spinal cord (*shown*) or in the brain stem (*not shown*) so that information from one side of the body is transmitted to the contralateral thalamus and cerebral cortex.

into electrochemical energy. The conversion process, called **sensory transduction,** is mediated through opening or closing specific ion channels. Opening or closing ion channels leads to a change in membrane potential, either depolarization or hyperpolarization, of the sensory receptor. Such a change in membrane potential of the sensory receptor is called the **receptor potential.**

After transduction and generation of the receptor potential, the information is transmitted to the CNS along a series of sensory afferent neurons, which are designated as first-order, second-order, third-order, and fourth-order neurons (see Fig. 3-3). First-order refers to those neurons closest to the sensory receptor, and the higher-order neurons are those closer to the CNS.

2. **First-order sensory afferent neurons.** The first-order neuron is the primary sensory afferent neuron; in some cases (somatosensory, olfaction), it also is the receptor cell. When the sensory receptor is

a specialized epithelial cell, it synapses on a first-order neuron. When the receptor is also the primary afferent neuron, there is no need for this synapse. The primary afferent neuron usually has its cell body in a dorsal root or spinal cord ganglion. (Exceptions are the auditory, olfactory, and visual systems.)

3. **Second-order sensory afferent neurons.** First-order neurons synapse on second-order neurons in **relay nuclei,** which are located in the spinal cord or in the brain stem. Usually, many first-order neurons synapse on a single second-order neuron within the relay nucleus. Interneurons, also located in the relay nuclei, may be excitatory or inhibitory. These interneurons process and modify the sensory information received from the first-order neurons. Axons of the second-order neurons leave the relay nucleus and ascend to the next relay, located in the thalamus, where they synapse on third-order neurons. En route to the thalamus, the axons of these second-order neurons **cross at the midline.**

Table 3-2 Types and Examples of Sensory Receptors

Type of Receptor	Modality	Receptor	Location
Mechanoreceptors	Touch	Pacinian corpuscle	Skin
	Audition	Hair cell	Organ of Corti
	Vestibular	Hair cell	Macula, semicircular canal
Photoreceptors	Vision	Rods and cones	Retina
Chemoreceptors	Olfaction	Olfactory receptor	Olfactory mucosa
	Taste	Taste buds	Tongue
	Arterial P_{O_2}		Carotid and aortic bodies
	pH of CSF		Ventrolateral medulla
Thermoreceptors	Temperature	Cold receptors	Skin
		Warm receptors	Skin
Nociceptors	Extremes of pain and temperature	Thermal nociceptors	Skin
		Polymodal nociceptors	Skin

CSF, Cerebrospinal fluid; P_{O_2}, partial pressure of oxygen.

The decussation, or crossing, may occur in the spinal cord (illustrated in Fig. 3-3) or in the brain stem (not illustrated).

4. **Third-order sensory afferent neurons.** Third-order neurons typically reside in relay nuclei in the **thalamus.** Again, many second-order neurons synapse on a single third-order neuron. The relay nuclei process the information they receive via local interneurons, which may be excitatory or inhibitory.

5. **Fourth-order sensory afferent neurons.** Fourth-order neurons reside in the appropriate sensory area of the cerebral cortex. For example, in the auditory pathway, fourth-order neurons are found in the primary auditory cortex; in the visual pathway, they reside in the primary visual cortex; and so forth. As noted, there are secondary and tertiary areas, as well as association areas in the cortex, all of which integrate complex sensory information.

Sensory Receptors

Consider again the first step in the sensory pathway in which an environmental stimulus is transduced into an electrical signal in the sensory receptor. This section discusses the various types of sensory receptors, mechanisms of sensory transduction, receptive fields of sensory neurons, sensory coding, and adaptation of sensory receptors.

Types of Receptors

Receptors are classified by the type of stimulus that activates them. The five types of receptors are mechanoreceptors, photoreceptors, chemoreceptors, thermoreceptors, and nociceptors. Table 3-2 summarizes the receptors and gives examples and locations of each type.

Mechanoreceptors are activated by pressure or changes in pressure. Mechanoreceptors include, but are not limited to, the pacinian corpuscles in subcutaneous tissue, Meissner's corpuscles in nonhairy skin (touch), baroreceptors in the carotid sinus (blood pressure), and hair cells on the organ of Corti (audition) and in the semicircular canals (vestibular system). **Photoreceptors** are activated by light and are involved in vision. **Chemoreceptors** are activated by chemicals and are involved in olfaction, taste, and detection of oxygen and carbon dioxide in the control of breathing. **Thermoreceptors** are activated by temperature or changes in temperature. **Nociceptors** are activated by extremes of pressure, temperature, or noxious chemicals.

Sensory Transduction and Receptor Potentials

Sensory transduction is the process by which an environmental stimulus (e.g., pressure, light, chemicals) activates a receptor and is converted into electrical energy. The conversion typically involves opening or closing of ion channels in the receptor membrane, which leads to a flow of ions (current flow) across the membrane. Current flow then leads to a change in membrane potential, called a **receptor potential,** which increases or decreases the likelihood that action potentials will occur. The following series of steps occurs when a stimulus activates a sensory receptor:

1. The environmental **stimulus** interacts with the sensory receptor and causes a change in its properties. A mechanical stimulus causes *movement* of the

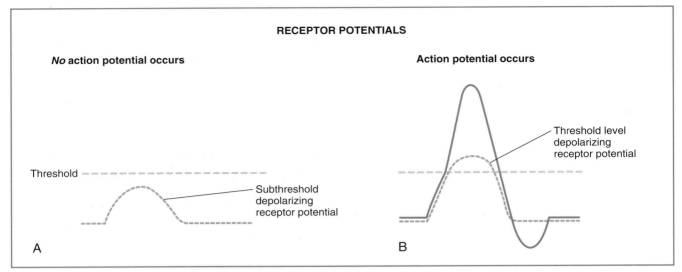

RECEPTOR POTENTIALS

No action potential occurs

Action potential occurs

Threshold level depolarizing receptor potential

Threshold

Subthreshold depolarizing receptor potential

A

B

Figure 3–4 **Receptor potentials in sensory receptor cells.** Receptor potentials may be either depolarizing (*shown*) or hyperpolarizing (*not shown*). **A,** If a depolarizing receptor potential does not bring the membrane potential to threshold, no action potential occurs. **B,** If a depolarizing receptor potential brings the membrane potential to threshold, then an action potential occurs in the sensory receptor.

*mechano*receptor (e.g., sound waves move the hair cells in the organ of Corti). Photons of light are absorbed by pigments in *photo*receptors on the retina, causing photoisomerization of rhodopsin (a chemical in the photoreceptor membrane). Chemical stimulants react with *chemo*receptors, which activate G_s proteins and adenylyl cyclase. In each case, a *change* occurs in the sensory receptor.

2. These changes cause **ion channels** in the sensory receptor membrane to open or close, which results in a change in current flow. If ionic current flow is inward (i.e., positive charges move into the receptor cell), then depolarization occurs. If current flow is outward (i.e., positive charges move out of the cell), then hyperpolarization occurs. The resulting change in membrane potential, either depolarization or hyperpolarization, is called the **receptor potential** or **generator potential.** The receptor potential is *not* an action potential. Rather, the receptor potential increases or decreases the likelihood that an action potential will occur, depending on whether it is depolarizing or hyperpolarizing. Receptor potentials are graded electronic potentials, whose amplitude correlates with the size of the stimulus.

3. If the receptor potential is **depolarizing,** it moves the membrane potential *toward* threshold and increases the likelihood that an action potential will occur (Fig. 3-4). Because receptor potentials are graded in amplitude, a small depolarizing receptor potential still may be subthreshold and, therefore, insufficient to produce an action potential. However, a larger stimulus will produce a larger depolarizing

receptor potential, and if it reaches or exceeds threshold, action potentials will occur. If the receptor potential is **hyperpolarizing** (not illustrated), it moves the membrane potential *away* from threshold, always decreasing the likelihood that action potentials will occur.

Receptive Fields

A receptive field defines an *area of the body that when stimulated results in a change in firing rate of a sensory neuron.* The change in firing rate can be an increase *or* a decrease; therefore, receptive fields are described as **excitatory** (producing an increase in the firing rate of a sensory neuron) or **inhibitory** (producing a decrease in the firing rate of a sensory neuron).

There are receptive fields for first-, second-, third-, and fourth-order sensory neurons. For example, the receptive field of a second-order neuron is the area of receptors in the periphery that causes a change in the firing rate of *that* second-order neuron.

Receptive fields vary in size (Fig. 3-5). The smaller the receptive field, the more precisely the sensation can be localized or identified. Typically, the higher the order of the CNS neuron, the more complex the receptive field, since more neurons converge in relay nuclei at each level. Thus, first-order sensory neurons have the simplest receptive fields, and fourth-order sensory neurons have the most complex receptive fields.

As noted, receptive fields can be excitatory or inhibitory, with the pattern of excitatory or inhibitory receptive fields conveying *additional* information to the CNS. Figure 3-6 illustrates one such pattern for a

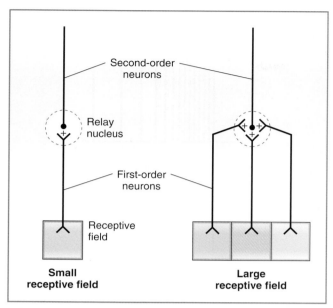

Figure 3–5 Size of receptive fields of sensory neurons.

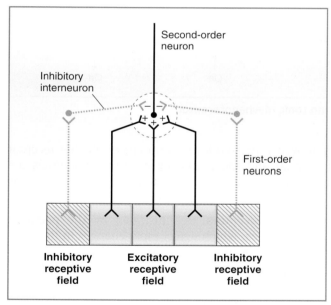

Figure 3–6 Excitatory and inhibitory receptive fields of sensory neurons.

second-order neuron. The receptive field on the skin for this particular neuron has a central region of excitation, bounded on either side by regions of inhibition. All of the incoming information is processed in relay nuclei of the spinal cord or brain stem. The areas of inhibition contribute to a phenomenon called **lateral inhibition** and aid in the precise localization of the stimulus by defining its boundaries and providing a contrasting border.

Sensory Coding

Sensory neurons are responsible for encoding stimuli in the environment. Coding begins when the stimulus is transduced by sensory receptors and continues as the information is transmitted to progressively higher levels of the CNS. One or more aspects of the stimulus are encoded and interpreted. For example, in seeing a red ball, its size, location, color, and depth all are encoded. The features that can be encoded include sensory modality, spatial location, frequency, intensity, threshold, and duration of stimulus.

♦ Stimulus **modality** is often encoded by **labeled lines,** which consist of pathways of sensory neurons *dedicated to that modality.* Thus, the pathway of neurons dedicated to vision begins with photoreceptors in the retina. This pathway is not activated by somatosensory, auditory, or olfactory stimuli. Those modalities have their *own* labeled lines.

♦ Stimulus **location** is encoded by the receptive field of sensory neurons and may be enhanced by lateral inhibition as previously described.

♦ **Threshold** is the minimum stimulus that can be detected. Threshold is best appreciated in the context of the receptor potential. If a stimulus is large enough to produce a depolarizing receptor potential that reaches threshold, it will be detected. Smaller subthreshold stimuli will not be detected.

♦ Stimulus **intensity** is encoded in three ways. (1) Intensity can be encoded by the number of receptors that are activated. Thus, large stimuli will activate more receptors and produce larger responses than will small stimuli. (2) Intensity can be encoded by differences in firing rates of sensory neurons in the pathway. (3) Intensity even may be encoded by activating different types of receptors. Thus, a light touch of the skin may activate only mechanoreceptors, whereas an intense damaging stimulus to the skin may activate mechanoreceptors *and* nociceptors. The intense stimulus would be detected not only as stronger, but also as a different modality.

♦ Stimulus information also is encoded in **neural maps** formed by arrays of neurons receiving information from different locations on the body (i.e., somatotopic maps), from different locations on the retina (i.e., retinotopic maps), or from different sound frequencies (i.e., tonotopic maps).

♦ Other stimulus information is encoded in the **pattern of nerve impulses.** Some of these codes are based on mean discharge frequency, others are based on the duration of firing, while others are based on a temporal firing pattern. The frequency of the stimulus may be encoded directly in the intervals between

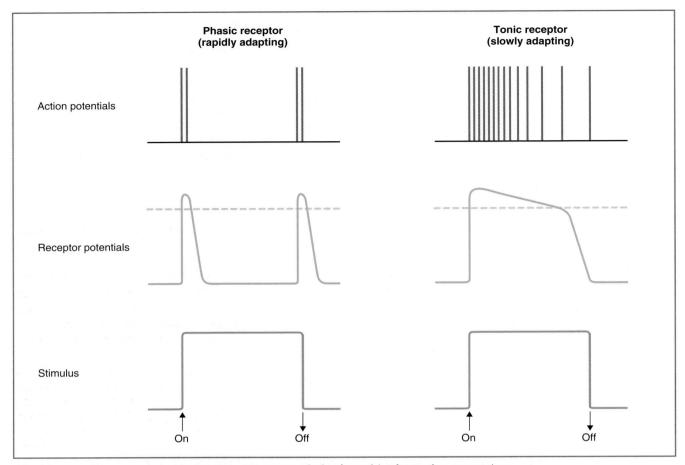

Figure 3-7 **Response of phasic and tonic mechanoreceptors.**

discharges of sensory neurons (called interspike intervals).

♦ Stimulus **duration** is encoded by the duration of firing of sensory neurons. However, during a prolonged stimulus, receptors "adapt" to the stimulus and change their firing rates. Sensory neurons may be rapidly adapting or slowly adapting.

Adaptation of Sensory Receptors

Sensory receptors "adapt" to stimuli. **Adaptation** is observed when a constant stimulus is applied for a period of time. Initially, the frequency of action potentials is high, but as time passes, this frequency declines even though the stimulus continues (Fig. 3-7). The pattern of adaptation differs among different types of receptors. Some receptors are **phasic,** meaning they adapt rapidly to the stimulus (e.g., pacinian corpuscles), and others are **tonic**, meaning they adapt slowly to the stimulus (e.g., Merkel's receptors).

The physiologic basis for adaptation also is illustrated in Figure 3-7. Two types of receptors are shown: a phasic receptor and a tonic receptor. A stimulus (e.g., pressure) is applied (*on*), and then the stimulus is

removed (*off*). While the stimulus is on, the receptor potential and the frequency of action potentials are measured. (In the figure, action potentials appear as "spikes.")

♦ **Phasic receptors** are illustrated by the **pacinian corpuscles,** which detect rapid changes in the stimulus or **vibrations.** These receptors adapt rapidly to a constant stimulus and primarily detect **onset** and **offset** of a stimulus and a changing stimulus. The phasic receptor responds promptly at the onset of the stimulus with a depolarizing receptor potential that brings the membrane potential above threshold. A short burst of action potential follows. After this burst, the receptor potential decreases below the threshold level, and although the stimulus continues, there are no action potentials (i.e., there is silence). When the stimulus is turned off, the receptor is once again activated, as the receptor potential depolarizes to threshold, causing a second short burst of action potentials.

♦ **Tonic receptors** are illustrated by mechanoreceptors (e.g., Merkel's receptors) in the skin, which detect **steady pressure.** When compared with the pacinian

Table 3-3 Types of Mechanoreceptors

Type of Mechanoreceptor	Location	Adaptation	Sensation Encoded
Pacinian corpuscle	Subcutaneous; intramuscular	Very rapidly	Vibration, tapping
Meissner's corpuscle	Nonhairy skin	Rapidly	Point discrimination, tapping, flutter
Hair follicles	Hairy skin	Rapidly	Velocity, direction of movement
Ruffini's corpuscle	Hairy skin	Slowly	Stretch, joint rotation
Merkel's receptors	Nonhairy skin	Slowly	Vertical indentation of skin
Tactile discs	Hairy skin	Slowly	Vertical indentation of skin

corpuscles (which detect vibration with their fast on-off response), tonic mechanoreceptors are designed to encode duration and intensity of stimulus. The tonic receptor responds to the onset of the stimulus with a depolarizing receptor potential that brings the membrane to threshold, resulting in a long series of action potentials. Unlike the pacinian corpuscle, whose receptor potential returns quickly to baseline, here the receptor potential remains depolarized for a longer portion of the stimulus period, and the action potentials continue. Once the receptor potential begins to repolarize, the rate of action potentials declines and eventually there is silence. Tonic receptors encode **stimulus intensity:** The greater the intensity, the larger the depolarizing receptor potential, and the more likely action potentials are to occur. Thus, tonic receptors also encode **stimulus duration:** The longer the stimulus, the longer the period in which the receptor potential exceeds threshold.

SOMATOSENSORY SYSTEM AND PAIN

The somatosensory system processes information about touch, position, pain, and temperature. The receptors involved in transducing these sensations are mechanoreceptors, thermoreceptors, and nociceptors. There are two pathways for transmission of somatosensory information to the CNS: the dorsal column system and the anterolateral system. The dorsal column system processes the sensations of fine touch, pressure, two-point discrimination, vibration, and proprioception (limb position). The anterolateral system processes the sensations of pain, temperature, and light touch.

Types of Somatosensory Receptors

Somatosensory receptors are categorized according to the specific sensation they encode. The major groups of receptors are **mechanoreceptors** (for touch and proprioception), **thermoreceptors** (for temperature), and **nociceptors** (for pain or noxious stimuli).

Mechanoreceptors

Mechanoreceptors are subdivided into different types of receptors, depending on which kind of pressure or proprioceptive quality they encode. Some types of mechanoreceptors are found in nonhairy skin and other types in hairy skin. Mechanoreceptors are described in Table 3-3 according to their location in the skin or muscle, the type of adaptation they exhibit, and the sensation they encode, and they are illustrated in Figure 3-8.

An important characteristic of each receptor is the type of adaptation that it exhibits. Among the various mechanoreceptors, adaptation varies from "very rapidly adapting" (e.g., pacinian corpuscle), to "rapidly adapting" (e.g., Meissner's corpuscle and hair follicles), to "slowly adapting" (e.g., Ruffini's corpuscle, Merkel's receptors, and tactile discs). **Very rapidly** and **rapidly adapting receptors** detect *changes in the stimulus* and, therefore, detect changes in velocity. **Slowly adapting receptors** respond to intensity and duration of the stimulus.

- **Pacinian corpuscle.** Pacinian corpuscles are encapsulated receptors found in the subcutaneous layers of nonhairy and hairy skin and in muscle. They are the most rapidly adapting of all mechanoreceptors. Because of their very rapid on-off response, they can detect changes in stimulus velocity and encode the sensation of **vibration.**

- **Meissner's corpuscle.** Meissner's corpuscles are also encapsulated receptors found in the dermis of nonhairy skin, most prominently on the fingertips, lips, and other locations where tactile discrimination is especially good. They have small receptive fields and can be used for **two-point discrimination.** Meissner's corpuscles are rapidly adapting receptors that encode point discrimination, precise location, tapping, and flutter.

- **Hair follicle.** Hair-follicle receptors are arrays of nerve fibers surrounding hair follicles in hairy skin. When the hair is displaced, it excites the hair-follicle receptors. These receptors are also rapidly adapting

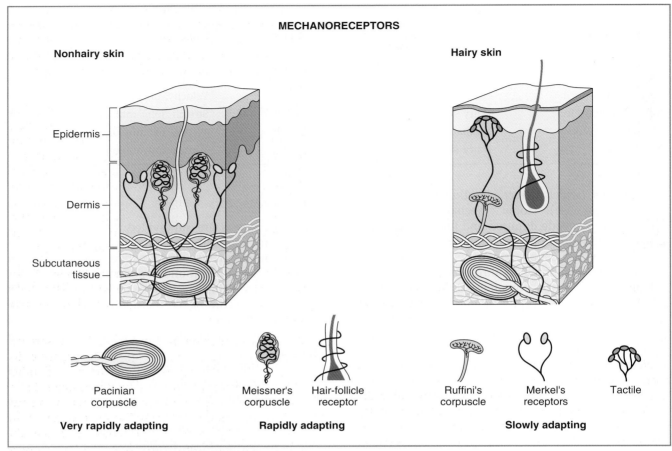

MECHANORECEPTORS

Nonhairy skin

Hairy skin

Epidermis

Dermis

Subcutaneous tissue

Pacinian corpuscle

Very rapidly adapting

Meissner's corpuscle

Hair-follicle receptor

Rapidly adapting

Ruffini's corpuscle

Merkel's receptors

Tactile

Slowly adapting

Figure 3–8 **Types of mechanoreceptors found in nonhairy skin and hairy skin.** (Modified from Schmidt RF: Fundamentals of Sensory Physiology, 3rd ed. Berlin, Springer-Verlag, 1986.)

and detect **velocity** and direction of movement across the skin.

♦ **Ruffini's corpuscle.** Ruffini's corpuscles are located in the dermis of nonhairy and hairy skin and in joint capsules. These receptors have large receptive fields and are stimulated when the skin is stretched. The stimulus may be located some distance from the receptors it activates. Ruffini's corpuscles are slowly adapting receptors. When the skin is stretched, the receptors fire rapidly, then slowly adapt to a new level of firing that corresponds to stimulus intensity. Ruffini's corpuscles detect **stretch** and joint rotation.

♦ **Merkel's receptors and tactile discs.** Merkel's receptors are slowly adapting receptors found in nonhairy skin and have very small receptive fields. These receptors detect vertical **indentations** of the skin, and their response is proportional to stimulus intensity. Tactile discs are similar to Merkel's receptors but are found in hairy, rather than nonhairy, skin.

Thermoreceptors

Thermoreceptors are slowly adapting receptors that detect changes in skin temperature. The two classes of thermoreceptors are cold receptors and warm receptors (Fig. 3-9). Each type of receptor functions over a broad range of temperatures, with some overlap in the moderate temperature range (e.g., at 36°C, both receptors are active). When the skin is warmed above 36°C, the cold receptors become quiescent, and when the skin is cooled below 36°C, the warm receptors become quiescent.

If skin temperature rises to damaging levels (above 45°C), warm receptors become inactive; thus, warm receptors do not signal pain from extreme heat. At temperatures above 45°C, polymodal nociceptors will be activated. Likewise, extremely cold (freezing) temperatures also activate nociceptors.

Transduction of warm temperatures involves **transient receptor potential (TRP) channels** in the family of vanilloid receptors (i.e., TRPV). These channels are activated by compounds in the vanilloid class, which includes capsaicin, an ingredient in spicy foods.

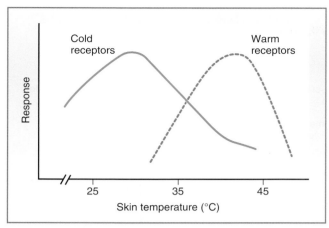

Figure 3-9 **The response profiles of skin temperature receptors.**

Transduction of cold temperatures involves a different TRP channel, TRPM8, which is also opened by compounds like menthol (which gives a cold sensation).

Nociceptors

Nociceptors respond to noxious stimuli that can produce tissue damage. There are two major classes of nociceptors: thermal or mechanical nociceptors and polymodal nociceptors. **Thermal or mechanical nociceptors** (TRPV or TRPM8 channels) are supplied by finely myelinated A-delta afferent nerve fibers and respond to mechanical stimuli such as sharp, pricking pain. **Polymodal nociceptors** are supplied by unmyelinated C fibers and respond to high-intensity mechanical or chemical stimuli and hot and cold stimuli.

Damaged skin releases a variety of chemicals including bradykinin, prostaglandins, substance P, K^+, and H^+, which initiate the **inflammatory response.** The blood vessels become permeable, and, as a result, there is local edema and redness of the skin. Mast cells near the site of injury release histamine, which directly activates nociceptors. In addition, axons of the nociceptors release substances that sensitize the nociceptors to stimuli that were not previously noxious or painful. This sensitization process, called **hyperalgesia,** is the basis for various phenomena including reduced threshold for pain.

Somatosensory Pathways

There are two pathways for transmission of somatosensory information to the CNS: the dorsal column system and the anterolateral or spinothalamic system (Fig. 3-10). Each pathway follows the general pattern already described for sensory systems.

1. The **first-order neuron** in the somatosensory pathway is the primary afferent neuron. Primary afferent neurons have their cell bodies in dorsal root or cranial ganglia, and their axons synapse on somatosensory receptor cells (i.e., mechanoreceptors). The signal is transduced by the receptor and transmitted to the CNS by the primary afferent neuron.

2. The **second-order neuron** is located in the spinal cord (anterolateral system) or in the brain stem (dorsal column system). The second-order neurons receive information from first-order neurons and transmit that information to the thalamus. Axons of the second-order neurons **cross the midline,** either in the spinal cord or in the brain stem, and ascend to the thalamus. This decussation means that somatosensory information from one side of the body is received in the contralateral thalamus.

3. The **third-order neuron** is located in one of the somatosensory nuclei of the thalamus. The thalamus has a somatotopic arrangement of somatosensory information.

4. The **fourth-order neuron** is located in the somatosensory cortex, called S1 and S2. Higher-order neurons in the somatosensory cortex and other associative cortical areas integrate complex information. The S1 somatosensory cortex has a somatotopic representation, or "map," similar to that in the thalamus. This map of the body is called the **somatosensory homunculus** (Fig. 3-11). The largest areas of representation of the body are the face, hands, and fingers, which are densely innervated by somatosensory nerves and where sensitivity is greatest. The sensory homunculus illustrates the "place" coding of somatosensory information.

Dorsal Column System

The dorsal column system is used for transmitting somatosensory information about **discriminative touch, pressure, vibration, two-point discrimination,** and **proprioception.** The dorsal column system consists mainly of group I and II nerve fibers. The first-order neurons have their cell bodies in the dorsal root ganglion cells or in cranial nerve ganglion cells and ascend ipsilaterally to the **nucleus gracilis** (lower body) or **nucleus cuneatus** (upper body) in the medulla of the brain stem. In the medulla, first-order neurons synapse on second-order neurons, which *cross the midline*. The second-order neurons ascend to the contralateral thalamus, where they synapse on third-order neurons, which ascend to the somatosensory cortex and synapse on fourth-order neurons.

Anterolateral System

The anterolateral (spinothalamic) system transmits somatosensory information about **pain, temperature,**

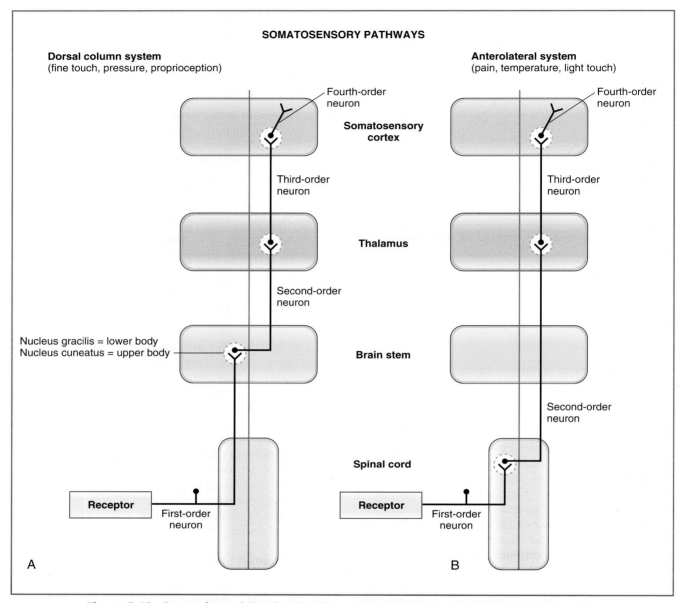

SOMATOSENSORY PATHWAYS

Dorsal column system
(fine touch, pressure, proprioception)

Anterolateral system
(pain, temperature, light touch)

Fourth-order neuron

Somatosensory cortex

Third-order neuron

Thalamus

Second-order neuron

Nucleus gracilis = lower body
Nucleus cuneatus = upper body

Brain stem

Spinal cord

Second-order neuron

Receptor

First-order neuron

Receptor

First-order neuron

A

B

Figure 3-10 **Comparison of the dorsal column (A) and the anterolateral (B) somatosensory systems.** The dorsal column system crosses the midline in the brain stem. The anterolateral system crosses the midline in the spinal cord.

and **light touch.** The anterolateral system consists mainly of group III and group IV fibers. (Recall that group IV fibers have the slowest conduction velocities of all the sensory nerves.) In the anterolateral system, first-order neurons have their cell bodies in the dorsal horn and synapse on thermoreceptors and nociceptors in the skin. The first-order neurons synapse on second-order neurons in the spinal cord. In the spinal cord, the second-order neurons *cross the midline* and ascend to the contralateral thalamus. In the thalamus, second-order neurons synapse on third-order neurons, which

ascend to the somatosensory cortex and synapse on fourth-order neurons.

Fast pain (e.g., pin prick) is carried on A delta, group II, and group III fibers, has a rapid onset and offset, and is precisely localized. **Slow pain** (e.g., burn) is carried on C fibers and is characterized as aching, burning, or throbbing pain that is poorly localized.

Referred pain is of visceral origin. The pain is "referred" according to the **dermatomal rule,** which states that sites on the skin are innervated by nerves

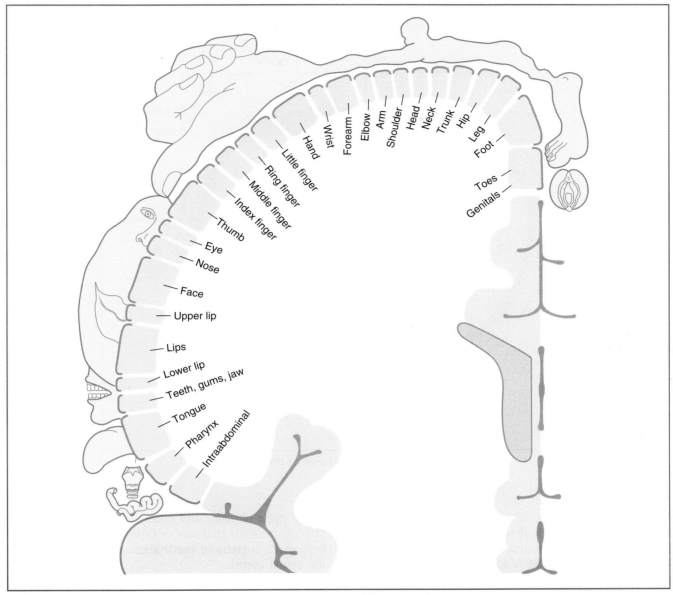

Figure 3–11 **The somatosensory homunculus.** (Modified from Wilder P, Rasmussen T: The Cerebral Cortex of Man. New York, Macmillan, 1950. Reprinted by permission of The Gale Group.)

arising from the same spinal cord segments as those innervating the visceral organs. Thus, according to the dermatomal rule, ischemic heart pain is referred to the chest and shoulder, gallbladder pain is referred to the abdomen, kidney pain is referred to the lower back, and so forth.

VISION

The visual system detects and interprets light stimuli, which are electromagnetic waves. The eye can distinguish two qualities of light: its brightness and its wavelength. For humans, the wavelengths between 400 and 750 nanometers are called **visible light.**

Structures of the Eye

The major structures of the eye are illustrated in Figure 3-12. The wall of the eye consists of three concentric layers: an outer layer, a middle layer, and an inner layer. The outer layer, which is fibrous, includes the cornea, corneal epithelium, conjunctiva, and sclera. The middle layer, which is vascular, includes the iris and the choroid. The inner layer, which is neural, contains the retina. The functional portions of the retina cover

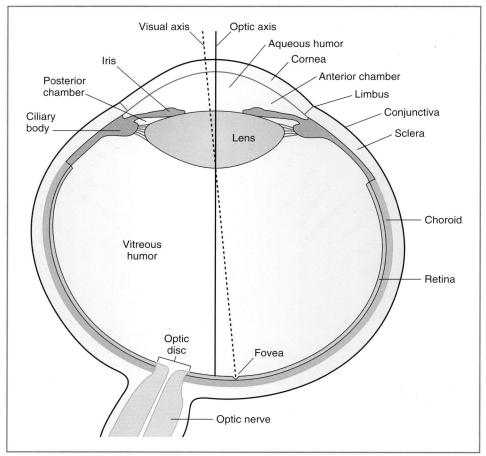

Figure 3–12 Structures of the eye.

the entire posterior eye, with the exception of the **blind spot,** which is the **optic disc** (head of the optic nerve). Visual acuity is highest at a central point of the retina, called the **macula;** light is focused at a depression in the macula, called the **fovea.** The eye also contains a lens, which focuses light; pigments, which absorb light and reduce scatter; and two fluids, aqueous and vitreous humors. **Aqueous humor** fills the anterior chamber of the eye, and **vitreous humor** fills the posterior chamber of the eye.

The sensory receptors for vision are **photoreceptors,** which are located on the retina. There are two types of photoreceptors, rods and cones (Table 3-4). **Rods** have low thresholds, are sensitive to low-intensity light, and function well in darkness. The rods have low acuity and do not participate in color vision. **Cones** have a higher threshold for light than the rods, operate best in daylight, provide higher visual acuity, and participate in color vision. The cones are not sensitive to low-intensity light.

Information is received and transduced by photoreceptors on the retina and then is carried to the CNS via axons of retinal ganglion cells. Some optic nerves cross

at the optic chiasm, and others continue ipsilaterally. The main visual pathway is through the dorsal lateral geniculate nucleus of the thalamus, which projects to the visual cortex.

Photoreception

Layers of the Retina

The retina is a specialized sensory epithelium that contains photoreceptors and other cell types arranged in layers. Retinal cells include photoreceptors, interneurons (bipolar cells, horizontal cells, and amacrine cells), and ganglion cells. Synapses are made between cells in two plexiform layers, an outer plexiform layer and an inner plexiform layer. The *layers of the retina* are described as follows and correspond with the circled numbers in Figure 3-13:

1. **Pigment cell layer.** The retina begins just inside the choroid with a layer of **pigment epithelium** (see Fig. 3-12). The pigment epithelial cells absorb stray light and have tentacle-like processes that extend into the photoreceptor layer to prevent scatter of

Table 3-4 Properties of Rods and Cones

Photoreceptor	Sensitivity to Light	Acuity	Dark Adaptation	Color Vision
Rods	Low threshold Sensitive to low-intensity light Night vision	Low acuity Not present on fovea	Adapt late	No
Cones	High threshold Sensitive to high-intensity light Day vision	High acuity Present on fovea	Adapt early	Yes

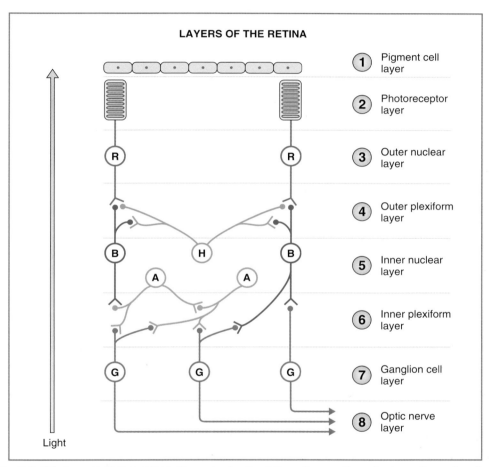

Figure 3-13 Layers of the retina. The output cells of the retina are the retinal ganglion cells, whose axons form the optic nerves. Circled numbers correspond to layers of the retina described in the text. *A,* Amacrine cells; *B,* bipolar cells; *G,* ganglion cells; *H,* horizontal cells; *R,* photoreceptors.

light between photoreceptors. The pigment cells also convert all-*trans*-retinal to 11-*cis*-retinal and deliver the 11-*cis* form to the photoreceptors (refer to the steps in photoreception).

2. **Photoreceptor layer.** The photoreceptors are rods and cones, which consist of a cell body, an outer segment, and an inner segment. Only rods are shown in this figure.

3. **Outer nuclear layer.** The nuclei of photoreceptors (*R*) are contained in the outer nuclear layer.

4. **Outer plexiform layer.** The outer plexiform layer is a synaptic layer containing presynaptic and postsynaptic elements of photoreceptors and interneurons of the retina. (The cell bodies of retinal interneurons are contained in the inner nuclear layer.) Synapses are made between photoreceptors and interneurons and also between the interneurons themselves.

5. **Inner nuclear layer.** The inner nuclear layer contains cell bodies of retinal interneurons including

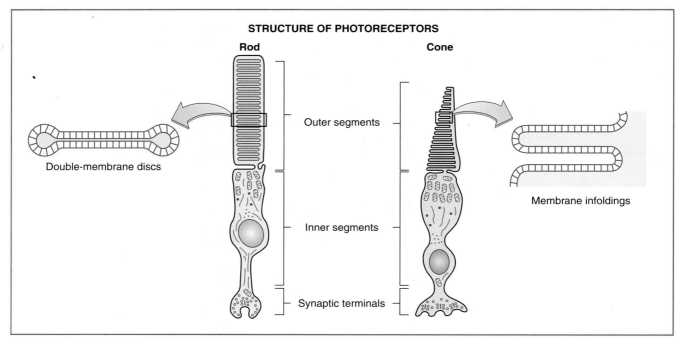

STRUCTURE OF PHOTORECEPTORS

Rod   Cone

Outer segments

Double-membrane discs

Membrane infoldings

Inner segments

Synaptic terminals

Figure 3–14   **Structure of photoreceptors.** The enlargements show a magnified view of the outer segments.

bipolar cells (B), horizontal cells (H), and amacrine cells (A).

6. **Inner plexiform layer.** The inner plexiform layer is the second synaptic layer. It contains presynaptic and postsynaptic elements of retinal interneurons. Synapses are made between retinal interneurons and ganglion cells.

7. **Ganglion cell layer.** The ganglion cell layer contains cell bodies of ganglion cells (G), which are the output cells of the retina.

8. **Optic nerve layer.** Axons of retinal ganglion cells form the optic nerve layer. These axons pass through the retina (avoiding the macula), enter the optic disc, and leave the eye in the optic nerve.

As mentioned, there are differences in acuity between rods and cones, which can be explained by differences in their retinal circuitry (see Table 3-4). Only a *few* **cones** synapse on a single bipolar cell, which synapses on a single ganglion cell. This arrangement accounts for the higher acuity and lower sensitivity of the cones. Acuity is highest in the fovea, where one cone synapses on one bipolar cell, which synapses on one ganglion cell. In contrast, *many* **rods** synapse on a single bipolar cell. This arrangement accounts for the lower acuity but the higher sensitivity of the rods—light striking any one of the rods will activate the bipolar cell.

Structure of the Photoreceptors

Photoreceptors, the rods and cones, span several layers of the retina, as previously described. The outer and inner segments of photoreceptors are located in the photoreceptor layer, the nuclei are located in the outer nuclear layer, and the synaptic terminals (on bipolar and horizontal cells) are located in the outer plexiform layer. The structures of the rods and cones are shown in Figure 3-14.

The **outer segments** of both rods and cones contain **rhodopsin,** a light-sensitive pigment (a photopigment). In rods, the outer segments are long and consist of stacks of free-floating double-membrane discs containing large amounts of rhodopsin. The cones have short, cone-shaped outer segments, which consist of infoldings of surface membrane. This infolded membrane also contains rhodopsin, but a smaller amount than is present in the rods. The greater the amount of photopigment, the greater the sensitivity to light, which accounts in part for the greater light sensitivity of the rods. *A single photon of light can activate a rod, whereas several hundred photons are required to activate a cone.*

The **inner segments** of the rods and cones are connected to the outer segments by a single cilium. The inner segments contain mitochondria and other organelles. Rhodopsin is synthesized in the inner segments and then incorporated in the membranes of the outer segments as follows: In the *rods,* rhodopsin is inserted in new membrane discs, which are displaced toward the outer segment; eventually they are shed and phagocytosed by the pigment cell epithelium, giving the outer segments their rodlike shape. In the *cones,* rhodopsin is incorporated randomly into membrane folds, with no shedding process.

Steps in Photoreception

Photoreception is the transduction process in rods and cones that converts light energy into electrical energy. **Rhodopsin,** the photosensitive pigment, is composed of opsin (a protein belonging to the superfamily of G protein–coupled receptors) and retinal (an aldehyde of vitamin A). When light strikes the photoreceptors, retinal is chemically transformed in a process called photoisomerization, which begins the transduction process. The steps in photoreception, discussed as follows, correspond to the circled numbers shown in Figure 3-15:

1. **Light** strikes the retina, which initiates **photoisomerization** of retinal. 11-*cis* Retinal is converted to all-*trans* retinal. From there, a series of conformational changes occur in the opsin that culminate in the production of **metarhodopsin II.** (Regeneration of 11-*cis* retinal requires **vitamin A,** and deficiency of vitamin A causes **night blindness.**)

2. Metarhodopsin II activates a G protein that is called **transducin,** or G_t. When activated, transducin stimulates a phosphodiesterase that catalyzes the conversion of cyclic guanosine monophosphate (GMP) to 5′-GMP. Consequently, there is increased breakdown of cyclic GMP, causing cyclic GMP levels to decrease.

3. and 4. In the photoreceptor membrane, **Na⁺ channels** that carry inward current are regulated by cyclic GMP. In the **dark,** there is an increase in cyclic GMP levels, which produces an Na⁺ inward current (or "**dark current**") and **depolarization** of the photoreceptor membrane. In the **light,** there is a decrease in cyclic GMP levels, as already described, which closes Na⁺ channels in the photoreceptor membrane, reduces inward Na⁺ current, and produces **hyperpolarization.**

5. **Hyperpolarization** of the photoreceptor membrane *decreases* **the release of glutamate,** an excitatory neurotransmitter, from the synaptic terminals of the photoreceptor. (Recall from Figure 3-13 that photoreceptors synapse on bipolar cells and horizontal cells in the outer plexiform layer.)

6. There are two **types of glutamate receptors** on bipolar and horizontal cells: ionotropic receptors, which are depolarizing (excitatory), and metabotropic receptors, which are hyperpolarizing (inhibitory). The type of receptor on the bipolar or horizontal cell determines whether the response will be depolarization (excitation) or hyperpolarization (inhibition). Thus, *decreased* release of glutamate that interacts with **ionotropic receptors** will result in hyperpolarization and inhibition of the bipolar or horizontal cell (i.e., decreased

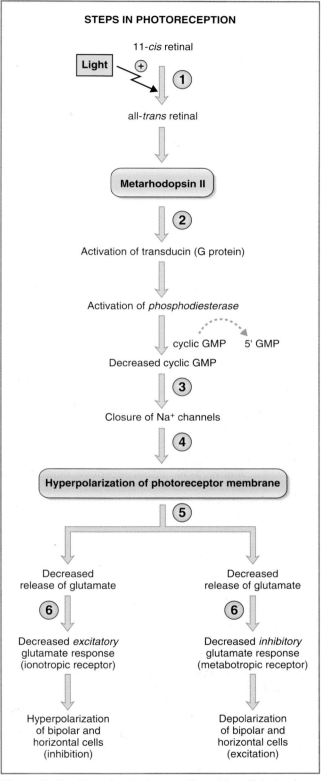

Figure 3–15 **Steps in photoreception.** When light impinges on the retina, the photoreceptors are hyperpolarized. In turn, the photoreceptors decrease their release of glutamate, leading to either hyperpolarization or depolarization of bipolar or horizontal cells. Circled numbers correlate with steps described in the text. Cyclic GMP, Cyclic guanosine monophosphate; GMP, guanosine monophosphate.

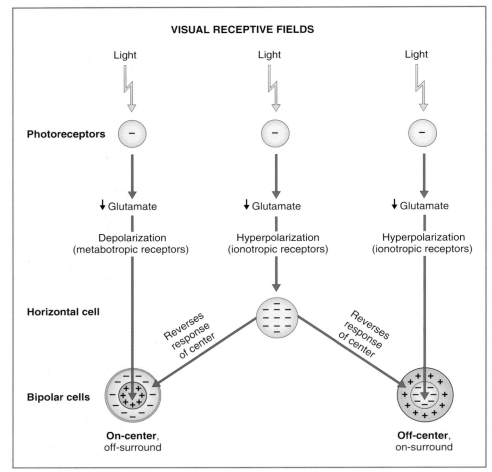

Figure 3-16 **Visual receptive fields of bipolar cells in the retina.** Two patterns are shown: on-center and off-center.

excitation). And *decreased* release of glutamate that interacts with **metabotropic receptors** will result in depolarization and excitation of the bipolar or horizontal cell (i.e., decreased inhibition causes excitation). This process will establish the **on-off patterns** for visual fields.

Visual Receptive Fields

Each level of the visual pathway can be described by its receptive fields. Thus, there are receptive fields for photoreceptors, bipolar and horizontal cells, ganglion cells, cells of the lateral geniculate body in the thalamus, and cells in the visual cortex. At each higher level, the receptive fields become increasingly complex.

PHOTORECEPTORS, HORIZONTAL CELLS, AND BIPOLAR CELLS

One simple arrangement of visual receptive fields is illustrated in Figure 3-16. The figure shows the receptive fields for three photoreceptors, for two bipolar cells, and for one horizontal cell positioned between

the bipolar cells. When light hits the photoreceptors, they are *always* hyperpolarized and release *decreased* amounts of glutamate (recall the steps in photoreception), as indicated by the minus signs on the photoreceptors. Photoreceptors synapse directly on bipolar cells in the outer plexiform layer of the retina. The receptive field of the bipolar cell is shown as two concentric circles: The inner circle is called the "center," and the outer circle is called the "surround." The center of the bipolar cell's receptive field represents direct connections from photoreceptors and can be either excited (*on*) or inhibited (*off*), depending on the type of glutamate receptor on the bipolar cell, as described earlier. If the center of the receptive field has metabotropic glutamate receptors, then the bipolar cell will be excited (+); if the center of the receptive field has ionotropic glutamate receptors, then the bipolar cell will be inhibited (-). The surround of the bipolar cell's receptive field receives input from adjacent photoreceptors via horizontal cells. The surround of the receptive field shows the *opposite* response of the center because the horizontal cells are inhibitory (i.e., they reverse the direct response of the photoreceptor on its bipolar cell). Two patterns for receptive fields of bipolar cells are illustrated in Figure 3-16 and explained as follows:

♦ **On-center, off-surround** (or "on-center"). This pattern is illustrated in the bipolar cell shown on the left of the figure. The center of its receptive field is excited (*on*) by light, and the surround of its receptive field is inhibited (*off*) by light. *How is this pattern achieved?* As always, light impinging on photoreceptors produces hyperpolarization and decreased release of glutamate. This photoreceptor is connected to the *center* of the bipolar cell's receptive field and glutamate binds to a metabotropic receptor. Thus, the center of the receptive field is excited (i.e., decreased inhibition produces excitation). Light also inhibits the adjacent photoreceptor, which binds to an ionotropic receptor in the horizontal cell, thus inhibiting the horizontal cell. The horizontal cell is connected to the *surround* of the bipolar cell's receptive field. Because the horizontal cell is inhibited, it reverses the direct action of the photoreceptors on the bipolar cell and produces inhibition in the surround.

♦ **Off-center, on-surround** (or "off-center"). This pattern is illustrated in the bipolar cell shown on the right of the figure. The center of its receptive field is inhibited (*off*) by light, and the surround is excited (*on*) by light. *How is this pattern achieved?* Again, light impinging on the photoreceptor produces inhibition. This photoreceptor is connected to the center of the bipolar cell's receptive field and binds to an ionotropic receptor. Thus, the *center* of the receptive field is inhibited. Light also inhibits the adjacent photoreceptor, which inhibits the horizontal cell. The horizontal cell is connected to the *surround* of the bipolar cell's receptive field. Because the horizontal cell is inhibited, it reverses the direct action of the photoreceptor on the bipolar cell and produces excitation in the surround.

AMACRINE CELLS

The amacrine cells receive input from different combinations of on-center and off-center bipolar cells. Thus, the receptive fields of the amacrine cells are mixtures of on-center and off-center patterns.

GANGLION CELLS

Ganglion cells receive input from both bipolar cells and amacrine cells (see Fig. 3-13). When input to the ganglion cells is primarily from bipolar cells, the ganglion cells retain the on-center and off-center patterns established at the level of the bipolar cells. When the input to a ganglion cell is primarily from amacrine cells, the receptive fields tend to be diffuse because there has been mixing of input at the amacrine cell level.

LATERAL GENICULATE CELLS OF THE THALAMUS

Cells of the lateral geniculate body of the thalamus retain the on-center or off-center patterns transmitted from the ganglion cells.

VISUAL CORTEX

Neurons of the visual cortex detect shape and orientation of figures. Three cell types are involved in this type of visual discrimination: simple cells, complex cells, and hypercomplex cells. **Simple cells** have receptive fields similar to those of the ganglion cells and lateral geniculate cells (i.e., on-center or off-center), although the patterns are elongated rods rather than concentric circles. Simple cells respond best to bars of light that have the "correct" position and orientation. **Complex cells** respond best to moving bars of light or edges of light with the correct orientation. **Hypercomplex cells** respond best to lines of particular length and to curves and angles.

Optic Pathways

The optic pathways from the retina to the CNS are shown in Figure 3-17. Axons from retinal ganglion cells form the optic nerves and optic tracts, synapse in the lateral geniculate body of the thalamus, and ascend to the visual cortex in the geniculocalcarine tract.

Notice that the temporal visual fields project onto the nasal retina, and the nasal fields project onto the temporal retina. Nerve fibers from each **nasal hemiretina** cross at the **optic chiasm** and ascend contralaterally. Nerve fibers from each **temporal hemiretina** remain uncrossed and ascend ipsilaterally. Thus, fibers from the *left* nasal hemiretina and fibers from the *right* temporal hemiretina form the *right* optic tract and synapse on the *right* lateral geniculate body. Conversely, fibers from the *right* nasal hemiretina and fibers from the *left* temporal hemiretina form the *left* optic tract and synapse on the *left* lateral geniculate body. Fibers from the lateral geniculate body form the **geniculocalcarine tract**, which ascends to the **visual cortex** (area 17 of the occipital lobe). Fibers from the right lateral geniculate body form the right geniculocalcarine tract; fibers from the left lateral geniculate body form the left geniculocalcarine tract.

Lesions at various points in the optic pathway cause deficits in vision, which can be predicted by tracing the pathway, as shown in Figure 3-18. **Hemianopia** is the loss of vision in half the visual field of one or both eyes. If the loss occurs on the same side of the body as the lesion, it is called ipsilateral; if the loss occurs on the opposite side of the body as the lesion, it is called contralateral. The following **lesions** correspond to the shaded bars and circled numbers on the figure:

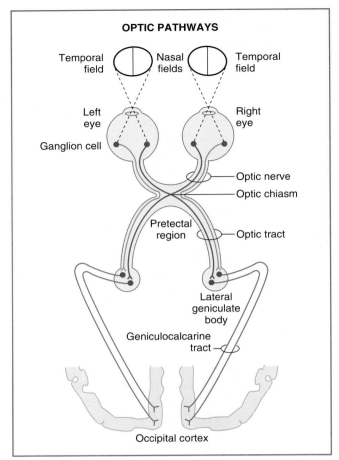

OPTIC PATHWAYS

Temporal field
Nasal fields
Temporal field
Left eye
Right eye
Ganglion cell
Optic nerve
Optic chiasm
Pretectal region
Optic tract
Lateral geniculate body
Geniculocalcarine tract
Occipital cortex

Figure 3–17   Optic pathways. Fibers from the temporal visual fields cross at the optic chiasm, but fibers from the nasal visual fields remain uncrossed. (Modified from Ganong WF: Review of Medical Physiology, 20th ed. Norwalk, Conn, Appleton & Lange, 2001.)

1. **Optic nerve.** Cutting the optic nerve causes blindness in the ipsilateral (same side) eye. Thus, cutting the left optic nerve causes blindness in the left eye. All sensory information coming from that eye is lost because the cut occurs before any fibers cross at the optic chiasm.

2. **Optic chiasm.** Cutting the optic chiasm causes heteronymous (both eyes) bitemporal (both temporal visual fields) hemianopia. In other words, *all information is lost from fibers that cross.* Thus, information from the temporal visual fields from *both* eyes is lost because these fibers cross at the optic chiasm.

3. **Optic tract.** Cutting the optic tract causes homonymous contralateral hemianopia. As shown in the figure, cutting the left optic tract results in loss of the temporal visual field from the right eye (crossed) and loss of the nasal visual field from the left eye (uncrossed).

4. **Geniculocalcarine tract.** Cutting the geniculocalcarine tract causes homonymous contralateral

hemianopia with **macular sparing** (the visual field from the macula is intact). Macular sparing occurs because lesions of the visual cortex do not destroy all neurons that represent the macula.

AUDITION

Audition, the sense of hearing, involves the transduction of sound waves into electrical energy, which then can be transmitted in the nervous system. Sound is produced by waves of compression and decompression, which are transmitted in elastic media such as air or water. These waves are associated with increases (compression) and decreases (decompression) in pressure. The units for expressing sound pressure are **decibels (dB),** which is a relative measure on a log scale. Sound frequency is measured in cycles per second or **hertz (Hz).** A pure tone results from sinusoidal waves of a single frequency.

Most sounds are mixtures of pure tones. The human ear is sensitive to tones with frequencies between **20 and 20,000 Hz** and is most sensitive between 2000 and 5000 Hz. A reference, 0 dB, is the average threshold for hearing at 1000 Hz. Sound pressure, in dB, is calculated as follows:

$$dB = 20 \log P/P_0$$

where

dB = Decibel
P = Sound pressure being measured
P_0 = Reference pressure measured at the threshold frequency

Therefore, if a sound pressure is 10 times the reference pressure, it is 20 dB (20 × log 10 = 20 × 1 = 20 dB). If a sound pressure is 100 times the reference pressure, it is 40 dB (20 × log 100 = 20 × 2 = 40 dB).

The usual range of frequencies in human speech is between 300 and 3500 Hz, and the sound intensity is about 65 dB. Sound intensities greater than 100 dB can damage the auditory apparatus, and those greater than 120 dB can cause pain.

Structures of the Ear

Structures of the external, middle, and inner ear are shown in Figure 3-19 and are described as follows:

♦ The **external ear** consists of the pinna and the external auditory meatus (auditory canal). The function of the external ear is to direct sound waves into the auditory canal. The external ear is air filled.

♦ The **middle ear** consists of the **tympanic membrane** and a chain of auditory ossicles called the

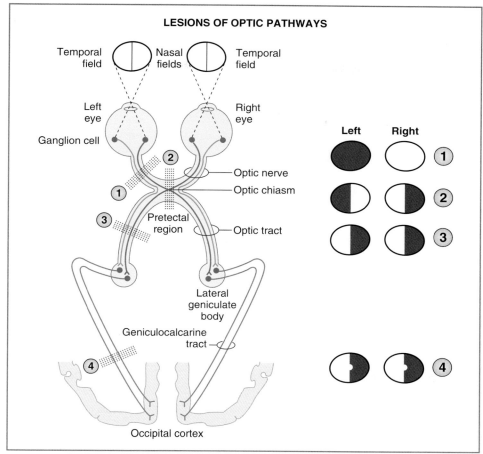

LESIONS OF OPTIC PATHWAYS

Figure 3–18 **Visual field defects produced by lesions at various levels of the visual pathway.** Circled numbers refer to deficits and are explained in the text. (Modified from Ganong WF: Review of Medical Physiology, 20th ed. Norwalk, Conn, Appleton & Lange, 2001.)

malleus, incus, and **stapes**. The tympanic membrane separates the external ear from the middle ear. An oval window and a round window lie between the middle ear and the inner ear. The stapes has a footplate, which inserts into the oval window and provides the interface between the middle ear and the inner ear. The middle ear is air filled.

♦ The **inner ear** consists of a bony labyrinth and a membranous labyrinth. The bony labyrinth consists of three **semicircular canals** (lateral, posterior, and superior). The membranous labyrinth consists of a series of ducts called the scala vestibuli, scala tympani, and scala media.

The cochlea and the vestibule are formed from the bony and membranous labyrinths. The **cochlea,** which is a spiral-shaped structure composed of three tubular canals or ducts, contains the organ of Corti. The **organ of Corti** contains the receptor cells and is the site of auditory transduction. The inner ear is fluid filled, and the fluid in each duct has a different composition. The fluid in the scala vestibuli and scala tympani is called **perilymph,** which is similar to extracellular fluid. The fluid in the scala media is called **endolymph,** which has a **high-potassium (K^+)** concentration and a low-sodium (Na^+) concentration. Thus, endolymph is unusual in that its composition is similar to that of intracellular fluid, even though, technically, it is extracellular fluid.

Auditory Transduction

Auditory transduction is the transformation of sound pressure into electrical energy. Many of the structures of the ear participate, directly or indirectly, in this transduction process. Recall that the external and middle ears are air filled, and the inner ear, which contains the organ of Corti, is fluid filled. Thus, before transduction can occur, sound waves traveling through air must be converted into pressure waves in fluid. The acoustic impedance of fluid is much greater than that of air. The combination of the tympanic membrane and the ossicles serves as an impedance-matching device

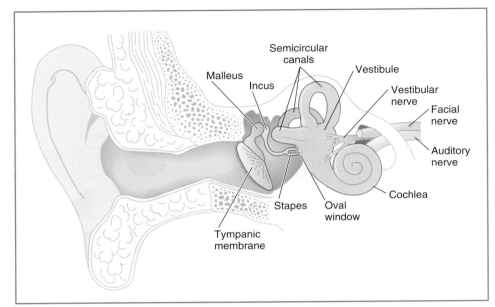

Figure 3–19 **Structures of the external, middle, and inner ear.** The cochlea has been turned slightly for visualization.

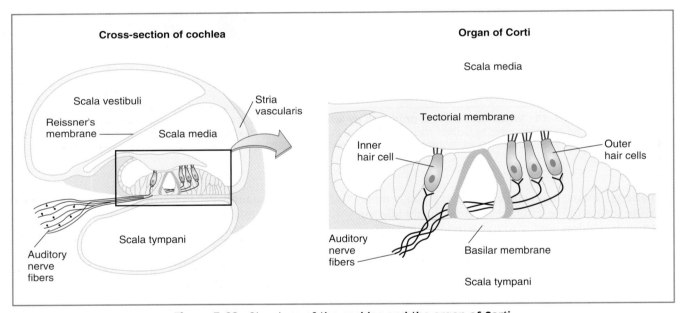

Figure 3–20 **Structure of the cochlea and the organ of Corti.**

that makes this conversion. Impedance matching is accomplished by the ratio of the large surface area of the tympanic membrane to the small surface area of the oval window and the mechanical advantage offered by the lever system of the ossicles.

The external ear directs sound waves into the auditory canal, which transmits the sound waves onto the tympanic membrane. When sound waves move the tympanic membrane, the chain of ossicles also moves, pushing the footplate of the stapes into the oval window and displacing the fluid in the inner ear.

Cochlea and Organ of Corti

The cochlea contains the sensory transduction apparatus, the organ of Corti. The structures of the cochlea and the organ of Corti are shown in Figure 3-20.

The **cross-section of the cochlea** shows its three chambers: scala vestibuli, scala media, and scala tympani. Each chamber is fluid filled, the scala vestibuli and scala tympani with perilymph and the scala media with endolymph. The scala vestibuli is separated from the scala media by Reissner's membrane. The basilar membrane separates the scala media from the scala tympani.

The **organ of Corti** lies on the basilar membrane of the cochlea and is bathed in the endolymph contained in the scala media. Auditory hair cells in the organ of Corti are the sites of auditory transduction. The organ of Corti contains two types of receptor cells: inner hair cells and outer hair cells. There are fewer **inner hair cells,** which are arranged in single rows. **Outer hair cells** are arranged in parallel rows and are more numerous than inner hair cells. Cilia, protruding from the hair cells, are embedded in the tectorial membrane. Thus, the bodies of the hair cells are in contact with the basilar membrane, and the cilia of the hair cells are in contact with the tectorial membrane.

The nerves that serve the organ of Corti are contained in the vestibulocochlear nerve (**CN VIII**). The cell bodies of these nerves are located in spiral ganglia, and their axons synapse at the base of the hair cells. These nerves will transmit information from the auditory hair cells to the CNS.

Steps in Auditory Transduction

Several important steps precede transduction of sound waves by the auditory hair cells on the organ of Corti. Sound waves are directed toward the tympanic membrane, and, as the tympanic membrane vibrates, it causes the ossicles to vibrate and the stapes to be pushed into the oval window. This movement displaces fluid in the cochlea. The sound energy is **amplified** by two effects: the lever action of the ossicles and the concentration of sound waves from the large tympanic membrane onto the small oval window. Thus, sound waves are transmitted and amplified from the air-filled external and middle ears to the fluid-filled inner ear, which contains the receptors.

Auditory transduction by hair cells on the **organ of Corti** then occurs in the following steps (Fig. 3-21):

1. Sound waves are transmitted to the inner ear and cause **vibration** of the organ of Corti.

2. The **auditory hair cells** are mechanoreceptors, which are located on the organ of Corti (see Fig. 3-20). The base of the hair cells sits on the basilar membrane, and the cilia of the hair cells are embedded in the tectorial membrane. The basilar membrane is more elastic than the tectorial membrane. Thus, vibration of the organ of Corti causes **bending of cilia** on the hair cells by a shearing force as the cilia push against the tectorial membrane.

3. Bending of the cilia produces a change in **K⁺ conductance** of the hair cell membrane. Bending in one direction produces an increase in K^+ conductance and hyperpolarization; bending in the other

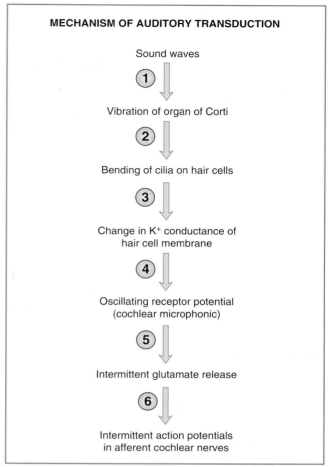

Figure 3–21 Steps in auditory transduction in hair cells. Circled numbers correspond to steps described in the text.

direction produces a decrease in K^+ conductance and depolarization.

4. These changes in membrane potential are the receptor potentials of the auditory hair cells. The oscillating receptor potential is called the **cochlear microphonic potential.**

5. When hair cells are *de*polarized, the depolarization opens voltage-gated Ca^{2+} channels in the presynaptic terminals of the hair cells. As a result, Ca^{2+} enters the presynaptic terminals and causes release of glutamate, which functions here as an excitatory neurotransmitter, causing action potentials in the afferent cochlear nerves that will transmit this information to the CNS. When the hair cells are *hyper*polarized, the opposite events occur, and there is decreased release of glutamate.

6. Thus, oscillating depolarizing and hyperpolarizing receptor potentials in the hair cells cause intermittent release of glutamate, which produces intermittent firing of afferent cochlear nerves.

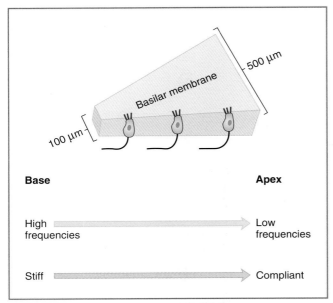

Figure 3-22 Frequency responses of the basilar membrane.

Encoding of Sound

Encoding of sound frequencies occurs because different auditory hair cells are activated by different frequencies. The frequency that activates a particular hair cell depends on the *position* of that hair cell along the **basilar membrane,** as illustrated in Figure 3-22. The **base** of the basilar membrane is nearest the stapes and is narrow and stiff. Hair cells located at the base respond best to high frequencies. The **apex** of the basilar membrane is wide and compliant. Hair cells located at the apex respond best to low frequencies. Thus, the basilar membrane acts as a sound frequency analyzer, with hair cells positioned along the basilar membrane responding to different frequencies. This spatial mapping of frequencies generates a **tonotopic map,** which then is transmitted to higher levels of the auditory system.

Auditory Pathways

Information is transmitted from the hair cells of the organ of Corti to the afferent cochlear nerves. The cochlear nerves synapse on neurons of the dorsal and ventral cochlear nuclei of the medulla, which send out axons that ascend in the CNS. Some of these axons cross to the contralateral side and ascend in the **lateral lemniscus** (the primary auditory tract) to the **inferior colliculus.** Other axons remain ipsilateral. The two inferior colliculi are connected via the commissure of the inferior colliculus. Fibers from nuclei of the inferior colliculus ascend to the **medial geniculate nucleus of the thalamus.** Fibers from the thalamus ascend to the

auditory cortex. The tonotopic map, generated at the level of the organ of Corti, is preserved at all levels of the CNS. Complex feature discrimination (e.g., the ability to recognize a patterned sequence) is the property of the auditory cortex.

Because some auditory fibers are crossed and some are uncrossed, a mixture of ascending nerve fibers represents *both* ears at all levels of the CNS. Thus, lesions of the cochlea of one ear will cause ipsilateral deafness. However, more central unilateral lesions do not cause deafness because some of the fibers transmitting information from that ear have already crossed to the undamaged side.

VESTIBULAR SYSTEM

The vestibular system is used to maintain **equilibrium** or **balance** by detecting angular and linear accelerations of the head. Sensory information from the vestibular system is then used to provide a stable visual image for the retina (while the head moves) and to make the adjustments in posture that are necessary to maintain balance.

Vestibular Organ

The vestibular organ is located within the temporal bone, adjacent to the auditory apparatus (the cochlea). The vestibular organ consists of a membranous labyrinth within the bony labyrinth (Fig. 3-23). The membranous labyrinth consists of three perpendicular semicircular canals (horizontal, superior, and posterior) and two otolith organs (utricle and saccule). The semicircular canals and otolith organs are filled with endolymph and are surrounded by perilymph, much like the auditory organ.

The **semicircular canals,** which are arranged perpendicular to each other, are used to detect *angular* or rotational acceleration of the head. (The perpendicular arrangement of canals ensures that they cover the three principal axes of head rotation.) Each canal, filled with endolymph, contains an enlargement at one end called an **ampulla.** Each ampulla contains **vestibular hair cells,** which are covered with a gelatinous mass called a **cupula** (Fig. 3-24). The cupula, which spans the cross-sectional area of the ampulla, has the same specific gravity as the endolymph in the canal. During angular acceleration of the head, the cupula is displaced, causing excitation or inhibition of the hair cells.

The **otolith organs,** the **utricle** and **saccule,** are used to detect *linear* acceleration (e.g., gravitational forces). Within the utricle and saccule, an otolith mass composed of mucopolysaccharides and calcium carbonate crystals overlies the vestibular hair cells (like a "pillow"). When the head is tilted, gravitational forces

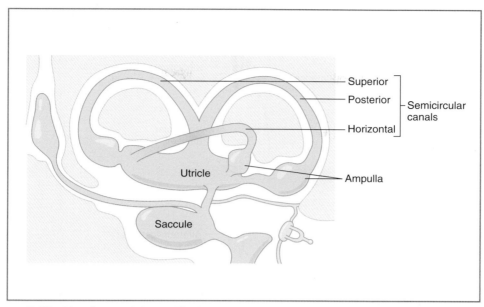

Figure 3–23 Structures of the vestibular organ, showing the three perpendicular semicircular canals and two otolith organs (utricle and saccule).

act on the otolith mass, moving it across the vestibular hair cells. The hair cells are either activated or inhibited, alerting the person to a change in the position of the head.

Vestibular Transduction

Semicircular Canals

The function of the horizontal semicircular canals is to detect **angular acceleration** of the head, as illustrated in Figure 3-24. In this figure, the left and right horizontal canals are shown with their attached ampullae. The ampulla contains the vestibular hair cells, which are embedded in the gelatinous mass of the cupula. The vestibular hair cells differ from auditory hair cells in that the vestibular hair cells have a large **kinocilium** and a cluster of stereocilia. Afferent nerve fibers from the hair cells carry vestibular information to the CNS.

For example, when the **head is rotated counterclockwise** (to the left), the following events occur in the horizontal semicircular canals:

1. When the head is rotated to the left, the horizontal semicircular canals and their attached ampullae also rotate left. Initially, the cupula (anchored to the ampulla) moves before the endolymph begins to flow. Thus, the cupula is displaced or dragged through the endolymph, causing bending of the cilia on the hair cells. Eventually, as rotation continues, the endolymph begins to move.

2. If the stereocilia are bent *toward* the kinocilium, the hair cell *depolarizes* and there is an increased firing rate in the afferent vestibular nerves. If the stereocilia are bent *away from* the kinocilium, the hair cell *hyperpolarizes* and there is a decreased firing rate in the afferent vestibular nerves. Therefore, during the initial leftward rotation of the head, the left horizontal canal is excited and the right horizontal canal is inhibited.

3. While the head is still rotating to the left, the endolymph eventually "catches up" with the movement of the head, the ampulla, and the cupula. The cilia now return to their original positions, and the hair cells are neither depolarized nor hyperpolarized.

4. When the head stops rotating, the events occur in reverse. For a brief period, the endolymph continues to move, pushing the cupula and kinocilia on the hair cells in the opposite direction. Thus, if the hair cell was depolarized in the initial rotation, it now will be hyperpolarized, with inhibition of afferent nerve output. If the hair cell was hyperpolarized in the initial rotation, it now will be depolarized, with excitation of afferent nerve output. Thus, when the head stops moving left, the left horizontal canal will be inhibited and the right canal will be excited.

In summary, rotation of the head to the left stimulates the left semicircular canals, and rotation to the right stimulates the right semicircular canals.

Otolith Organs

The maculae are sensitive to **linear acceleration** (e.g., acceleration due to gravitational forces). Recall that the

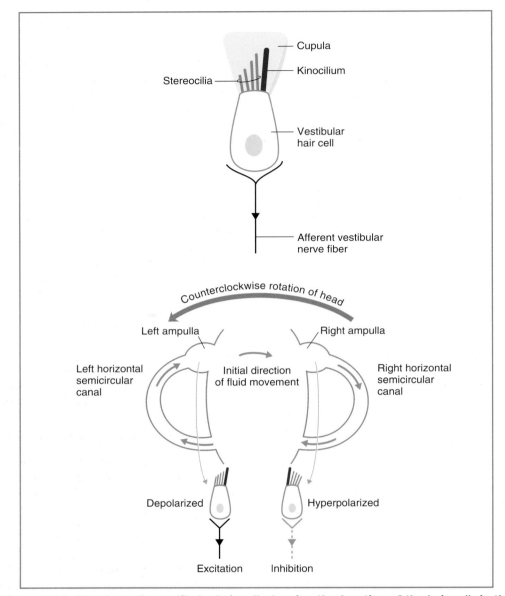

Figure 3–24 **Structure of a vestibular hair cell, showing the function of the hair cells in the horizontal semicircular canal.** Counterclockwise (*left*) rotation of the head causes excitation of the left semicircular canals and inhibition of the right semicircular canals.

hair cells of the maculae are embedded in the otolith mass. When the head is tilted, gravitational forces cause the otolith mass to slide across the vestibular hair cells, bending the stereocilia toward or away from the kinocilium. Movement of the stereocilia *toward* the kinocilium causes *depolarization* of the hair cell and excitation. Movement of the stereocilia *away from* the kinocilium causes *hyperpolarization* of the hair cell and inhibition.

When the head is upright, the macula of the utricle is oriented horizontally and the saccule is oriented vertically. In the **utricle,** tilting the head forward or laterally causes excitation of the ipsilateral utricle; tilting the head backward or medially causes inhibition

of the ipsilateral utricle. The **saccule** responds to head movements in all directions. Hair cells of the saccule are excited with both forward and backward movements (called "pitch") and lateral and medial movements (called "roll"). The saccule also responds to up and down movements of the head.

Because of the bilateral arrangement of the otolith organs, every possible orientation of the head can be encoded by excitation or inhibition of the vestibular hair cells. For each position of the head, there is a unique pattern of activity from the afferent nerves innervating the otolith organs that provides detailed information to the CNS about the position of the head in space.

Vestibular Pathways

Afferent nerves from vestibular hair cells terminate in vestibular nuclei of the medulla: the superior, medial, lateral (Deiters' nucleus), and inferior nuclei. **Medial and superior nuclei** receive their input from the semicircular canals and project to nerves innervating extraocular muscles via the medial longitudinal fasciculus. The **lateral vestibular nucleus** receives input from the utricles and projects to spinal cord motoneurons via the lateral vestibulospinal tract. Projections of the lateral vestibular nucleus play a role in maintaining postural reflexes. The **inferior vestibular nucleus** receives its input from the utricles, saccules, and semicircular canals. It projects to the brain stem and the cerebellum via the medial longitudinal fasciculus.

Vestibulo-Ocular Reflexes

Several vestibular reflexes are produced in response to movement of the head. One reflex, called **nystagmus,** occurs in response to angular or rotational acceleration of the head. When the head is rotated, the eyes initially move in the opposite direction of the rotation, attempting to maintain a constant direction of gaze. This initial movement is the slow component of nystagmus. Once the eyes approach the limit of their lateral movement, there is a rapid eye movement in the same direction as the head's rotation. This movement is the rapid component of nystagmus, in which the eyes "jump ahead" to fix on a new position in space. Nystagmus is defined by the direction of the rapid component: *The nystagmus is in the direction of the head's rotation.*

If the rotation is stopped abruptly, the eyes will move in the direction opposite that of the original rotation. This eye movement is called **postrotatory nystagmus.** During the postrotatory period, the person tends to fall in the direction of the original rotation (due to stimulation of contralateral extensor muscles) because the person *thinks* he or she is spinning in the opposite direction.

Testing Vestibulo-ocular Reflexes

Vestibular function can be tested using the phenomena of nystagmus and postrotatory nystagmus.

The **Bárány test** involves rotating a person on a special chair for about 10 revolutions. In a person with normal vestibular function, rotation to the right causes a right *rotatory* nystagmus, a left *postrotatory* nystagmus, and the person falls to the right during the postrotatory period. Likewise, rotation to the left causes a left rotatory nystagmus, a right postrotatory nystagmus, and the person falls to the left during the postrotatory period.

The **caloric test** involves thermal stimulation of the inner ears, in which the right and left horizontal semicircular canals can be stimulated separately. In this test, the head is tilted back 60 degrees so that the horizontal canals have a vertical orientation. Rinsing the ear with warm or cold water causes endolymph to flow, which deflects the cupula as if the head were rotated. A nystagmus occurs, lasting approximately 2 minutes. **Warm water** produces a nystagmus toward the treated side; **cold water** produces a nystagmus toward the untreated side.

OLFACTION

The chemical senses involve detection of chemical stimuli and transduction of those stimuli into electrical energy that can be transmitted in the nervous system. Olfaction, the sense of smell, is one of the chemical senses. In humans, olfaction is not necessary for survival, yet it improves the quality of life and even protects against hazards.

Anosmia is the absence of the sense of smell, **hyposmia** is impaired sense of smell, and **dysosmia** is a distorted sense of smell. Head injury, upper respiratory infections, tumors of the anterior fossa, and exposure to toxic chemicals (which destroy the olfactory epithelium) all can cause olfactory impairment.

Olfactory Epithelium and Receptors

Odorant molecules, which are present in the gas phase, reach the olfactory receptors via the nasal cavity: Air enters the nostril, crosses the nasal cavity, and exits into the nasopharynx. The nasal cavity contains structures called turbinates, some of which are lined with olfactory epithelium containing the olfactory receptor cells. (The remainder of the nasal cavity is lined by respiratory epithelium.) The turbinates act as baffles, causing air flow to become turbulent and, thereby, to reach the upper regions of the nasal cavity.

The **olfactory epithelium** consists of three cell types: supporting cells, basal cells, and olfactory receptor cells (Fig. 3-25).

♦ **Supporting cells** are columnar epithelial cells lined with microvilli at their mucosal border and filled with secretory granules.

♦ **Basal cells** are located at the base of the olfactory epithelium and are undifferentiated stem cells that give rise to the olfactory receptor cells. These stem cells undergo mitosis, producing a continuous turnover of receptor cells.

♦ **Olfactory receptor cells,** which are also **primary afferent neurons,** are the site of odorant binding, detection, and transduction. Odorant molecules

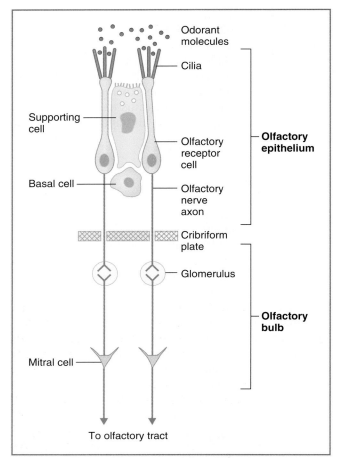

Figure 3-25 Olfactory pathways, showing the olfactory epithelium and olfactory bulb.

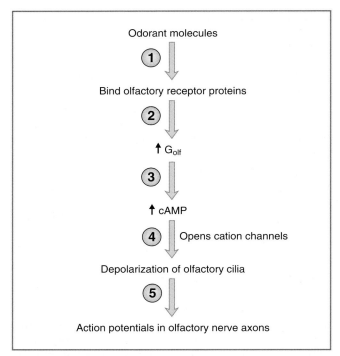

Figure 3-26 Steps in olfactory transduction. Circled numbers correspond to steps described in the text. cAMP, cyclic adenosine monophosphate.

bind to receptors on the cilia, which extend into the nasal mucosa. Axons from olfactory receptor cells leave the olfactory epithelium and travel centrally to the olfactory bulb. These axons must pass through the **cribriform plate** at the base of the skull to reach the olfactory bulb. Thus, fractures of the cribriform plate can sever olfactory neurons, leading to olfactory disorders (e.g., anosmia). Olfactory nerve axons are unmyelinated and are among the smallest and slowest fibers in the nervous system (recall the relationships between fiber diameter, myelination, and conduction velocity discussed in Chapter 1).

Because the olfactory receptor cells are also primary afferent neurons, the continuous replacement of receptor cells from basal cells means that there is **continuous neurogenesis.**

Olfactory Transduction

Transduction in the olfactory system involves the conversion of a chemical signal into an electrical signal that can be transmitted to the CNS. The steps in olfactory transduction are as follows (Fig. 3-26):

1. Odorant molecules bind to specific **olfactory receptor proteins** located on the cilia of olfactory receptor cells. There are at least 1000 different olfactory receptor proteins (members of the superfamily of G protein–coupled receptors), each encoded by a different gene and each found on a different olfactory receptor cell.

2. The olfactory receptor proteins are coupled to adenylyl cyclase via a G protein called G_{olf}. When the odorant is bound, G_{olf} is activated, which activates **adenylyl cyclase.**

3. Adenylyl cyclase catalyzes the conversion of ATP to cAMP. Intracellular levels of cAMP increase, which **opens cation channels** in the cell membrane of the olfactory receptor that are permeable to Na^+, K^+, and Ca^{2+}.

4. The receptor cell membrane depolarizes (i.e., the membrane potential is driven toward a value in between the equilibrium potentials for the three cations, which is depolarization). This depolarizing receptor potential brings the membrane potential closer to threshold and depolarizes the initial segment of the olfactory nerve axon.

5. Action potentials are then generated and propagated along the olfactory nerve axons toward the olfactory bulb.

Encoding Olfactory Stimuli

It is not known exactly how olfactory stimuli are encoded; that is, how do we *recognize* the scent of a rose or a gardenia or a special person, and how do we *distinguish* a rose from a gardenia?

The following information is known: (1) Olfactory receptor proteins are *not* dedicated to a single odorant, and each protein can respond to a variety of odorants. (2) Still, olfactory receptor proteins are selective, responding to some odorants more than others, and to some not at all. (3) Different olfactory receptor proteins have different responses to the same odorant. For example, receptor protein "A" has a much stronger response to "apple" than does receptor protein "B." (4) If the response to a given odorant is examined across many receptors, different patterns emerge for different odorants. This is called an **across-fiber pattern code.** Each odorant produces a unique pattern of activity across a population of receptors, which is projected onto targeted glomeruli in the olfactory bulb ("odor map"). The CNS then interprets these odor maps (e.g., a rose or a gardenia or a special person).

Olfactory Pathways

As noted, olfactory receptor cells are the primary afferent neurons in the olfactory system. Axons from the receptor cells leave the olfactory epithelium, pass through the cribriform plate, and synapse on apical dendrites of **mitral cells** (the second-order neurons) in the **olfactory bulb.** These synapses occur in clusters called **glomeruli** (see Fig. 3-25). In the glomeruli, approximately 1000 olfactory receptor axons converge onto 1 mitral cell. The mitral cells are arranged in a single layer in the olfactory bulb and have lateral dendrites in addition to the apical dendrites. The olfactory bulb also contains granule cells and periglomerular cells (not shown). The granule and periglomerular cells are inhibitory interneurons that make **dendrodendritic synapses** on neighboring mitral cells. The inhibitory inputs serve a function similar to that of the horizontal cells of the retina and may provide lateral inhibition that "sharpens" the information projected to the CNS.

Mitral cells of the olfactory bulb project to higher centers in the CNS. As the olfactory tract approaches the base of the brain, it divides into two major tracts, a lateral tract and a medial tract. The **lateral olfactory tract** synapses in the primary olfactory cortex, which includes the prepiriform cortex. The **medial olfactory tract** projects to the anterior commissure and the contralateral olfactory bulb.

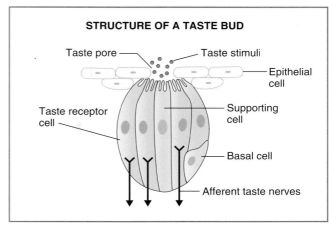

Figure 3–27 **Structure of a taste bud.**

TASTE

The second chemical sense is **gestation,** or taste. For the sense of taste, chemicals called tastants are detected and transduced by chemoreceptors located in taste buds. Tastes are mixtures of five elementary taste qualities: salty, sweet, sour, bitter, and umami (savory, including monosodium glutamate).

Disorders associated with the sense of taste are not life threatening, but they can impair the quality of life, impair nutritional status, and increase the possibility of accidental poisoning. Taste disorders include **ageusia** (absence of taste), **hypogeusia** (decreased taste sensitivity), **hypergeusia** (increased taste sensitivity), and **dysgeusia** (distortion of taste, including taste sensation in the absence of taste stimuli).

Taste Buds and Receptors

Taste receptor cells are located within taste buds on the tongue, palate, pharynx, and larynx. The taste buds on the tongue are found in taste papillae, which include as many as several hundred taste buds. The taste buds are anatomically similar to the olfactory epithelium and consist of three cell types: supporting cells, basal cells, and receptor cells (Fig. 3-27).

♦ **Supporting cells** are found among the taste receptor cells. These cells do not respond to taste stimuli, and their function is not known.

♦ **Basal cells** are undifferentiated stem cells that serve as precursors to taste receptor cells (just as basal cells serve as precursors to olfactory receptor cells). Basal cells undergo **continuous replacement.** New cells, which are generated approximately every 10 days, migrate toward the center of the taste bud and differentiate into new receptor cells. New receptor cells are needed to replace those cells that are sloughed from the tongue.

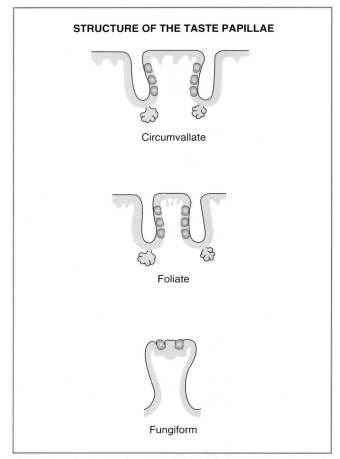

STRUCTURE OF THE TASTE PAPILLAE

Circumvallate

Foliate

Fungiform

Figure 3–28 **Structure of taste papillae lined with taste buds.**

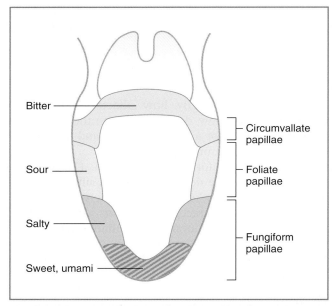

Bitter

Sour

Salty

Sweet, umami

Circumvallate papillae

Foliate papillae

Fungiform papillae

Figure 3–29 **Organization of taste papillae on the tongue.** The circumvallate, foliate, and fungiform papillae and the chemicals they detect are shown.

♦ **Taste receptor cells** are the chemoreceptors of the taste system. They line the taste buds and extend microvilli into the taste pores. These **microvilli** provide a large surface area for detection of chemical stimuli. In contrast to the olfactory system (in which the receptor cells are the primary afferent neurons), in the gustatory system, the receptor cells *are not neurons.* They are specialized epithelial cells that function as chemoreceptors, transducing chemical stimuli into electrical signals. Afferent fibers innervate the taste receptor cells and transmit this information to the CNS.

Taste buds on the tongue are organized in specialized **papillae** (Fig. 3-28). Three types of papillae contain taste buds: circumvallate, foliate, and fungiform.

♦ **Circumvallate papillae** are the largest in size but fewest in number. They are arranged in rows at the base of the tongue. Each circumvallate papilla is surrounded by a trench, with taste buds located along the sides of the trenches. Because of their large size, approximately half the total number of taste buds are found in circumvallate papillae. The taste cells in circumvallate papillae are innervated by CN VII and IX.

♦ **Foliate papillae** are located on the lateral borders of the tongue. Taste buds are located in folds on the sides of the papillae.

♦ **Fungiform papillae** are scattered on the dorsal surface of the tongue and are most numerous near the anterior tip. They are mushroom shaped ("fungiform"), with each papilla containing anywhere from three to five taste buds. The fungiform papillae are translucent with a dense blood supply, making them appear as red spots on the surface of the tongue. The taste cells in fungiform papillae are innervated exclusively by the chorda tympani branch of CN VII.

Taste Transduction

Detection of the five basic taste qualities involves differential sensitivity of areas of the tongue (Fig. 3-29). Although all five taste qualities can be detected over the full surface of the tongue, different regions of the tongue do have different thresholds. The tip of the tongue is most responsive to sweet, salty, and umami, whereas the posterior tongue is most responsive to bitter, and the sides of the tongue are most responsive to sour.

The chemical signals for the five taste qualities are transduced by the mechanisms shown in Figure 3-30. In most cases, transduction ultimately results in

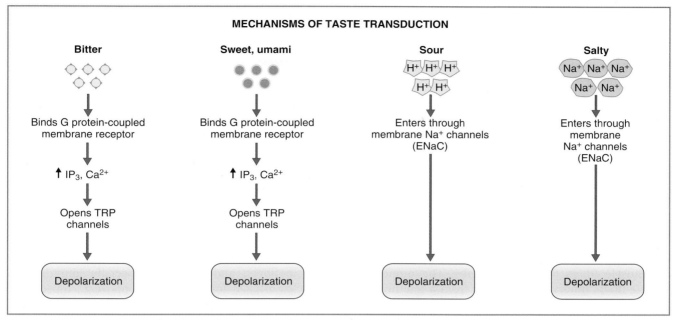

Figure 3–30 **Mechanisms of transduction in taste receptor cells.** ENaC, Epithelial Na$^+$ channel; IP$_3$, inositol 1,4,5-triphosphate; TRP, transient receptor potential.

depolarization of the taste receptor membrane (i.e., a depolarizing generator potential). This depolarization leads to action potentials in afferent nerves innervating that portion of the tongue. For **bitter** sensation, the tastant molecules bind to G protein–coupled receptors on the taste receptor membrane and, mediated by an inositol 1,4,5-triphosphate (IP$_3$)/Ca^{2+} mechanism, opens so-called transient receptor potential (TRP) channels and results in depolarization. For **sweet and umami** sensations, molecules bind to a different class of G protein–coupled receptors on the taste receptor cell membrane and, mediated by IP$_3$/Ca^{2+}, open TRP channels and cause depolarization. For **sour** sensation (mediated by H$^+$), H$^+$ enters the taste receptor through epithelial *Na$^+$* channels (**ENaC**), leading to depolarization. For **salty** sensation (mediated by Na$^+$), Na$^+$ enters the taste receptor through the same epithelial Na$^+$ channels, leading directly to depolarization.

Encoding Taste Stimuli

How taste qualities are encoded in the CNS is not precisely known. One theory states there is an **across-fiber pattern code** in which each taste fiber responds best to one stimulus but also responds to a lesser extent to other stimuli. Thus, an afferent taste fiber might respond best to salt but also responds to acid. Another taste fiber might respond best to acid but also responds to bitter. Thus, each afferent taste fiber receives input from a population of taste receptors with a distinctive *pattern* of responses. The response pattern *across* many fibers then encodes for a particular taste sensation.

Taste Pathways

As noted, taste begins with transduction of chemical signals in the taste receptor cells, which are located in taste buds. Transduction leads to depolarizing receptor potentials, which lead to action potentials in primary afferent neurons innervating specific regions of the tongue. Different regions of the tongue are innervated by branches of three cranial nerves. The posterior one third of the tongue (where bitter and sour sensations are most sensitive) is innervated by the glossopharyngeal nerve (CN IX). The anterior two thirds of the tongue (where sweet, umami, and salty sensations are most sensitive) is innervated by the facial nerve (CN VII). The back of the throat and epiglottis are innervated by the vagus nerve (CN X). These three cranial nerves (CN VII, IX, and X) enter the brain stem, ascend in the **solitary tract,** and terminate on second-order neurons in the **solitary nucleus** of the medulla. The second-order neurons project ipsilaterally to the ventral posteromedial nucleus of the thalamus. Third-order neurons leave the thalamus and terminate in the taste cortex.

MOTOR SYSTEMS

Posture and movement depend on a combination of involuntary reflexes coordinated by the spinal cord and voluntary actions controlled by higher brain centers.

Organization of Motor Function by the Spinal Cord

Posture and movement ultimately depend on contraction of some skeletal muscles while, simultaneously, other muscles remain relaxed. Recall that activation and contraction of skeletal muscles is under the control of the motoneurons that innervate them. The motor system is designed to execute this coordinated response largely through reflexes integrated in the spinal cord.

Motor Units

A **motor unit** is defined as a *single* motoneuron and the muscle fibers that it innervates. The number of muscle fibers innervated can vary from a few fibers to thousands of fibers, depending on the nature of the motor activity. Thus, for eye movements requiring fine control, motoneurons innervate only a few muscle fibers. For postural muscles involved in large movements, motoneurons innervate thousands of muscle fibers. A **motoneuron pool** is the set of motoneurons innervating fibers within the same muscle.

The force of contraction of a muscle is graded by **recruitment** of motor units (size principle). For example, small motoneurons innervate a few muscle fibers, and, because they have the lowest thresholds, they fire first. Small motoneurons also generate the smallest amounts of force. On the other hand, large motoneurons innervate many muscle fibers. They have the highest thresholds to fire action potentials; thus, they fire last. Because large motoneurons innervate many muscle fibers, they also generate the greatest amounts of force. The **size principle** states that as more motor units are recruited, progressively larger motoneurons are involved and greater tension will be generated.

Types of Motoneurons

There are two types of motoneurons: α motoneurons and γ motoneurons. **α Motoneurons** innervate extrafusal skeletal muscle fibers. Action potentials in α motoneurons lead to action potentials in the extrafusal muscle fibers they innervate, which results in contraction (see Chapter 1). **γ Motoneurons** innervate specialized intrafusal muscle fibers, a component of the muscle spindles. The overall function of the muscle spindle is to sense muscle length; the function of the γ motoneurons innervating them is to adjust the sensitivity of the muscle spindles (so that they respond appropriately as the extrafusal fibers contract and shorten). α Motoneurons and γ motoneurons are coactivated (activated simultaneously) so that muscle

spindles remain sensitive to changes in muscle length even as the muscle contracts and shortens.

Types of Muscle Fibers

As already noted, there are two types of muscle fibers: extrafusal fibers and intrafusal fibers. **Extrafusal fibers** constitute the majority of skeletal muscle, are innervated by α motoneurons, and are used to generate force. **Intrafusal fibers** are specialized fibers that are innervated by γ motoneurons and are too small to generate significant force. Intrafusal fibers are encapsulated in sheaths, forming muscle spindles that run parallel to the extrafusal fibers.

Muscle Spindles

Muscle spindles are distributed among the extrafusal muscle fibers, and they are especially abundant in muscles utilized for fine movements (e.g., muscles of the eye). Muscle spindles are spindle-shaped organs composed of intrafusal muscle fibers and innervated by sensory and motor nerve fibers, as illustrated in Figure 3-31. Muscle spindles are attached to connective tissue and arranged in parallel with the extrafusal muscle fibers.

Intrafusal Muscle Fibers of Muscle Spindles

There are two types of intrafusal fibers present in muscle spindles: nuclear bag fibers and nuclear chain fibers (see Fig. 3-31). Generally, both types of fibers are present in every muscle spindle, but nuclear chain fibers are more plentiful than nuclear bag fibers. (There are five or six nuclear chain fibers per muscle spindle, compared with two nuclear bag fibers.) **Nuclear bag fibers** are larger, and their nuclei are accumulated in a central ("bag") region. **Nuclear chain fibers** are smaller, and their nuclei are arranged in rows ("chains").

Innervation of Muscle Spindles

Muscle spindles are innervated by both sensory (afferent) and motor (efferent) nerves.

♦ **Sensory innervation** of the muscle spindle consists of a single **group Ia afferent nerve,** which innervates the central region of both the nuclear bag fibers and the nuclear chain fibers, and **group II afferent nerves,** which primarily innervate the nuclear chain fibers. Recall that group Ia fibers are among the largest nerves in the body; thus, they have among the fastest conduction velocities. These fibers form primary endings in a spiral-shaped terminal around the central region of the nuclear bag and nuclear chain fibers. Group II fibers have intermediate diameters and intermediate conduction velocities. Group II fibers form secondary endings primarily on the nuclear chain fibers.

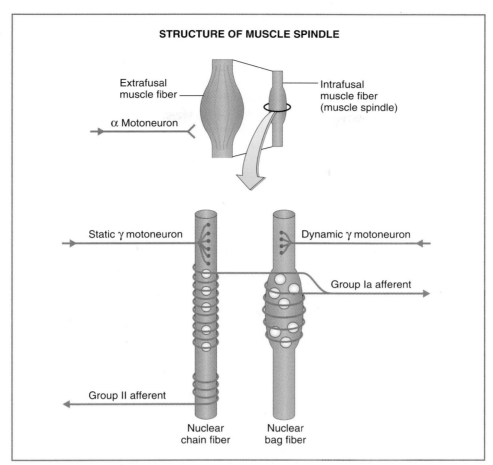

STRUCTURE OF MUSCLE SPINDLE

Extrafusal muscle fiber

α Motoneuron

Intrafusal muscle fiber (muscle spindle)

Static γ motoneuron

Dynamic γ motoneuron

Group Ia afferent

Group II afferent

Nuclear chain fiber

Nuclear bag fiber

Figure 3–31 **Structure of the muscle spindle.** An intrafusal muscle fiber is shown in relation to an extrafusal muscle fiber.

♦ **Motor innervation** of the muscle spindle consists of two types of γ motoneurons: dynamic and static. **Dynamic γ motoneurons** synapse on nuclear bag fibers in "plate endings." **Static γ motoneurons** synapse on nuclear chain fibers in "trail endings," which spread out over longer distances. γ Motoneurons are smaller and slower than the α motoneurons that innervate the extrafusal fibers. Again, the function of the γ motoneurons (either static or dynamic) is to regulate the sensitivity of the intrafusal muscle fibers they innervate.

Function of Muscle Spindles

Muscle spindles are **stretch receptors** whose function is to correct for changes in muscle length when extrafusal muscle fibers are either shortened (by contraction) or lengthened (by stretch). Thus, muscle spindle reflexes operate to return muscle to its resting length after it has been shortened or lengthened. To illustrate the function of the muscle spindle reflex, consider the events that occur when a muscle is stretched.

1. When a muscle is stretched, the extrafusal muscle fibers are lengthened. Because of their parallel arrangement in the muscle, the intrafusal muscle fibers also are lengthened.

2. The increase in length of the intrafusal fibers is detected by the sensory afferent fibers innervating them. The **group Ia afferent fibers** (innervating the central region of nuclear bag and nuclear chain fibers) detect the *velocity* of length change, and the **group II afferent fibers** (innervating the nuclear chain fibers) detect the *length* of the muscle fiber. Thus, when the muscle is stretched, the increase in the length of the intrafusal fibers activates both group Ia and group II sensory afferent fibers.

3. Activation of the group Ia afferent fibers stimulates α motoneurons in the spinal cord. These α motoneurons innervate extrafusal fibers in the homonymous (same) muscle and, when activated, cause the muscle to contract (i.e., to shorten). Thus, the original stretch (lengthening) is opposed when the

Table 3-5 Muscle Reflexes

Type of Reflex (Example)	Number of Synapses	Stimulus for Reflex	Sensory Afferent Fibers	Responses
Stretch reflex (knee jerk)	One	Stretch (lengthening) of the muscle	Ia	Contraction of the muscle
Golgi tendon reflex (clasp knife)	Two	Contraction (shortening) of the muscle	Ib	Relaxation of the muscle
Flexor-withdrawal reflex (touching a hot stove)	Many	Pain; temperature	II, III, and IV	Flexion on ipsilateral side; extension on contralateral side

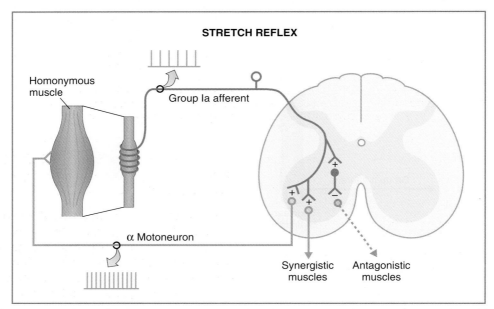

Figure 3-32 **Operation of the stretch reflex.** *Solid lines* show excitatory pathways; *dashed lines* show inhibitory steps. *Open* neurons are excitatory; *filled* neurons are inhibitory.

reflex causes the muscle to contract and shorten. γ Motoneurons are coactivated with the α motoneurons, ensuring that the muscle spindle will remain sensitive to changes in muscle length even during the contraction.

Spinal Cord Reflexes

Spinal cord reflexes are **stereotypical** motor responses to specific kinds of stimuli, such as stretch of the muscle. The neuronal circuit that directs this motor response is called the **reflex arc.** The reflex arc includes the sensory receptors; the sensory afferent nerves, which carry information to the spinal cord; the interneurons in the spinal cord; and the motoneurons, which direct the muscle to contract or relax.

The stretch reflex is the simplest of all spinal cord reflexes, having only one synapse between sensory afferent nerves and motor efferent nerves. The Golgi

tendon reflex is of intermediate complexity and has two synapses. The most complex of the spinal cord reflexes is the flexor-withdrawal reflex, which has multiple synapses. Characteristics of the three types of spinal cord reflexes are summarized in Table 3-5.

Stretch Reflex

The stretch (**myotatic**) reflex is exemplified by the knee-jerk reflex (Fig. 3-32). The following steps occur in the stretch reflex, which has only one synapse between the sensory afferent nerves (group Ia afferents) and the motor efferent nerves (α motoneurons):

1. When the muscle is stretched, group Ia afferent fibers in the muscle spindle are activated and their firing rate increases. These group Ia afferents enter the spinal cord and synapse *directly* on and activate α motoneurons. This pool of α motoneurons innervates the homonymous muscle.

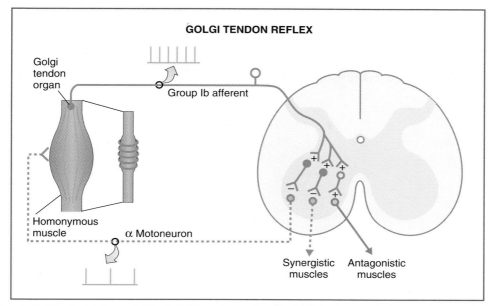

Figure 3-33 **Operation of the Golgi tendon reflex.** *Solid lines* show excitatory pathways; *dashed lines* show inhibitory steps. *Open* neurons are excitatory; *filled* neurons are inhibitory.

2. When these α motoneurons are activated, they cause contraction of the muscle that was originally stretched (the homonymous muscle). When the muscle contracts, it shortens, thereby decreasing stretch on the muscle spindle. The muscle spindle returns to its original length, and the firing rate of the group Ia afferents returns to baseline.

3. Simultaneously, information is sent from the spinal cord to cause contraction of synergistic muscles and relaxation of antagonistic muscles.

The stretch reflex is illustrated by the **knee-jerk reflex,** which is initiated by tapping the patellar tendon, causing the quadriceps muscle to stretch. When the quadriceps and its muscle spindles are stretched, group Ia afferent fibers are stimulated. These group Ia afferent fibers synapse on and activate α motoneurons in the spinal cord. These α motoneurons innervate and cause contraction of the quadriceps (the muscle that originally was stretched). As the quadriceps muscle contracts and shortens, it forces the lower leg to extend in the characteristic knee-jerk reflex.

Golgi Tendon Reflex

The Golgi tendon reflex is a disynaptic spinal cord reflex, which is also called the **inverse myotatic reflex** (inverse or opposite of the stretch reflex).

The **Golgi tendon organ** is a stretch receptor found in tendons, which senses contraction (shortening) of muscle and activates group Ib afferent nerves. Golgi tendon organs are arranged in series with the extrafusal muscle fibers (contrasting the parallel arrangement of

muscle spindles in the stretch reflex). The steps in the Golgi tendon reflex are shown in Figure 3-33 and are described as follows:

1. When the muscle contracts, the extrafusal muscle fibers shorten, activating the Golgi tendon organs attached to them. In turn, the group Ib afferent fibers that synapse on inhibitory interneurons in the spinal cord are activated. These inhibitory interneurons synapse on the α motoneurons.

2. When the inhibitory interneurons are activated (i.e., activated to *inhibit*), they inhibit firing of the α motoneurons, producing relaxation of the homonymous muscle (the muscle that originally was contracted).

3. As the homonymous muscle relaxes, the reflex also causes synergistic muscles to relax and antagonistic muscles to contract.

An exaggerated form of the Golgi tendon reflex is illustrated by the **clasp-knife reflex.** This reflex is abnormal and occurs when there is an increase in muscle tone (e.g., hypertonicity or spasticity of muscle). When a joint is passively flexed, the opposing muscles initially resist this passive movement. However, if the flexion continues, tension increases in the opposing muscle and activates the Golgi tendon reflex, which then causes the opposing muscles to relax and the joint to close rapidly. The initial resistance to flexion followed by a rapid flexion is similar to the way a pocket knife closes: At first the knife closes slowly against high resistance, and then it quickly snaps shut.

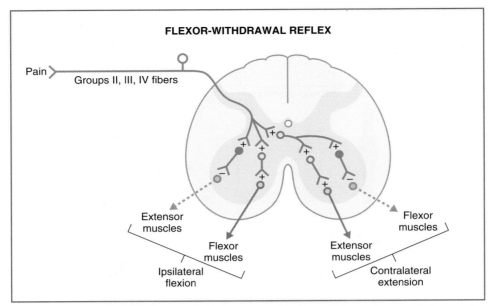

FLEXOR-WITHDRAWAL REFLEX

Pain

Groups II, III, IV fibers

Extensor
muscles

Flexor
muscles

Extensor
muscles

Flexor
muscles

Ipsilateral
flexion

Contralateral
extension

Figure 3-34 Operation of the flexor-withdrawal reflex. *Solid lines* show excitatory pathways; *dashed lines* show inhibitory steps. *Open* neurons are excitatory; *filled* neurons are inhibitory.

Flexor-Withdrawal Reflex

The flexor-withdrawal reflex is a polysynaptic reflex that occurs in response to tactile, painful, or noxious stimulus. Somatosensory and pain afferent fibers initiate a flexion reflex that causes withdrawal of the affected part of the body from the painful or noxious stimulus (e.g., touching a hand to a hot stove and then rapidly withdrawing the hand). The reflex produces **flexion** on the ipsilateral side (i.e., side of the stimulus) and **extension** on the contralateral side (Fig. 3-34). The steps involved in the flexor-withdrawal reflex are explained as follows:

1. When a limb touches a painful stimulus (e.g., hand touches a hot stove), flexor reflex afferent fibers (groups II, III, and IV) are activated. These afferent fibers synapse on multiple interneurons in the spinal cord (i.e., polysynaptic reflex).

2. On the ipsilateral side of the pain stimulus, reflexes are activated that cause flexor muscles to contract and extensor muscles to relax. This portion of the reflex produces flexion on the ipsilateral side (e.g., withdrawal of the hand from the hot stove).

3. On the contralateral side of the pain stimulus, reflexes are activated that cause extensor muscles to contract and flexor muscles to relax. This portion of the reflex produces extension on the contralateral side and is called the **crossed-extension reflex.** Thus, if the painful stimulus occurs on the left side, the left arm and leg will flex or withdraw and the right arm and leg will extend to maintain balance.

4. A persistent neural discharge, called an **afterdischarge,** occurs in the polysynaptic reflex circuits.

As a result of the afterdischarge, the contracted muscles remain contracted for a period of time after the reflex is activated.

Control of Posture and Movement by the Brain Stem

Descending motor pathways (i.e., those descending from the cerebral cortex and brain stem) are divided among the pyramidal tract and the extrapyramidal tract. **Pyramidal tracts** are corticospinal and corticobulbar tracts that pass through the medullary pyramids and descend directly onto lower motoneurons in the spinal cord. All others are **extrapyramidal tracts.** The extrapyramidal tracts originate in the following structures of the brain stem:

♦ The **rubrospinal tract** originates in the red nucleus and projects to motoneurons in the lateral spinal cord. Stimulation of the red nucleus produces activation of flexor muscles and inhibition of extensor muscles.

♦ The **pontine reticulospinal tract** originates in nuclei of the pons and projects to the ventromedial spinal cord. Stimulation has a generalized activating effect on *both* flexor and extensor muscles, with its predominant effect on extensors.

♦ The **medullary reticulospinal tract** originates in the medullary reticular formation and projects to motoneurons in the spinal cord. Stimulation has a generalized inhibitory effect on *both* flexor and extensor muscles, with the predominant effect on extensors.

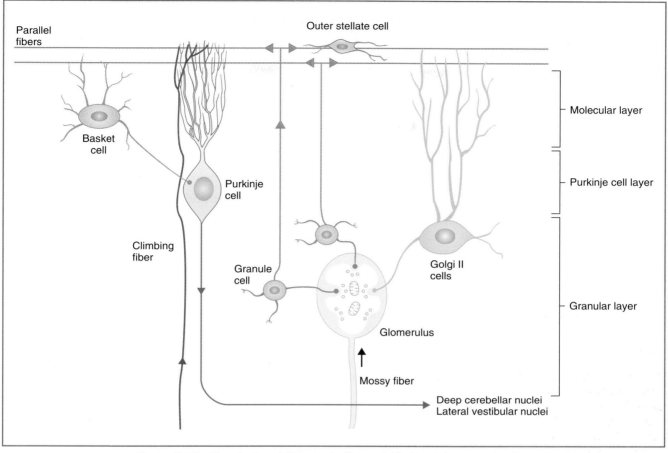

Figure 3-35 **Structures of the cerebellar cortex shown in cross section.**

♦ The **lateral vestibulospinal tract** originates in the lateral vestibular nucleus (Deiters' nucleus) and projects to ipsilateral motoneurons in the spinal cord. Stimulation produces activation of extensors and inhibition of flexors.

♦ The **tectospinal tract** originates in the superior colliculus (tectum or "roof" of the brain stem) and projects to the cervical spinal cord. It is involved in control of neck muscles.

Both the pontine reticular formation and the lateral vestibular nucleus have powerful excitatory effects on extensor muscles. Therefore, lesions of the brain stem *above* the pontine reticular formation and lateral vestibular nucleus, but *below* the midbrain, cause a dramatic increase in extensor tone, called **decerebrate rigidity.** Lesions *above* the midbrain *do not* cause decerebrate rigidity.

Cerebellum

The cerebellum, or "little brain," regulates movement and posture and plays a role in certain kinds of motor learning. The cerebellum helps control the rate, range, force, and direction of movements (collectively known as **synergy**). Damage to the cerebellum results in lack of coordination.

The cerebellum is located in the posterior fossa just below the occipital lobe. It is connected to the brain stem by three cerebellar peduncles, which contain both afferent and efferent nerve fibers.

There are three main divisions of the cerebellum: the vestibulocerebellum, the spinocerebellum, and the pontocerebellum. The **vestibulocerebellum** is dominated by vestibular input and controls balance and eye movements. The **spinocerebellum** is dominated by spinal cord input and controls synergy of movement. The **pontocerebellum** is dominated by cerebral input, via pontine nuclei, and controls the planning and initiation of movements.

Layers of the Cerebellar Cortex

The cerebellar cortex has three layers, which are described in relation to its output cells, the Purkinje cells (Fig. 3-35). The layers of the cerebellar cortex are as follows:

- The **granular layer** is the innermost layer. It contains granule cells, Golgi II cells, and glomeruli. In the glomeruli, axons of mossy fibers from the spinocerebellar and pontocerebellar tracts synapse on dendrites of granule and Golgi type II cells.

- The **Purkinje cell layer** is the middle layer. It contains Purkinje cells, and its output is *always inhibitory.*

- The **molecular layer** is the outermost layer. It contains outer stellate cells, basket cells, dendrites of Purkinje and Golgi II cells, and axons of granule cells. The axons of granule cells form parallel fibers, which synapse on the dendrites of Purkinje cells, basket cells, outer stellate cells, and Golgi type II cells.

Input to the Cerebellar Cortex

Two systems provide **excitatory input** to the cerebellar cortex: the climbing fiber system and the mossy fiber system. Each system also sends collateral branches directly to deep cerebellar nuclei, in addition to their projections to the cerebellar cortex. Excitatory projections from the cerebellar cortex then activate secondary circuits, which modulate the output of the cerebellar nuclei via the Purkinje cells.

- **Climbing fibers** originate in the inferior olive of the medulla and project directly onto Purkinje cells. These fibers make multiple synaptic connections along the dendrites of Purkinje cells, although each Purkinje cell receives input from only *one* climbing fiber. These synaptic connections are powerful! A single action potential from a climbing fiber can elicit multiple excitatory bursts, called **complex spikes,** in the dendrites of the Purkinje cell. It is believed that climbing fibers "condition" the Purkinje cells and modulate their responses to mossy fiber input. Climbing fibers also may play a role in cerebellar learning.

- **Mossy fibers** constitute the majority of the cerebellar input. These fibers include vestibulocerebellar, spinocerebellar, and pontocerebellar afferents. Mossy fibers project to granule cells, which are excitatory interneurons located in collections of synapses called glomeruli. Axons from these granule cells then ascend to the molecular layer, where they bifurcate and give rise to parallel fibers. **Parallel fibers** from the granule cells contact the dendrites of *many* Purkinje cells, producing a "beam" of excitation along the row of Purkinje cells. The dendritic tree of each Purkinje cell may receive input from as many as 250,000 parallel fibers! In contrast to the climbing fiber input to the Purkinje dendrites (which produce complex spikes), the mossy fiber input produces single action potentials called **simple spikes.**

These parallel fibers also synapse on cerebellar interneurons (basket, stellate, and Golgi II).

Interneurons of the Cerebellum

The function of cerebellar interneurons is to **modulate** Purkinje cell output. With the exception of granule cells, all of the cerebellar interneurons are inhibitory. Granule cells have excitatory input to basket cells, stellate cells, Golgi II cells, and Purkinje cells. Basket cells and stellate cells inhibit Purkinje cells (via parallel fibers). Golgi II cells inhibit granule cells, thereby reducing their excitatory effect on Purkinje cells.

Output of the Cerebellar Cortex

The only output of the cerebellar cortex is via **axons of Purkinje cells.** The output of the Purkinje cells is *always* **inhibitory** because the neurotransmitter released at these synapses is γ-aminobutyric acid (**GABA**) (see Chapter 1). Axons of Purkinje cells project topographically to deep cerebellar nuclei and to lateral vestibular nuclei. This inhibitory output of the cerebellar cortex regulates the rate, range, force, and direction of movement (synergy).

Disorders of the Cerebellum

Cerebellar lesions result in an abnormality of movement called **ataxia.** Cerebellar ataxia is a lack of coordination due to errors in rate, range, force, and direction of movement. Ataxia can be exhibited in one of several ways. There may be a **delayed onset** of movement or poor execution of the sequence of a movement, causing the movement to appear uncoordinated. A limb may **overshoot** its target or stop before reaching its target. Ataxia may be expressed as **dysdiadochokinesia,** in which a person is unable to perform rapid, alternating movements. **Intention tremors** may occur perpendicular to the direction of a voluntary movement, increasing near the end of the movement. (Intention tremors seen in cerebellar disease differ from the resting tremors seen in Parkinson disease.) The **rebound phenomenon** is the inability to stop a movement; for example, if a person with cerebellar disease flexes his forearm against a resistance, he may be unable to stop the flexion when the resistance is removed.

Basal Ganglia

The basal ganglia are the deep nuclei of the telencephalon: **caudate nucleus, putamen, globus pallidus,** and **amygdala.** There also are associated nuclei including the ventral anterior and ventral lateral nuclei of the thalamus, the subthalamic nucleus of the diencephalon, and the substantia nigra of the midbrain.

The main function of the basal ganglia is to influence the motor cortex via pathways through the thalamus. The role of the basal ganglia is to aid in planning

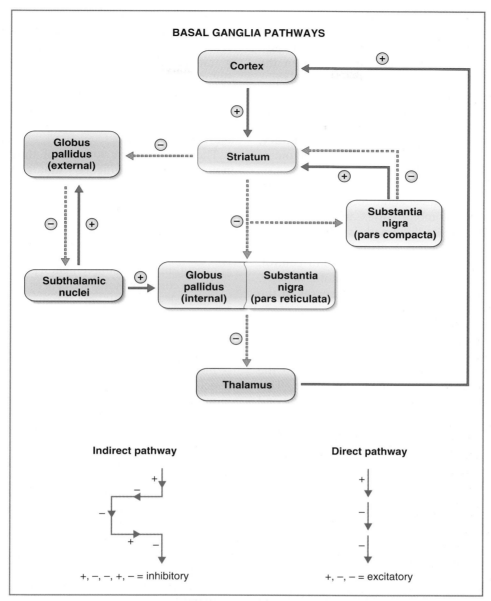

BASAL GANGLIA PATHWAYS

Indirect pathway

+, −, −, +, − = inhibitory

Direct pathway

+, −, − = excitatory

Figure 3–36 **Pathways in the basal ganglia.** The relationship between the cerebral cortex, the basal ganglia, and the thalamus are shown. *Solid blue lines* show excitatory pathways; *dashed brown lines* show inhibitory pathways. The overall output of the indirect pathway is inhibition, and the overall output of the direct pathway is excitation. (Modified from Kandel ER, Schwartz JH, Jessell TM: Principles of Neural Science, 4th ed. New York, McGraw-Hill, 2000.)

and execution of smooth movements. The basal ganglia also contribute to affective and cognitive functions.

The pathways into and out of the basal ganglia are complex, as illustrated in Figure 3-36. Almost all areas of the cerebral cortex project topographically onto the striatum including a critical input from the motor cortex. The striatum then communicates with the thalamus and then back to the cortex via two different pathways.

♦ **Indirect pathway.** In the indirect pathway, the striatum has inhibitory input to the external segment of the globus pallidus, which has inhibitory input to the subthalamic nuclei. The subthalamic nuclei project excitatory input to the internal segment of the globus pallidus and the pars reticulata of the substantia nigra, which send inhibitory input to the thalamus. The thalamus then sends excitatory input back to the motor cortex. In this pathway, the inhibitory neurotransmitter is **GABA,** and the excitatory neurotransmitter is **glutamate.** The overall output of the indirect pathway is **inhibitory,** as illustrated in the summary diagram at the bottom of the figure.

♦ **Direct pathway.** In the direct pathway, the striatum sends inhibitory input to the internal segment of the globus pallidus and the pars reticulata of the substantia nigra, which send inhibitory input to the thalamus. As in the indirect pathway, the thalamus sends excitatory input back to the motor cortex. Again, the inhibitory neurotransmitter is **GABA,** and the excitatory neurotransmitter is **glutamate.** The overall output of the direct pathway is **excitatory,** as shown in the summary diagram at the bottom of the figure.

The outputs of the indirect and direct pathways from the basal ganglia to the motor cortex are opposite and carefully balanced: The indirect path is inhibitory, and the direct path is excitatory. A disturbance in one of the pathways will upset this balance of motor control, with either an increase or a decrease in motor activity. Such an imbalance is characteristic of diseases of the basal ganglia.

In addition to the basic circuitry of the indirect and direct pathways, there is an additional connection, *back and forth,* between the striatum and the pars compacta of the substantia nigra. The neurotransmitter for the connection back to the striatum is **dopamine.** This additional connection between the substantia nigra and the striatum means that dopamine will be inhibitory (via D_2 receptors) in the indirect pathway and excitatory (via D_1 receptors) in the direct pathway.

Diseases of the Basal Ganglia

Diseases of the basal ganglia include Parkinson disease and Huntington disease. In **Parkinson disease,** cells of the pars compacta of the substantia nigra degenerate, reducing inhibition via the indirect pathway and reducing excitation via the direct pathway. The characteristics of Parkinson disease are explainable by dysfunction of the basal ganglia: resting tremor, slowness and delay of movement, and shuffling gait. Treatment of Parkinson disease includes replacement of dopamine by treatment with **L-dopa** (the precursor to dopamine) or administration of dopamine agonists such as bromocriptine. **Huntington disease** is a hereditary disorder caused by destruction of striatal and cortical cholinergic neurons and inhibitory GABAergic neurons. The neurologic symptoms of Huntington disease are choreic (writhing) movements and dementia. There is no cure.

Motor Cortex

Voluntary movements are directed by the motor cortex, via descending pathways. The motivation and ideas necessary to produce voluntary motor activity are first organized in multiple associative areas of the cerebral cortex and then transmitted to the supplementary motor and premotor cortices for the development of a **motor plan.** The motor plan will identify the specific muscles that need to contract, how much they need to contract, and in what sequence. The plan then is transmitted to upper motoneurons in the primary motor cortex, which send it through descending pathways to lower motoneurons in the spinal cord. The planning and execution stages of the plan are also influenced by motor control systems in the cerebellum and basal ganglia.

The motor cortex consists of three areas: primary motor cortex, supplementary motor cortex, and premotor cortex.

♦ **Premotor cortex and supplementary motor cortex (area 6)** are the regions of the motor cortex responsible for **generating a plan** of movement, which then is transferred to the primary motor cortex for execution. The supplementary motor cortex programs complex motor sequences and is active during "mental rehearsal" of a movement, even in the absence of movement.

♦ **Primary motor cortex (area 4)** is the region of the motor cortex responsible for **execution** of a movement. Programmed patterns of motoneurons are activated from the primary motor cortex. As upper motoneurons in the motor cortex are excited, this activity is transmitted to the brain stem and spinal cord, where lower motoneurons are activated and produce coordinated contraction of the appropriate muscles (i.e., the voluntary movement). The primary motor cortex is topographically organized and is described as the **motor homunculus.** This topographic organization is dramatically illustrated in **jacksonian seizures,** which are epileptic events originating in the primary motor cortex. The epileptic event usually begins in the fingers of one hand, progresses to the hand and arms, and eventually spreads over the entire body (i.e., the "jacksonian march").

HIGHER FUNCTIONS OF THE NERVOUS SYSTEM

Electroencephalogram

The electroencephalogram (EEG) records electrical activity of the cerebral cortex via electrodes placed on the skull. The EEG waves originate from alternating excitatory and inhibitory synaptic potentials that produce sufficient extracellular current flow across the cortex to be detected by surface electrodes. (EEG waves are not action potentials. Electrodes on the surface of the skull are not sufficiently sensitive to detect the small voltage changes of single action potentials.)

The normal EEG (Fig. 3-37) comprises waves with various amplitudes and frequencies. In a normal,

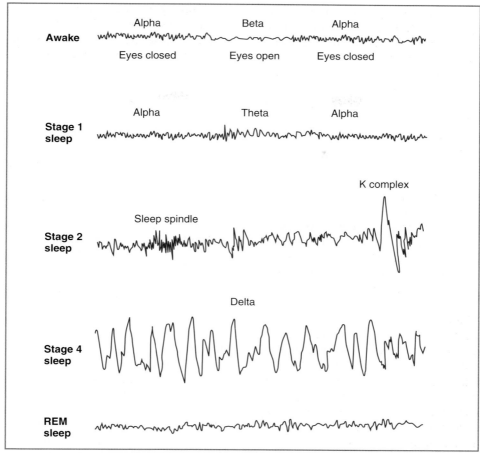

Figure 3–37 **Electroencephalogram of an awake subject and of subjects in Stages 1, 2, 4, and REM sleep.**

awake adult with **eyes open,** the dominant frequency recorded over the parietal and occipital lobes is the beta rhythm (13–30 Hz), which consists of desynchronous low-voltage, high-frequency waves. With **eyes closed,** the dominant frequency is the alpha rhythm (8–13 Hz), which has more synchronous waves of higher voltage and lower frequency.

As a person falls asleep, he or she passes through four stages of **slow-wave sleep.** In Stage 1, the alpha waves seen in an awake adult with eyes closed are interspersed with lower-frequency theta waves. In Stage 2, these low-frequency waves are interspersed with high-frequency bursts called **sleep spindles** and large, slow potentials called **K complexes.** In Stage 3 (not shown in the figure), there are very low-frequency delta waves and occasional sleep spindles. Stage 4 is characterized by delta waves. Approximately every 90 minutes, the slow-wave sleep pattern changes to **rapid eye movement (REM) sleep,** in which the EEG becomes desynchronized, with low-voltage, high-frequency waves that resemble those in an awake person. REM sleep is sometimes called paradoxical sleep: Even though the EEG is most similar to that of the awake state, the person is

(paradoxically) most difficult to awaken. REM sleep is characterized by loss of muscle tone, notably in the eye muscles resulting in rapid eye movements, loss of temperature regulation, pupillary constriction, penile erection, and fluctuations in heart rate, blood pressure, and respiration. Most dreams occur during REM sleep. The proportion of slow-wave sleep and REM sleep varies over the life span. Newborns spend half of their sleep in REM sleep; young adults spend about 25% of sleep in REM sleep; and the elderly have little REM sleep.

Learning and Memory

Learning and memory are higher-level functions of the nervous system. **Learning** is the neural mechanism by which a person changes his or her behavior as a result of experiences. **Memory** is the mechanism for storing what is learned.

Learning is categorized as either nonassociative or associative. In **nonassociative** learning, exemplified by habituation, a repeated stimulus causes a response, but that response gradually diminishes as it is "learned" that the stimulus is not important. For example, a newcomer to New York City may be awakened at first by street noises, but eventually the noises will be ignored as it is learned they are not relevant. The opposite of habituation is sensitization, where a stimulus results in a greater probability of a subsequent response when it is learned that the stimulus is important. In **associative** learning, there is a consistent relationship in the timing of stimuli. In **classic conditioning,** there is a temporal relationship between a conditioned stimulus and an unconditioned stimulus that elicits an unlearned response. When the combination is repeated, provided the temporal relationship is maintained, the association is learned; once learned (e.g., by Pavlov's dog), the stimulus alone (e.g., the bell) elicits the unlearned response (e.g., salivation). In **operant conditioning,** the response to a stimulus is reinforced, either positively or negatively, causing the probability of a response to change.

Synaptic plasticity is the fundamental mechanism that underlies learning. That is, synaptic function is variable and depends on the prior level of activity or "traffic" through the synapse. The responsiveness of postsynaptic neurons (called **synaptic strength**) is not fixed, but rather depends on the previous level of synaptic traffic. For example, in the phenomenon of **potentiation,** repeated activation of a neuronal pathway leads to increased responsiveness of the postsynaptic neurons in that pathway. The period of enhanced responsiveness may be brief, lasting for only milliseconds, or it may last for days or weeks (i.e., **long-term potentiation**). Conversely, in habituation, increased synaptic activity causes decreased responsiveness of the postsynaptic neuron.

The mechanism of long-term potentiation involves synaptic pathways that use the excitatory neurotransmitter **glutamate** and its *N*-**methyl-D-aspartate** (**NMDA**) **receptor.** When the presynaptic neurons are activated, they release glutamate, which diffuses across the synapse and activates NMDA receptors on the postsynaptic membranes. The NMDA receptors are ligand-gated ion Ca^{2+} channels that, when open, allow Ca^{2+} to enter the postsynaptic cells. With high-frequency stimulation (increased activity of the pathway), more Ca^{2+} accumulates in the postsynaptic cells; the higher intracellular Ca^{2+} concentration leads to an increase in protein kinase activity and, by mechanisms that are not fully understood, increased responsiveness of those synapses.

CEREBROSPINAL FLUID

The human brain is composed of 80% fluid, most of which is cerebrospinal fluid (CSF). CSF is formed at a rate of 500 milliliters (mL) per day by the epithelial cells of the choroid plexus (located in the lateral, third,

and fourth ventricles). Once produced by the choroid plexus, CSF flows into the ventricles and the subarachnoid spaces, which surround the brain and spinal cord. Distended regions of the subarachnoid space are called subarachnoid cisterns. Fluid is transferred from CSF to venous blood by one-way bulk flow and is returned to the systemic circulation. In the steady state, the movement of fluid from CSF to venous blood should equal the rate of CSF formation (i.e., 500 mL/day). For diagnostic purposes, CSF can be sampled using a **lumbar puncture** in the lumbar cistern.

The relationships between the arterial blood supply of the brain, the choroid plexus, and the blood-brain barrier are shown in Figure 3-38. Note that substances can be exchanged between brain cells (which are bathed in interstitial fluid), the interstitial fluid, and CSF.

The barrier between cerebral capillary blood and CSF is the **choroid plexus.** This barrier consists of three layers: capillary endothelial cells and basement membrane, neuroglial membrane, and epithelial cells of the choroid plexus. The choroid plexus epithelial cells are similar to those of the renal distal tubule and contain transport mechanisms that move solutes and fluid from capillary blood into CSF.

The barrier between cerebral capillary blood and interstitial fluid of the brain is the **blood-brain barrier.** Anatomically, the blood-brain barrier consists of capillary endothelial cells and basement membrane, neuroglial membrane, and glial end feet (projections of astrocytes from the brain side of the barrier). Functionally, the blood-brain barrier differs in two ways from the analogous barrier in other tissues. (1) The junctions between endothelial cells in the brain are so "tight" that few substances can cross *between* the cells. (2) Only a few substances can pass *through* the endothelial cells: Lipid-soluble substances (e.g., oxygen and carbon dioxide) can cross the blood-brain barrier, but water-soluble substances are excluded.

Formation of Cerebrospinal Fluid

CSF is formed by the epithelial cells of the choroid plexus. Transport mechanisms in these cells secrete some substances from blood into CSF (e.g., Na^+, Cl^-, water) and absorb other substances from CSF into blood. Molecules such as protein and cholesterol are excluded from CSF because of their large molecular size. On the other hand, lipid-soluble substances such as oxygen and carbon dioxide move freely and equilibrate between the two compartments. Thus, depending on the transport mechanisms and the characteristics of the barrier, some substances are present in higher concentration in CSF than in blood, some are present at approximately the same concentration, and some are present in lower concentration in CSF than in blood.

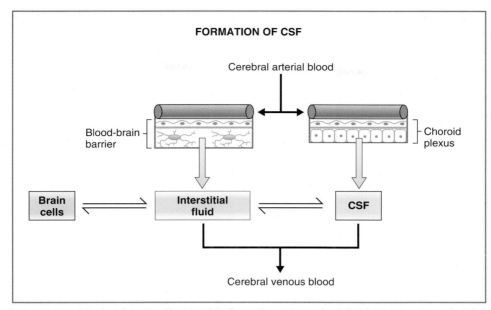

FORMATION OF CSF

Figure 3-38 **Mechanism for the production of cerebrospinal fluid.** CSF, Cerebrospinal fluid.

Table 3-6 Composition of Cerebrospinal Fluid

[CSF] ≈ [Blood]	[CSF] < [Blood]	[CSF] > [Blood]
Na$^+$	K$^+$	Mg^{2+}
Cl$^-$	Ca^{2+}	Creatinine
HCO$_3^-$	Glucose	
Osmolarity	Amino acids	
	pH	
	Cholesterol*	
	Protein*	

CSF, Cerebrospinal fluid.
*Negligible in CSF.

Many substances readily exchange between brain interstitial fluid and CSF (see Fig. 3-38); thus, the compositions of interstitial fluid and CSF are similar to each other but different from blood. Table 3-6 compares the composition of CSF and blood.

Functions of Cerebrospinal Fluid

The functions of CSF are to provide a constant, controlled environment for the brain cells and to protect the brain from endogenous or exogenous toxins. CSF also may function to prevent escape of local neurotransmitters into the general circulation. Depending on their lipid solubility, drugs penetrate the blood-brain barrier in varying degrees. Thus, nonionized (lipid-soluble) drugs penetrate the brain readily, whereas ionized (non–lipid-soluble) drugs do not penetrate. Inflammation, irradiation, and tumors may increase the permeability of the blood-brain barrier and allow substances normally excluded to enter the brain. These substances include cancer chemotherapeutic drugs, antibiotics, and radiolabeled markers.

SUMMARY

■ Sensory systems transmit information from the environment to the CNS via specialized sensory receptors and a series of first-, second-, third-, and fourth-order neurons in the CNS. Sensory receptors include mechanoreceptors, photoreceptors, chemoreceptors, thermoreceptors, and nociceptors. A stimulus (e.g., light) is converted to electrical energy in the sensory receptors via transduction processes, which result in receptor potentials.

■ Somatosensory and pain systems process information about touch, position, pain, and temperature using the dorsal column and anterolateral systems.

■ The visual system detects and interprets light stimuli. Photoreceptors are rods and cones of the retina, which hyperpolarize in response to light. Photoreceptors synapse on bipolar cells and horizontal cells of the retina, where they produce either excitation or inhibition, depending on the type of receptor on the bipolar and horizontal cells. The output cells of the retina are ganglion cells, whose axons form the optic nerves. The optic nerves synapse in the lateral geniculate nucleus of the thalamus. Fibers from each nasal hemiretina cross at the optic chiasm and ascend contralaterally; fibers from each temporal hemiretina ascend ipsilaterally.

■ The auditory system involves transduction of sound waves. The mechanoreceptors are auditory hair cells located in the organ of Corti of the inner ear. Bending of cilia on the hair cells produces an oscillating receptor potential. Location of the hair cells along the basilar membrane encodes frequency.

■ The vestibular system is used to maintain equilibrium and balance. Vestibular hair cells are mechanoreceptors located in ampullae of semicircular canals and in otolith organs. The semicircular canals detect angular acceleration of the head, and the otolith organs detect linear acceleration.

■ The chemical senses are olfaction and gustation. Olfactory epithelium contains olfactory receptor cells, which are also primary afferent neurons. Axons from these neurons pass through the cribriform plate and synapse in glomeruli of the olfactory bulb. Taste receptors are found on taste buds, which are organized in papillae.

■ Muscle spindles are composed of intrafusal fibers and are arranged in parallel with extrafusal muscle fibers. Muscle spindles are stretch receptors, which detect changes in muscle length when extrafusal fibers contract or relax.

■ Spinal cord reflexes include the stretch reflex (monosynaptic), the Golgi tendon reflex (disynaptic), and the flexor-withdrawal reflex (multisynaptic).

■ Descending motor pathways from the cerebral cortex and brain stem are divided among the pyramidal tract and extrapyramidal tract. Pyramidal tracts pass through the medulla and synapse on lower motoneurons in the spinal cord. Extrapyramidal tracts include rubrospinal, pontine reticulospinal, medullary reticulospinal, lateral vestibulospinal, and tectospinal tracts.

■ The cerebellum regulates movement by controlling synergy. The cerebellar cortex includes a granular layer, a Purkinje cell layer, and a molecular layer. The output of the cerebellar cortex is via axons of Purkinje cells and is always inhibitory. Disorders of the cerebellum cause ataxia.

■ Basal ganglia are deep nuclei of the telencephalon, which are involved in planning and execution of smooth movements.

■ The motor cortex includes premotor and supplementary cortices, which are responsible for generating a motor plan. The primary motor cortex is responsible for execution of the motor plan.

Challenge Yourself

Answer each question with a word, phrase, sentence, or numerical solution. When a list of possible answers is supplied with the question, one, more than one, or none of the choices may be correct. Correct answers are provided at the end of the book.

1 *Cutting which of the following leads to total blindness in the right eye: optic chiasm, left optic tract, right optic tract, right optic nerve, left optic nerve?*

2 *A ballerina spins to the right. When she suddenly stops spinning, which way will her eyes move?*

3 *How many motoneurons are in a motor unit?*

4 *Which of the following reflexes comprise(s) only one synapse: knee-jerk reflex, Golgi tendon reflex, stretch reflex, the reflex involved when one removes a hand from a hot stove?*

5 *In which type of receptor, phasic or tonic, does the receptor potential fall below threshold, even as the stimulus continues?*

6 *Put these photoreception events in their correct order: release of neurotransmitter, decreased cyclic GMP, light, conversion of 11-cis rhodopsin to all-trans rhodopsin, transducin, hyperpolarization, closure of Na^+ channels.*

7 *A hyperpolarizing receptor potential makes the membrane potential _____ (more or less) negative and _____ (increases or decreases) the likelihood of action potentials occurring.*

8 *Indicate whether each of the following is activated (increased), inhibited (decreased), or unchanged in the operation of the Golgi tendon reflex:*

Golgi tendon organs
Ia afferent fibers
Ib afferent fibers
Inhibitory interneurons
α motoneurons

9 *Which of the following is/are found in higher concentration in blood than in CSF: protein, osmolarity, Mg^{2+}, glucose, Na^+, K^+?*

10 *If the head is rotated to the right, which horizontal semicircular canal (right or left) is activated during the initial rotation? When the head stops rotating, which canal (right or left) is activated?*

11 *Compared with the base, the apex of the basilar membrane is _____ (wider/narrower), is _____ (more compliant/less compliant), and responds to _____ (higher/lower) frequencies.*

SELECTED READINGS

Adrian ED, Zotterman Y: The impulses produced by sensory nerve endings. Part 2. The response of a single end-organ. J Physiol 61:151–171, 1926.

Boyd IA: The isolated mammalian muscle spindle. Trends Neurosci 3:258–265, 1980.

Finger TE, Silver WL: Neurobiology of Taste and Smell. New York, John Wiley, 1987.

Hille B: Ionic Channels of Excitable Membranes, 2nd ed. Sunderland, Mass, Sinauer, 1991.

Hubel DH, Wiesel TN: Brain mechanisms of vision. Sci Am 242:150–162, 1979.

Ito M: The Cerebellum and Neural Control. New York, Raven Press, 1984.

Kandel ER, Schwartz JH, Jessell TM: Principles of Neural Science, 4th ed. New York, McGraw-Hill, 2000.

Katz B: Nerve, Muscle, and Synapse. New York, McGraw-Hill, 1966.

Schnapf JL, Baylor DA: How photoreceptor cells respond to light. Sci Am 256:40–47, 1987.

Cardiovascular Physiology

The primary function of the cardiovascular system is to deliver blood to the tissues, providing essential nutrients *to* the cells for metabolism and removing waste products *from* the cells. The heart serves as the pump, which, by contracting, generates the pressure to drive blood through a series of blood vessels. The vessels that carry blood from the heart to the tissues are the arteries, which are under high pressure and contain a relatively small percentage of the blood volume. The veins, which carry blood from the tissues back to the heart, are under low pressure and contain the largest percentage of the blood volume. Within the tissues, thin-walled blood vessels, called capillaries, are interposed between the arteries and veins. Exchange of nutrients, wastes, and fluid occurs across the capillary walls.

The cardiovascular system also is involved in several homeostatic functions: It participates in the regulation of arterial blood pressure; it delivers regulatory hormones from the endocrine glands to their sites of action in target tissues; it participates in the regulation of body temperature; and it is involved in the homeostatic adjustments to altered physiologic states such as hemorrhage, exercise, and changes in posture.

CIRCUITRY OF THE CARDIOVASCULAR SYSTEM

Left and Right Sides of the Heart

Figure 4-1 is a schematic diagram of the circuitry of the cardiovascular system. The left and right sides of the heart and the blood vessels are shown in relation to each other. Each side of the heart has two chambers, an **atrium** and a **ventricle,** connected by one-way valves, called **atrioventricular (AV) valves.** The AV valves are designed so that blood can flow only in one direction, from the atrium to the ventricle.

The left heart and right heart have different functions. The left heart and the systemic arteries, capillaries, and veins are collectively called the **systemic circulation.** The left ventricle pumps blood to all organs of the body except the lungs. The right heart and the pulmonary arteries, capillaries, and veins are collectively called the **pulmonary circulation.** The right ventricle pumps blood to the lungs. The left heart and right heart function in series so that blood is pumped sequentially from the left heart to the systemic

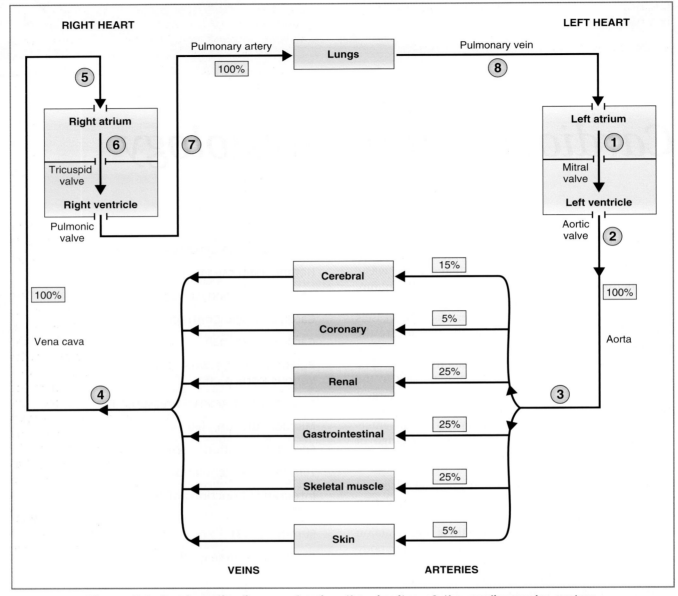

Figure 4–1 A schematic diagram showing the circuitry of the cardiovascular system. The *arrows* show the direction of blood flow. Percentages represent the percent (%) of cardiac output. See the text for an explanation of the circled numbers.

circulation, to the right heart, to the pulmonary circulation, and then back to the left heart.

The rate at which blood is pumped from either ventricle is called the **cardiac output.** Because the two sides of the heart operate in series, the cardiac output of the left ventricle equals the cardiac output of the right ventricle in the steady state. The rate at which blood is returned to the atria from the veins is called the **venous return.** Again, because the left heart and the right heart operate in series, venous return to the left heart equals venous return to the right heart in the steady state. Finally, in the steady state, cardiac output *from* the heart equals venous return *to* the heart.

Blood Vessels

The blood vessels have several functions. They serve as a closed system of passive conduits, delivering blood to and from the tissues where nutrients and wastes are exchanged. The blood vessels also participate actively in the regulation of blood flow to the organs. When resistance of the blood vessels, particularly of the arterioles, is altered, blood flow to that organ is altered.

Circuitry

The steps in one complete circuit through the cardiovascular system are shown in Figure 4-1. The circled numbers in the figure correspond with the steps described here.

1. **Oxygenated blood fills the left ventricle.** Blood that has been oxygenated in the lungs returns to the left atrium via the pulmonary vein. This blood then flows from the left atrium to the left ventricle through the **mitral valve** (the AV valve of the left heart).

2. **Blood is ejected from the left ventricle into the aorta.** Blood leaves the left ventricle through the **aortic valve** (the semilunar valve of the left side of the heart), which is located between the left ventricle and the aorta. When the left ventricle contracts, the pressure in the ventricle increases, causing the aortic valve to open and blood to be ejected forcefully into the aorta. (As noted previously, the amount of blood ejected from the left ventricle per unit time is called the **cardiac output.**) Blood then flows through the arterial system, driven by the pressure created by contraction of the left ventricle.

3. **Cardiac output is distributed among various organs.** The total cardiac output of the left heart is distributed among the organ systems via sets of parallel arteries. Thus, simultaneously, 15% of the cardiac output is delivered to the brain via the cerebral arteries, 5% is delivered to the heart via the coronary arteries, 25% is delivered to the kidneys via the renal arteries, and so forth. Given this **parallel arrangement** of the organ systems, it follows that the total systemic blood flow must equal the cardiac output.

   The percentage distribution of cardiac output among the various organ systems is not fixed, however. For example, during strenuous exercise, the percentage of the cardiac output going to skeletal muscle increases, compared with the percentage at rest. There are three major mechanisms for achieving such a change in blood flow to an organ system. In the *first* mechanism, the cardiac output remains constant, but the blood flow is redistributed among the organ systems by the selective alteration of arteriolar resistance. In this scenario, blood flow to one organ can be increased at the expense of blood flow to other organs. In the *second* mechanism, the cardiac output increases or decreases, but the percentage distribution of blood flow among the organ systems is kept constant. Finally, in a *third* mechanism, a combination of the first two mechanisms occurs in which *both* cardiac output *and* the percentage distribution of blood flow are altered. This third mechanism is used, for example, in the response to strenuous exercise: Blood flow to skeletal muscle increases to meet the increased metabolic demand by a combination of increased cardiac output and increased percentage distribution to skeletal muscle.

4. **Blood flow from the organs is collected in the veins.** The blood leaving the organs is venous blood and contains waste products from metabolism, such as carbon dioxide (CO_2). This mixed venous blood is collected in veins of increasing size and finally in the largest vein, the **vena cava.** The vena cava carries blood to the right heart.

5. **Venous return to the right atrium.** Because the pressure in the vena cava is higher than in the right atrium, the right atrium fills with blood, the venous return. In the steady state, venous return to the right atrium equals cardiac output from the left ventricle.

6. **Mixed venous blood fills the right ventricle.** Mixed venous blood flows from the right atrium to the right ventricle through the AV valve in the right heart, the **tricuspid valve.**

7. **Blood is ejected from the right ventricle into the pulmonary artery.** When the right ventricle contracts, blood is ejected through the pulmonic valve (the semilunar valve of the right side of the heart) into the pulmonary artery, which carries blood to the lungs. Note that the cardiac output ejected from the right ventricle is identical to the cardiac output that was ejected from the left ventricle. In the capillary beds of the lungs, oxygen (O_2) is added to the blood from alveolar gas, and CO_2 is removed from the blood and added to the alveolar gas. Thus, the blood leaving the lungs has more O_2 and less CO_2 than the blood that entered the lungs.

8. **Blood flow from the lungs is returned to the heart via the pulmonary vein.** Oxygenated blood is returned to the left atrium via the pulmonary vein to begin a new cycle.

HEMODYNAMICS

The term **hemodynamics** refers to the principles that govern blood flow in the cardiovascular system. These basic principles of physics are the same as those applied to the movement of fluids in general. The concepts of flow, pressure, resistance, and capacitance are applied to blood flow to and from the heart and within the blood vessels.

Types and Characteristics of Blood Vessels

Blood vessels are the conduits through which blood is carried from the heart to the tissues and from the tissues back to the heart. In addition, some blood vessels (capillaries) are so thin walled that substances can exchange across them. The size of the various

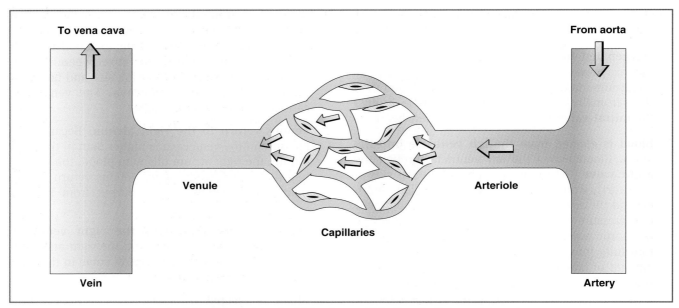

Figure 4–2 **Arrangement of blood vessels in the cardiovascular system.**

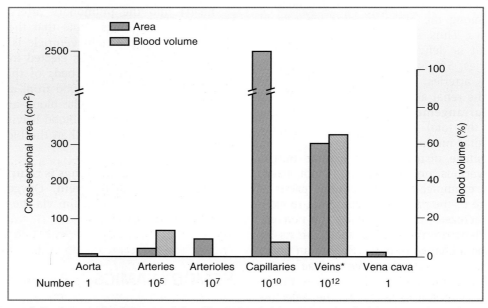

Figure 4–3 **Area and volume contained in systemic blood vessels.** The blood vessels are described by the number of each type, total cross-sectional area, and percentage (%) of blood volume contained. (Pulmonary blood vessels are not included in this figure.) *Total number includes veins and venules.

types of blood vessels and the histologic characteristics of their walls vary. These variations have profound effects on their resistance and capacitance properties.

Figure 4-2 is a schematic drawing of a vascular bed. The direction of blood flow through the vascular bed is from artery to arteriole, to capillaries, to venule, to vein. Figure 4-3, a companion figure, is a graph showing the total cross-sectional area, the number of blood vessels at each level of the vasculature, and the

percentage of the blood volume contained in each type of vessel.

♦ **Arteries.** The aorta is the largest artery of the systemic circulation. Medium- and small-sized arteries branch off the aorta. The function of the arteries is to deliver oxygenated blood to the organs. The arteries are **thick-walled** structures with extensive development of **elastic tissue,** smooth muscle, and connective tissue. The thickness of the arterial wall is a significant feature: The arteries receive blood directly from the heart and are under the highest pressure in the vasculature. The volume of blood contained in the arteries is called the **stressed volume** (meaning the blood volume under *high* pressure).

♦ **Arterioles.** The arterioles are the smallest branches of the arteries. Their walls have an extensive development of **smooth muscle,** and they are the **site of highest resistance** to blood flow.

The smooth muscle in the walls of the arterioles is tonically active (i.e., always contracted). It is extensively innervated by sympathetic adrenergic nerve fibers. α_1-**Adrenergic receptors** are found on the arterioles of several vascular beds (e.g., skin and splanchnic vasculature). When activated, these receptors cause contraction or constriction of the vascular smooth muscle. Constriction produces a decrease in the diameter of the arteriole, which increases its resistance to blood flow. Less common, β_2-**adrenergic receptors** are found in arterioles of skeletal muscle. When activated, these receptors cause relaxation of the vascular smooth muscle, which increases the diameter and decreases the resistance of these arterioles to blood flow.

Thus, arterioles are not only the site of highest resistance in the vasculature, but they also are the site where resistance can be changed by alterations in sympathetic nerve activity, by circulating catecholamines, and by other vasoactive substances.

♦ **Capillaries.** The capillaries are thin-walled structures lined with a **single layer of endothelial cells,** which is surrounded by a basal lamina. Capillaries are the site where nutrients, gases, water, and solutes are exchanged between the blood and the tissues and, in the lungs, between the blood and the alveolar gas. **Lipid-soluble substances** (e.g., O_2 and CO_2) cross the capillary wall by dissolving in and diffusing across the endothelial cell membranes. In contrast, **water-soluble substances** (e.g., ions) cross the capillary wall either through water-filled clefts (spaces) between the endothelial cells or through large pores in the walls of some capillaries (e.g., fenestrated capillaries).

Not all capillaries are perfused with blood at all times. Rather, there is selective perfusion of capillary beds, depending on the metabolic needs of the tissues. This selective perfusion is determined by the degree of dilation or constriction of the arterioles and precapillary sphincters (smooth muscle bands that lie "before" the capillaries). The degree of dilation or constriction is, in turn, controlled by the sympathetic innervation of vascular smooth muscle and by vasoactive metabolites produced in the tissues.

♦ **Venules and veins.** Like the capillaries, the venules are thin-walled structures. The walls of the veins are composed of the usual endothelial cell layer and a modest amount of elastic tissue, smooth muscle, and connective tissue. Because the walls of the veins contain much less elastic tissue than the arteries, the veins have a large capacitance (capacity to hold blood). In fact, the veins contain the *largest percentage of blood in the cardiovascular system.* The volume of blood contained in the veins is called the **unstressed volume** (meaning the blood volume under *low* pressure). The smooth muscle in the walls of the veins is, like that in the walls of the arterioles, innervated by sympathetic nerve fibers. Increases in sympathetic nerve activity, via α_1 **adrenergic receptors,** cause contraction of the veins, which reduces their capacitance, and, therefore, reduces the unstressed volume.

Velocity of Blood Flow

The velocity of blood flow is the rate of displacement of blood per unit time. The blood vessels of the cardiovascular system vary in terms of diameter and cross-sectional area. These differences in diameter and area, in turn, have profound effects on velocity of flow. The relationship between velocity, flow, and cross-sectional area (which depends on vessel radius or diameter) is as follows:

$$v = Q/A$$

where

  v = Velocity of blood flow (cm/sec)
  Q = Flow (mL/sec)
  A = Cross-sectional area (cm^2)

Velocity of blood flow (v) is *linear* velocity and refers to the rate of displacement of blood per unit time. Thus, velocity is expressed in units of distance per unit time (e.g., cm/sec).

Flow (Q) is *volume* flow per unit time and is expressed in units of volume per unit time (e.g., mL/sec).

Area (A) is the cross-sectional area of a blood vessel (e.g., aorta) or a group of blood vessels (e.g., all of the capillaries). Area is calculated as $A = \pi r^2$, where r is the radius of a single blood vessel (e.g., aorta) or the total radius of a group of blood vessels (e.g., all of the capillaries).

Figure 4-4 illustrates how changes in diameter alter the velocity of flow through a vessel. In this figure, three blood vessels are shown in order of increasing diameter and cross-sectional area. The flow through each blood vessel is identical, at 10 mL/sec. However, because of the inverse relationship between velocity and cross-sectional area, as vessel diameter increases, the velocity of flow through the vessel decreases.

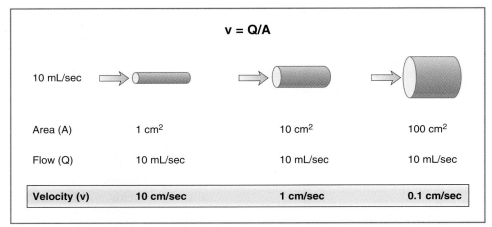

Figure 4-4 **Effect of the diameter of the blood vessel on the velocity of blood flow.**

This example can be extrapolated to the cardio-vascular system. Imagine that the smallest vessel represents the aorta, the medium-sized vessel represents *all* of the arteries, and the largest vessel represents *all* of the capillaries. The total blood flow at each level of blood vessels is the same and is equal to the cardiac output. Because of the inverse relationship between velocity and total cross-sectional area, the velocity of blood flow will be highest in the aorta and lowest in the capillaries. From the standpoint of capillary function (i.e., exchange of nutrients, solutes, and water), the low velocity of blood flow is advantageous: It maximizes the time for exchange across the capillary wall.

SAMPLE PROBLEM. A man has a cardiac output of 5.5 L/min. The diameter of his aorta is estimated to be 20 mm, and the total cross-sectional area of his systemic capillaries is estimated to be 2500 cm². *What is the velocity of blood flow in the aorta relative to the velocity of blood flow in the capillaries?*

SOLUTION. To compare the velocity of blood flow in the aorta with the velocity in the capillaries, two values are needed for each type of blood vessel: the total blood flow (Q) and the total cross-sectional area (cm²). The total flow at each level is the same and is equal to the cardiac output. The total cross-sectional area of the capillaries is given in the problem, and the cross-sectional area of the aorta must be calculated from its radius, which is 10 mm. Area = πr^2 = 3.14 × (10 mm)² = 3.14 × (1 cm)² = 3.14 cm². Thus,

$$V_{capillaries} = Q/A$$
$$= \frac{5.5 \text{ L/min}}{2500 \text{ cm}^2}$$
$$= \frac{5500 \text{ mL/min}}{2500 \text{ cm}^2}$$
$$= \frac{5500 \text{ cm}^3/\text{min}}{2500 \text{ cm}^2}$$
$$= 2.2 \text{ cm/min}$$

$$V_{aorta} = Q/A$$
$$= \frac{5500 \text{ cm}^3/\text{min}}{3.14 \text{ cm}^2}$$
$$= 1752 \text{ cm/min}$$

Hence, velocity in the aorta is 800-fold that in the capillaries (1752 cm/min in the aorta compared with 2.2 cm/min in the capillaries). These calculations confirm the previous discussion concerning velocity of blood flow. The velocity of flow should be lowest in vessels with the largest total cross-sectional area (the capillaries) and highest in the vessels with the smallest total cross-sectional area (the aorta).

Relationships between Blood Flow, Pressure, and Resistance

Blood flow through a blood vessel or a series of blood vessels is determined by two factors: the **pressure difference** between the two ends of the vessel (the inlet and the outlet) and the **resistance** of the vessel to blood flow. The pressure difference is the driving force for blood flow, and the resistance is an impediment to flow.

The relationship of flow, pressure, and resistance is analogous to the relationship of current (I), voltage (ΔV), and resistance (R) in electrical circuits, as expressed by **Ohm's law** (Ohm's law states that ΔV = I × R or I = ΔV/R). Blood flow is analogous to current flow, the pressure difference or driving force is analogous to the voltage difference, and hydrodynamic resistance is analogous to electrical resistance. The equation for blood flow is expressed as follows:

$$Q = \Delta P/R$$

where

$$Q = \text{Flow (mL/min)}$$
$$\Delta P = \text{Pressure difference (mm Hg)}$$
$$R = \text{Resistance (mm Hg/mL/min)}$$

The *magnitude* of **blood flow (Q)** is directly proportional to the size of the **pressure difference (ΔP)** or pressure gradient. The *direction* of blood flow is determined by the direction of the pressure gradient and always is from *high to low pressure*. For example, during ventricular ejection, blood flows from the left ventricle into the aorta and not in the other direction, because pressure in the ventricle is higher than pressure in the aorta. For another example, blood flows from the vena cava to the right atrium because pressure in the vena cava is slightly higher than in the right atrium.

Furthermore, blood flow is inversely proportional to **resistance (R).** Increasing resistance (e.g., by arteriolar vasoconstriction) decreases flow, and decreasing resistance (e.g., by arteriolar vasodilation) increases flow. *The major mechanism for changing blood flow in the cardiovascular system is by changing the resistance of blood vessels, particularly the arterioles.*

The flow, pressure, and resistance relationship also can be rearranged to determine resistance. If the blood flow and the pressure gradient are known, the resistance is calculated as $R = \Delta P/Q$. This relationship can be used to measure the resistance of the entire systemic vasculature (i.e., total peripheral resistance), or it can be used to measure resistance in a single organ or single blood vessel.

♦ **Total peripheral resistance.** The resistance of the entire systemic vasculature is called the total peripheral resistance (TPR) or the systemic vascular resistance (SVR). TPR can be measured with the flow, pressure, and resistance relationship by substituting cardiac output for flow (Q) and the difference in pressure between the aorta and the vena cava for ΔP.

♦ **Resistance in a single organ.** The flow, pressure, and resistance relationship also can be applied on a smaller scale to determine the resistance of a single organ. As illustrated in the following sample problem, the resistance of the renal vasculature can be determined by substituting renal blood flow for flow (Q) and the difference in pressure between the renal artery and the renal vein for ΔP:

SAMPLE PROBLEM. Renal blood flow is measured by placing a flow meter on a woman's left renal artery. Simultaneously, pressure probes are inserted in her left renal artery and left renal vein to measure pressure. Renal blood flow measured by the flow meter is 500 mL/min. The pressure probes measure renal arterial pressure as 100 mm Hg and renal venous pressure as 10 mm Hg. *What is the vascular resistance of the left kidney in this woman?*

SOLUTION. Blood flow to the left kidney, as measured by the flow meter, is Q. The difference in pressure

---

between the renal artery and renal vein is ΔP. The resistance to flow in the renal vasculature is calculated by rearranging the blood flow equation:

$$Q = \Delta P/R$$

Rearranging and solving for R,

$R = \Delta P/Q$
   = (Pressure in renal artery – Pressure in renal vein)/ Renal blood flow
R = (100 mm Hg – 10 mm Hg)/500 mL/min
   = 90 mm Hg/500 mL/min
   = 0.18 mm Hg/mL/min

Resistance to Blood Flow

The blood vessels and the blood itself constitute resistance to blood flow. The relationship between resistance, blood vessel diameter (or radius), and blood viscosity is described by the **Poiseuille equation.** The total resistance offered by a set of blood vessels also depends on whether the vessels are arranged in series (i.e., blood flows sequentially from one vessel to the next) or in parallel (i.e., the total blood flow is distributed simultaneously among parallel vessels).

Poiseuille Equation

The factors that determine the resistance of a blood vessel to blood flow are expressed by the **Poiseuille equation:**

$$R = \frac{8\eta l}{\pi r^4}$$

where

R = Resistance
η = Viscosity of blood
l = Length of blood vessel
r^4 = Radius of blood vessel raised to the fourth power

The most important concepts expressed in the Poiseuille equation are as follows: First, resistance to flow is directly proportional to **viscosity (η)** of the blood; for example, as viscosity increases (e.g., if the hematocrit increases), the resistance to flow also increases. Second, resistance to flow is directly proportional to the **length (l)** of the blood vessel. Third, and most important, resistance to flow is inversely proportional to the **fourth power of the radius (r^4)** of the blood vessel. This is a powerful relationship, indeed! When the radius of a blood vessel decreases, its resistance increases, not in a linear fashion but magnified by the fourth power relationship. For example, if the radius of a blood vessel decreases by one half, resistance does not simply increase twofold—it increases by 16-fold (2^4)!

SAMPLE PROBLEM. A man suffers a stroke caused by partial occlusion of his left internal carotid artery. An evaluation of the carotid artery using magnetic resonance imaging (MRI) shows a 75% reduction in its radius. *Assuming that blood flow through the left internal carotid artery is 400 mL/min prior to the occlusion, what is blood flow through the artery after the occlusion?*

SOLUTION. The variable in this example is the diameter (or radius) of the left internal carotid artery. Blood flow is inversely proportional to the resistance of the artery ($Q = \Delta P/R$), and resistance is inversely proportional to the radius raised to the fourth power (Poiseuille equation). The internal carotid artery is occluded, and its radius is decreased by 75%. Another way of expressing this reduction is to say that the radius is decreased to one fourth its original size.

The first question is *How much would resistance increase with 75% occlusion of the artery?* The answer is found in the Poiseuille equation. After the occlusion, the radius of the artery is one fourth its original radius; thus, resistance has increased by $1/(1/4)^4$, or 256-fold.

The second question is *What would the flow be if resistance were to increase by 256-fold?* The answer is found in the flow, pressure, resistance relationship ($Q = \Delta P/R$). Because resistance increased by 256-fold, flow decreased to 1/256, or 0.0039, or 0.39% of the original value. The flow is 0.39% of 400 mL/min, or 1.56 mL/min. Clearly, this is a dramatic decrease in blood flow to the brain, all based on the fourth-power relationship between resistance and vessel radius.

Series and Parallel Resistances

Resistances in the cardiovascular system, as in electrical circuits, can be arranged in series or in parallel (Fig. 4-5). Whether the arrangement is series or parallel produces different values for total resistance.

♦ **Series resistance** is illustrated by the arrangement of blood vessels *within* a given organ. Each organ is supplied with blood by a major artery and drained by a major vein. Within the organ, blood flows from the major artery to smaller arteries, to arterioles, to capillaries, to venules, to veins. **The total resistance**

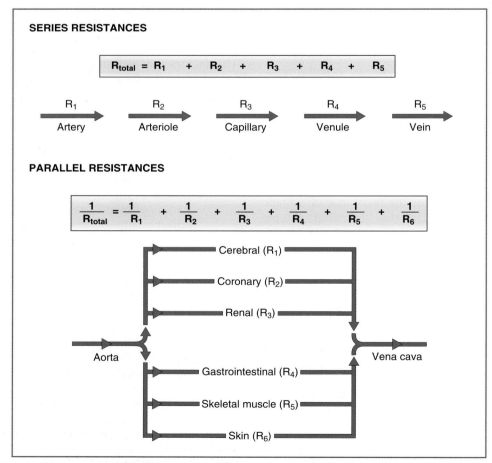

Figure 4-5 Arrangements of blood vessels in series and in parallel. The *arrows* show the direction of blood flow. R, Resistance (subscripts refer to individual resistances).

of the system arranged in series is equal to the sum of the individual resistances, as shown in the following equation and in Figure 4-5. Of the various resistances in series, arteriolar resistance is by far the greatest. The total resistance of a vascular bed is determined, therefore, in large part by the arteriolar resistance. Series resistance is expressed as follows:

$$R_{total} = R_{artery} + R_{arterioles} + R_{capillaries} + R_{venules} + R_{vein}$$

When resistances are arranged in series, the total flow through each level of the system is the same. For example, blood flow through the aorta equals blood flow through all the large systemic arteries, equals blood flow through all the systemic arterioles, equals blood flow through all the systemic capillaries. For another example, blood flow through the renal artery equals blood flow through all the renal capillaries, equals blood flow through the renal vein (less a small volume lost in urine). Although total flow is constant at each level in the series, the pressure decreases progressively as blood flows through each sequential component (remember $Q = \Delta P/R$ or $\Delta P = Q \times R$). The **greatest decrease in pressure occurs in the arterioles** because they contribute the largest portion of the resistance.

◆ **Parallel resistance** is illustrated by the distribution of blood flow *among* the various major arteries branching off the aorta (see Figs. 4-1 and 4-5). Recall that the cardiac output flows through the aorta and then is distributed, on a percentage basis, among the various organ systems. Thus, there is parallel, simultaneous blood flow through each of the circulations (e.g., renal, cerebral, and coronary). The venous effluent from the organs then collects in the vena cava and returns to the heart. As shown in the following equation and in Figure 4-5, the total **resistance in a *parallel* arrangement is less than any of the individual resistances.** The subscripts 1, 2, 3, and so forth refer to the resistances of cerebral, coronary, renal, gastrointestinal, skeletal muscle, and skin circulations. Parallel resistance is expressed as follows:

$$\frac{1}{R_{total}} = \frac{1}{R_1} + \frac{1}{R_2} + \frac{1}{R_3} + \frac{1}{R_4} + \frac{1}{R_5} + \frac{1}{R_6}$$

When blood flow is distributed through a set of parallel resistances, the flow through each organ is a fraction of the total blood flow. The effects of this arrangement are that there is **no loss of pressure** in the major arteries and that mean pressure in each major artery will be approximately the same as mean pressure in the aorta.

Another predictable consequence of a parallel arrangement is that adding a resistance to the circuit causes total resistance to decrease, *not to increase.*

Mathematically, this can be demonstrated as follows: Four resistances, each with a numeric value of 10, are arranged in parallel. According to the equation, the total resistance is 2.5 ($1/R_{total} = 1/10 + 1/10 + 1/10 + 1/10 = 2.5$). If a fifth resistance with a value of 10 is added to the parallel arrangement, the total resistance decreases to 2 ($1/R_{total} = 1/10 + 1/10 + 1/10 + 1/10 + 1/10 = 2$).

On the other hand, if the resistance of one of the individual vessels in a parallel arrangement increases, then total resistance *increases*. This can be shown by returning to the parallel arrangement of four blood vessels where each individual resistance is 10 and the total resistance is 2.5. If one of the four blood vessels is completely occluded, its individual resistance becomes infinite. The total resistance of the parallel arrangement then increases to 3.333 ($1/R_{total} = 1/10 + 1/10 + 1/10 + 1/\infty$).

Laminar Flow and Reynolds Number

Ideally, blood flow in the cardiovascular system is **laminar,** or streamlined. In laminar flow, there is a parabolic profile of velocity within a blood vessel, with the velocity of blood flow highest in the center of the vessel and lowest toward the vessel walls (Fig. 4-6). The parabolic profile develops because the layer of blood next to the vessel wall adheres to the wall and, essentially, does not move. The next layer of blood (toward the center) slips past the motionless layer and moves a bit faster. Each successive layer of blood

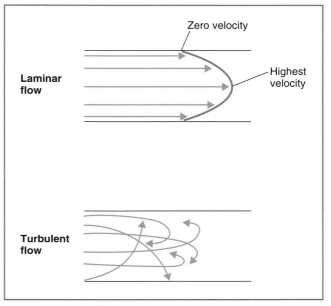

Figure 4–6 Comparison of laminar flow to turbulent blood flow. The length of the *arrows* shows the approximate velocity of blood flow. Laminar blood flow has a parabolic profile, with velocity lowest at the vessel wall and highest in the center of the stream. Turbulent blood flow exhibits axial and radial flow.

toward the center moves faster yet, with less adherence to adjacent layers. Thus, *the velocity of flow at the vessel wall is zero, and the velocity at the center of the stream is maximal.* Laminar blood flow conforms to this orderly parabolic profile.

When an irregularity occurs in a blood vessel (e.g., at the valves or at the site of a blood clot), the laminar stream is disrupted and blood flow may become **turbulent.** In turbulent flow (see Fig. 4-6), the fluid streams do not remain in the parabolic profile; instead, the streams mix radially and axially. Because energy is wasted in propelling blood radially and axially, more energy (pressure) is required to drive turbulent blood flow than laminar blood flow. Turbulent flow is often accompanied by audible vibrations called **murmurs.**

The **Reynolds number** is a dimensionless number that is used to predict whether blood flow will be laminar or turbulent. It considers a number of factors including diameter of the blood vessel, mean velocity of flow, and viscosity of the blood. Thus,

$$N_R = \frac{\rho d v}{\eta}$$

where

N_R = Reynolds number
ρ = Density of blood
d = Diameter of blood vessel
v = Velocity of blood flow
η = Viscosity of blood

If Reynolds number (N_R) is less than 2000, blood flow will be laminar. If Reynolds number is greater than 2000, there is increasing likelihood that blood flow will be turbulent. Values greater than 3000 always predict turbulent flow.

The major influences on Reynolds number in the cardiovascular system are changes in blood **viscosity** and changes in the **velocity** of blood flow. Inspection of the equation shows that decreases in viscosity (e.g., decreased hematocrit) cause an increase in Reynolds number. Likewise, narrowing of a blood vessel, which produces an increase in velocity of blood flow, causes an increase in Reynolds number.

The effect of narrowing a blood vessel (i.e., decreased diameter and radius) on Reynolds number is initially puzzling because, according to the equation, decreases in vessel diameter should *decrease* Reynolds number (diameter is in the numerator). Recall, however, that the velocity of blood flow also depends on diameter (radius), according to the earlier equation, $v = Q/A$ or $v = Q/\pi r^2$. Thus, velocity (also in the numerator of the equation for Reynolds number) *increases* as radius *decreases,* raised to the *second power.* Hence, the dependence of Reynolds number on velocity is more powerful than the dependence on diameter.

Two common clinical situations, anemia and thrombi, illustrate the application of Reynolds number in predicting turbulence.

♦ **Anemia** is associated with a decreased hematocrit (decreased mass of red blood cells) and, because of turbulent blood flow, causes functional murmurs. Reynolds number, the predictor of turbulence, is increased in anemia due to decreased blood viscosity. A second cause of increased Reynolds number in patients with anemia is a high cardiac output, which causes an increase in the velocity of blood flow ($v = Q/A$).

♦ **Thrombi** are blood clots in the lumen of a vessel. Thrombi narrow the diameter of the blood vessel, which causes an increase in blood velocity at the site of the thrombus, thereby increasing Reynolds number and producing turbulence.

Shear

Shear is a consequence of the fact that blood travels at different velocities within a blood vessel (see Fig. 4-6). Shear occurs if adjacent layers of blood travel at different velocities; when adjacent layers travel at the same velocity, there is no shear. Thus, **shear is highest** at the blood vessel wall, according to the following reasoning. Right at the wall, there is a motionless layer of blood (i.e., velocity is zero); the adjacent layer of blood *is* moving and therefore has a velocity. The greatest relative difference in velocity of blood is between the motionless layer of blood right at the wall and the next layer in. **Shear is lowest** at the center of the blood vessel, where the velocity of blood is highest, but where the adjacent layers of blood are essentially moving at the same velocity. One consequence of shear is that it breaks up aggregates of red blood cells and decreases blood viscosity. Therefore, at the wall, where shear rate is normally highest, red blood cell aggregation and viscosity are lowest.

Compliance of Blood Vessels

The compliance or **capacitance** of a blood vessel describes the volume of blood the vessel can hold at a given pressure. Compliance is related to **distensibility** and is given by the following equation:

$$C = V/P$$

where

C = Compliance or capacitance (mL/mm Hg)
V = Volume (mL)
P = Pressure (mm Hg)

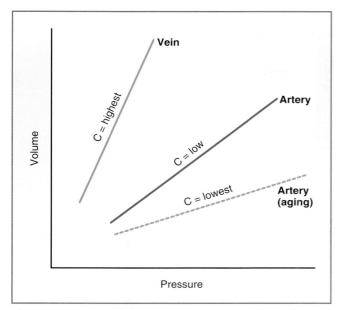

Figure 4–7 Capacitance of veins and arteries. Volume is plotted as a function of pressure. The slopes of the curves are capacitance (C).

Table 4–1 Pressures in the Cardiovascular System

Location	Mean Pressure (mm Hg)
Systemic	
Aorta	100
Large arteries	100 (systolic, 120; diastolic, 80)
Arterioles	50
Capillaries	20
Vena cava	4
Right atrium	0–2
Pulmonary	
Pulmonary artery	15 (systolic, 25; diastolic, 8)
Capillaries	10
Pulmonary vein	8
Left atrium*	2–5

*Pressures on the left side of the heart are difficult to measure directly. However, left atrial pressure can be measured by the *pulmonary wedge pressure.* With this technique, a catheter is inserted into the pulmonary artery and advanced into a small branch of the pulmonary artery. The catheter *wedges* and blocks all blood flow from that branch. Once the flow is stopped, the catheter senses the pressure in the left atrium almost directly.

The equation for compliance states that the higher the compliance of a vessel, the more volume it can hold at a given pressure. Or, stated differently, compliance describes how the volume of blood contained in a vessel changes for a given change in pressure ($\Delta V/\Delta P$).

Figure 4-7 illustrates the principle of compliance and shows the relative compliance of veins and arteries. For each type of blood vessel, volume is plotted as a function of pressure. The **slope** of each curve is the **compliance.** Compliance of the veins is high; in other words, the veins hold large volumes of blood at low pressure. Compliance of the arteries is much lower than that of the veins; the arteries hold much less blood than the veins, and they do so at high pressure.

The difference in the compliance of the veins and the arteries underlies the concepts of unstressed volume and stressed volume. The veins are most compliant and contain the unstressed volume (large volume under low pressure). The arteries are much less compliant and contain the stressed volume (low volume under high pressure). The total volume of blood in the cardiovascular system is the sum of the unstressed volume plus the stressed volume (plus whatever volume is contained in the heart).

Changes in compliance of the veins cause redistribution of blood between the veins and the arteries (i.e., the blood shifts between the unstressed and stressed volumes). For example, if the compliance of the veins decreases (e.g., due to venoconstriction), there is a decrease in the volume the veins can hold and, consequently, a shift of blood from the veins to the arteries: unstressed volume decreases and stressed volume

increases. If the compliance of the veins increases, there is an increase in the volume the veins can hold and, consequently, a shift of blood from the arteries to the veins: unstressed volume increases and stressed volume decreases. Such redistributions of blood between the veins and arteries have consequences for arterial pressure, as discussed later in this chapter.

Figure 4-7 also illustrates the effect of **aging** on **compliance of the arteries.** The characteristics of the arterial walls change with increasing age: The walls become stiffer, less distensible, and less compliant. At a given arterial pressure, the arteries can hold less blood. Another way to think of the decrease in compliance associated with aging is that in order for an "old artery" to hold the same volume as a "young artery," the pressure in the "old artery" must be higher than the pressure in the "young artery." Indeed, arterial pressures are increased in the elderly due to decreased arterial compliance.

Pressures in the Cardiovascular System

Blood pressures are not equal throughout the cardiovascular system. If they were equal, blood would not flow, since flow requires a driving force (i.e., a pressure difference). The pressure differences that exist between the heart and blood vessels are the driving force for blood flow. Table 4-1 provides a summary of pressures in the systemic and pulmonary circulations.

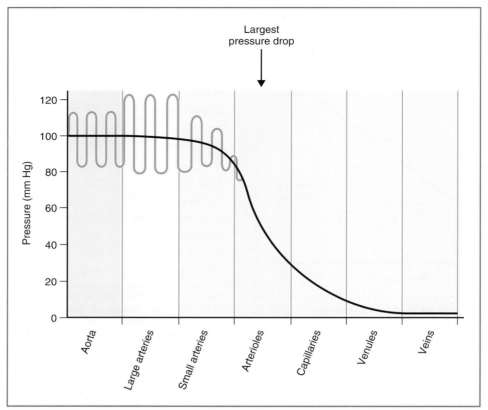

Figure 4–8 **Pressure profile in the vasculature.** The smooth curve is the mean pressure. Pulsations, when present, are superimposed on the mean pressure.

Pressure Profile in the Vasculature

Figure 4-8 is a profile of pressures within the systemic vasculature. First, examine the smooth profile, ignoring the pulsations. The smooth curve gives mean pressure, which is highest in the aorta and large arteries and decreases progressively as blood flows from the arteries, to the arterioles, to the capillaries, to the veins, and back to the heart. This decrease in pressure occurs as blood flows through the vasculature because energy is consumed in overcoming the frictional resistances.

Mean pressure in the **aorta** is high, averaging 100 mm Hg (see Table 4-1 and Fig. 4-8). This high mean arterial pressure is a result of two factors: the large volume of blood pumped from the left ventricle into the aorta (cardiac output) and the low compliance of the arterial wall. (Recall that a given volume causes greater pressure when compliance of the vessel is low.) The pressure remains high in the **large arteries,** which branch off the aorta, because of the high elastic recoil of the arterial walls. Thus, little energy is lost as blood flows from the aorta through the arterial tree.

Beginning in the **small arteries,** arterial pressure decreases, with the most significant decrease occurring in the arterioles. At the end of the **arterioles,** mean pressure is approximately 30 mm Hg. This dramatic decrease in pressure occurs because the arterioles constitute a high resistance to flow. Since total blood flow is constant at all levels of the cardiovascular system, as resistance increases, downstream pressure must necessarily decrease ($Q = \Delta P/R$, or $\Delta P = Q \times R$).

In the **capillaries,** pressure decreases further for two reasons: frictional resistance to flow and filtration of fluid out of the capillaries (refer to the discussion on microcirculation). When blood reaches the **venules** and **veins,** pressure has decreased even further. (Recall that because capacitance of the veins is high, the veins can hold large volumes of blood at this low pressure.) Pressure in the vena cava is only 4 mm Hg and in the right atrium is even lower at 0 to 2 mm Hg.

Arterial Pressure in the Systemic Circulation

Further examination of Figure 4-8 reveals that although *mean* pressure in the arteries is high and constant, there are oscillations or pulsations of arterial pressure. These **pulsations** reflect the pulsatile activity of the heart: ejecting blood during systole, resting during diastole, ejecting blood, resting, and so forth. Each cycle of pulsation in the arteries coincides with one cardiac cycle.

Figure 4-9 shows an expanded version of two such pulsations in a large artery.

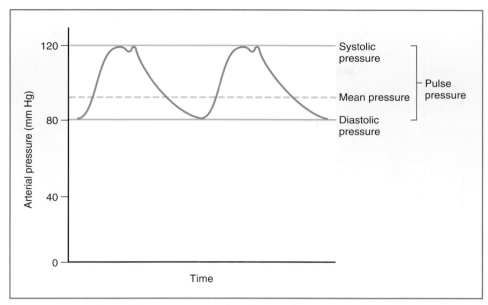

Figure 4–9 **Systemic arterial pressure during the cardiac cycle.** Systolic pressure is the highest pressure measured during systole. Diastolic pressure is the lowest pressure measured during diastole. Pulse pressure is the difference between systolic pressure and diastolic pressure. (See the text for a discussion of mean arterial pressure.)

♦ **Diastolic pressure** is the lowest arterial pressure measured during a cardiac cycle and is the pressure in the arteries during ventricular relaxation when no blood is being ejected from the left ventricle.

♦ **Systolic pressure** is the highest arterial pressure measured during a cardiac cycle. It is the pressure in the arteries after blood has been ejected from the left ventricle during systole. The "blip" in the arterial pressure curve, called the **dicrotic notch** (or **incisura**), is produced when the aortic valve closes. Aortic valve closure produces a brief period of retrograde flow from the aorta back toward the valve, briefly decreasing the aortic pressure below the systolic value.

♦ **Pulse pressure** is the difference between systolic pressure and diastolic pressure. If all other factors are equal, the magnitude of the pulse pressure reflects the volume of blood ejected from the left ventricle on a single beat, or the **stroke volume.**

Pulse pressure can be used as an indicator of stroke volume because of the relationships between pressure, volume, and compliance. Recall that compliance of a blood vessel is the volume the vessel can hold at a given pressure (C = V/P). Thus, assuming that arterial compliance is constant, arterial pressure depends on the volume of blood the artery contains at any moment in time. For example, the volume of blood in the aorta at a given time is determined by the balance between inflow and outflow of blood. When the left ventricle contracts, it rapidly ejects a stroke volume into the aorta, and

the pressure rises rapidly to its highest level, the systolic pressure. Blood then begins to flow from the aorta into the rest of the arterial tree. Now, as the volume in the aorta decreases, the pressure also decreases. Arterial pressure reaches its lowest level, the diastolic pressure, when the ventricle is relaxed and blood is returning from the arterial system back to the heart.

♦ **Mean arterial pressure** is the average pressure in a complete cardiac cycle and is calculated as follows:

Mean arterial pressure
= Diastolic pressure + 1/3 Pulse pressure

Notice that mean arterial pressure is not the simple mathematical average of diastolic and systolic pressures. This is because a greater fraction of each cardiac cycle is spent in diastole than in systole. Thus, the calculation of mean arterial pressure gives more weight to diastolic pressure than systolic pressure.

Interestingly, the **pulsations in large arteries** are even greater than the pulsations in the aorta (see Fig. 4-8). In other words, systolic pressure and pulse pressure are higher in the large arteries than in the aorta. It is not immediately obvious why pulse pressure should increase in the "downstream" arteries. The explanation resides in the fact that, following ejection of blood from the left ventricle, the pressure wave travels at a higher velocity than the blood itself travels (due to the inertia of the blood), augmenting the

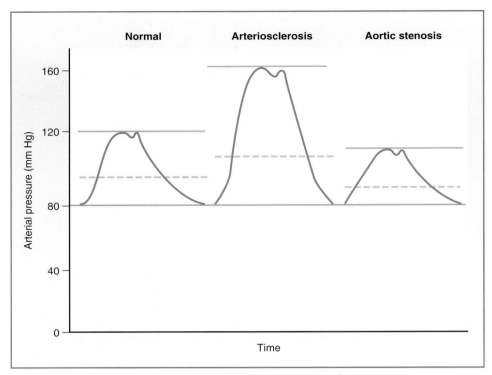

Figure 4–10 **Effect of arteriosclerosis and aortic stenosis on arterial pressures.**

downstream pressure. Furthermore, at branch points of arteries, pressure waves are reflected backward, which also tends to augment pressure at those sites. (Given that blood flows from the aorta to the large arteries, it may seem odd that systolic pressure and pulse pressure are higher in the downstream arteries. We know that the direction of blood flow must be from high to low pressure, and not the other way around! The explanation is that the driving force for blood flow in the arteries is the *mean* arterial pressure, which is influenced more by diastolic pressure than by systolic pressure (because a greater proportion of each cardiac cycle is spent in diastole). Note in Figure 4-8 that while systolic pressure is higher in the large arteries than in the aorta, diastolic pressure is lower; thus, mean arterial pressure is lower downstream.)

Although systolic pressure and pulse pressure are augmented in the large arteries (compared with the aorta), from that point on, there is damping of the oscillations. The pulse pressure is still evident, but decreased, in the smaller arteries; it is virtually absent in the arterioles; and it is completely absent in the capillaries, venules, and veins. This damping and loss of pulse pressure occurs for two reasons. (1) The resistance of the blood vessels, particularly the arterioles, makes it difficult to transmit the pulse pressure. (2) The compliance of the blood vessels, particularly of the veins, damps the pulse pressure—the more compliant the blood vessel, the more volume that can be added to it without causing an increase in pressure.

Several pathologic conditions alter the arterial pressure curve in a predictable way (Fig. 4-10). As previously noted, pulse pressure is the change in arterial pressure that occurs when a stroke volume is ejected from the left ventricle into the aorta. Logically, then, pulse pressure will change if stroke volume changes, *or* if the compliance of the arteries changes.

♦ **Arteriosclerosis** (see Fig. 4-10). In arteriosclerosis, plaque deposits in the arterial walls decrease the diameter of the arteries and make them stiffer and less compliant. Because arterial compliance is decreased, ejection of a stroke volume from the left ventricle causes a much greater change in arterial pressure than it does in normal arteries ($C = \Delta V/\Delta P$ or $\Delta P = \Delta V/C$). Thus, in arteriosclerosis, systolic pressure, pulse pressure, and mean pressure all will be increased.

♦ **Aortic stenosis** (see Fig. 4-10). If the aortic valve is stenosed (narrowed), the size of the opening through which blood can be ejected from the left ventricle into the aorta is reduced. Thus, stroke volume is decreased, and less blood enters the aorta on each beat. Systolic pressure, pulse pressure, and mean pressure all will be decreased.

♦ **Aortic regurgitation** (*not shown*). When the aortic valve is incompetent (e.g., due to a congenital abnormality), the normal one-way flow of blood from the left ventricle into the aorta is disrupted.

Instead, blood that was ejected into the aorta flows backward into the ventricle. Such retrograde flow can occur because the ventricle is relaxed (is at low pressure) and because the incompetent aortic valve cannot prevent it, as it normally does.

Venous Pressures in the Systemic Circulation

By the time blood reaches the venules and veins, pressure is less than 10 mm Hg; pressure will decrease even further in the vena cava and the right atrium. The reason for the continuing decrease in pressure is now familiar: The resistance provided by the blood vessels at each level of the systemic vasculature causes a fall in pressure. Table 4-1 and Figure 4-8 show the mean values for venous pressures in the systemic circulation.

Pressures in the Pulmonary Circulation

Table 4-1 also compares pressures in the pulmonary circulation with pressures in the systemic circulation. As the table shows, the entire pulmonary vasculature is at much **lower pressure** than the systemic vasculature. The *pattern* of pressures within the pulmonary circulation is analogous to the systemic circulation, however. Blood is ejected from the right ventricle into the pulmonary artery, where pressure is highest. Thereafter, the pressure decreases as blood flows through the pulmonary arteries, arterioles, capillaries, venules, and veins and back to the left atrium.

An important implication of these lower pressures on the pulmonary side is that **pulmonary vascular resistance is much lower than systemic vascular resistance.** This conclusion can be reached by recalling that the total flow through the systemic and pulmonary circulations must be equal (i.e., cardiac output of the left and right hearts is equal). Because pressures on the pulmonary side are much lower than pressures on the systemic side, to achieve the same flow, pulmonary resistance must be lower than systemic resistance (Q = ΔP/R). (The pulmonary circulation is discussed in more detail in Chapter 5.)

CARDIAC ELECTROPHYSIOLOGY

Cardiac electrophysiology includes all of the processes involved in the electrical activation of the heart: the cardiac action potentials; the conduction of action potentials along specialized conducting tissues; excitability and the refractory periods; the modulating effects of the autonomic nervous system on heart rate, conduction velocity, and excitability; and the electrocardiogram (ECG).

Ultimately, the function of the heart is to pump blood through the vasculature. To serve as a pump, the ventricles must be electrically activated and then contract. In cardiac muscle, electrical activation is the cardiac action potential, which normally originates in the sinoatrial (SA) node. The action potentials initiated in the SA node then are conducted to the entire myocardium in a specific, timed sequence. Contraction follows, also in a specific sequence. "Sequence" is especially critical because the atria must be activated and contract before the ventricles, and the ventricles must contract from apex to base for efficient ejection of blood.

Cardiac Action Potentials

Origin and Spread of Excitation within the Heart

The heart consists of two kinds of muscle cells: contractile cells and conducting cells. **Contractile cells** constitute the majority of atrial and ventricular tissues and are the working cells of the heart. Action potentials in contractile cells lead to contraction and generation of force or pressure. **Conducting cells** constitute the tissues of the SA node, the atrial internodal tracts, the AV node, the bundle of His, and the Purkinje system. Conducting cells are specialized muscle cells that do not contribute significantly to generation of force; instead, they function to rapidly spread action potentials over the entire myocardium. Another feature of the specialized conducting tissues is their capacity to generate action potentials spontaneously. Except for the SA node, however, this capacity normally is suppressed.

Figure 4-11 is a schematic drawing showing the relationships of the SA node, atria, ventricles, and specialized conducting tissues. The action potential spreads throughout the myocardium in the following sequence:

1. **SA node.** Normally, the action potential of the heart is initiated in the specialized tissue of the SA node, which serves as the **pacemaker.** After the action potential is initiated in the SA node, there is a specific sequence and timing for the conduction of action potentials to the rest of the heart.

2. **Atrial internodal tracts and atria.** The action potential spreads from the SA node to the right and left atria via the atrial internodal tracts. Simultaneously, the action potential is conducted to the AV node.

3. **AV node.** Conduction velocity through the AV node is considerably slower than in the other cardiac tissues. **Slow conduction** through the AV node ensures that the ventricles have sufficient time to fill with blood before they are activated and contract. Increases in conduction velocity of the AV node can lead to decreased ventricular filling and decreased stroke volume and cardiac output.

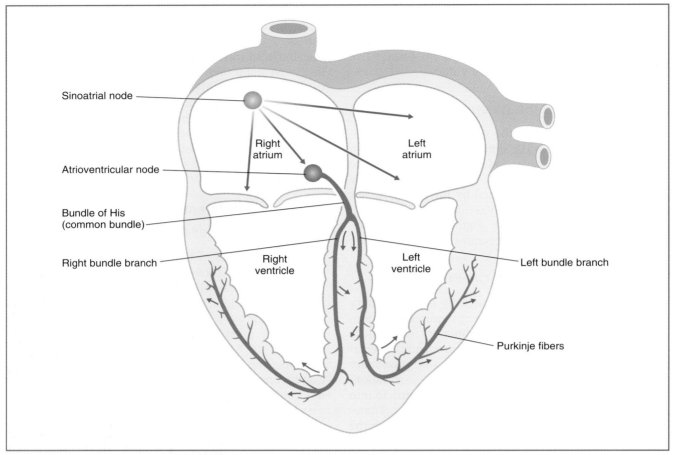

Figure 4–11   Schematic diagram showing the sequence of activation of the myocardium.
The cardiac action potential is initiated in the sinoatrial node and spreads throughout the myocardium, as shown by the *arrows*.

4. **Bundle of His, Purkinje system, and ventricles.** From the AV node, the action potential enters the specialized conducting system of the ventricles. The action potential is first conducted to the bundle of His through the common bundle. It then invades the left and right bundle branches and then the smaller bundles of the Purkinje system. Conduction through the His-Purkinje system is extremely fast, and it rapidly distributes the action potential to the ventricles. The action potential also spreads from one ventricular muscle cell to the next, via low-resistance pathways between the cells. Rapid conduction of the action potential throughout the ventricles is essential and allows for efficient contraction and ejection of blood.

The term **normal sinus rhythm** has a specific meaning. It means that the pattern and timing of the electrical activation of the heart are normal. To qualify as normal sinus rhythm, the following three criteria must be met: (1) The action potential must originate in the SA node. (2) The SA nodal impulses must occur regularly at a rate of 60 to 100 impulses per minute. (3) The activation of the myocardium must occur in the correct sequence and with the correct timing and delays.

Concepts Associated with Cardiac Action Potentials

The concepts applied to cardiac action potentials are the same concepts that are applied to action potentials in nerve, skeletal muscle, and smooth muscle. The following section is a summary of those principles, which are discussed in Chapter 1:

1. The **membrane potential** of cardiac cells is determined by the relative conductances (or permeabilities) to ions and the concentration gradients for the permeant ions.

2. If the cell membrane has a high conductance or permeability to an ion, that ion will flow down its electrochemical gradient and attempt to drive the membrane potential toward its **equilibrium potential** (calculated by the Nernst equation). If the cell

Table 4–2 Comparison of Action Potentials in Cardiac Tissues

Cardiac Tissue	Action Potential Duration (msec)	Upstroke	Plateau	Phase 4 Depolarization
Sinoatrial node	150	Inward Ca^{2+} current Ca^{2+} channels	None	Inward Na^+ current (I_f) Normal pacemaker
Atrium	150	Inward Na^+ current	Inward Ca^{2+} current (slow inward current) L-type Ca^{2+} channels	None
Ventricle	250	Inward Na^+ current	Inward Ca^{2+} current (slow inward current) L-type Ca^{2+} channels	None
Purkinje fibers	300	Inward Na^+ current	Inward Ca^{2+} current (slow inward current) L-type Ca^{2+} channels	Latent pacemaker

membrane is impermeable to an ion, that ion will make little or no contribution to the membrane potential.

3. By convention, membrane potential is expressed in millivolts (mV), and intracellular potential is expressed relative to extracellular potential; for example, a membrane potential of −85 mV means 85 mV, cell interior negative.

4. The **resting membrane potential** of cardiac cells is determined primarily by potassium ions (K^+). The conductance to K^+ at rest is high, and the resting membrane potential is close to the K^+ equilibrium potential. Since the conductance to sodium (Na^+) at rest is low, Na^+ contributes little to the resting membrane potential.

5. The role of **Na^+-K^+ ATPase** is primarily to maintain Na^+ and K^+ concentration gradients across the cell membrane, although it makes a small direct electrogenic contribution to the membrane potential.

6. **Changes in membrane potential** are caused by the flow of ions into or out of the cell. For ion flow to occur, the cell membrane must be permeable to that ion. **Depolarization** means the membrane potential has become *less negative.* Depolarization occurs when there is net movement of positive charge into the cell, which is called an **inward current. Hyperpolarization** means the membrane potential has become *more negative,* and it occurs when there is net movement of positive charge out of the cell, which is called an **outward current.**

7. Two basic mechanisms can produce a change in membrane potential. In one mechanism, there is a **change in the electrochemical gradient for a permeant ion,** which changes the equilibrium potential for that ion. The permeant ion then will flow into or out of the cell in an attempt to reestablish

electrochemical equilibrium, and this current flow will alter the membrane potential. For example, consider the effect of decreasing the extracellular K^+ concentration on the resting membrane potential of a myocardial cell. The K^+ equilibrium potential, calculated by the Nernst equation, will become more negative. K^+ ions will then flow out of the cell and down the now larger electrochemical gradient, driving the resting membrane potential toward the new, more negative K^+ equilibrium potential.

In the other mechanism, there is a **change in conductance to an ion.** For example, the resting permeability of ventricular cells to Na^+ is quite low, and Na^+ contributes minimally to the resting membrane potential. However, during the upstroke of the ventricular action potential, Na^+ conductance dramatically increases, Na^+ flows into the cell down its electrochemical gradient, and the membrane potential is briefly driven toward the Na^+ equilibrium potential (i.e., is depolarized).

8. **Threshold potential** is the potential difference at which there is a net inward current (i.e., inward current becomes greater than outward current). At threshold potential, the depolarization becomes self-sustained and gives rise to the upstroke of the action potential.

Action Potentials of Ventricles, Atria, and the Purkinje System

The ionic basis for the action potentials in the ventricles, atria, and Purkinje system is identical. The action potential in these tissues shares the following characteristics (Table 4-2):

♦ **Long duration.** In each of these tissues, the action potential is of long duration. Action potential duration varies from 150 msec in atria, to 250 msec in

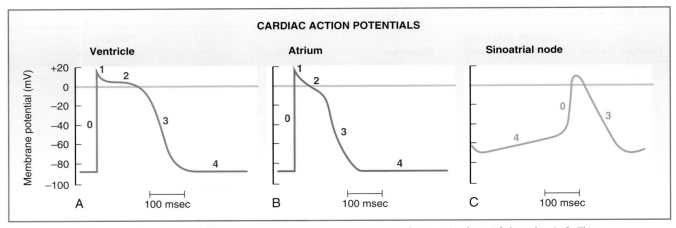

Figure 4-12 **Cardiac action potentials in the ventricle, atrium, and sinoatrial node. A–C,** The numbers correspond to the phases of the action potentials.

ventricles, to 300 msec in Purkinje fibers. These durations can be compared with the brief duration of the action potential in nerve and skeletal muscle (1 to 2 msec). Recall that the duration of the action potential also determines the duration of the refractory periods: The longer the action potential, the longer the cell is refractory to firing another action potential. Thus, atrial, ventricular, and Purkinje cells have **long refractory periods** compared with other excitable tissues.

♦ **Stable resting membrane potential.** The cells of the atria, ventricles, and Purkinje system exhibit a stable, or constant, resting membrane potential. (AV nodal and Purkinje fibers *can* develop unstable resting membrane potentials, and under special conditions, they can become the heart's pacemaker, as discussed in the section on latent pacemakers.)

♦ **Plateau.** The action potential in cells of the atria, ventricles, and Purkinje system is characterized by a plateau. The plateau is a sustained period of depolarization, which accounts for the long duration of the action potential and, consequently, the long refractory periods.

Figure 4-12*A* and *B* illustrate the action potential in a ventricular muscle fiber and an atrial muscle fiber. An action potential in a Purkinje fiber (not shown) would look similar to that in the ventricular fiber, but its duration would be slightly longer. The **phases of the action potential** are described subsequently and correspond to the numbered phases shown in Figure 4-12*A* and *B*. The ventricular action potential has also been redrawn in Figure 4-13 to show the ionic currents responsible for each phase. Some of this information also is summarized in Table 4-2.

1. **Phase 0, upstroke.** In ventricular, atrial, and Purkinje fibers, the action potential begins with a phase

of **rapid depolarization,** called the upstroke. As in nerve and skeletal muscle, the upstroke is caused by a transient increase in Na^+ conductance (g_{Na}), produced by depolarization-induced opening of activation gates on the Na^+ channels. When g_{Na} increases, there is an **inward Na^+ current** (influx of Na^+ into the cell), or I_{Na}, which drives the membrane potential toward the Na^+ equilibrium potential of approximately +65 mV. The membrane potential does not quite reach the Na^+ equilibrium potential because, as in nerve, the inactivation gates on the Na^+ channels close in response to depolarization (albeit more slowly than the activation gates open). Thus, the Na^+ channels open briefly and then close. At the peak of the upstroke, the membrane potential is depolarized to a value of about +20 mV.

The **rate of rise of the upstroke** is called **dV/dT.** dV/dT is the rate of change of the membrane potential as a function of time, and its units are volts per second (V/sec). dV/dT varies, depending on the value of the **resting membrane potential.** This dependence is called the **responsiveness relationship.** Thus, dV/dT is greatest (the rate of rise of the upstroke is fastest) when the resting membrane potential is most negative, or hyperpolarized (e.g., −90 mV), and dV/dT is lowest (the rate of rise of the upstroke is slowest) when the resting membrane potential is less negative, or depolarized (e.g., −60 mV). This correlation is based on the relationship between membrane potential and the position of the inactivation gates on the Na^+ channel (see Chapter 1). When the resting membrane potential is relatively hyperpolarized (e.g., −90 mV), the voltage-dependent inactivation gates are open and many Na^+ channels are available for the upstroke. When the resting membrane potential is relatively depolarized (e.g., −60 mV), the inactivation gates

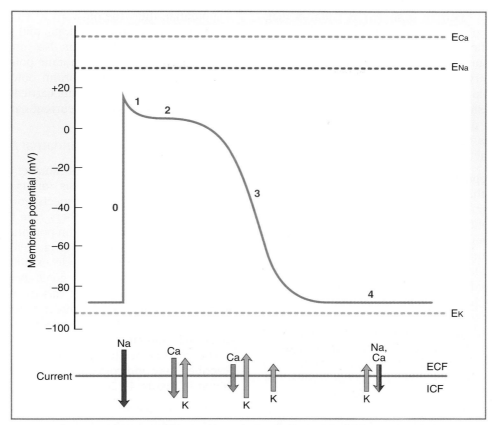

Figure 4–13 Currents responsible for ventricular action potential. The length of the *arrows* shows the relative size of each ionic current. E, Equilibrium potential; ECF, extracellular fluid; ICF, intracellular fluid.

on the Na⁺ channels tend to be closed and fewer Na⁺ channels are available to open during the upstroke. dV/dT also correlates with the **size of the inward current** (i.e., in ventricular, atrial, and Purkinje fibers, the size of the inward Na⁺ current).

2. **Phase 1, initial repolarization.** Phase 1 in ventricular, atrial, and Purkinje fibers is a brief period of repolarization, which immediately follows the upstroke. Recall that, for repolarization to occur, there must be a **net outward current.** There are two explanations for the occurrence of the net outward current during phase 1. First, the inactivation gates on the Na⁺ channels close in response to depolarization. When these gates close, g_{Na} decreases and the inward Na⁺ current (which caused the upstroke) ceases. Second, there is an outward K⁺ current, caused by the large driving force on K⁺ ions: At the peak of the upstroke, *both* the chemical and the electrical driving forces favor K⁺ movement *out* of the cell (the intracellular K⁺ concentration is higher than extracellular K⁺ concentration, and the cell interior is electrically positive). Because the K⁺ conductance (g_K) is high, K⁺ flows out of the cell, down this steep electrochemical gradient.

3. **Phase 2, plateau.** During the plateau, there is a long period (150 to 200 msec) of relatively **stable, depolarized membrane potential,** particularly in ventricular and Purkinje fibers. (In atrial fibers, the plateau is shorter than in ventricular fibers.) Recall that for the membrane potential to be stable, inward and outward currents must be equal such that there is no net current flow across the membrane.

    How is such a balance of inward and outward currents achieved during the plateau? There is an increase in Ca²⁺ conductance (g_{Ca}), which results in an **inward Ca²⁺ current.** Inward Ca²⁺ current is also called **slow inward current,** reflecting the slower kinetics of these channels (compared with the fast Na⁺ channels of the upstroke). The Ca²⁺ channels that open during the plateau are **L-type channels** and are inhibited by the **Ca²⁺ channel blockers** nifedipine, diltiazem, and verapamil. To balance the inward Ca²⁺ current, there is an **outward K⁺ current,** driven by the electrochemical driving force on K⁺ ions (as described for phase 1). Thus, during the plateau, the inward Ca²⁺ current is balanced by the outward K⁺ current, the net current is zero, and the membrane potential remains at a stable depolarized value. (See Fig. 4-13, where during phase 2, the inward Ca^{2+} current is shown as equal in magnitude to the outward K^+ current.)

The significance of the inward Ca^{2+} current extends beyond its effect on membrane potential. This Ca^{2+} entry during the plateau of the action potential initiates the release of more Ca^{2+} from intracellular stores for excitation-contraction coupling. This process of so-called **Ca^{2+}-induced Ca^{2+}release** is discussed in the section on cardiac muscle contraction.

4. **Phase 3, repolarization.** Repolarization begins gradually at the end of phase 2, and then there is rapid repolarization to the resting membrane potential during phase 3. Recall that repolarization is produced when outward currents are greater than inward currents. During phase 3, repolarization results from a combination of a decrease in g_{Ca} (previously increased during the plateau) and an increase in g_K (to even higher levels than at rest). The reduction in g_{Ca} results in a decrease in the inward Ca^{2+} current, and the increase in g_K results in an increase in the outward K^+ current (I_K), with K^+ moving down a steep electrochemical gradient (as described for phase 1). At the end of phase 3, the outward K^+ current is reduced because repolarization brings the membrane potential closer to the K^+ equilibrium potential, thus decreasing the driving force on K^+.

5. **Phase 4, resting membrane potential, or electrical diastole.** The membrane potential fully repolarizes during phase 3 and returns to the resting level of approximately −85 mV. During phase 4, the membrane potential is stable again, and inward and outward currents are equal. The resting membrane potential approaches, but does not fully reach, the K^+ equilibrium potential, reflecting the high resting conductance to K^+. The K^+ channels, and the resulting K^+ current, responsible for phase 4 are different from those responsible for repolarization in phase 3. In phase 4, the K^+ conductance is called g_{K1} and the K^+ current is called, accordingly, I_{K1}.

The stable membrane potential in phase 4 means that inward and outward currents are equal. The high conductance to K^+ produces an outward K^+ current (I_{K1}), which has already been described. The inward current that balances this outward current is carried by Na^+ and Ca^{2+} (see Fig. 4-13), even though the conductances to Na^+ and Ca^{2+} are low at rest. The question may arise: *How can the sum of inward Na^+ and Ca^{2+} currents be the same magnitude as the outward K^+ current, given that g_{Na} and g_{Ca} are very low, and g_{K1} is very high?* The answer lies in the fact that, for each ion, current = conductance × driving force. Although g_{K1} is high, the driving force on K^+ is low because the resting membrane potential is close to the K^+ equilibrium

potential; thus, the outward K^+ current is relatively small. On the other hand, g_{Na} and g_{Ca} are both low, but the driving forces on Na^+ and Ca^{2+} are high because the resting membrane potential is far from the Na^+ and Ca^{2+} equilibrium potentials; thus, the sum of the inward currents carried by Na^+ and Ca^{2+} is equal to the outward current carried by K^+.

Action Potentials in the Sinoatrial Node

The SA node is the normal pacemaker of the heart. The configuration and ionic basis for its action potential differ in several important aspects from those in atrial, ventricular, and Purkinje fibers (see Fig. 4-12C). The following features of the action potential of the SA node are different from those in atria, ventricles, and Purkinje fibers: (1) The SA node exhibits **automaticity;** that is, it can spontaneously generate action potentials without neural input. (2) It has an **unstable resting membrane potential,** in direct contrast to cells in atrial, ventricular, and Purkinje fibers. (3) It has **no sustained plateau.**

The phases of the SA node action potential are described here and correspond to the numbered phases shown in Figure 4-12C.

1. **Phase 0, upstroke.** Phase 0 (as in the other cardiac cells) is the upstroke of the action potential. Note that the upstroke is not as rapid or as steep as in the other types of cardiac tissues. The ionic basis for the upstroke in the SA node differs as well. In the other myocardial cells, the upstroke is the result of an increase in g_{Na} and an inward Na^+ current. In the SA nodal cells, the upstroke is the result of an **increase in g_{Ca} and an inward Ca^{2+} current** carried primarily by L-type Ca^{2+} channels. There are also T-type Ca^{2+} channels in SA node, which carry part of the inward Ca^{2+} current of the upstroke.

2. **Phases 1 and 2 are absent.**

3. **Phase 3, repolarization.** As in the other myocardial tissues, repolarization in the SA node is due to an increase in g_K. Because the electrochemical driving forces on K^+ are large (both chemical and electrical driving forces favor K^+ leaving the cell), there is an outward K^+ current, which repolarizes the membrane potential.

4. **Phase 4, spontaneous depolarization or pacemaker potential.** Phase 4 is the longest portion of the SA node action potential. This phase accounts for the **automaticity** of SA nodal cells (the ability to spontaneously generate action potentials without neural input). During phase 4, the most negative value of the membrane potential (called the **maximum diastolic potential**) is approximately −65 mV, but the membrane potential does not

remain at this value. Rather, there is a slow depolarization, produced by the opening of Na$^+$ channels and an **inward Na$^+$ current** called **I$_f$**. The "f," which stands for *funny,* denotes that this Na$^+$ current differs from the fast Na$^+$ current responsible for the upstroke in ventricular cells. *I$_f$ is turned on by repolarization from the preceding action potential,* thus ensuring that each action potential in the SA node will be followed by another action potential. Once I$_f$ and slow depolarization bring the membrane potential to threshold, the T-type Ca^{2+} channels are opened for the upstroke.

The rate of phase 4 depolarization sets the heart rate. If the rate of phase 4 depolarization increases, threshold is reached more quickly, the SA node will fire more action potentials per time, and heart rate will increase. Conversely, if the rate of phase 4 depolarization decreases, threshold is reached more slowly, the SA node will fire fewer action potentials per time, and heart rate will decrease. The effects of the autonomic nervous system on heart rate are based on such changes in the rate of phase 4 depolarization and are discussed later in the chapter.

Latent Pacemakers

The cells in the SA node are not the only myocardial cells with intrinsic automaticity; other cells, called **latent pacemakers,** also have the capacity for spontaneous phase 4 depolarization. Latent pacemakers include the cells of the **AV node**, **bundle of His**, and **Purkinje fibers.** Although each of these cells has the potential for automaticity, it normally is not expressed.

The rule is that *the pacemaker with the fastest rate of phase 4 depolarization controls the heart rate.* Normally, the SA node has the fastest rate of phase 4 depolarization, and therefore, it sets the heart rate (Table 4-3). Recall also that, of all myocardial cells, the SA nodal cells have the shortest action potential duration (i.e., the shortest refractory periods). Therefore, SA nodal cells recover faster and are ready to fire another action potential before the other cell types are ready.

When the SA node drives the heart rate, the latent pacemakers are suppressed, a phenomenon called **overdrive suppression,** which is explained as follows: The SA node has the fastest firing rate of all the potential pacemakers, and impulses spread from the SA node to the other myocardial tissues in the sequence illustrated in Figure 4-11. Although some of these tissues are potential pacemakers themselves (AV node, bundle of His, Purkinje fibers), as long as their firing rate is driven by the SA node, their own capacity to spontaneously depolarize is suppressed.

The latent pacemakers have an opportunity to drive the heart rate *only* if the SA node is suppressed or if the intrinsic firing rate of a latent pacemaker becomes faster than that of the SA node. Since the intrinsic rate of the latent pacemakers is slower than that of the SA node, the heart will beat at the slower rate if it is driven by a latent pacemaker (see Table 4-3).

Under the following conditions a latent pacemaker takes over and becomes *the* pacemaker of the heart, in which case it is called an **ectopic pacemaker,** or **ectopic focus.** (1) If the SA node firing rate decreases (e.g., due to vagal stimulation) or stops completely (e.g., because the SA node is destroyed, removed, or suppressed by drugs), then one of the latent sites will assume the role of pacemaker in the heart. (2) Or, if the intrinsic rate of firing of one of the latent pacemakers should become faster than that of the SA node, then it will assume the pacemaker role. (3) Or, if the conduction of action potentials from the SA node to the rest of the heart is blocked because of disease in the conducting pathways, then a latent pacemaker can appear in addition to the SA node.

Conduction Velocity

Conduction of the Cardiac Action Potential

In the heart, **conduction velocity** has the same meaning that it has in nerve and skeletal muscle fibers: It is the speed at which action potentials are propagated within the tissue. The units for conduction velocity are meters per second (m/sec). Conduction velocity is not the same in all myocardial tissues: It is slowest in the AV node (0.01 to 0.05 m/sec) and fastest in the Purkinje fibers (2 to 4 m/sec), as shown in Figure 4-14.

Conduction velocity determines how long it takes the action potential to spread to various locations in the myocardium. These times, in milliseconds, are superimposed on the diagram in Figure 4-14. The action potential originates in the SA node at what is called time zero. It then takes a total of 220 msec for the action potential to spread through the atria, AV node, and His-Purkinje system to the farthest points in the ventricles. Conduction through the AV node (called **AV delay**) requires almost one half of the total conduction time through the myocardium. The reason for the AV delay is that, of all the myocardial tissues, conduction

Table 4-3 Firing Rate of Sinoatrial Node and Latent Pacemakers in the Heart

Location	Intrinsic Firing Rate (impulses/min)
Sinoatrial node	70–80
Atrioventricular node	40–60
Bundle of His	40
Purkinje fibers	15–20

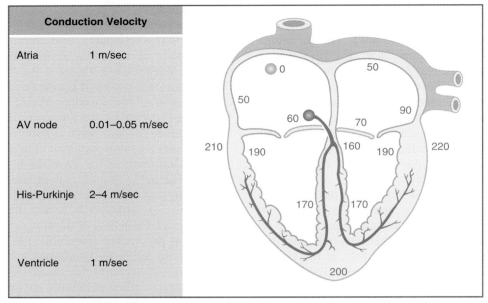

Conduction Velocity	
Atria	1 m/sec
AV node	0.01–0.05 m/sec
His-Purkinje	2–4 m/sec
Ventricle	1 m/sec

Figure 4–14 Timing of activation of the myocardium. The numbers superimposed on the myocardium indicate the cumulative time, in msec, from the initiation of the action potential in the sinoatrial node.

velocity in the AV node is slowest (0.01 to 0.05 m/sec), making conduction time the longest (100 msec).

Differences in conduction velocity among the cardiac tissues have implications for their physiologic functions. For example, the slow conduction velocity of the AV node ensures that the ventricles do not activate too early (i.e., before they have time to fill with blood from the atria). On the other hand, the rapid conduction velocity of the Purkinje fibers ensures that the ventricles can be activated quickly and in a smooth sequence for efficient ejection of blood.

Mechanism of Propagation of Cardiac Action Potential

As in nerve and skeletal muscle fibers, the physiologic basis for conduction of cardiac action potentials is the spread of **local currents** (see Chapter 1). Action potentials at one site generate local currents at adjacent sites; the adjacent sites are depolarized to threshold as a result of this local current flow and fire action potentials themselves. This local current flow is the result of the inward current of the upstroke of the action potential. Recall that, in atrial, ventricular, and Purkinje fibers, this inward current of the upstroke is carried by Na^+, and in the SA node, the inward current of the upstroke is carried by Ca^{2+}.

Conduction velocity depends on the **size of the inward current** during the upstroke of the action potential. The larger the inward current, the more rapidly local currents will spread to adjacent sites and depolarize them to threshold. Conduction velocity also correlates with **dV/dT,** the rate of rise of the upstroke

of the action potential, because dV/dT *also* correlates with the size of the inward current, as discussed previously.

Propagation of the action potential depends not only upon the inward current of the upstroke to establish local currents, but also on the **cable properties** of the myocardial fibers. Recall that these cable properties are determined by cell membrane resistance (R_m) and internal resistance (R_i). For example, in myocardial tissue, R_i is particularly low because of low-resistance connections between the cells called **gap junctions.** Thus, myocardial tissue is especially well suited to fast conduction.

Conduction velocity *does not* depend on action potential duration, a point that can be confusing. Recall, however, that action potential duration is simply the time it takes a given site to go from depolarization to complete repolarization (e.g., action potential duration in a ventricular cell is 250 msec). Action potential duration implies nothing about how long it takes for that action potential to spread to neighboring sites.

Excitability and Refractory Periods

Excitability is the capacity of myocardial cells to generate action potentials in response to inward, depolarizing current. Strictly speaking, excitability is the amount of inward current required to bring a myocardial cell to the threshold potential. The excitability of a myocardial cell varies over the course of the action potential, and these changes in excitability are reflected in the refractory periods.

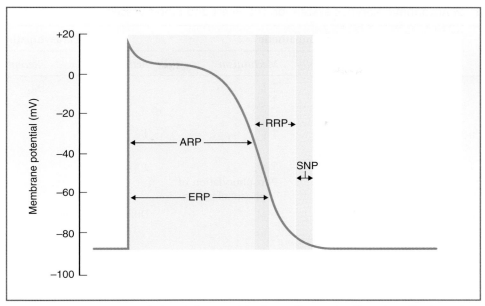

Figure 4-15 Refractory periods of the ventricular action potential. The effective refractory period (ERP) includes the absolute refractory period (ARP) and the first half of the relative refractory period (RRP). The RRP begins when the absolute refractory period ends and includes the last portion of the effective refractory period. The supranormal period (SNP) begins when the relative refractory period ends.

The physiologic basis for the **refractory periods** in myocardial cells is similar to that in nerve cells. Recall from Chapter 1 that activation gates on Na⁺ channels *open* when the membrane potential is depolarized to threshold, permitting a rapid influx of Na⁺ into the cell, which causes further depolarization toward the Na⁺ equilibrium potential. This rapid depolarization is the upstroke of the action potential. However, inactivation gates on the Na⁺ channels also *close* with depolarization (although they close more slowly than the activation gates open). Therefore, during those phases of the action potential when the membrane potential is depolarized, a portion of the Na⁺ channels will be closed because the inactivation gates are closed. When the Na⁺ channels are closed, inward depolarizing current cannot flow through them, and there can be no upstroke. Without an upstroke, a normal action potential cannot occur and the cell is *refractory*. Once repolarization occurs, the inactivation gates on the Na⁺ channels open, and the cell is once again excitable.

Figure 4-15 is a familiar diagram showing an action potential in ventricular muscle, with the refractory periods now superimposed on it. The following refractory periods reflect differences in excitability over the duration of the action potential:

♦ **Absolute refractory period.** For most of the duration of the action potential, the ventricular cell is completely refractory to fire another action potential. No matter how large a stimulus (i.e., inward current) might be applied, the cell is incapable of generating a second action potential during the absolute refractory period (ARP), because most of the Na⁺ channels are closed. The absolute refractory period includes the upstroke, the entire plateau, and a portion of the repolarization. This period concludes when the cell has repolarized to approximately −50 mV.

♦ **Effective refractory period.** The effective refractory period (ERP) includes, and is slightly longer than, the absolute refractory period. At the end of the effective refractory period, the Na⁺ channels start to recover (i.e., become available to carry inward current). The distinction between the absolute and effective refractory periods is that *absolute* means *absolutely* no stimulus is large enough to generate another action potential; *effective* means that a *conducted* action potential cannot be generated (i.e., there is not enough inward current to conduct to the next site).

♦ **Relative refractory period.** The relative refractory period (RRP) begins at the end of the absolute refractory period and continues until the cell membrane has almost fully repolarized. During the relative refractory period, even more Na⁺ channels have recovered and it is possible to generate a second action potential, although a *greater-than-normal stimulus is required*. If a second action potential is generated during the relative refractory period, it will have an abnormal configuration and a shortened plateau phase.

Table 4–4   Effects of Autonomic Nervous System on the Heart and Blood Vessels

	Sympathetic			Parasympathetic		
	Action	*Receptor*	*Mechanism*	*Action*	*Receptor*	*Mechanism*
Heart rate	↑	β_1	↑ I_f ↑ I_{Ca}	↓	M_2	↓ I_f ↑ $I_{K\text{-}ACh}$ ↓ I_{Ca}
Conduction velocity	↑	β_1	↑ I_{Ca}	↓	M_2	↓ I_{Ca} ↑ $I_{K\text{-}ACh}$
Contractility	↑	β_1	↑ I_{Ca} Phosphorylation of phospholamban	↓ (atria only)	M_2	↓ I_{Ca} ↑ $I_{K\text{-}ACh}$
Vascular smooth muscle (skin, renal, and splanchnic)	Constriction	α_1	—	Dilation (releases EDRF)	M_3	—
Vascular smooth muscle (skeletal muscle)	Dilation	β_2	—	Dilation (releases EDRF)	M_3	—
	Constriction	α_1	—			

AV, Atrioventricular; EDRF, endothelial-derived relaxing factor; M, muscarinic.

♦ **Supranormal period.** The supranormal period (SNP) follows the relative refractory period. It begins when the membrane potential is −70 mV and continues until the membrane is fully repolarized back to −85 mV. As the name suggests, the cell is *more excitable than normal* during this period. In other words, less inward current is required to depolarize the cell to the threshold potential. The physiologic explanation for this increased excitability is that the Na$^+$ channels are recovered (i.e., the inactivation gates are open again), and because the membrane potential is closer to threshold than it is at rest, it is easier to fire an action potential than when the cell membrane is at the resting membrane potential.

Autonomic Effects on the Heart and Blood Vessels

Table 4-4 summarizes the effects of the autonomic nervous system on the heart and blood vessels. For convenience, the autonomic effects on heart rate, conduction velocity, myocardial contractility, and vascular smooth muscle are combined into one table. The effects on cardiac electrophysiology (i.e., heart rate and conduction velocity) are discussed in this section, and the other autonomic effects are discussed in later sections.

Autonomic Effects on Heart Rate

The effects of the autonomic nervous system on heart rate are called **chronotropic effects.** The effects of the sympathetic and parasympathetic nervous systems on heart rate are summarized in Table 4-4 and are illustrated in Figure 4-16. Briefly, sympathetic stimulation increases heart rate and parasympathetic stimulation decreases heart rate.

Figure 4-16*A* shows the normal firing pattern of the SA node. Recall that phase 4 depolarization is produced by opening Na$^+$ channels, which leads to a slow depolarizing, inward Na$^+$ current called I_f. Once the membrane potential is depolarized to the threshold potential, an action potential is initiated.

♦ **Positive chronotropic effects** are increases in heart rate. The most important example is that of stimulation of the **sympathetic nervous system,** as illustrated in Figure 4-16*B*. Norepinephrine, released from sympathetic nerve fibers, activates β_1 receptors in the SA node. These **β_1 receptors** are coupled to adenylyl cyclase through a Gs protein (see also Chapter 2). Activation of β_1 receptors in the SA node produces **an increase in I_f,** which increases the rate of phase 4 depolarization. In addition, there is an increase in I_{Ca}, which means there are more functional Ca^{2+} channels and thus less depolarization is required to reach threshold (i.e., threshold potential decreases). Increasing the rate of phase 4 depolarization and decreasing the threshold potential means that the SA node is depolarized to threshold potential more frequently and, as a consequence, fires more action potentials per unit time (i.e., increased heart rate).

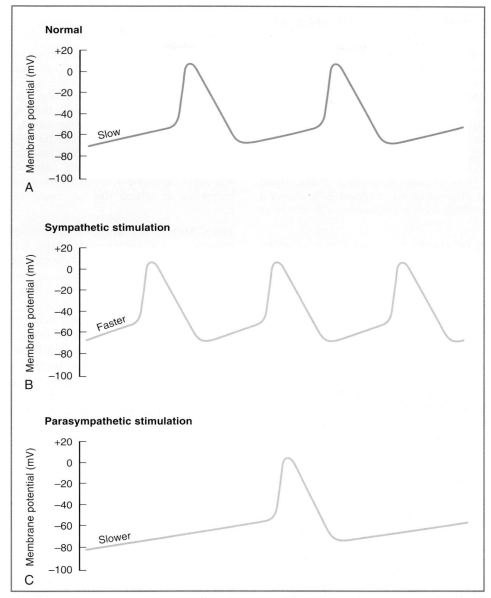

Figure 4-16 **Effect of sympathetic and parasympathetic stimulation on the SA node action potential. A,** The normal firing pattern of the SA node is shown. **B,** Sympathetic stimulation increases the rate of phase 4 depolarization and increases the frequency of action potentials. **C,** Parasympathetic stimulation decreases the rate of phase 4 depolarization and hyperpolarizes the maximum diastolic potential to decrease the frequency of action potentials.

♦ **Negative chronotropic effects** are decreases in heart rate. The most important example is that of stimulation of the **parasympathetic nervous system,** illustrated in Figure 4-16C. Acetylcholine (ACh), released from parasympathetic nerve fibers, activates **muscarinic (M₂)** receptors in the SA node. Activation of muscarinic receptors in the SA node has two effects that combine to produce a decrease in heart rate. First, these muscarinic receptors are coupled to a type of **G_i protein** called **G_K** that inhibits adenylyl cyclase and produces a **decrease in I_f.** A decrease in I_f decreases the rate of phase 4

depolarization. Second, G_k *directly* increases the conductance of a K⁺ channel called **K⁺-ACh** and increases an outward K⁺ current (similar to I_{K1}) called **I_{K-ACh}.** Enhancing this outward K⁺ current hyperpolarizes the maximum diastolic potential so that the SA nodal cells are further from threshold potential. In addition, there is a decrease in I_{Ca}, which means there are fewer functional Ca²⁺ channels and thus more depolarization is required to reach threshold (i.e., threshold potential increases). In sum, the parasympathetic nervous system decreases heart rate through three effects on the SA

BOX 4–1 Clinical Physiology: Sinus Bradycardia

DESCRIPTION OF CASE. A 72-year-old woman with hypertension is being treated with propranolol, a β-adrenergic blocking agent. She has experienced several episodes of light-headedness and syncope (fainting). An ECG shows sinus bradycardia: normal, regular P waves, followed by normal QRS complexes; however, the frequency of P waves is decreased, at 45/min. The physician tapers off and eventually discontinues the propranolol and then changes the woman's medication to a different class of antihypertensive drugs. Upon discontinuation of propranolol, a repeat ECG shows a normal sinus rhythm with a frequency of P waves of 80/min.

EXPLANATION OF CASE. The heart rate is given by the frequency of P waves. During treatment with

propranolol, her heart rate was only 45 beats/min. The presence of P waves on the ECG indicates that the heart is being activated in the SA node, which is the normal pacemaker. However, the frequency of depolarization of the SA node is much lower than normal because she is being treated with propranolol, a β-adrenergic blocking agent. Recall that β-adrenergic agonists *increase* the rate of phase 4 depolarization in the SA node by increasing I_f. β-Adrenergic antagonists, therefore, will *decrease* phase 4 depolarization and decrease the frequency at which the SA nodal cells fire action potentials.

TREATMENT. The woman's sinus bradycardia was an adverse effect of propranolol therapy. When propranolol was discontinued, her heart rate returned to normal.

---

node: (1) slowing the rate of phase 4 depolarization, (2) hyperpolarizing the maximum diastolic potential so that more inward current is required to reach threshold potential, and (3) increasing the threshold potential. As a result, the SA node is depolarized to threshold less frequently and fires fewer action potentials per unit time (i.e., decreased heart rate) (Box 4-1).

Autonomic Effects on Conduction Velocity in the Atrioventricular Node

The effects of the autonomic nervous system on conduction velocity are called **dromotropic effects.** Increases in conduction velocity are called positive dromotropic effects, and decreases in conduction velocity are called negative dromotropic effects. The most important physiologic effects of the autonomic nervous system on conduction velocity are those on the AV node, which, in effect, alter the rate at which action potentials are conducted from the atria to the ventricles. Recall, in considering the mechanism of these autonomic effects, that conduction velocity correlates with the size of the inward current of the upstroke of the action potential and the rate of rise of the upstroke, dV/dT.

Stimulation of the **sympathetic nervous system** produces an **increase in conduction velocity** through the AV node (positive dromotropic effect), which increases the rate at which action potentials are conducted from the atria to the ventricles. The mechanism of the sympathetic effect is increased I_{Ca}, which is responsible for the upstroke of the action potential in the AV node (as it is in the SA node). Thus, increased I_{Ca} means increased inward current and increased conduction velocity. In a supportive role, the increased I_{Ca} shortens the ERP so

that the AV nodal cells recover earlier from inactivation and can conduct the increased firing rate.

Stimulation of the **parasympathetic nervous system** produces a **decrease in conduction velocity** through the AV node (negative dromotropic effect), which decreases the rate at which action potentials are conducted from the atria to the ventricles. The mechanism of the parasympathetic effect is a combination of decreased I_{Ca} (decreased inward current) and increased I_{K-ACh} (increased outward K^+ current, which further reduces net inward current). Additionally, the ERP of AV nodal cells is prolonged. If conduction velocity through the AV node is slowed sufficiently (e.g., by increased parasympathetic activity or by damage to the AV node), some action potentials may not be conducted at all from the atria to the ventricles, producing **heart block.** The degree of heart block may vary: In the milder forms, conduction of action potentials from atria to ventricles is simply slowed; in more severe cases, action potentials may not be conducted to the ventricles at all.

Electrocardiogram

The electrocardiogram (ECG or EKG) is a measurement of tiny potential differences on the surface of the body that reflect the electrical activity of the heart. Briefly, these potential differences or voltages are measurable on the body's surface because of the timing and sequence of depolarization and repolarization of the heart. Recall that the entire myocardium is not depolarized at once: The atria depolarize before the ventricles; the ventricles depolarize in a specific sequence; the atria repolarize while the ventricles are depolarizing; and the ventricles repolarize in a specific sequence. As a result of the sequence and the timing of the spread

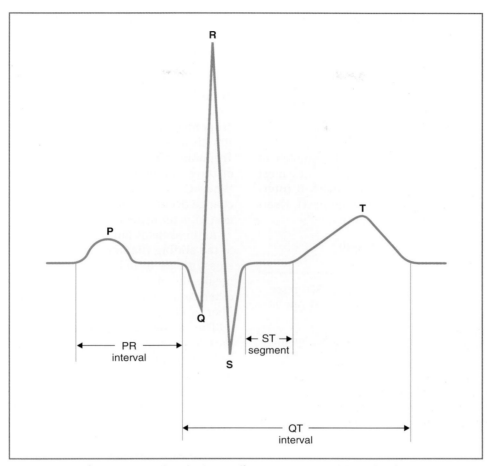

Figure 4–17 **The electrocardiogram measured from lead II.**

of depolarization and repolarization in the myocardium, potential differences are established between different portions of the heart, which can be detected by electrodes placed on the body surface.

The configuration of a normal ECG is shown in Figure 4-17. The nomenclature of the ECG is as follows: The various waves represent depolarization or repolarization of different portions of the myocardium and are given lettered names. Intervals and segments between the waves also are named. The difference between intervals and segments is that intervals include the waves, and segments do not. The following waves, intervals, and segments are seen on the ECG:

1. **P wave.** The P wave represents depolarization of the atria. The duration of the P wave correlates with conduction time through the atria; for example, if conduction velocity through the atria decreases, the P wave will spread out. Atrial repolarization is not seen on a normal ECG because it is "buried" in the QRS complex.

2. **PR interval.** The PR interval is the time from initial depolarization of the atria to initial depolarization of the ventricles. Thus, the PR interval includes the P wave and the PR segment, an isoelectric (flat) portion of the ECG that corresponds to **AV node conduction.** Because the PR interval includes the PR segment, it also *correlates with conduction time through the AV node.*

Normally, the PR interval is 160 msec, which is the cumulative time from first depolarization of the atria to first depolarization of the ventricles (see Fig. 4-14). Increases in conduction velocity through the AV node *decrease* the PR interval (e.g., due to sympathetic stimulation), and decreases in conduction velocity through the AV node *increase* the PR interval (e.g., due to parasympathetic stimulation).

3. **QRS complex.** The QRS complex consists of three waves: Q, R, and S. Collectively, these waves represent depolarization of the ventricles. Note that the total duration of the QRS complex is similar to that of the P wave. This fact may seem surprising because the ventricles are so much larger than the atria; however, the ventricles depolarize just as quickly as the atria because conduction velocity in the His-Purkinje system is much faster than in the atrial conducting system.

4. **T wave.** The T wave represents repolarization of the ventricles.

5. **QT interval.** The QT interval includes the QRS complex, the ST segment, and the T wave. It represents first ventricular depolarization to last ventricular repolarization. The ST segment is an isoelectric portion of the QT interval that correlates with the plateau of the ventricular action potential.

Heart rate is measured by counting the number of QRS complexes (or R waves because they are most prominent) per minute. **Cycle length** is the **R-R interval** (the time between one R wave and the next). Heart rate is related to cycle length as follows:

$$\text{Heart rate} = 1/\text{Cycle length}$$

SAMPLE PROBLEM. If the R-R interval is 800 msec (0.8 sec), what is the heart rate? If the heart rate is 90 beats/min, what is the cycle length?

SOLUTION. The R-R interval is the cycle length. If the cycle length is 0.8 sec, then the heart rate = 1/cycle length or 1.25 beats/sec or 75 beats/min (1 beat/0.8 sec). If the heart rate is 90 beats/min, then the cycle length = 1/heart rate or 0.66 sec or 660 msec. A longer cycle length signifies a slower heart rate, and a shorter cycle length signifies a faster heart rate.

Changes in heart rate (and cycle length) change the duration of the action potential and, as a result, change the durations of the refractory periods and excitability. For example, if heart rate increases (and cycle length decreases), there is a decrease in the duration of the action potential. Not only will there be more action potentials per time, but those action potentials will have a shorter duration and shorter refractory periods. Because of the relationship between heart rate and refractory period, increases in heart rate may be a factor in producing **arrhythmias** (abnormal heart rhythms). As heart rate increases and refractory periods shorten, the myocardial cells are excitable earlier and more often.

CARDIAC MUSCLE CONTRACTION

Myocardial Cell Structure

There are several morphologic and functional differences between cardiac muscle and skeletal muscle, but the basic contractile machinery in the two cell types is similar.

As in skeletal muscle, the cardiac muscle cell is composed of **sarcomeres.** The sarcomeres, which run from Z line to Z line, are composed of thick and thin filaments. The **thick filaments** are composed of **myosin,** whose globular heads have actin-binding sites and ATPase activity. The **thin filaments** are composed of three proteins: actin, tropomyosin, and troponin. **Actin** is a globular protein with a myosin-binding site, which, when polymerized, forms two twisted strands. **Tropomyosin** runs along the groove of the twisted actin strands and functions to block the myosin-binding site. **Troponin** is a globular protein composed of a complex of three subunits; the troponin C subunit binds Ca^{2+}. When Ca^{2+} is bound to troponin C, a conformational change occurs, which removes the tropomyosin inhibition of actin-myosin interaction.

As in skeletal muscle, contraction occurs according to the **sliding filament model,** which states that when cross-bridges form between myosin and actin and then break, the thick and thin filaments move past each other. As a result of this cross-bridge cycling, the muscle fiber produces tension.

The **transverse (T) tubules** invaginate cardiac muscle cells at the Z lines, are continuous with the cell membranes, and function to carry action potentials to the cell interior. The T tubules form dyads with the **sarcoplasmic reticulum,** which is the site of storage and release of Ca^{2+} for excitation-contraction coupling.

Excitation-Contraction Coupling

As in skeletal and smooth muscle, excitation-contraction coupling in cardiac muscle translates the action potential into the production of tension. The following steps are involved in excitation-contraction coupling in cardiac muscle. These steps correlate with the circled numbers shown in Figure 4-18.

1. The cardiac **action potential** is initiated in the myocardial cell membrane, and the depolarization spreads to the interior of the cell via the T tubules. Recall that a unique feature of the cardiac action potential is its plateau (phase 2), which results from an increase in g_{Ca} and an **inward Ca^{2+} current** in which Ca^{2+} flows through L-type Ca^{2+} channels (**dihydropyridine receptors**) from extracellular fluid (ECF) to intracellular fluid (ICF).

2. Entry of Ca^{2+} into the myocardial cell produces an increase in intracellular Ca^{2+} concentration. This increase in intracellular Ca^{2+} concentration is *not* sufficient *alone* to initiate contraction, but it triggers the release of *more* Ca^{2+} from stores in the sarcoplasmic reticulum through Ca^{2+} release channels (**ryanodine receptors**). This process is called **Ca^{2+}-induced Ca^{2+} release**, and the Ca^{2+} that enters during the plateau of the action potential is called the **trigger Ca^{2+}**. Two factors determine how much

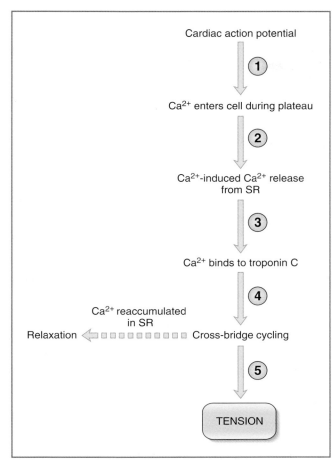

Figure 4–18 Excitation-contraction coupling in myocardial cells. See the text for an explanation of the circled numbers. SR, Sarcoplasmic reticulum.

Ca²⁺ is released from the sarcoplasmic reticulum in this step: the amount of Ca²⁺ previously stored and the size of the inward Ca²⁺ current during the plateau of the action potential.

3. and 4. Ca²⁺ release from the sarcoplasmic reticulum causes the intracellular Ca²⁺ concentration to increase even further. Ca²⁺ now binds to **troponin C,** tropomyosin is moved out of the way, and the interaction of actin and myosin can occur. Actin and myosin bind, **cross-bridges** form and then break, the thin and thick filaments move past each other, and tension is produced. Cross-bridge cycling continues as long as intracellular Ca²⁺ concentration is high enough to occupy the Ca²⁺-binding sites on troponin C.

5. A critically important concept is that *the magnitude of the tension developed by myocardial cells is proportional to the intracellular Ca²⁺ concentration.* Therefore, it is reasonable that hormones, neurotransmitters, and drugs that alter the inward Ca²⁺ current during the action potential plateau *or* that

alter sarcoplasmic reticulum Ca²⁺ stores would be expected to change the amount of tension produced by myocardial cells.

Relaxation occurs when Ca²⁺ is reaccumulated in the sarcoplasmic reticulum by the action of the **Ca²⁺ ATPase.** This reaccumulation causes the intracellular Ca²⁺ concentration to decrease to resting levels. In addition, Ca²⁺, which entered the cell during the plateau of the action potential, is extruded from the cell by Ca²⁺ ATPase and Ca²⁺-Na⁺ exchange in the sarcolemmal membrane. These sarcolemmal transporters pump Ca²⁺ out of the cell against its electrochemical gradient, with the Ca²⁺ ATPase using ATP directly and the Ca²⁺-Na⁺ exchanger using energy from the inward Na⁺ gradient.

Contractility

Contractility, or **inotropism,** is the intrinsic ability of myocardial cells to develop force at a given muscle cell length. Agents that produce an increase in contractility are said to have **positive inotropic effects.** Positive inotropic agents increase both the rate of tension development and the peak tension. Agents that produce a decrease in contractility are said to have **negative inotropic effects.** Negative inotropic agents decrease both the rate of tension development and the peak tension.

Mechanisms for Changing Contractility

Contractility correlates directly with the **intracellular Ca²⁺ concentration,** which in turn depends on the amount of Ca²⁺ released from sarcoplasmic reticulum stores during excitation-contraction coupling. The amount of Ca²⁺ released from the sarcoplasmic reticulum depends on two factors: the **size of the inward Ca²⁺ current** during the plateau of the myocardial action potential (the size of the trigger Ca²⁺) and the **amount of Ca²⁺ previously stored in the sarcoplasmic reticulum** for release. Therefore, the larger the inward Ca²⁺ current and the larger the intracellular stores, the greater the increase in intracellular Ca²⁺ concentration and the greater the contractility.

Effects of the Autonomic Nervous System on Contractility

The effects of the autonomic nervous system on contractility are summarized in Table 4-4. Of these effects, the most important is the positive inotropic effect of the sympathetic nervous system.

♦ **Sympathetic nervous system.** Stimulation of the sympathetic nervous system and circulating catecholamines have a **positive inotropic effect** on the myocardium (i.e., increased contractility). This positive inotropic effect has three important features:

increased peak tension, increased rate of tension development, and faster rate of relaxation. Faster relaxation means that the contraction (twitch) is shorter, allowing more time for refilling. This effect, like the sympathetic effect on heart rate, is mediated via activation of β_1 **receptors,** which are coupled via a G_s protein to adenylyl cyclase. Activation of adenylyl cyclase leads to the production of cyclic adenosine monophosphate (cAMP), activation of protein kinases, and phosphorylation of proteins that produce the physiologic effect of increased contractility.

Two different proteins are phosphorylated to produce the increase in contractility. The coordinated actions of these phosphorylated proteins then produce an increase in intracellular Ca^{2+} concentration. (1) There is phosphorylation of the sarcolemmal **Ca^{2+} channels** that carry inward Ca^{2+} current during the plateau of the action potential. As a result, there is increased inward Ca^{2+} current during the plateau and increased trigger Ca^{2+}, which increases the amount of Ca^{2+} released from the sarcoplasmic reticulum. (2) There is phosphorylation of **phospholamban,** a protein that regulates Ca^{2+} ATPase in the sarcoplasmic reticulum. When phosphorylated, phospholamban stimulates the Ca^{2+} ATPase, resulting in greater uptake and storage of Ca^{2+} by the sarcoplasmic reticulum. Increased Ca^{2+} uptake by the sarcoplasmic reticulum has two effects: It causes faster relaxation (i.e., briefer contraction), and it increases the amount of stored Ca^{2+} for release on subsequent beats.

♦ **Parasympathetic nervous system.** Stimulation of the parasympathetic nervous system and ACh have a **negative inotropic effect** on the *atria*. This effect is mediated via **muscarinic receptors,** which are coupled via a G_i protein called G_K to adenylyl cyclase. Because the G protein in this case is inhibitory, contractility is decreased (opposite of the effect of activation of β_1 receptors by catecholamines). Two factors are responsible for the decrease in atrial contractility caused by parasympathetic stimulation. (1) ACh decreases inward Ca^{2+} current during the plateau of the action potential. (2) ACh increases I_{K-ACh}, thereby shortening the duration of action potential and, indirectly, decreasing the inward Ca^{2+} current (by shortening the plateau phase). Together, these two effects decrease the amount of Ca^{2+} entering atrial cells during the action potential, decrease the trigger Ca^{2+}, and decrease the amount of Ca^{2+} released from the sarcoplasmic reticulum.

Effect of Heart Rate on Contractility

Perhaps surprisingly, changes in heart rate produce changes in contractility: When the heart rate increases, contractility increases; when the heart rate decreases, contractility decreases. The mechanism can be understood by recalling that contractility correlates directly with intracellular Ca^{2+} concentration during excitation-contraction coupling.

For example, an **increase in heart rate** produces an **increase in contractility,** which can be explained as follows: (1) When heart rate increases, there are more action potentials per unit time and an increase in the *total* amount of trigger Ca^{2+} that enters the cell during the plateau phases of the action potentials. Furthermore, if the increase in heart rate is caused by sympathetic stimulation or by catecholamines, then the size of the inward Ca^{2+} current with each action potential also is increased. (2) Because there is greater influx of Ca^{2+} into the cell during the action potentials, the sarcoplasmic reticulum accumulates more Ca^{2+} for subsequent release (i.e., increased stored Ca^{2+}). Again, if the increase in heart rate is caused by sympathetic stimulation, then phospholamban, which augments Ca^{2+} uptake by the sarcoplasmic reticulum, will be phosphorylated, further increasing the uptake process. Two specific examples of the effect of heart rate on contractility, the positive staircase effect and postextrasystolic potentiation, are illustrated in Figure 4-19.

♦ **Positive staircase effect.** The positive staircase effect is also called the **Bowditch staircase,** or Treppe (see Fig. 4-19A). When heart rate doubles, for example, the tension developed on each beat increases in a stepwise fashion to a maximal value. This increase in tension occurs because there are more action potentials per unit time, more total Ca^{2+} entering the cell during the plateau phases, and more Ca^{2+} for accumulation by the sarcoplasmic reticulum (i.e., more stored Ca^{2+}). Notice that the *very first beat* after the increase in heart rate shows *no increase in tension* because extra Ca^{2+} has not yet accumulated. On subsequent beats, the effect of the extra accumulation of Ca^{2+} by the sarcoplasmic reticulum becomes evident. Tension rises stepwise, *like a staircase:* With each beat, more Ca^{2+} is accumulated by the sarcoplasmic reticulum, until a maximum storage level is achieved.

♦ **Postextrasystolic potentiation.** When an **extrasystole** occurs (an anomalous "extra" beat generated by a latent pacemaker), the tension developed on the next beat is greater than normal (see Fig. 4-19B). Although the tension developed on the extrasystolic beat *itself* is less than normal, the *very next beat* exhibits increased tension. An unexpected or "extra" amount of Ca^{2+} entered the cell during the extrasystole and was accumulated by the sarcoplasmic reticulum (i.e., increased stored Ca^{2+}).

Effect of Cardiac Glycosides on Contractility

Cardiac glycosides are a class of drugs that act as **positive inotropic agents.** These drugs are derived from

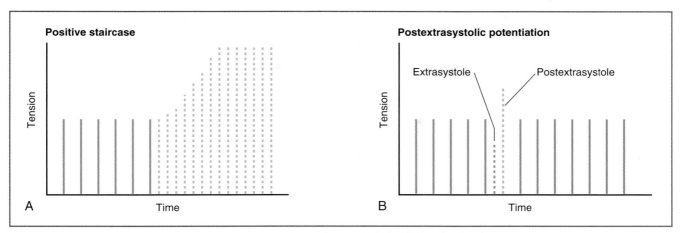

Figure 4–19 **Examples of the effect of heart rate on contractility. A,** Positive staircase; **B,** postextrasystolic potentiation. Tension is used as a measure of contractility. The frequency of the bars shows the heart rate, and the height of the bars shows the tension produced on each beat.

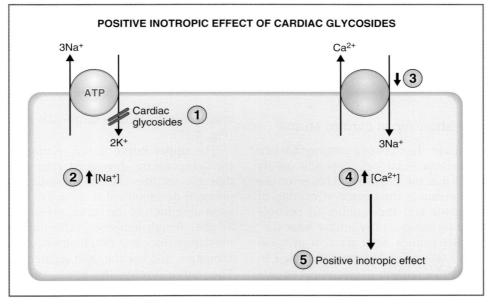

Figure 4–20 **Mechanism of the positive inotropic effect of cardiac glycosides.** See the text for an explanation of the circled numbers.

extracts of the foxglove plant, *Digitalis purpurea.* The prototype drug is **digoxin;** other drugs in this class include digitoxin and ouabain.

The well-known action of the cardiac glycosides is inhibition of Na^+-K^+ ATPase. In the myocardium, inhibition of Na^+-K^+ ATPase underlies the positive inotropic effect of the cardiac glycosides, as explained in Figure 4-20. The circled numbers in the figure correlate with the following steps:

1. The Na^+-K^+ ATPase is located in the cell membrane of the myocardial cell. Cardiac glycosides **inhibit Na^+-K^+ ATPase** at the extracellular K^+-binding site.

2. When the Na^+-K^+ ATPase is inhibited, less Na^+ is pumped out of the cell, increasing the **intracellular Na^+ concentration.**

3. The increase in intracellular Na^+ concentration alters the Na^+ gradient across the myocardial cell membrane, thereby altering the function of a **Ca^{2+}-Na^+ exchanger.** This exchanger pumps Ca^{2+} out of the cell against an electrochemical gradient in exchange for Na^+ moving into the cell down an electrochemical gradient. (Recall that Ca^{2+}-Na^+ exchange is one of the mechanisms that extrudes the Ca^{2+} that entered the cell during the plateau of the myocardial cell action potential.) The energy for pumping Ca^{2+}*uphill* comes from the *downhill* Na^+ gradient, which is normally maintained by the Na^+-K^+ ATPase. When the intracellular Na^+ concentration increases, the inwardly directed Na^+ gradient decreases. As a result, Ca^{2+}-Na^+ exchange decreases because it depends on the Na^+ gradient for its energy source.

4. As less Ca^{2+} is pumped out of the cell by the Ca^{2+}-Na^+ exchanger, the **intracellular Ca^{2+} concentration increases.**

5. Since tension is directly proportional to the intracellular Ca^{2+} concentration, cardiac glycosides produce an increase in tension by increasing intracellular Ca^{2+} concentration—a **positive inotropic effect.**

The major therapeutic use of cardiac glycosides is in the treatment of **congestive heart failure,** a condition characterized by decreased contractility of ventricular muscle (i.e., negative inotropism). When the failure occurs on the left side of the heart, the left ventricle is unable to develop normal tension when it contracts and is unable to eject a normal stroke volume into the aorta. When the failure occurs on the right side of the heart, the right ventricle is unable to develop normal tension and is unable to eject a normal stroke volume into the pulmonary artery. Either situation is serious and potentially life threatening. By increasing the intracellular Ca^{2+} concentration of the ventricular cells, cardiac glycosides have a positive inotropic action, which may counteract the negative inotropism of the failed ventricle.

Length-Tension Relationship in Cardiac Muscle

Just as in skeletal muscle, the maximal tension that can be developed by a myocardial cell depends on its resting length. Recall that the physiologic basis for the length-tension relationship is the degree of overlap of thick and thin filaments and the number of *possible* sites for cross-bridge formation. (The intracellular Ca^{2+} concentration then determines what fraction of these possible cross-bridges will *actually* form and cycle.) In myocardial cells, maximal tension development occurs at cell lengths of about 2.2 µm, or L_{max}. At this length, there is maximal overlap of thick and thin filaments; at either shorter or longer cell lengths, the tension developed will be less than maximal. In addition to the degree of overlap of thick and thin filaments, there are two additional length-dependent mechanisms in cardiac muscle that alter the tension developed: Increasing muscle length increases the Ca^{2+}-sensitivity of troponin C and increasing muscle length increases Ca^{2+} release from the sarcoplasmic reticulum.

The length-tension relationship for single myocardial cells can be extended to a **length-tension relationship for the ventricles.** For example, consider the left ventricle. The *length* of a single left ventricular muscle fiber just prior to contraction corresponds to left ventricular end-diastolic volume. The *tension* of a single left ventricular muscle fiber corresponds to the tension or pressure developed by the entire left ventricle. When these substitutions are made, a curve can be developed that shows ventricular pressure during

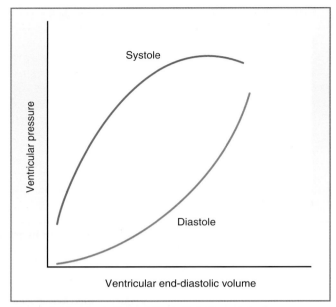

Figure 4–21 **Systolic and diastolic left ventricular pressure-volume curves.** The systolic curve shows active pressure as a function of end-diastolic volume (fiber length). The diastolic curve shows passive pressure as a function of end-diastolic volume.

systole as a function of ventricular end-diastolic volume (Fig. 4-21).

The **upper curve** is the relationship between ventricular pressure developed during systole and end-diastolic volume (or end-diastolic fiber length). This pressure development is an active mechanism. On the ascending limb of the curve, pressure increases steeply as fiber length increases, reflecting greater degrees of overlap of thick and thin filaments, greater cross-bridge formation and cycling, and greater tension developed. The curve eventually levels off when overlap is maximal. If end-diastolic volume were to increase further and the fibers were stretched to even longer lengths, overlap would decrease and the pressure would decrease (descending limb of the curve). In contrast to skeletal muscle, which operates over the entire length-tension curve (see Chapter 1, Fig. 1-26), cardiac muscle normally operates only on the **ascending limb** of the curve. The reason for this difference is that cardiac muscle is much stiffer than skeletal muscle. Thus, cardiac muscle has high resting tension, and small increases in length produce large increases in resting tension. For this reason, cardiac muscle is "held" on the ascending limb of its length-tension curve, and it is difficult to lengthen cardiac muscle fibers beyond L_{max}. For example, the "working length" of cardiac muscle fibers (the length at the end of diastole) is 1.9 µm ($<L_{max}$, which is 2.2 µm). This systolic pressure-volume (i.e., length-tension) relationship for the ventricle is the basis for the **Frank-Starling relationship** in the heart.

The **lower curve** is the relationship between ventricular pressure and ventricular volume during diastole, when the heart is not contracting. As end-diastolic volume increases, ventricular pressure increases through passive mechanisms. The increasing pressure in the ventricle reflects the increasing tension of the muscle fibers as they are stretched to longer lengths.

The terms "preload" and "afterload" can be applied to cardiac muscle just as they are applied to skeletal muscle.

♦ The **preload** for the left ventricle is **left ventricular end-diastolic volume,** or end-diastolic fiber length; that is, preload is the resting length from which the muscle contracts. The relationship between preload and developed tension or pressure, illustrated in the upper (systolic) curve in Figure 4-21, is based on the degree of overlap of thick and thin filaments.

♦ The **afterload** for the left ventricle is **aortic pressure.** The velocity of shortening of cardiac muscle is maximal when afterload is zero, and velocity of shortening decreases as afterload increases. (The relationship between the ventricular pressure developed and aortic pressure or afterload is discussed more fully in the section on ventricular pressure-volume loops.)

Stroke Volume, Ejection Fraction, and Cardiac Output

The function of the ventricles is described by the following three parameters: (1) **Stroke volume** is the volume of blood ejected by the ventricle on each beat; (2) **Ejection fraction** is the fraction of the end-diastolic volume ejected in each stroke volume, which is a measure of ventricular efficiency; and (3) **Cardiac output** is the total volume ejected by the ventricle per unit time.

Stroke Volume

The volume of blood ejected on one ventricular contraction is the stroke volume. Stroke volume is the difference between the volume of blood in the ventricle *before ejection* (end-diastolic volume) and the volume remaining in the ventricle *after ejection* (end-systolic volume). Typically, stroke volume is about **70 mL.** Thus,

Stroke volume
= End-diastolic volume – End-systolic volume

where

Stroke volume = Volume ejected on one
beat (mL)
End-diastolic volume = Volume in the ventricle
before ejection (mL)
End-systolic volume = Volume in the ventricle
after ejection (mL)

Ejection Fraction

The effectiveness of the ventricles in ejecting blood is described by the ejection fraction, which is the *fraction of the end-diastolic volume that is ejected in one stroke volume.* Normally, ejection fraction is approximately **0.55, or 55%.** The ejection fraction is an indicator of **contractility,** with increases in ejection fraction reflecting an increase in contractility and decreases in ejection fraction reflecting a decrease in contractility. Thus,

$$\text{Ejection fraction} = \frac{\text{Stroke volume}}{\text{End-diastolic volume}}$$

Cardiac Output

The total volume of blood ejected per unit time is the cardiac output. Thus, cardiac output depends on the volume ejected on a single beat (stroke volume) and the number of beats per minute (heart rate). Cardiac output is approximately **5000 mL/min** in a 70-kg man (based on a stroke volume of 70 mL and a heart rate of 72 beats/min). Thus,

$$\text{Cardiac output} = \text{Stroke volume} \times \text{Heart rate}$$

where

Cardiac output = Volume ejected per minute
(mL/min)
Stroke volume = Volume ejected in one beat (mL)
Heart rate = Beats per minute (beats/min)

SAMPLE PROBLEM. A man has an end-diastolic volume of 140 mL, an end-systolic volume of 70 mL, and a heart rate of 75 beats/min. *What is his stroke volume, his cardiac output, and his ejection fraction?*

SOLUTION. These calculations are basic and important. The stroke volume is the volume ejected from the ventricle on a single beat; therefore, it is the difference between the volume in the ventricle before and after it contracts. Cardiac output is stroke volume multiplied by heart rate. The ejection fraction is the efficiency of the ventricle in ejecting blood, and it is the stroke volume divided by the end-diastolic volume.

Stroke volume = End-diastolic volume –
End-systolic volume
= 140 mL – 70 mL
= 70 mL
Cardiac output = Stroke volume × Heart rate
= 70 mL × 75 beats/min
= 5250 mL/min
Ejection fraction = Stroke volume/End-diastolic volume
= 70 mL/140 mL = 0.50

Frank-Starling Relationship

The length-tension relationship for ventricular systole has already been described. This relationship now can be understood, using the parameters of stroke volume, ejection fraction, and cardiac output.

The German physiologist Otto Frank first described the relationship between the pressure developed during systole in a frog ventricle and the volume present in the ventricle just prior to systole. Building on Frank's observations, the British physiologist Ernest Starling demonstrated, in an isolated dog heart, that the volume the ventricle ejected in systole was determined by the end-diastolic volume. Recall that the principle underlying this relationship is the length-tension relationship in cardiac muscle fibers.

The Frank-Starling law of the heart, or the **Frank-Starling relationship**, is based on these landmark experiments. It states that the *volume of blood ejected by the ventricle depends on the volume present in the ventricle at the end of diastole.* The volume present at the end of diastole, in turn, depends on the volume returned to the heart, or the venous return. Therefore, stroke volume and cardiac output correlate directly with end-diastolic volume, which correlates with venous return. The Frank-Starling relationship governs normal ventricular function and ensures that the volume the heart *ejects* in systole equals the volume it *receives* in venous return. Recall from a previous discussion that, in the steady state, **cardiac output equals venous return.** It is the Frank-Starling law of the heart that underlies and ensures this equality.

The Frank-Starling relationship is illustrated in Figure 4-22. Cardiac output and stroke volume are plotted as a function of ventricular end-diastolic volume or right atrial pressure. (Right atrial pressure may be substituted for end-diastolic volume because both parameters are related to venous return.) There is a curvilinear relationship between stroke volume or cardiac output and ventricular end-diastolic volume. As venous return increases, end-diastolic volume increases, and because of the length-tension relationship in the ventricles, stroke volume increases accordingly. In the physiologic range, the relationship between stroke

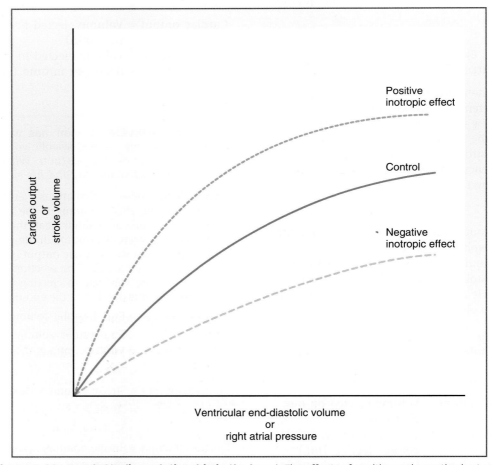

Figure 4–22 Frank-Starling relationship in the heart. The effects of positive and negative inotropic agents are shown with respect to the normal Frank-Starling relationship.

volume and end-diastolic volume is nearly linear. Only when end-diastolic volume becomes high does the curve start to bend: At these high levels, the ventricle reaches a limit and simply is not able to "keep up" with venous return.

Also illustrated in Figure 4-22 are the effects of changing contractility on the Frank-Starling relationship. Agents that increase contractility have a **positive inotropic effect** (*uppermost curve*). Positive inotropic agents (e.g., digoxin) produce increases in stroke volume and cardiac output for a given end-diastolic volume. The result is that a larger fraction of the end-diastolic volume is ejected per beat and there is an increase in ejection fraction.

Agents that decrease contractility have a **negative inotropic effect** (*lowermost curve*). Negative inotropic agents produce decreases in stroke volume and cardiac output for a given end-diastolic volume. The result is that a smaller fraction of the end-diastolic volume is ejected per beat and there is a decrease in ejection fraction.

Ventricular Pressure-Volume Loops

Normal Ventricular Pressure-Volume Loop

The function of the left ventricle can be observed over an entire cardiac cycle (diastole plus systole) by combining the two pressure-volume relationships from Figure 4-21. By connecting these two pressure-volume curves, it is possible to construct a so-called **ventricular pressure-volume loop** (Fig. 4-23). Recall that the systolic pressure-volume relationship in Figure 4-21 shows the maximum developed ventricular pressure for a given ventricular volume. To facilitate understanding, a portion of that systolic pressure-volume curve is

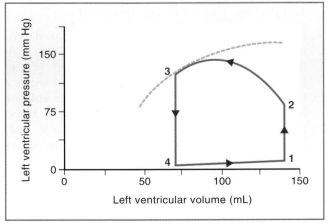

Figure 4–23 Left ventricular pressure-volume loop. One complete left ventricular cycle is shown. (Refer to the text for a complete explanation.) The *dashed line* shows a portion of the systolic pressure-volume curve from Figure 4-21.

superimposed as a gold dashed line on the ventricular pressure-volume loop. The dashed line shows the maximum possible pressure that can be developed for a given ventricular volume during systole (i.e., when the ventricle is contracting). Note that point 3 on the pressure-volume loop touches the systolic pressure-volume curve (*dashed line*). Also, it may not be evident that the portion of the loop between points 4 and 1 corresponds to a portion of the diastolic pressure-volume curve from Figure 4-21.

The ventricular pressure-volume loop describes one complete cycle of ventricular contraction, ejection, relaxation, and refilling as follows:

♦ **Isovolumetric contraction (1 → 2).** Begin the cycle at point 1, which marks the end of diastole. The left ventricle has filled with blood from the left atrium, and its volume is the end-diastolic volume, 140 mL. The corresponding pressure is quite low because the ventricular muscle is relaxed. At this point, the ventricle is activated, it contracts, and ventricular pressure increases dramatically. Because all valves are closed, no blood can be ejected from the left ventricle, and ventricular volume is constant, although ventricular pressure becomes quite high (point 2). Thus, this phase of the cycle is called *isovolumetric* contraction.

♦ **Ventricular ejection (2 → 3).** At point 2, left ventricular pressure becomes higher than aortic pressure, causing the aortic valve to open. (You may wonder why the pressure at point 2 does not reach the systolic pressure-volume curve shown by the dashed gold line. The simple reason is that *it does not have to*. The pressure at point 2 is determined by aortic pressure. Once ventricular pressure reaches the value of aortic pressure, the aortic valve opens and the rest of the contraction is used for ejection of the stroke volume through the open aortic valve.) Once the valve is open, blood is rapidly ejected, driven by the pressure gradient between the left ventricle and the aorta. During this phase, left ventricular pressure remains high because the ventricle is still contracting. Ventricular volume decreases dramatically, however, as blood is ejected into the aorta. The volume remaining in the ventricle at point 3 is the end-systolic volume, 70 mL. The **width of the pressure-volume loop** is the volume of blood ejected, or the **stroke volume.** The stroke volume in this ventricular cycle is 70 mL (140 mL − 70 mL).

♦ **Isovolumetric relaxation (3 → 4).** At point 3, systole ends and the ventricle relaxes. Ventricular pressure decreases below aortic pressure and the aortic valve closes. Although ventricular pressure decreases rapidly during this phase, ventricular volume remains constant (*isovolumetric*) at the

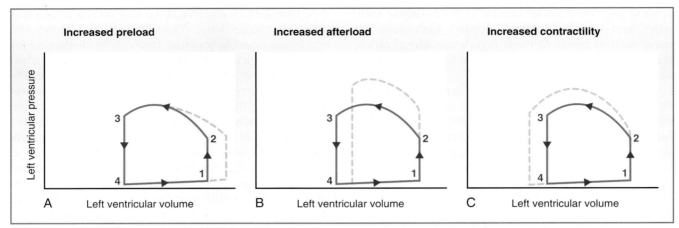

Figure 4-24 Changes in the left ventricular pressure-volume loop. A, Increased preload; **B,** increased afterload; **C,** increased contractility. The normal ventricular cycle is shown by the *solid lines,* and the effect of the change is shown by the *dashed lines.*

end-systolic value of 70 mL because all valves are closed again.

♦ **Ventricular filling (4 → 1).** At point 4, ventricular pressure has fallen to a level that now is less than left atrial pressure, causing the mitral (AV) valve to open. The left ventricle fills with blood from the left atrium passively and also actively, as a result of atrial contraction in the next cycle. Left ventricular volume increases back to the end-diastolic volume of 140 mL. During this last phase, the ventricular muscle is relaxed, and pressure increases only slightly as the compliant ventricle fills with blood.

Changes in Ventricular Pressure-Volume Loops

Ventricular pressure-volume loops can be used to visualize the effects of changes in preload (i.e., changes in venous return or end-diastolic volume), changes in afterload (i.e., changes in aortic pressure), or changes in contractility (Fig. 4-24). The solid lines depict a single, normal ventricular cycle and are identical to the pressure-volume loop shown in Figure 4-23. The dashed lines demonstrate the effects of various changes on a single ventricular cycle (but they do not include any compensatory responses that may occur later).

♦ Figure 4-24*A* illustrates the effect of **increased preload** on the ventricular cycle. Recall that preload is end-diastolic volume. In this example, preload is increased because venous return is increased, which increases end-diastolic volume (point 1). Afterload and contractility remain constant. As the ventricle proceeds through its cycle of contraction, ejection, relaxation, and refilling, the effect of this increase in preload can be appreciated: Stroke volume, as measured by the width of the pressure-volume loop, increases. This **increase in stroke volume** is based

on the Frank-Starling relationship, which states that the greater the end-diastolic volume (end-diastolic fiber length), the greater the stroke volume ejected in systole.

♦ Figure 4-24*B* illustrates the effect of **increased afterload** or increased aortic pressure on the ventricular cycle. In this example, the left ventricle must eject blood against a greater-than-normal pressure. To eject blood, ventricular pressure must rise to a greater than normal level during isovolumetric contraction (point 2) and during ventricular ejection (i.e., 2 → 3). A consequence of the increased afterload is that less blood is ejected from the ventricle during systole; thus, **stroke volume decreases,** more blood remains in the ventricle at the end of systole, and **end-systolic volume increases.** One can envision the effect of increased afterload as follows: if more of the contraction is "spent" in isovolumetric contraction to match the higher afterload, then less of the contraction is "leftover" and available for ejection of the stroke volume.

♦ Figure 4-24*C* illustrates the effect of **increased contractility** on the ventricular cycle. When contractility increases, the ventricle can develop greater tension and pressure during systole and eject a larger volume of blood than normal. **Stroke volume increases**, as does ejection fraction; less blood remains in the ventricle at the end of systole, and, consequently, **end-systolic volume decreases** (points 3 and 4).

Cardiac Work

Work is defined as force times distance. In terms of myocardial function, "work" is **stroke work** or the work the heart performs on each beat. For the left ventricle, stroke work is stroke volume multiplied by aortic pressure, where aortic pressure corresponds to force and stroke volume corresponds to distance. The work of the left ventricle can also be thought of as the area within the pressure-volume loop, such as the loop illustrated in Figure 4-23.

Minute work or power is defined as work per unit time. In terms of myocardial function, **cardiac minute work** is cardiac output multiplied by aortic pressure. Therefore, cardiac minute work can be considered to have two components: **volume work** (i.e., cardiac output) and **pressure work** (i.e., aortic pressure).

Sometimes the volume work component is called "external" work, and the pressure work component is called "internal" work. Thus, increases in cardiac output (due to an increase in stroke volume and/or an increase in heart rate) *or* increases in aortic pressure will increase the work of the heart.

Myocardial Oxygen Consumption

Myocardial O_2 consumption correlates directly with cardiac minute work. Of the two components of cardiac minute work, in terms of O_2 consumption, *pressure work is far more costly than volume work.* In other words, pressure work constitutes a large percentage of the total cardiac work, and volume work contributes a small percentage. These observations explain why overall myocardial O_2 consumption correlates poorly with cardiac output: The largest percentage of the O_2 consumption is for pressure work (or internal work), which is not cardiac output.

It can be further concluded that, in conditions where a larger than normal percentage of the total cardiac work is pressure work, the cost in terms of O_2 consumption increases. For example, in **aortic stenosis,** myocardial O_2 consumption is greatly increased because the left ventricle must develop extremely high pressures to pump blood through the stenosed aortic valve (even though cardiac output actually is reduced).

On the other hand, during **strenuous exercise** when cardiac output becomes very high, volume work contributes a greater-than-normal percentage of the total cardiac work (up to 50%). Although myocardial O_2 consumption increases during exercise, it does not increase as much as when pressure work increases.

Another consequence of the greater O_2 consumption of pressure work is that the *left ventricle must work harder than the right ventricle.* Although cardiac output is the same on both sides of the heart, mean aortic pressure (100 mm Hg) is much higher than mean pulmonary artery pressure (15 mm Hg). Thus, the pressure work of the left ventricle is much greater than the pressure work of the right ventricle, although the volume work is the same. In fact, the left ventricular wall is thicker than the right ventricular wall as a compensatory mechanism for performing more pressure work.

In pathologic conditions such as **systemic hypertension** (elevated arterial pressure in the systemic circulation), the left ventricle must perform even more pressure work than it does normally. Because aortic pressure is elevated, the left ventricular wall hypertrophies (thickens) as a compensation for the increased workload.

The greater thickness of the normal left ventricular wall and the compensatory hypertrophy of the left ventricular wall in systemic hypertension are adaptive mechanisms for performing more pressure work. These adaptive mechanisms are explained by the **law of Laplace.** The law of Laplace for a sphere (i.e., the approximate shape of the heart) states that pressure correlates directly with tension and wall thickness and correlates inversely with radius. Thus,

$$P = \frac{2HT}{r}$$

where

P = Pressure
H = Thickness (height)
T = Tension
r = Radius

In words, the law of Laplace for a sphere states that the greater the thickness of the wall of the sphere (e.g., left ventricle), the greater the pressure that can be developed. Illustrating this point, the left ventricular wall is thicker than the right ventricular wall because the left ventricle must develop greater pressure to eject blood.

It can be further concluded that ventricular wall thickness will increase as a compensatory mechanism if the ventricle has to pump against increased aortic pressure (e.g., hypertension). Thus, in systemic hypertension, the left ventricle hypertrophies; in pulmonary hypertension, the right ventricle hypertrophies. Unfortunately, this type of compensatory ventricular hypertrophy also may lead to ventricular failure and, eventually, be harmful or even fatal.

Measurement of Cardiac Output—Fick Principle

Cardiac output has previously been *defined* as the volume ejected by the left ventricle per unit time and is *calculated* as the product of stroke volume and heart rate. Cardiac output can be *measured* using the Fick principle, whose fundamental assumption is that, in the steady state, the cardiac output of the left and right ventricles is equal.

The **Fick principle** states that there is *conservation of mass,* a concept that can be applied to the utilization of O_2 by the body. In the steady state, the rate of O_2 consumption by the body must equal the amount of O_2 leaving the lungs in the pulmonary vein minus the amount of O_2 returning to the lungs in the pulmonary artery. Each of these parameters can be measured. Total O_2 consumption can be measured directly. The amount of O_2 in the pulmonary veins is pulmonary blood flow multiplied by the O_2 content of pulmonary venous blood. Likewise, the amount of O_2 returned to the lungs via the pulmonary artery is pulmonary blood flow multiplied by the O_2 content of pulmonary arterial blood. Recall that pulmonary blood flow is the cardiac output of the right heart and is equal to the cardiac output of the left heart. Thus, stating these equalities mathematically,

$$O_2 \text{ consumption} = \text{Cardiac output} \times [O_2]_{\text{pulmonary vein}}$$
$$- \text{Cardiac output} \times [O_2]_{\text{pulmonary artery}}$$

or, *rearranging to solve for cardiac output:*

$$\text{Cardiac output} = \frac{O_2 \text{ consumption}}{[O_2]_{\text{pulmonary vein}} - [O_2]_{\text{pulmonary artery}}}$$

where

$$\text{Cardiac output} = \text{Cardiac output (mL/min)}$$
$$O_2 \text{ consumption} = O_2 \text{ consumption by whole body}$$
$$\text{(mL } O_2/\text{min)}$$
$$[O_2]_{\text{pulmonary vein}} = O_2 \text{ content of pulmonary venous}$$
$$\text{blood (mL } O_2/\text{mL blood)}$$
$$[O_2]_{\text{pulmonary artery}} = O_2 \text{ content of pulmonary arterial}$$
$$\text{blood (mL } O_2/\text{mL blood)}$$

The total O_2 consumption of the body typically is 250 mL/min in a 70-kg man. The O_2 content of pulmonary venous blood can be measured by sampling blood from a peripheral artery (because none of the O_2 added to blood in the lungs has been consumed by the tissues yet). The O_2 content of pulmonary arterial blood is equal to that of mixed venous blood and can be sampled either in the pulmonary artery itself or in the right ventricle.

SAMPLE PROBLEM. A man has a resting O_2 consumption of 250 mL O_2/min, a femoral arterial O_2 content of 0.20 mL O_2/mL blood, and a pulmonary arterial O_2 content of 0.15 mL O_2/mL blood. *What is his cardiac output?*

SOLUTION. To calculate cardiac output using the Fick principle, the following values are required: total body O_2 consumption, pulmonary venous O_2 content (in this example, femoral arterial O_2 content), and pulmonary arterial O_2 content.

$$\text{Cardiac output} = \frac{O_2 \text{ consumption}}{[O_2]_{\text{pulmonary vein}} - [O_2]_{\text{pulmonary artery}}}$$

$$\text{Cardiac output} = \frac{250 \text{ mL } O_2/\text{min}}{0.20 \text{ mL } O_2/\text{mL blood} - 0.15 \text{ mL } O_2/\text{mL blood}}$$

$$= 5000 \text{ mL/min}$$

Not only is the Fick principle applicable to measurement of cardiac output (essentially the blood flow to the whole body), but it also can be applied to the measurement of blood flow to individual organs. For example, renal blood flow can be measured by dividing the O_2 consumption of the kidneys by the difference in O_2 content of renal arterial blood and renal venous blood.

CARDIAC CYCLE

Figure 4-25 illustrates the mechanical and electrical events that occur during a **single cardiac cycle.** The cycle is divided into seven phases (Fig. 4-25, letters *A* through *G*), which are separated by vertical lines in the figure. The ECG marks the electrical events of the cardiac cycle. Left ventricular pressure and volume, aortic and left atrial pressures, venous pulse, and heart sounds are all plotted simultaneously. The points at which the mitral and aortic valves open and close are shown by arrows.

Figure 4-25 is best studied vertically, one phase at a time, so that all of the cardiovascular parameters in a given phase of the cycle can be correlated. The ECG can be used as a time/event marker. The cycle begins with depolarization and contraction of the atria. Table 4-5 can be used in conjunction with Figure 4-25 to learn the events of the cardiac cycle.

Atrial Systole (A)

Atrial systole is atrial contraction. It is preceded by the **P wave** on the ECG, which marks depolarization of the atria. **Contraction of the left atrium** causes an increase in left atrial pressure. When this increase in atrial pressure is reflected back to the veins, it appears on the venous pulse record as the **a wave.** The left ventricle is relaxed during this phase, and because the mitral valve (AV valve of the left side of the heart) is open, the ventricle is filling with blood from the atrium, even prior to atrial systole. Atrial systole causes a further increase in ventricular volume as blood is actively ejected from the left atrium to the left ventricle through the open mitral valve. The corresponding "blip" in left ventricular pressure reflects this additional volume added to the ventricle from atrial systole. The **fourth heart sound (S_4)** is not audible in normal adults, although it may be heard in ventricular hypertrophy, where ventricular compliance is decreased. When present, S_4 coincides with atrial contraction. The sound is caused by the atrium contracting against, and trying to fill, a stiffened ventricle.

Isovolumetric Ventricular Contraction (B)

Isovolumetric ventricular contraction begins during the QRS complex, which represents the electrical activation

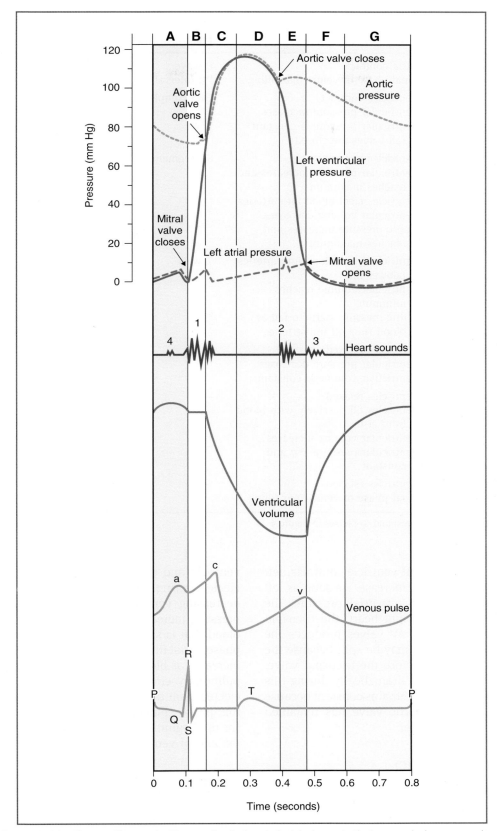

Figure 4–25 **The cardiac cycle.** The mechanical and electrical events that occur during one cycle are shown. Atrial systole (*A*); isovolumetric ventricular contraction (*B*); rapid ventricular ejection (*C*); reduced ventricular ejection (*D*); isovolumetric ventricular relaxation (*E*); rapid ventricular filling (*F*); reduced ventricular filling (diastasis) (*G*).

Table 4–5 Events of the Cardiac Cycle

Phase of Cardiac Cycle*	Major Events	Electrocardiogram	Valves	Heart Sounds
Atrial Systole (A)	Atria contract Final phase of ventricular filling	P wave PR interval	—	Fourth heart sound
Isovolumetric Ventricular Contraction (B)	Ventricles contract Ventricular pressure increases Ventricular pressure is constant (all valves are closed)	QRS complex	Mitral valve closes	First heart sound
Rapid Ventricular Ejection (C)	Ventricles contract Ventricular pressure increases and reaches maximum Ventricles eject blood into arteries Ventricular volume decreases Aortic pressure increases and reaches maximum	ST segment	Aortic valve opens	—
Reduced Ventricular Ejection (D)	Ventricles eject blood into arteries (slower rate) Ventricular volume reaches minimum Aortic pressure starts to fall as blood runs off into arteries	T wave	—	—
Isovolumetric Ventricular Relaxation (E)	Ventricles relaxed Ventricular pressure decreases Ventricular volume is constant	—	Aortic valve closes	Second heart sound
Rapid Ventricular Filling (F)	Ventricles relaxed Ventricles fill passively with blood from atria Ventricular volume increases Ventricular pressure low and constant	—	Mitral valve opens	Third heart sound
Reduced Ventricular Filling, or Diastasis (G)	Ventricles relaxed Final phase of ventricular filling	—	—	—

*Lettered phases of cardiac cycle correspond to phases in Figure 4-25.

of the ventricles. When the left ventricle contracts, left ventricular pressure begins to increase. As soon as left ventricular pressure exceeds left atrial pressure, the **mitral valve closes**. (In the right heart, the tricuspid valve closes.) Closure of the AV valves produces the **first heart sound (S_1)**, which may be split because the mitral valve closes slightly before the tricuspid valve. Ventricular pressure increases dramatically during this phase, but ventricular volume remains constant because all valves are closed (the aortic valve has remained closed from the previous cycle).

Rapid Ventricular Ejection (C)

The ventricle continues to contract, and ventricular pressure reaches its highest value. When ventricular pressure becomes greater than aortic pressure, the **aortic valve opens.** Now blood is rapidly ejected from the left ventricle into the aorta through the open aortic valve, driven by the pressure gradient between the left ventricle and the aorta. Most of the stroke volume is ejected during rapid ventricular ejection, dramatically decreasing ventricular volume. Concomitantly, aortic pressure increases as a result of the large volume of blood that is suddenly added to the aorta. During this phase, atrial filling begins and left atrial pressure slowly increases as blood is returned to the left heart from the pulmonary circulation. This blood will, of course, be ejected from the left heart in the *next cycle.* The end of this phase coincides with the end of the ST segment (or the beginning of the T wave) on the ECG and with the end of ventricular contraction.

Reduced Ventricular Ejection (D)

During reduced ventricular ejection, the ventricles begin to repolarize, which is marked by the beginning of the **T wave** on the ECG. Ventricular pressure falls because the ventricles are no longer contracting. Because the aortic valve is still open, blood continues to be ejected from the left ventricle into the aorta, albeit at a reduced rate; ventricular volume also continues to fall, but at a reduced rate. Even though blood continues to be added to the aorta from the left ventricle, blood is "running off" into the arterial tree at an even faster rate, causing aortic pressure to fall. Left atrial pressure continues to increase as blood returns to the left heart from the lungs.

Isovolumetric Ventricular Relaxation (E)

Isovolumetric ventricular relaxation begins after the ventricles are fully repolarized, marked by the end of the T wave on the ECG. Because the left ventricle is relaxed, left ventricular pressure decreases dramatically. When left ventricular pressure falls below aortic pressure, the **aortic valve closes.** The aortic valve closes slightly before the pulmonic valve, producing the **second heart sound** (S_2). Inspiration delays closure of the pulmonic valve and causes **splitting** of the second heart sound; that is, during inspiration, the pulmonic valve closes *distinctly after* the aortic valve. Splitting occurs during inspiration because the associated decrease in intrathoracic pressure produces an increase in venous return to the right side of the heart. The resulting increase in right ventricular end-diastolic volume causes an increase in right ventricular stroke volume by the Frank-Starling mechanism and prolongs right ventricular ejection time; the prolongation of ejection time delays closure of the pulmonic valve relative to the aortic valve. At the point where the aortic valve closes, the aortic pressure curve shows a "blip," called the **dicrotic notch** or **incisura.** Because all valves are closed again, no blood can be ejected from the left ventricle, nor can the left ventricle fill with blood from the atria. Therefore, during this phase, ventricular volume is constant (isovolumetric).

Rapid Ventricular Filling (F)

When ventricular pressure falls to its lowest level (and slightly below left atrial pressure), the **mitral valve opens.** Once the mitral valve opens, the ventricle begins to fill with blood from the left atrium, and ventricular volume increases rapidly. Ventricular pressure remains low, however, because the ventricle is still relaxed and compliant. (The high compliance of the ventricle means that volume can be added to it without changing pressure.) The rapid flow of blood from the atria to the ventricles produces the **third heart sound** (S_3), which is normal in children but is not heard in normal adults; in middle-aged or older adults, the presence of S_3 indicates volume overload, as in congestive heart failure or advanced mitral or tricuspid regurgitation. During this phase (and for the remainder of the cardiac cycle),

aortic pressure decreases as blood runs off from the aorta into the arterial tree, to the veins, and then back to the heart.

Reduced Ventricular Filling (Diastasis) (G)

Reduced ventricular filling, or **diastasis,** is the longest phase of the cardiac cycle and includes the final portion of ventricular filling, which occurs at a slower rate than in the previous phase. Atrial systole marks the end of diastole, at which point ventricular volume is equal to end-diastolic volume.

Changes in heart rate alter the time available for diastasis because it is the longest phase of the cardiac cycle. For example, increases in heart rate reduce the time interval before the next P wave (i.e., the next cycle) and reduce, or even eliminate, this final portion of ventricular filling. If diastasis is reduced by such an increase in heart rate, ventricular filling will be compromised, end-diastolic volume will be reduced, and, as a consequence, stroke volume also will be reduced (recall the Frank-Starling relationship).

RELATIONSHIPS BETWEEN CARDIAC OUTPUT AND VENOUS RETURN

It should be clear from the previous discussion that one of the most important factors determining cardiac output is left ventricular end-diastolic volume. In turn, left ventricular end-diastolic volume depends on venous return, which also determines right atrial pressure. Thus, it follows that there is *not only* a relationship between cardiac output and end-diastolic volume but *also* a relationship between cardiac output and right atrial pressure.

Cardiac output and venous return each can be examined separately as a function of right atrial pressure. These separate relationships also can be combined in a single graph to visualize the normal interrelationship between cardiac output and venous return (see Fig. 4-25). The combined graphs can be used to predict the effects of changes in various cardiovascular parameters on cardiac output, venous return, and right atrial pressure.

Cardiac Function Curve

The cardiac function curve or cardiac output curve, shown in Figure 4-26, is based on the **Frank-Starling relationship** for the left ventricle. The cardiac function curve is a plot of the relationship between cardiac output of the left ventricle and right atrial pressure. Again, recall that right atrial pressure is related to venous return, end-diastolic volume, and end-diastolic

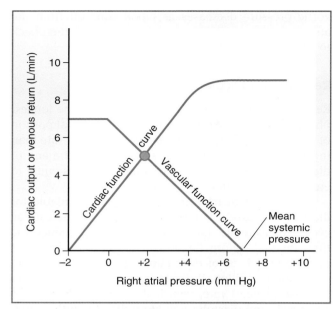

Figure 4–26 **Cardiac and vascular function curves.** The cardiac function curve is cardiac output as a function of right atrial pressure. The vascular function curve is venous return as a function of right atrial pressure. The curves intersect at the steady state operating point (*filled circle*) where cardiac output and venous return are equal.

fiber length: As venous return increases, right atrial pressure increases, and end-diastolic volume and end-diastolic fiber length increase. Increases in end-diastolic fiber length produce increases in cardiac output. Thus, in the steady state, the volume of blood the left ventricle ejects as cardiac output equals or matches the volume it receives in venous return.

Increases in end-diastolic volume (i.e., right atrial pressure) produce increases in cardiac output by the Frank-Starling mechanism. However, this "matching" occurs only *up to a point:* When right atrial pressure reaches a value of approximately 4 mm Hg, cardiac output can no longer keep up with venous return and the cardiac function curve levels off. This maximum level of cardiac output is approximately 9 L/min.

Vascular Function Curve

The vascular function curve or venous return curve, shown in Figure 4-26, depicts the relationship between venous return and right atrial pressure. Venous return is blood flow through the systemic circulation and back to the right heart. The *inverse relationship* between venous return and right atrial pressure is explained as follows: Venous return back to the heart, like all blood flow, is driven by a pressure gradient. The lower the pressure in the right atrium, the higher the pressure gradient between the systemic arteries and the right atrium and the greater the venous return. Thus, as right

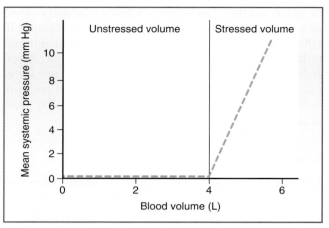

Figure 4–27 **Effect of changes in stressed volume on mean systemic pressure.** Total blood volume is the sum of unstressed volume (in the veins) and stressed volume (in the arteries). Increases in stressed volume produce increases in mean systemic pressure.

atrial pressure increases, this pressure gradient decreases and venous return also decreases.

The **knee** (flat portion) of the vascular function curve occurs at negative values of right atrial pressure. At such negative values, the veins collapse, impeding blood flow back to the heart. Although the pressure gradient has increased (i.e., as right atrial pressure becomes negative), venous return levels off because the veins have collapsed.

Mean Systemic Pressure

The value for right atrial pressure at which venous return is zero is called the mean systemic pressure. It is the point at which the vascular function curve intersects the X-axis (i.e., where venous return is zero and right atrial pressure is at its highest value). **Mean systemic pressure** or mean circulatory pressure is the pressure that would be measured throughout the cardiovascular system if the heart were stopped. Under these conditions, pressure would be the same throughout the vasculature and, by our definition, would be equal to the mean systemic pressure. When pressures are equal throughout the vasculature, there is no blood flow, and therefore, venous return is zero (because there is no pressure gradient or driving force).

Two factors influence the value for mean systemic pressure: (1) the **blood volume** and (2) the **distribution of blood** between the unstressed volume and the stressed volume. In turn, the value for mean systemic pressure determines the intersection point (zero flow) of the vascular function curve with the X-axis.

Figure 4-27 reviews the concepts of unstressed volume and stressed volume and relates them to mean systemic pressure. The **unstressed volume** (thought of as the *volume of blood that the veins can hold*) is the volume of blood in the vasculature that produces no pressure. The **stressed volume** (thought of as the *volume in the arteries*) is the volume that produces pressure by stretching the elastic fibers in the blood vessel walls.

♦ Consider the effect of **changing blood volume** on mean systemic pressure. When the blood volume ranges from 0 to 4 L, all of the blood will be in the unstressed volume (the veins), producing no pressure, and the mean systemic pressure will be zero. When blood volume is greater than 4 L, some of the blood will be in the stressed volume (the arteries) and produce pressure. For example, if the total blood volume is 5 L, 4 L is in the unstressed volume, producing no pressure, and 1 L is in the stressed volume, producing a pressure of approximately 7 mm Hg (on the graph, read mean systemic pressure as 7 mm Hg at a blood volume of 5 L).

It now should be clear how changes in blood volume can alter the mean systemic pressure (see Fig. 4-26). If **blood volume increases,** the amount of blood in the unstressed volume will be unaffected (if it is already full), but the amount of blood in the stressed volume will increase. When stressed volume increases, mean systemic pressure increases and the vascular function curve and its intersection point with the X-axis shift to the right. If **blood volume decreases,** then stressed volume decreases, mean systemic pressure decreases, and the vascular function curve and its intersection point with the X-axis shift to the left.

♦ **Redistribution of blood** between the unstressed volume and the stressed volume also produces changes in mean systemic pressure. For example, if the **compliance of the veins decreases** (e.g., venoconstriction), the veins can hold less blood and blood shifts from the unstressed volume to the stressed volume. Although total blood volume is unchanged, the shift of blood increases the mean systemic pressure and shifts the vascular function curve to the right. Conversely, if **the compliance of the veins increases** (e.g., venodilation), the veins can hold more blood. Hence, the unstressed volume will increase, the stressed volume and mean systemic pressure will decrease and the vascular function curve shifts to the left.

In summary, increased blood volume and decreased compliance of the veins produce an increase in mean systemic pressure and shift the vascular function curve to the right. Decreased blood volume and increased compliance of the veins produce a decrease in mean systemic pressure and shift the vascular function curve to the left.

Slope of the Vascular Function Curve

If mean systemic pressure is fixed or constant, the slope of the vascular function curve can be changed by rotating it. The slope of the vascular function curve is determined by **total peripheral resistance (TPR).** Recall that TPR is determined primarily by the resistance of the arterioles. The effect of TPR on venous return and the vascular function curve is explained as follows (see Fig. 4-26):

♦ A **decrease in TPR** causes a *clockwise* rotation of the vascular function curve. A clockwise rotation means that, for a given right atrial pressure, venous return is increased. In other words, decreased resistance of the arterioles (decreased TPR) makes it *easier* for blood to flow from the arterial to the venous side of the circulation and back to the heart.

♦ An **increase in TPR** causes a *counterclockwise* rotation of the vascular function curve. A counterclockwise rotation means that, for a given right atrial pressure, venous return is decreased. In other words, increased resistance of the arterioles (increased TPR) makes it *more difficult* for blood to flow from the arterial to the venous side of the circulation and back to the heart.

Combining Cardiac and Vascular Function Curves

The interaction between cardiac output and venous return can be visualized by combining the cardiac and vascular function curves (see Fig. 4-26). The point at which the two curves intersect is the unique operating or equilibrium point of the system in the **steady state.** In the steady state, cardiac output and venous return are, by definition, equal at the point of intersection. Why then do the cardiac and vascular function curves go in opposite directions and why do they have opposite relationships with right atrial pressure?

The answers lie in the way the two curves are determined. The cardiac function curve is determined as follows: as right atrial pressure and end-diastolic volume are increased, there is increased ventricular fiber length, which leads to increased stroke volume and cardiac output. The higher the right atrial pressure, the higher the cardiac output—this is the Frank-Starling relationship for the heart.

The vascular function curve is determined as follows: as right atrial pressure is decreased, venous return increases because of the greater pressure gradient driving blood flow back to the heart. The lower the right atrial pressure, the higher the venous return.

Now, to the questions! We have established that cardiac and vascular function curves have opposite

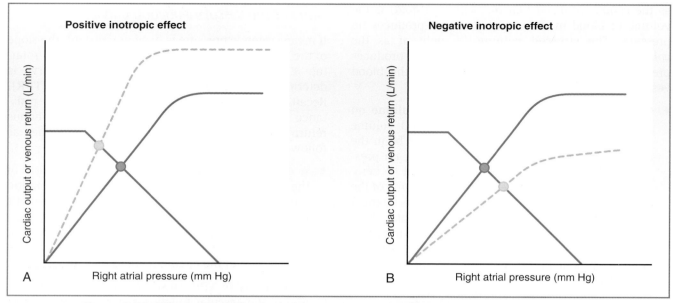

Figure 4-28 **Effects of positive inotropic agents (A) and negative inotropic agents (B) on the cardiac and vascular function curves.** The *solid lines* show the normal relationships, and the *dashed lines* show changes. The *circle* intersecting the dashed line shows the new steady state operating point.

relationships with right atrial pressure. But how can this be true if cardiac output and venous return are always equal? When cardiac output and venous return are plotted simultaneously as a function of right atrial pressure, they intersect at a single value of right atrial pressure (see Fig. 4-26). At this one value of right atrial pressure, cardiac output equals venous return and, by definition, is the steady state operating point of the system. That one value of right atrial pressure satisfies both cardiac output and venous return relationships.

Combining these curves provides a useful tool for predicting the **changes in cardiac output** that will occur when various cardiovascular parameters are altered. Cardiac output can be altered by changes in the cardiac function curve, by changes in the vascular function curve, or by simultaneous changes in both curves. The basic premise of this approach is that, after such a change, the system will move to a **new steady state.** In the new steady state, the operating point at which the cardiac and the vascular function curves intersect will have changed. This new operating point tells what the *new* cardiac output and the *new* venous return are in the *new* steady state.

Changes in cardiac output can be produced by any of the following mechanisms: (1) positive or negative inotropic effects that alter the cardiac function curve; (2) changes in blood volume or venous compliance that alter the vascular function curve by changing mean systemic pressure; and (3) changes in TPR that alter both the cardiac and vascular function curves.

Inotropic Effects

Inotropic agents alter the cardiac function curve (Fig. 4-28). Recall that positive inotropic agents cause an increase in contractility for a given end-diastolic volume (or right atrial pressure), and negative inotropic agents produce a decrease in contractility.

♦ The effect of a **positive inotropic agent** (e.g., ouabain, digitalis, or digoxin) on the cardiac function curve is shown in Figure 4-28A. Positive inotropic agents produce an increase in contractility, an increase in stroke volume, and an increase in cardiac output for any level of right atrial pressure. Thus, the cardiac function curve shifts upward, but the vascular function curve is unaffected. The point of intersection (the steady state point) of the two curves now has shifted upward and to the left. In the new steady state, **cardiac output is increased** and **right atrial pressure is decreased**. The decrease in right atrial pressure reflects the fact that *more* blood is ejected from the heart on each beat as a result of the increased contractility and increased stroke volume.

♦ Figure 4-28B shows the effect of a **negative inotropic agent**. The effect is just the opposite of a positive inotropic agent: There is a decrease in contractility and a decrease in cardiac output for any level of right atrial pressure. The cardiac function curve shifts downward, and the vascular function curve is unchanged. In the new steady state, **cardiac output is decreased** and **right atrial pressure is increased**.

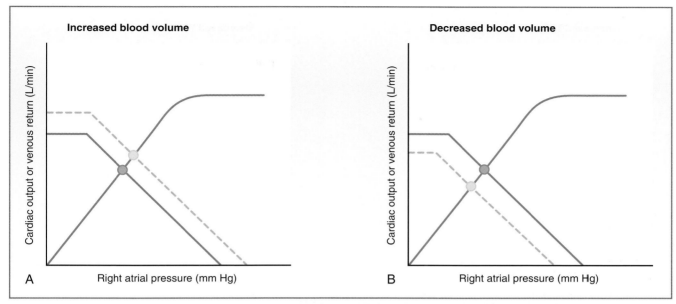

Figure 4-29 **Effects of increased blood volume (A) and decreased blood volume (B) on the cardiac and vascular function curves.** The *solid lines* show the normal relationships, and the *dashed lines* show changes. The *circle* intersecting the dashed line shows the new steady state operating point.

Right atrial pressure is increased because *less* blood is ejected from the heart on each beat, due to decreased contractility and decreased stroke volume.

Effects of Changes in Blood Volume

Changes in blood volume alter mean systemic pressure and, thereby, alter the vascular function curve (Fig. 4-29).

♦ The effects of **increases in blood volume** (e.g., transfusion) are shown in Figure 4-29*A*. Increases in blood volume increase the amount of blood in the stressed volume and, therefore, increase the mean systemic pressure. Mean systemic pressure is the point on the vascular function curve where venous return is zero. Increases in blood volume shift this intersection point to the right and, therefore, shift the curve to the right in a parallel manner. (The shift is parallel because there is no accompanying change in TPR, which determines the slope of the vascular function curve.) In the new steady state, the cardiac and vascular function curves intersect at a new point at which **cardiac output is increased** and **right atrial pressure is increased**.

♦ The effects of **decreases in blood volume** (e.g., hemorrhage) are shown in Figure 4-29*B*. The decrease in blood volume decreases the amount of blood in the stressed volume and mean systemic pressure, which shifts the vascular function curve to the left in a parallel manner. In the new steady state, **cardiac output is decreased** and **right atrial pressure is decreased**.

♦ Changes in venous compliance produce effects similar to those produced by changes in blood volume. **Decreases in venous compliance** cause a shift of blood *out of* the unstressed volume and *into* the stressed volume and produce changes similar to those caused by increases in blood volume, a parallel shift to the right. Likewise, **increases in venous compliance** cause a shift of blood *into* the unstressed volume and *out of* the stressed volume and produce changes similar to those caused by decreased blood volume, a parallel shift to the left.

Effects of Changes in Total Peripheral Resistance

Changes in TPR reflect changes in the degree of constriction of the arterioles. Such changes alter the extent to which blood is "held" on the arterial side of the circulation (i.e., in the stressed volume). Thus, changes in TPR alter both arterial blood pressure and venous return to the heart. For example, an increase in TPR, by restricting the flow of blood out of the arteries, produces an increase in arterial blood pressure and, concomitantly, a decrease in venous return.

The effects of changes in TPR on the cardiac and vascular function curves are, therefore, more complicated than those produced by changes in contractility or blood volume. Changes in TPR alter *both* curves: The cardiac function curve changes because of a change in afterload (arterial blood pressure), and the vascular function curve changes because of a change in venous return (Fig. 4-30).

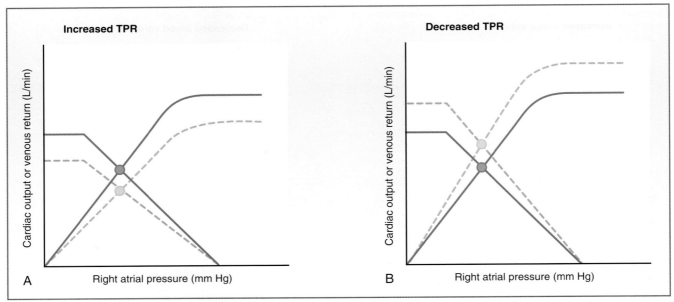

Figure 4–30 **Effects of increased total peripheral resistance (TPR) (A) and decreased TPR (B) on the cardiac and vascular function curves.** The *solid lines* show the normal relationships, and the *dashed lines* show the changes. The *circle* intersecting the *dashed lines* shows the new steady state operating point.

♦ The effects of an **increase in TPR** (i.e., constriction of the arterioles) are shown in Figure 4-30A. (1) Increases in TPR cause an increase in arterial pressure by "holding" blood in the arteries. This increase in arterial pressure produces an increase in afterload on the heart, which decreases cardiac output. The cardiac function curve shifts downward as a result of the increased afterload. (2) The increase in TPR produces a counterclockwise rotation of the vascular function curve. This rotation means that less blood returns to the heart for a given right atrial pressure—venous return is decreased. (3) The combination of these two changes is shown in Figure 4-30A. The curves intersect at a new steady state point at which both cardiac output and venous return are decreased.

In the figure, right atrial pressure is shown as unchanged. Actually, the final effect of increased TPR on right atrial pressure is not predictable because TPR has different directional effects via the cardiac and vascular function curves. An increase in TPR decreases cardiac output, which *increases* right atrial pressure (less blood is pumped out of the heart). And, an increase in TPR decreases venous return, which *decreases* right atrial pressure (less flow back to the heart). Depending on the relative magnitude of the effects on the cardiac and vascular function curves, right atrial pressure can be slightly increased, slightly decreased, or unchanged. The figure shows it as unchanged—the compromise position.

♦ The effects of a **decrease in TPR** (i.e., dilation of the arterioles) are shown in Figure 4-30B. (1)

Decreases in TPR cause a decrease in arterial pressure and a decrease in afterload, causing the cardiac function curve to shift upward. (2) The decrease in TPR produces a clockwise rotation of the vascular function curve, which means that more blood returns to the heart for a given right atrial pressure—venous return is increased. The curves intersect at a new steady state point at which both cardiac output and venous return are increased.

In the figure, right atrial pressure is shown as unchanged. However, the effect of decreased TPR on right atrial pressure is not easily predicted because a change in TPR has different effects via the cardiac and vascular function curves. A decrease in TPR increases cardiac output, which *decreases* right atrial pressure (more blood is pumped out of the heart). And a decrease in TPR increases venous return, which *increases* right atrial pressure (increased flow back to the heart). Depending on the relative magnitude of the effects, right atrial pressure can be slightly increased, slightly decreased, or unchanged. In the figure, it is shown as the compromise, or unchanged.

REGULATION OF ARTERIAL PRESSURE

The overall function of the cardiovascular system is to deliver blood to the tissues so that O_2 and nutrients can be provided and waste products carried away. Blood flow to the tissues is driven by the difference in pressure between the arterial and venous sides of the circulation. **Mean arterial pressure (P_a)** is the driving force for blood flow, and it must be maintained at a high, constant level of approximately **100 mm Hg.** Because of the parallel arrangement of arteries off the aorta, the pressure in the major artery serving each organ is equal to P_a. (The blood flow to each organ is then independently regulated by changing the resistance of its arterioles through local control mechanisms.)

The mechanisms that help to maintain P_a at a constant value are discussed in this section. The basis for this regulation can be appreciated by examining the equation for P_a:

$$P_a = \text{Cardiac output} \times TPR$$

where

$$P_a = \text{Mean arterial pressure (mm Hg)}$$
$$\text{Cardiac output} = \text{Cardiac output (mL/min)}$$
$$TPR = \text{Total peripheral resistance}$$
$$\text{(mm Hg/mL/min)}$$

Notice that the equation for P_a is simply a variation of the familiar equation for pressure, flow, and resistance, used previously in this chapter. Inspection of the equation reveals that P_a can be changed by altering the cardiac output (or any of its parameters), altering the TPR (or any of its parameters), or altering both cardiac output and TPR.

Be aware that this equation is *deceptively simple,* because cardiac output and TPR are *not* independent variables. In other words, changes in TPR can alter cardiac output and changes in cardiac output can alter TPR. Therefore, it cannot be stated that if TPR doubles, P_a also doubles. (In fact, when TPR doubles, cardiac output simultaneously is almost halved and P_a will increase only modestly.) Likewise, it cannot be stated that if cardiac output is halved, P_a also will be halved. (Rather, if cardiac output is halved, there is a compensatory increase in TPR and P_a will decrease but not be halved.)

This section discusses the mechanisms responsible for maintaining a constant value for arterial pressure. These mechanisms closely monitor P_a and compare it with the **set-point** value of approximately 100 mm Hg. If P_a increases above the set point or decreases below the set point, the cardiovascular system makes adjustments in cardiac output, in TPR, or in both, attempting to return P_a to the set-point value.

P_a is regulated by two major systems. The first system is neurally mediated and known as the **baroreceptor reflex.** The baroreceptor reflex attempts to restore P_a to its set-point value in a matter of seconds. The second system is hormonally mediated and includes the **renin-angiotensin-aldosterone** system, which regulates P_a more slowly, primarily by its effect on blood volume.

Baroreceptor Reflex

The baroreceptor mechanisms are fast, neurally mediated reflexes that attempt to keep arterial pressure constant via changes in the output of the sympathetic and parasympathetic nervous systems to the heart and blood vessels (Fig. 4-31). Pressure sensors, the **baroreceptors,** are located within the walls of the carotid sinus and the aortic arch and relay information about blood pressure to cardiovascular vasomotor centers in the brain stem. The vasomotor centers, in turn, coordinate a change in output of the autonomic nervous system to effect the desired change in P_a. Thus, the reflex arc consists of sensors for blood pressure; afferent neurons, which carry the information to the brain stem; brain stem centers, which process the information and coordinate an appropriate response; and efferent neurons, which direct changes in the heart and blood vessels.

Baroreceptors

The baroreceptors are located in the walls of the **carotid sinus,** where the common carotid artery bifurcates into the internal and external carotid arteries, and in the **aortic arch.** The carotid sinus baroreceptors are responsive to increases or decreases in arterial pressure, whereas the aortic arch baroreceptors are primarily responsive to increases in arterial pressure.

The baroreceptors are **mechanoreceptors,** which are sensitive to pressure or stretch. Thus, changes in arterial pressure cause more or less stretch on the mechanoreceptors, resulting in a change in their membrane potential. Such a change in membrane potential is a receptor potential, which increases or decreases the likelihood that action potentials will be fired in the afferent nerves that travel from the baroreceptors to the brain stem. (If the receptor potential is depolarizing, then action potential frequency increases; if the receptor potential is hyperpolarizing, then action potential frequency decreases.)

Increases in arterial pressure cause increased stretch on the baroreceptors and increased firing rate in the afferent nerves. Decreases in arterial pressure cause decreased stretch on the baroreceptors and decreased firing rate in the afferent nerves.

Although the baroreceptors are sensitive to the absolute level of pressure, they are even more sensitive to *changes in pressure* and the *rate of change of pressure.* The strongest stimulus for the baroreceptors is a rapid change in arterial pressure!

The sensitivity of the baroreceptors can be altered by disease. For example, in **chronic hypertension** (elevated blood pressure), the baroreceptors do not "see" the elevated blood pressure as abnormal. In such cases, the hypertension will be maintained, rather than corrected, by the baroreceptor reflex. The mechanism of

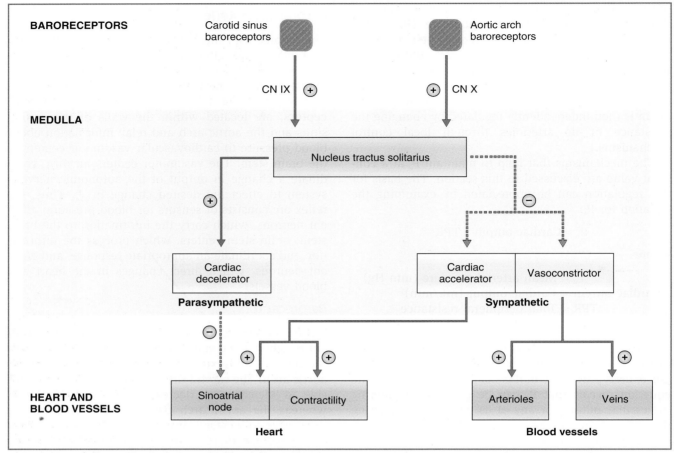

Figure 4–31 **Response of baroreceptor reflex to increased arterial pressure.** The + symbol shows increases in activity; the – symbol shows decreases in activity; the *dashed lines* show inhibitory pathways.

this defect is either decreased sensitivity of the baroreceptors to increases in arterial pressure or an increase in the blood pressure set point of the brain stem centers.

Information from the carotid sinus baroreceptors is carried to the brain stem on the **carotid sinus nerve,** which joins the glossopharyngeal nerve (cranial nerve [CN] IX). Information from the aortic arch baroreceptors is carried to the brain stem on the **vagus nerve (CN X).**

Brain Stem Cardiovascular Centers

Brain stem cardiovascular centers are located in the reticular formations of the **medulla** and in the lower one third of the **pons.** These centers function in a coordinated fashion, receiving information about blood pressure from the baroreceptors and then directing changes in output of the sympathetic and parasympathetic nervous systems to correct the blood pressure as needed.

As described, blood pressure is sensed by baroreceptors in the carotid sinus and aortic arch. Afferent information about blood pressure is then sent to the medulla

via the glossopharyngeal (CN IX) and vagus (CN X) nerves. This information is integrated in the **nucleus tractus solitarius,** which then directs changes in the activity of several cardiovascular centers. These cardiovascular centers are tonically active, and the nucleus tractus solitarius simply directs, via the centers, increases or decreases in outflow from the sympathetic and parasympathetic nervous systems.

The **parasympathetic** outflow is the effect of the vagus nerve on the SA node to decrease the heart rate. The **sympathetic** outflow has four components: an effect on the SA node to increase heart rate, an effect on cardiac muscle to increase contractility and stroke volume, an effect on the arterioles to produce vasoconstriction and increase TPR, and an effect on veins to produce venoconstriction and decrease unstressed volume.

The cardiovascular brain stem centers are as follows:

◆ The **vasoconstrictor center** (also called C1) is located in the upper medulla and the lower pons. Efferent neurons from this vasomotor center are part of the sympathetic nervous system and synapse in the spinal cord, then in sympathetic ganglia, and finally on the target organs, producing vasoconstriction in the arterioles and venules.

♦ The **cardiac accelerator center.** Efferent neurons from the cardiac accelerator center are also part of the sympathetic nervous system and synapse in the spinal cord, in sympathetic ganglia, and finally in the heart. In the heart, the effects of this activity are an increased firing rate of the SA node (to increase heart rate), increased conduction velocity through the AV node, and increased contractility.

♦ The **cardiac decelerator center.** Efferent fibers from the cardiac decelerator center are part of the parasympathetic nervous system: They travel in the vagus nerve and synapse on the SA node to decrease heart rate.

Integrated Function of the Baroreceptor Reflex

The function of the baroreceptor reflex can be illustrated by examining its **response to an increase in arterial pressure** as follows (see Fig. 4-31):

1. An **increase in P_a** is detected by baroreceptors in the carotid sinus and in the aortic arch. This increase in pressure results in increased firing rate of the **carotid sinus nerve** (glossopharyngeal nerve, CN IX) and in afferent fibers in the vagus nerve (CN X).

2. The glossopharyngeal and vagus nerve fibers synapse in the **nucleus tractus solitarius** of the medulla, where they transmit information about blood pressure. In this example, the P_a sensed by the baroreceptors is higher than the set-point pressure in the medulla.

3. The nucleus tractus solitarius directs a series of coordinated responses, using the medullary cardiovascular centers, to reduce P_a back to normal. These responses include an increase in parasympathetic outflow to the heart and a decrease in sympathetic outflow to the heart and blood vessels.

4. The increase in parasympathetic activity to the SA node (via the vagus nerve) results in a **decrease in heart rate.** The decrease in sympathetic activity to the SA node complements the increase in parasympathetic activity and also decreases heart rate. Decreased sympathetic activity also **decreases cardiac contractility.** Together, the decreased heart rate and decreased cardiac contractility produce a **decrease in cardiac output,** which tends to reduce P_a back to normal. (Recall that P_a = Cardiac output × TPR.)

The decrease in sympathetic activity also affects the tone of the blood vessels. First, there is decreased constriction of arterioles, or arteriolar vasodilation, which **decreases TPR** and reduces P_a. (Again, recall that P_a = Cardiac output × TPR.) Second, there is decreased constriction of veins, which increases the compliance of the veins, thereby **increasing the unstressed volume.** When unstressed volume increases, stressed volume decreases, which further contributes to a reduction in P_a.

5. Once these coordinated reflexes reduce P_a back to the set-point pressure (i.e., to 100 mm Hg), then activity of the baroreceptors and the cardiovascular brain stem centers will return to the tonic (baseline) level.

Response of the Baroreceptor Reflex to Hemorrhage

A second example of the operation of the baroreceptor reflex is the response to loss of blood volume or hemorrhage. **Hemorrhage** produces a decrease in P_a because, as blood volume decreases, stressed volume also decreases (see Fig. 4-27). In response to an acute reduction in P_a, the baroreceptor reflex is activated and attempts to restore blood pressure back toward normal (Fig. 4-32).

The responses of the baroreceptor reflex to a decrease in P_a are the exact opposite of those described previously for the response to an increase in P_a. Decreases in P_a produce decreased stretch on the baroreceptors and decreased firing rate of the carotid sinus nerve. This information is received in the nucleus tractus solitarius of the medulla, which produces a coordinated decrease in parasympathetic activity to the heart and an increase in sympathetic activity to the heart and blood vessels. Heart rate and contractility increase, which, together, produce an **increase in cardiac output.** There is increased constriction of arterioles, which produces an **increase in TPR,** and increased constriction of the veins, which **decreases unstressed volume.** The constriction of the veins increases venous return to contribute to the increase in cardiac output (Frank-Starling mechanism).

Test of Baroreceptor Reflex: Valsalva Maneuver

The integrity of the baroreceptor reflex can be tested with the **Valsalva maneuver,** which is expiring against a closed glottis as during coughing, defecation, or heavy lifting. When the subject expires against a closed glottis, there is an increase in intrathoracic pressure, which decreases venous return to the heart. This decrease in venous return produces a decrease in cardiac output (Frank-Starling mechanism) and a consequent decrease in arterial pressure. If the

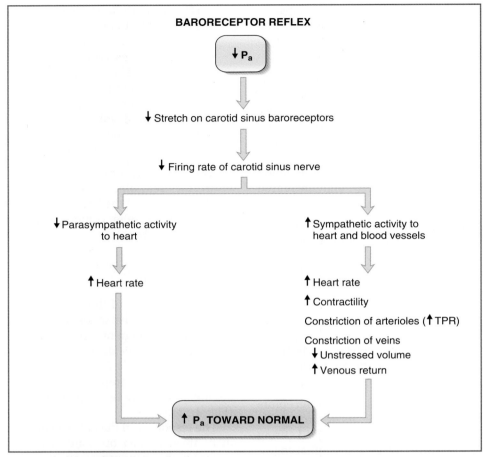

Figure 4–32 Response of the baroreceptor reflex to acute hemorrhage. The reflex is initiated by a decrease in mean arterial pressure (P_a). The compensatory responses attempt to increase P_a back to normal. TPR, Total peripheral resistance.

baroreceptor reflex is intact, the decrease in arterial pressure is sensed by the baroreceptors, and the nucleus tractus solitarius directs an increase in sympathetic outflow and a decrease in parasympathetic outflow to the heart and blood vessels. In the test, an increase in heart rate is noted. When the subject stops the maneuver, there is a rebound increase in venous return, cardiac output, and arterial pressure. The increase in arterial pressure is sensed by the baroreceptors, and they direct a decrease in heart rate.

Renin–Angiotensin II–Aldosterone System

The renin–angiotensin II–aldosterone system regulates P_a primarily by regulating blood volume. This system is much slower than the baroreceptor reflex because it is hormonally, rather than neurally, mediated.

The renin–angiotensin II–aldosterone system is activated in response to a decrease in the P_a. Activation of this system, in turn, produces a series of responses that attempt to restore arterial pressure to normal. This mechanism, shown in Figure 4-33, has the following steps:

1. A decrease in P_a causes a decrease in renal perfusion pressure, which is sensed by mechanoreceptors in afferent arterioles of the kidney. The decrease in P_a causes **prorenin** to be converted to **renin** in the juxtaglomerular cells (by mechanisms not entirely understood). Renin secretion by the juxtaglomerular cells is also increased by stimulation of renal sympathetic nerves and by β_1 agonists such as isoproterenol; renin secretion is decreased by β_1 antagonists such as propranolol.

2. Renin is an enzyme. In plasma, renin catalyzes the conversion of **angiotensinogen** (renin substrate) to **angiotensin I,** a decapeptide. Angiotensin I has little biologic activity, other than to serve as a precursor to angiotensin II.

3. In the lungs and kidneys, angiotensin I is converted to **angiotensin II,** catalyzed by **angiotensin-converting enzyme** (**ACE**). Angiotensin-converting enzyme inhibitors (**ACEi**), such as **captopril,** block the production of angiotensin II and all of its physiologic actions.

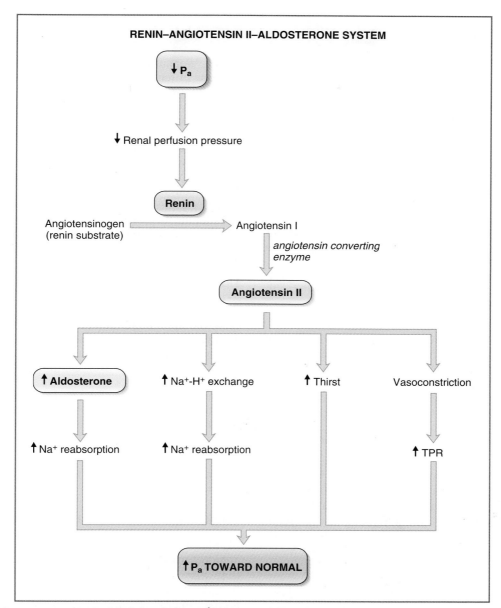

Figure 4-33 **Renin–angiotensin II–aldosterone system.** The system is described in terms of the response to a decrease in P_a. TPR, Total peripheral resistance.

4. **Angiotensin II** is an octapeptide with the following biologic actions in the adrenal cortex, vascular smooth muscle, kidneys, and brain, where it activates Type 1 G protein–coupled angiotensin II receptors (**AT$_1$ receptors**). Inhibitors of AT$_1$ receptors, such as **losartan,** block the actions of angiotensin II at the level of the target tissues.

♦ Angiotensin II acts on the zona glomerulosa cells of the **adrenal cortex** to stimulate the synthesis and secretion of aldosterone. **Aldosterone** then acts on the principal cells of the renal distal tubule and collecting duct to **increase Na$^+$ reabsorption** and, thereby, to increase ECF volume and blood volume. The actions of aldosterone require gene transcription and new protein synthesis in the kidney. These processes require hours to days to occur and account for the slow response time of the renin–angiotensin II–aldosterone system.

♦ Angiotensin II also has its own direct action on the **kidney,** independent of its actions through aldosterone. Angiotensin II **stimulates Na$^+$-H$^+$ exchange** in the renal proximal tubule and increases the reabsorption of Na$^+$ and HCO$_3^-$.

♦ Angiotensin II acts on the hypothalamus to increase **thirst** and water intake. It also

---

BOX 4-2 Clinical Physiology: Renal Vascular Hypertension

DESCRIPTION OF CASE. A 65-year-old woman visits her physician complaining of "not feeling well" and decreased urination. Her diastolic blood pressure is elevated at 115 mm Hg, and she has abdominal bruits (sounds). She is immediately admitted to the hospital and has a workup for hypertension.

Laboratory tests reveal the following information: Her blood pressure continues to be dangerously elevated, and her glomerular filtration rate (GFR) is significantly decreased, at 30 mL/min. Renal vascular disease is suspected. Renal angiography shows 90% stenosis of the right renal artery. Her plasma renin activity is elevated, and renin levels are much higher in right renal venous blood than in left renal venous blood.

An attempt to dilate the right renal artery with angioplasty is unsuccessful. The woman is treated with captopril, an ACE inhibitor.

EXPLANATION OF CASE. The woman has stenosis of her right renal artery, which reduces blood flow to her right kidney. The abdominal bruits are heard because blood flow through the stenosed renal artery is turbulent (i.e., Reynolds number is increased). As a result of the decreased renal blood flow, her GFR and her urine output are decreased.

The woman's hypertension is secondary to the decrease in renal blood flow. Renal perfusion pressure to the right kidney is significantly decreased. The right kidney "thinks" that arterial pressure is low and that aldosterone is needed. Thus, renin secretion by the right kidney increases, which results in renin levels in the right renal vein higher than those in the left renal vein. Increased circulating renin activity results in increased production of angiotensin II and aldosterone. Angiotensin II causes vasoconstriction of arterioles, which elevates TPR and mean arterial pressure. Aldosterone increases renal Na^+ reabsorption, elevating total body Na^+ content, ECF volume, and blood volume. The increase in blood volume leads to the increased diastolic blood pressure.

TREATMENT. Because an attempt to dilate the stenosed renal artery is unsuccessful, the woman is treated with an ACE inhibitor to interrupt the cycle that produced the hypertension (i.e., to block the conversion of angiotensin I to angiotensin II). Although the right kidney will continue to secrete high levels of renin and plasma renin activity will continue to be elevated, angiotensin II will not be produced if the angiotensin converting enzyme is inhibited. Likewise, aldosterone secretion will decrease, and Na^+ reabsorption also will decrease.

---

stimulates secretion of **antidiuretic hormone,** which increases water reabsorption in collecting ducts. By increasing total body water, these effects complement the increases in Na^+ reabsorption (caused by aldosterone and Na^+-H^+ exchange), thereby increasing ECF volume, blood volume, and blood pressure.

♦ Angiotensin II also acts directly on the **arterioles** by binding to G protein–coupled receptors and activating an IP_3/Ca^{2+} second messenger system to cause vasoconstriction. The resulting **increase in TPR** leads to an increase in P_a.

In summary, a decrease in P_a activates the renin–angiotensin II–aldosterone system, producing a set of responses that attempt to increase P_a back to normal. The most important of these responses is the effect of aldosterone to increase renal Na^+ reabsorption. When Na^+ reabsorption is increased, total body Na^+ content increases, which increases ECF volume and blood volume. Increases in blood volume produce an increase in venous return and, through the Frank-Starling mechanism, an increase in cardiac output. The increase in cardiac output produces an increase in P_a. There also is a direct effect of angiotensin II to constrict arterioles,

increasing TPR and contributing to the increase in P_a (Box 4-2).

Other Regulatory Mechanisms

In addition to the baroreceptor reflex and the renin–angiotensin II–aldosterone system, other mechanisms that may aid in regulating mean arterial pressure include chemoreceptors for O_2 in the carotid and aortic bodies, chemoreceptors for CO_2 in the brain, antidiuretic hormone, and atrial natriuretic peptide.

Peripheral Chemoreceptors in Carotid and Aortic Bodies

Peripheral chemoreceptors for O_2 are located in the **carotid bodies** near the bifurcation of the common carotid arteries and in the **aortic bodies** along the aortic arch. The carotid and aortic bodies have high blood flow, and their chemoreceptors are primarily sensitive to decreases in the partial pressure of O_2 (Po_2). The chemoreceptors also are sensitive to increases in the partial pressure of CO_2 (Pco_2) and decreases in pH, particularly when Po_2 is simultaneously decreased. In other words, the response of the peripheral chemoreceptors to decreased arterial Po_2 is greater when the Pco_2 is increased or the pH is decreased.

When **arterial Po$_2$** decreases, there is an increased firing rate of afferent nerves from the carotid and aortic bodies that activates sympathetic vasoconstrictor centers. As a result, there is **arteriolar vasoconstriction** in skeletal muscle, renal, and splanchnic vascular beds. In addition, there is an increase in parasympathetic outflow to the heart that produces a transient **decrease in heart rate.** The slowing of the heart rate is only transient, however, because these peripheral chemoreceptors are primarily involved in control of breathing (see Chapter 5). The decrease in arterial Po$_2$ also produces an increase in ventilation that independently decreases parasympathetic outflow to the heart, which increases the heart rate (the lung inflation reflex).

Central Chemoreceptors

The brain is intolerant of decreases in blood flow, and therefore, it is not surprising that chemoreceptors are located in the medulla itself. These chemoreceptors are most sensitive to CO$_2$ and pH and less sensitive to O$_2$. Changes in **Pco$_2$** or **pH** stimulate the medullary chemoreceptors, which then direct changes in outflow of the medullary cardiovascular centers.

The reflex that involves cerebral chemoreceptors operates as follows: If the **brain becomes ischemic** (i.e., there is decreased cerebral blood flow), cerebral Pco$_2$ immediately increases and pH decreases. The medullary chemoreceptors detect these changes and direct an **increase in sympathetic outflow** that causes intense arteriolar vasoconstriction in many vascular beds and an increase in TPR. Blood flow is thereby redirected to the brain to maintain its perfusion. As a result of this vasoconstriction, P$_a$ increases dramatically, even to life-threatening levels.

The **Cushing reaction** illustrates the role of the cerebral chemoreceptors in maintaining cerebral blood flow. When intracranial pressure increases (e.g., tumors, head injury), there is compression of cerebral arteries, which results in decreased perfusion of the brain. There is an immediate increase in Pco$_2$ and a decrease in pH because CO$_2$ generated from brain tissue is not adequately removed by blood flow. The medullary chemoreceptors respond to these changes in Pco$_2$ and pH by directing an increase in sympathetic outflow to the blood vessels. Again, the overall effect of these changes is to increase TPR and dramatically increase P$_a$.

Antidiuretic Hormone

Antidiuretic hormone (ADH), a hormone secreted by the posterior lobe of the pituitary gland, regulates body fluid osmolarity and participates in the regulation of arterial blood pressure.

There are two types of receptors for ADH: **V$_1$ receptors,** which are present in vascular smooth muscle, and **V$_2$ receptors,** which are present in principal cells of the renal collecting ducts. When activated, the V$_1$ receptors cause vasoconstriction of arterioles and increased TPR. The V$_2$ receptors are involved in water reabsorption in the collecting ducts and the maintenance of body fluid osmolarity.

ADH secretion from the posterior pituitary is increased by two types of stimuli: by increases in serum osmolarity and by decreases in blood volume and blood pressure. The blood volume mechanism is discussed at this time, and osmoregulation is discussed in Chapter 6.

Cardiopulmonary (Low-Pressure) Baroreceptors

In addition to the high-pressure baroreceptors that regulate arterial pressure (i.e., baroreceptor reflex), there are also low-pressure baroreceptors located in the veins, **atria,** and pulmonary arteries. These so-called cardiopulmonary baroreceptors sense changes in **blood volume,** or the "fullness" of the vascular system. They are located on the venous side of the circulation because that is where most of the blood volume is held.

For example, when there is an **increase in blood volume,** the resulting increase in venous and atrial pressure is detected by the cardiopulmonary baroreceptors. The function of the cardiopulmonary baroreceptors is then coordinated to return blood volume to normal, primarily by increasing the excretion of Na$^+$ and water. The responses to an increase in blood volume include the following:

♦ **Increased secretion of atrial natriuretic peptide (ANP).** ANP is secreted by the atria in response to increased atrial pressure. ANP has multiple effects, but the most important is to cause relaxation of vascular smooth muscle, which results in **vasodilation** and decreased TPR. In the kidneys, this vasodilation leads to **increased Na$^+$ and water excretion,** thereby decreasing total body Na$^+$ content, ECF volume, and blood volume.

♦ **Decreased secretion of ADH.** Pressure receptors in the atria also project to the hypothalamus, where the cell bodies of neurons that secrete ADH are located. In response to increased atrial pressure, ADH secretion is inhibited and, as a consequence, there is decreased water reabsorption in collecting ducts, resulting in increased water excretion.

♦ **Renal vasodilation.** There is inhibition of sympathetic vasoconstriction in renal arterioles, leading to renal vasodilation and increased Na$^+$ and water excretion, complementing the action of ANP on the kidneys.

♦ **Increased heart rate.** Information from the low-pressure atrial receptors travels in the vagus nerve to the nucleus tractus solitarius (as does information from the high-pressure arterial receptors involved in the baroreceptor reflex). The difference lies in the response of the medullary cardiovascular centers to the low- and high-pressure receptors. Whereas an increase in pressure at the *arterial* high-pressure receptors produces a *decrease* in heart rate (trying to lower arterial pressure back to normal), an increase in pressure at the *venous* low-pressure receptors produces an *increase* in heart rate (**Bainbridge reflex**). The low-pressure atrial receptors, sensing that blood volume is too high, direct an increase in heart rate and, thus, an increase in cardiac output; the increase in cardiac output leads to increased renal perfusion and increased Na^+ and water excretion.

MICROCIRCULATION

The term "microcirculation" refers to the functions of the smallest blood vessels, the capillaries and the neighboring lymphatic vessels. Delivery of blood to and from the capillaries is critically important because the capillaries are the site of exchange of nutrients and waste products in the tissues, as well as the site of fluid exchange between the vascular and interstitial compartments.

The anatomy of capillary beds has been discussed previously. To briefly review, blood is delivered to the capillary beds via the arterioles. The capillaries merge into venules, which carry effluent blood from the tissues to the veins. The capillaries are the site of the exchange of nutrients, wastes, and fluid. Capillaries are thin walled and are composed of a single layer of endothelial cells with water-filled clefts between the cells.

The degree of constriction or relaxation of the arterioles markedly affects blood flow to the capillaries (in addition to determining TPR). The capillaries themselves branch off metarterioles; a band of smooth muscle, called the precapillary sphincters, precedes the capillaries. The precapillary sphincters function like "switches": By opening or closing, these switches determine blood flow to the capillary bed.

Exchange of Substances Across the Capillary Wall

The exchange of solutes and gases across the capillary wall occurs by **simple diffusion.** Some solutes can diffuse *through* the endothelial cells, and others must diffuse *between the cells.* Generally, the route for diffusion depends on whether the solute or gas is lipid soluble.

Gases such as O_2 and CO_2 are highly **lipid soluble.** These gases readily cross the capillary wall by diffusing through the endothelial cells; diffusion is driven by

the partial pressure gradient for the individual gas. Recall that the rate of diffusion depends on the driving force (in the case of O_2 and CO_2, the partial pressure difference for the gas) and the surface area available for diffusion. Thus, the greater number of open capillaries, the greater the surface area for diffusion.

Water-soluble substances such as water itself, ions, glucose, and amino acids are not lipid soluble; thus, they cannot cross the endothelial cell membranes. The diffusion of water-soluble substances is limited to the aqueous clefts between endothelial cells; hence, the surface area for their diffusion is much less than that for the lipid-soluble gases.

By far, the most important mechanism for fluid transfer across the capillary wall is **osmosis,** driven by hydrostatic and osmotic pressures. These pressures are called the Starling pressures or **Starling forces.**

Proteins are generally too large to cross the capillary walls via the clefts between endothelial cells and are retained in the vascular compartment. In some tissues, such as brain, the clefts are particularly "tight," and little protein leaves these capillaries. In the kidney and intestine, the capillaries are **fenestrated** or perforated, which permits the passage of limited amounts of protein. In other capillaries, proteins may cross in **pinocytotic vesicles.**

Fluid Exchange Across Capillaries

Fluid movement by osmosis is described in Chapter 1. Briefly, fluid will flow by osmosis across a biologic membrane (or the capillary wall) if the membrane has aqueous pores (i.e., permits the passage of water) and if there is a pressure difference across the membrane. The pressure difference can be a hydrostatic pressure difference, an effective osmotic pressure difference, or a combination of hydrostatic and effective osmotic pressures. In capillaries, fluid movement is driven by the sum of hydrostatic and effective osmotic pressures.

Recall that solutes with reflection coefficients of 1.0 contribute most to the **effective osmotic pressure.** When the reflection coefficient is 1.0, the solute cannot cross the membrane and it exerts its full osmotic pressure. In capillary blood, *only protein* contributes to the effective osmotic pressure because it is the only solute whose reflection coefficient at the capillary wall is approximately 1.0. The effective osmotic pressure contributed by protein is called the **colloidosmotic pressure** or **oncotic pressure.**

Starling Equation

Fluid movement across a capillary wall is driven by the Starling pressures across the wall and is described by the **Starling equation** as follows:

$$J_v = K_f[(P_c - P_i) - (\pi_c - \pi_i)]$$

where

J_v = Fluid movement (mL/min)
K_f = Hydraulic conductance (mL/min • mm Hg)
P_c = Capillary hydrostatic pressure (mm Hg)
P_i = Interstitial hydrostatic pressure (mm Hg)
π_c = Capillary oncotic pressure (mm Hg)
π_i = Interstitial oncotic pressure (mm Hg)

The Starling equation states that fluid movement (J_v) across a capillary wall is determined by the net pressure across the wall, which is the sum of hydrostatic pressure and oncotic pressures. The **direction of fluid movement** can be either into or out of the capillary. When net fluid movement is *out of* the capillary into the interstitial fluid, it is called **filtration;** when net fluid movement is from the interstitium *into* the capillary, it is called **absorption.** The **magnitude of fluid movement** is determined by the hydraulic conductance, K_f (water permeability), of the capillary wall. The hydraulic conductance determines how much fluid movement will be produced for a given pressure difference.

Figure 4-34 is a pictorial presentation of the Starling pressures. Each of the four Starling pressures is represented by an arrow. The *direction* of the arrow indicates whether that pressure favors filtration out of the capillary or absorption into the capillary. The *size* of the arrow shows the relative magnitude of the pressure. The numerical value of the pressure, in mm Hg, has a plus (+) sign if the pressure favors filtration and a minus (−) sign if the pressure favors absorption.

The **net pressure,** which is the net driving force, is the algebraic sum of the four pressures. In the example in Figure 4-34*A*, the sum of the four Starling pressures is a net pressure of +6 mm Hg, indicating that there will be net filtration out of the capillary. In the example in Figure 4-34*B*, the sum of the four pressures is a net pressure of −5 mm Hg, indicating that there will be net absorption into the capillary.

By understanding how each parameter of the Starling equation affects fluid movement across the capillary wall, it is possible to predict the effects of changes in these parameters. Each of the parameters in the Starling equation is described as follows:

♦ **K_f, hydraulic conductance,** is the water permeability of the capillary wall. It varies among different types of tissues, depending on the anatomic characteristics of the capillary wall (e.g., the size of the clefts between endothelial cells; whether the capillaries are fenestrated). Therefore, the magnitude of fluid movement for a given pressure difference is largest in capillaries with the highest K_f (e.g., glomerular capillaries), and it is lowest in capillaries with the lowest K_f (e.g., cerebral capillaries). K_f is *not influenced* by such factors as changes in arteriolar resistance, hypoxia, or buildup of metabolites. However, K_f is increased in **capillary injury** (e.g., toxins or in burns). Such increases in K_f will increase the capillary permeability to water and also will result in the loss of protein from the capillary.

♦ **P_c, capillary hydrostatic pressure,** is a force favoring filtration out of the capillary. The value for P_c is determined by both arterial and venous pressures (the capillary being interposed between the arteries and veins), although the value for P_c is closer to arterial pressure than to venous pressure. Furthermore, P_c is more affected by changes in venous pressure than by changes in arterial pressure. Except in glomerular capillaries, P_c declines along the length

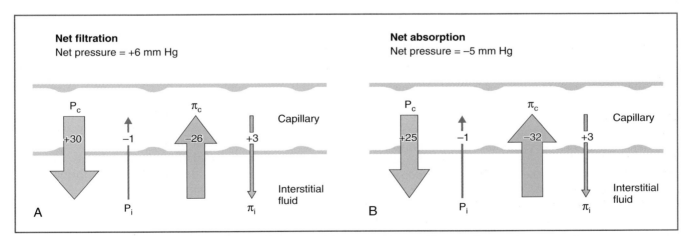

Figure 4–34 **Examples of Starling pressures across the capillary wall. A,** Net pressure favors filtration; **B,** net pressure favors absorption. *Arrows* pointing *out of* the capillary show the Starling pressures that favor filtration (+). *Arrows* pointing *into* the capillary show the Starling pressures that oppose filtration (−). Numbers give the magnitude of each pressure.

of the capillary because of the filtration of fluid. Therefore, P_c is highest at the arteriolar end of the capillary and lowest at the venous end.

♦ **P_i, interstitial hydrostatic pressure,** is a force opposing filtration. Normally, P_i is nearly zero, or it may be slightly negative.

♦ **π_c, capillary oncotic pressure,** is a force opposing filtration. As previously noted, π_c is the effective osmotic pressure of capillary blood due to the presence of plasma proteins, and according to the van't Hoff equation (see Chapter 1), it is determined by the **protein concentration** of capillary blood. Therefore, increases in protein concentration of blood cause increases in π_c and decrease filtration, and decreases in protein concentration of blood cause decreases in π_c and increase filtration.

♦ **π_i, interstitial oncotic pressure,** is a force favoring filtration. π_i is determined by the interstitial fluid protein concentration. Normally, because there is little loss of protein from capillaries, there is little protein in interstitial fluid, making π_i quite low.

SAMPLE PROBLEM. In a skeletal muscle capillary, the following Starling pressures were measured:

P_c, 30 mm Hg

P_i, 1 mm Hg

π_c, 26 mm Hg

π_i, 3 mm Hg

Assuming that K_f is 0.5 mL/min • mm Hg, what is the direction and magnitude of fluid movement across this capillary?

SOLUTION. There are two approaches to solving this problem. One is to apply the Starling equation directly by substituting the values for the Starling pressures and K_f. The other is to use the pictorial approach shown in Figure 4-34 to calculate the net pressure and determine its direction, and then to multiply the net pressure by K_f to obtain the magnitude of fluid movement. The pictorial approach is preferred because there is no equation to memorize and the student must understand how each pressure affects fluid movement.

The numerical values in this problem are identical to those in Figure 4-34A. Use the figure to solve the problem pictorially. If the pressure favors filtration, the arrow points out of the capillary and the numerical value is assigned a plus sign. If the pressure favors absorption, the arrow points into the capillary and the numerical value is assigned a minus sign. Two pressures, P_c and π_i, are assigned a plus sign because they favor filtration. Two pressures, π_c and P_i, are assigned a minus sign because they favor absorption. The four pressures are now added algebraically to

calculate the net pressure of +6 mm Hg (i.e., net pressure = +30 − 1 − 26 + 3 mm Hg = +6 mm Hg). The direction of the net pressure favors filtration because it carries a plus sign. The magnitude of fluid movement is calculated as K_f multiplied by the net pressure:

$$\text{Fluid movement} = K_f \times \text{net pressure}$$
$$= 0.5 \text{ mL/min} \bullet \text{mm Hg} \times 6 \text{ mm Hg}$$
$$= 3 \text{ mL/min}$$

Changes in Starling Forces

Changes in Starling forces can influence the direction and magnitude of fluid movement across capillaries. For example, consider the various changes that would produce increased filtration out of capillaries. In principle, increases in filtration will be caused by an increase in any of the Starling forces that favor filtration *or* by a decrease in any of the Starling forces that favor absorption. Thus, **increases in filtration** would be produced by **increases in P_c** resulting from increases in arterial pressure or venous pressure (but more so from increases in venous pressure). Increases in filtration also would be produced by **decreases in π_c** resulting from dilution of plasma protein concentration.

Lymph

The lymphatic system is responsible for returning interstitial fluid and proteins to the vascular compartment. The **lymphatic capillaries** lie in the interstitial fluid, close to the vascular capillaries. The lymphatic capillaries possess **one-way flap valves,** which permit interstitial fluid and protein to enter, but not leave, the capillaries. These capillaries merge into larger lymphatic vessels and eventually into the largest lymphatic vessel, the **thoracic duct,** which empties lymph into the large veins. The lymphatic vessels have a smooth muscle wall, which has intrinsic contractile ability. Lymph flow back to the thoracic duct is promoted by contraction of the smooth muscle in the lymph vessels and by compression of the lymph vessels by activity of the surrounding skeletal muscle.

An increase in interstitial fluid volume is called **edema** (swelling). By definition, edema forms when the volume of interstitial fluid (due to filtration out of the capillaries) exceeds the ability of the lymphatics to return it to the circulation. Thus, edema can form when there is increased filtration or when lymphatic drainage is impaired (Table 4-6).

Various mechanisms for producing increased filtration have been discussed previously in this chapter

Table 4–6 Causes and Examples of Edema Formation

Cause	Examples
↑ P_c (capillary hydrostatic pressure)	Arteriolar dilation Venous constriction Increased venous pressure Heart failure Extracellular fluid volume expansion
↓π_c (capillary oncotic pressure)	Decreased plasma protein concentration Severe liver failure (failure to synthesize protein) Protein malnutrition Nephrotic syndrome (loss of protein in urine)
↑ K_f (hydraulic conductance)	Burn Inflammation (release of histamine; cytokines)
Impaired lymphatic drainage	Standing (lack of skeletal muscle compression of lymphatics) Removal or irradiation of lymph nodes Parasitic infection of lymph nodes

(e.g., increased P_c; decreased π_c; increased K_f due to destruction of the capillary wall). Lymphatic drainage is impaired when the lymph nodes are surgically removed or irradiated (e.g., in malignancy); in filariasis, a parasitic infection of the lymph nodes; or when there is lack of muscular activity (e.g., a soldier standing at attention).

SPECIAL CIRCULATIONS

Blood flow is variable between one organ and another, depending on the overall demands of each organ system (see Fig. 4-1). For example, blood flow to the lungs is equal to the cardiac output because *all* blood must pass through the lungs, allowing O_2 to be added to it and CO_2 to be removed from it. No other organ receives the entire cardiac output! The kidneys, gastrointestinal tract, and skeletal muscle all have high blood flow, each receiving approximately 25% of cardiac output. Other organs receive smaller percentages of the cardiac output. These interorgan differences in blood flow are the result of differences in vascular resistance.

Furthermore, blood flow to a specific organ or organ system can increase or decrease, depending on its metabolic demands. For example, exercising skeletal muscle has greater demand for O_2 than does resting skeletal muscle. To meet the greater demand for O_2, blood flow to skeletal muscle must temporarily increase above the resting level.

Changes in blood flow to an individual organ are achieved by altering arteriolar resistance. The mechanisms that regulate blood flow to the various organs are broadly categorized as local (intrinsic) control and neural or hormonal (extrinsic) control. **Local control** of blood flow is the primary mechanism utilized for matching blood flow to the metabolic needs of a tissue. Local control is exerted through the direct action of local metabolites on arteriolar resistance. **Neural or hormonal control** of blood flow includes such mechanisms as the action of the sympathetic nervous system on vascular smooth muscle and the actions of vasoactive substances such as histamine, bradykinin, and prostaglandins.

Mechanisms for Control of Regional Blood Flow

Local Control of Blood Flow

There are several examples of local (intrinsic) control of blood flow including autoregulation, active hyperemia, and reactive hyperemia. Each example of local control is discussed generally, followed by a more detailed explanation of the mechanism.

♦ **Autoregulation** is the maintenance of a constant blood flow to an organ in the face of changing arterial pressure. Several organs exhibit autoregulation of blood flow including the kidneys, brain, heart, and skeletal muscle. For example, if arterial pressure in a coronary artery suddenly decreases, an attempt will be made to maintain constant blood flow through this coronary artery. Such autoregulation can be achieved by an immediate compensatory vasodilation of the coronary arterioles, decreasing the resistance of the coronary vasculature and keeping flow constant in the face of decreased pressure.

♦ **Active hyperemia** illustrates the concept that blood flow to an organ is proportional to its metabolic activity. As noted previously, if metabolic activity in skeletal muscle increases as a result of strenuous exercise, then blood flow to the muscle will increase proportionately to meet the increased metabolic demand.

♦ **Reactive hyperemia** is an increase in blood flow *in response* to or *reacting* to a prior period of decreased blood flow. For example, reactive hyperemia is the increase in blood flow to an organ that occurs following a period of arterial occlusion. During the occlusion, an O_2 debt is accumulated. The longer the period of occlusion, the greater the O_2 debt and the greater the subsequent increase in blood flow above the preocclusion levels. The increase in blood flow continues until the O_2 debt is "repaid."

Two basic mechanisms are proposed to explain the phenomena of autoregulation and active and reactive hyperemia: the myogenic hypothesis and the metabolic hypothesis.

♦ **Myogenic hypothesis.** The myogenic hypothesis can be invoked to explain **autoregulation**, but it does not explain active or reactive hyperemia. The myogenic hypothesis states that when vascular smooth muscle is stretched, it contracts. Thus, if arterial pressure is suddenly increased, the arterioles are stretched and the vascular smooth muscle in their walls contracts in response to this stretch. Contraction of arteriolar vascular smooth muscle causes constriction (i.e., increased resistance), thereby maintaining a constant flow in the face of increased pressure (recall that $Q = \Delta P/R$). Conversely, if arterial pressure suddenly decreases, there is less stretch on the arterioles, causing them to relax and arteriolar resistance to decrease. Thus, constant flow can be maintained in the face of increased or decreased arterial pressure by changing arteriolar resistance.

One can also think about the myogenic mechanism in terms of maintaining arteriolar **wall tension.** Blood vessels, such as arterioles, are built to withstand the wall tensions they normally "see." In the example of a sudden increase in arterial pressure, the increased pressure, if unopposed, will cause an increase in arteriolar wall tension. Such an increase in wall tension is undesirable for the arteriole. Thus, in response to the stretch, arteriolar vascular smooth muscle contracts, decreasing the arteriolar radius and returning wall tension back to normal. This relationship is explained by the **law of Laplace for a cylinder,** which states that $T = P \times r$. If pressure (P) increases and radius (r) decreases, then wall tension (T) can remain constant. (Of course, the other consequence of the decreased radius, discussed previously, is increased arteriolar resistance; in the face of increased pressure, increased resistance allows blood flow to be maintained constant, i.e., autoregulation.)

♦ **Metabolic hypothesis.** The metabolic hypothesis can be invoked to explain each of the phenomena of local control of blood flow. The basic premise of this hypothesis is that O_2 delivery to a tissue can be matched to O_2 consumption of the tissue by altering the resistance of the arterioles, which in turn alters blood flow. As a result of metabolic activity, the tissues produce various **vasodilator metabolites** (e.g., CO_2, H^+, K^+, **lactate**, and **adenosine**). The greater the level of metabolic activity, the greater the production of vasodilator metabolites. These metabolites produce **vasodilation of arterioles,** which decreases resistance and, therefore, increases flow to meet the increased demand for O_2. The tissues vary according to which vasodilator metabolite is primarily responsible for vasodilation; for example, the coronary circulation is most sensitive to P_{O_2} and adenosine, whereas the cerebral circulation is most sensitive to P_{CO_2} (Table 4-7).

The following two examples illustrate how the metabolic hypothesis explains **active hyperemia**: (1) The first example considers strenuous exercise. During strenuous exercise, metabolic activity in the exercising skeletal muscle increases and production of vasodilator metabolites, such as lactate, increases. These metabolites cause local vasodilation of skeletal muscle arterioles, which increases local blood flow and increases O_2 delivery to meet the increased demand of the exercising muscle. (2) The second example considers a scenario in which there is a spontaneous increase in arterial pressure to an organ. Initially, the increased pressure will increase blood flow, which will deliver *more* O_2 for metabolic activity and "wash out" vasodilator metabolites. As a result of this washout, there will be a local dilution of vasodilator metabolites, resulting in arteriolar vasoconstriction, increased resistance, and a compensatory decrease in blood flow back to the normal level.

Neural and Hormonal Control of Blood Flow

The most important example of neural (extrinsic) control of regional blood flow involves the **sympathetic innervation** of vascular smooth muscle in some tissues. The density of such sympathetic innervation varies widely from tissue to tissue. For example, blood vessels of the **skin and skeletal muscle** have a high density of sympathetic nerve fibers, whereas coronary, pulmonary, and cerebral vessels have little sympathetic innervation. It is important to note whether sympathetic innervation is absent or present and also, when present, whether it produces vasoconstriction or vasodilation (see Table 2-2). In skin, the sympathetic innervation produces vasoconstriction via α_1 receptors. In skeletal muscle, when the sympathetic nervous system is activated, there can be vasoconstriction (sympathetic nerve fibers, α_1 receptors) or vasodilation (epinephrine from adrenal medulla, β_2 receptors).

Other vasoactive substances include histamine, bradykinin, serotonin, and prostaglandins. **Histamine** is released in response to trauma and has powerful vascular effects. Simultaneously, it causes dilation of arterioles and constriction of venules, with the net effect

Table 4-7 Control of Special Circulations

Circulation	Local Metabolic Control	Vasoactive Metabolites	Sympathetic Control	Mechanical Effects
Coronary	Most important mechanism	Hypoxia Adenosine	Least important mechanism	Mechanical compression during systole
Cerebral	Most important mechanism	CO_2 H^+	Least important mechanism	Increases in intracranial pressure decrease cerebral blood flow
Skeletal Muscle	Most important mechanism during exercise	Lactate K^+ Adenosine	Most important mechanism at rest (α_1 receptors, vasoconstriction; β_2 receptors, vasodilation)	Muscular activity compresses blood vessels
Skin	Least important mechanism	—	Most important mechanism for temperature regulation (α_1 receptors, vasoconstriction)	—
Pulmonary	Most important mechanism	Hypoxia vasoconstricts	Least important mechanism	Lung inflation
Renal	Most important mechanism (myogenic; tubuloglomerular feedback)	—	Least important mechanism	—

being a large increase in P_c, which increases filtration out of capillaries, and local edema. **Bradykinin,** like histamine, causes dilation of arterioles and constriction of venules, resulting in increased filtration out of capillaries and local edema. **Serotonin** is released in response to blood vessel damage and causes local vasoconstriction (in an attempt to reduce blood flow and blood loss). Serotonin has been implicated in the pathophysiology of vascular spasms that occur in migraine headache. The **prostaglandins** produce various effects on vascular smooth muscle. Prostacyclin and the prostaglandin-E series are vasodilators in many vascular beds. Thromboxane A_2 and the prostaglandin-F series are vasoconstrictors. **Angiotensin II** and **vasopressin** (via V_1 receptors) are potent vasoconstrictors that increase TPR. **Atrial natriuretic peptide** is a vasodilator hormone that is secreted by the atria in response to increases in atrial pressure.

Coronary Circulation

Blood flow through the coronary circulation is controlled almost entirely by **local metabolites**, with sympathetic innervation playing only a minor role. The most important local metabolic factors are **hypoxia** and **adenosine.** For example, if there is an increase in myocardial contractility, there is increased O_2 demand by the cardiac muscle and increased O_2 consumption, causing local hypoxia. This local hypoxia causes vasodilation of the coronary arterioles, which then produces a compensatory increase in coronary blood flow and O_2 delivery to meet the demands of the cardiac muscle (i.e., active hyperemia).

An unusual feature of the coronary circulation is the effect of **mechanical compression** of the blood vessels during systole in the cardiac cycle. This compression causes a brief period of occlusion and reduction of blood flow. When the period of occlusion (i.e., systole) is over, reactive hyperemia occurs to increase blood flow and O_2 delivery and to repay the O_2 debt that was incurred during the compression.

Cerebral Circulation

The cerebral circulation is controlled almost entirely by **local metabolites** and exhibits autoregulation and active and reactive hyperemia. The most important local vasodilator in the cerebral circulation is **CO_2** (or H^+). An increase in cerebral P_{CO_2} (producing an increase in H^+ concentration and a decrease in pH) causes vasodilation of the cerebral arterioles, which results in an increase in blood flow to assist in removal of the excess CO_2.

It is interesting that many circulating vasoactive substances *do not affect* the cerebral circulation because their large molecular size prevents them from crossing the blood-brain barrier.

Pulmonary Circulation

The regulation of pulmonary circulation is discussed fully in Chapter 5. Briefly, the pulmonary circulation is controlled by O_2. The effect of O_2 on pulmonary arteriolar resistance is the *exact opposite* of its effect in other vascular beds: In the pulmonary circulation, **hypoxia causes vasoconstriction.** This seemingly counterintuitive effect of O_2 also is explained in Chapter 5. Briefly, regions of hypoxia in the lung cause local vasoconstriction, which effectively shunts blood *away from* poorly ventilated areas where the blood flow would be "wasted" and *toward* well-ventilated areas where gas exchange can occur.

Renal Circulation

The regulation of renal blood flow is discussed in detail in Chapter 6. Briefly, renal blood flow is tightly **autoregulated** so that flow remains constant even when renal perfusion pressure changes. Renal autoregulation is independent of sympathetic innervation, and it is retained even when the kidney is denervated (e.g., in a transplanted kidney). Autoregulation is presumed to result from a combination of the myogenic properties of the renal arterioles and tubuloglomerular feedback (see Chapter 6).

Skeletal Muscle Circulation

Blood flow to skeletal muscle is controlled both by **local metabolites** *and* by **sympathetic innervation** of its vascular smooth muscle. Incidentally, the degree of vasoconstriction of skeletal muscle arterioles is a major determinant of **TPR** because the mass of skeletal muscle is so large, compared with that of other organs.

♦ At **rest,** blood flow to skeletal muscle is regulated primarily by its **sympathetic innervation.** Vascular smooth muscle in the arterioles of skeletal muscle is densely innervated by sympathetic nerve fibers that are vasoconstricting (α_1 receptors). There are also β_2 receptors on the vascular smooth muscle of skeletal muscle that are activated by epinephrine and cause vasodilation. Thus, activation of α_1 receptors causes vasoconstriction, increased resistance, and decreased blood flow. Activation of β_2 receptors causes vasodilation, decreased resistance, and increased blood flow. Usually, vasoconstriction predominates because norepinephrine, released from sympathetic adrenergic neurons, stimulates primarily α_1 receptors. On the other hand, epinephrine released from the adrenal gland during the fight-or-flight response or during exercise activates β_2 receptors and produces vasodilation.

♦ During **exercise,** blood flow to skeletal muscle is controlled primarily by **local metabolites.** Each of the phenomena of local control is exhibited: autoregulation and active and reactive hyperemia. During exercise, the demand for O_2 in skeletal muscle varies with the activity level, and, accordingly, blood flow is increased or decreased to deliver sufficient O_2 to meet the demand. The local vasodilator substances in skeletal muscle are **lactate, adenosine, and K^+.**

Mechanical compression of the blood vessels in skeletal muscle can also occur during exercise and cause brief periods of occlusion. When the period of occlusion is over, a period of reactive hyperemia will occur, which increases blood flow and O_2 delivery to repay the O_2 debt.

Skin Circulation

The skin has blood vessels with dense **sympathetic innervation,** which controls its blood flow. The principal function of the sympathetic innervation is to alter blood flow to the skin for **regulation of body temperature.** For example, during exercise, as body temperature increases, sympathetic centers controlling cutaneous blood flow are *inhibited.* This selective inhibition produces vasodilation in cutaneous arterioles so that warm blood from the body core can be shunted to the skin surface for dissipation of heat. Local vasodilator metabolites have little effect on cutaneous blood flow.

The effects of vasoactive substances such as histamine have been discussed previously. In skin, the effects of histamine on blood vessels are visible. **Trauma to the skin releases histamine,** which produces a **triple response** in skin: a red line, a red flare, and a wheal. The **wheal** is local edema and results from histaminic actions that vasodilate arterioles and vasoconstrict veins. Together, these two effects produce increased P_c, increased filtration, and local edema.

TEMPERATURE REGULATION

Humans maintain a normal body temperature at a set point of 37° C (98.6° F). Because environmental temperatures vary greatly, the body has mechanisms, coordinated in the anterior hypothalamus, for both heat generation and heat loss to keep body temperature constant. When the environmental temperature decreases, the body generates and conserves heat. When the environmental temperature increases, the body reduces heat production and dissipates heat.

Mechanisms for Generating Heat

When environmental temperature is less than body temperature, mechanisms are activated that **increase heat production** and **reduce heat loss.** These mechanisms include stimulation of thyroid hormone production, activation of the sympathetic nervous system, and shivering. Behavioral components also may contribute by reducing the exposure of skin to the cold (e.g., wrapping arms around oneself, curling up in a ball, adding more clothing).

Thyroid Hormones

Thyroid hormones are **thermogenic:** Their actions on target tissues result in heat production. Major actions of thyroid hormone are **stimulation of Na$^+$-K$^+$ ATPase,** increased O_2 consumption, increased metabolic rate, and increased heat production. Therefore, it is logical that exposure to cold temperatures activates thyroid hormones. The mechanism for this activation is not entirely clear, but it includes increased conversion of thyroxine (T_4) to the active form, triiodothyronine (T_3), in target tissues.

Because thyroid hormones are thermogenic, it follows that an excess or deficit of thyroid hormones would cause disturbances in the regulation of body temperature. In **hyperthyroidism** (e.g., Graves disease, thyroid tumor), metabolic rate increases, O_2 consumption increases, and heat production increases. In **hypothyroidism** (e.g., thyroiditis, surgical removal of the thyroid, iodine deficiency), there is a decreased metabolic rate, decreased O_2 consumption, decreased heat production, and extreme sensitivity to cold. (For a complete discussion of this topic, refer to Chapter 9.)

Sympathetic Nervous System

Cold environmental temperatures **activate the sympathetic nervous system.** One consequence of this activation is stimulation of β receptors in **brown fat,** which increases metabolic rate and heat production. This action of the sympathetic nervous system is synergistic with the actions of thyroid hormones: For thyroid hormones to produce maximal thermogenesis, the sympathetic nervous system must be simultaneously activated by cold temperatures.

A second consequence of activation of the sympathetic nervous system is stimulation of α_1 receptors in vascular smooth muscle of skin blood vessels, producing vasoconstriction. Vasoconstriction reduces blood flow to the surface of the skin and, consequently, **reduces heat loss.**

Shivering

Shivering, which involves rhythmic contraction of skeletal muscle, is the most potent mechanism for increasing heat production in the body. Cold environmental temperatures activate centers in the **posterior hypothalamus,** which then activate the **α and γ motoneurons** innervating skeletal muscle. The skeletal muscle contracts rhythmically, generating heat and raising body temperature.

Mechanisms for Dissipating Heat

When the environmental temperature increases, mechanisms are activated that result in **increased heat loss** from the body by radiation and convection. Since heat is a normal byproduct of metabolism, the body must dissipate this heat just to maintain body temperature at the set point. When the environmental temperature is increased, more heat than usual must be dissipated.

Mechanisms for dissipating heat are coordinated in the **anterior hypothalamus.** Increased body temperature **decreases sympathetic activity in skin blood vessels.** This decrease in sympathetic tone results in increased blood flow through skin arterioles and greater arteriovenous **shunting of blood to venous plexuses** near the surface of skin. In effect, warm blood from the body core is shunted to the body surface, and heat is then lost by radiation and convection. Shunting of blood to the surface is evidenced by redness and warmth of the skin. There also is increased activity of the sympathetic cholinergic fibers innervating thermoregulatory sweat glands to produce increased sweating (cooling). The behavioral components to dissipate heat include increasing the exposure of skin to the air (e.g., removing clothing, fanning).

Regulation of Body Temperature

The temperature-regulating center is located in the **anterior hypothalamus.** This center receives information about environmental temperature from thermoreceptors in the skin and about core temperature from thermoreceptors in the anterior hypothalamus itself. The anterior hypothalamus then orchestrates the appropriate responses, which may involve heat-generating or heat-dissipating mechanisms.

If **core temperature is below the set-point temperature,** then heat-generating and heat-retaining mechanisms are activated. As previously discussed, these mechanisms include increased metabolic rate (thyroid hormones, sympathetic nervous system), shivering, and vasoconstriction of blood vessels of the skin (increased sympathetic tone).

If **core temperature is above the set-point temperature,** then heat-dissipating mechanisms are activated. These mechanisms include vasodilation of blood vessels of the skin (decreased sympathetic tone) and increased activity of sympathetic cholinergic fibers to sweat glands.

Fever

Fever is an abnormal elevation of body temperature. **Pyrogens** produce fever by increasing the hypothalamic set-point temperature. The result of such a change in set point is that a normal core temperature is "seen" by the hypothalamic center as *too low* relative to the new set point. The anterior hypothalamus then activates heat-generating mechanisms (e.g., shivering) to raise body temperature to the new set point.

At the cellular level, the mechanism of pyrogen action is increased production of **interleukin-1** (IL-1) in phagocytic cells. IL-1 then acts on the anterior hypothalamus to increase local production of prostaglandins, which increase the set-point temperature.

Fever can be reduced by **aspirin,** which inhibits the **cyclooxygenase** enzyme, necessary for the synthesis of prostaglandins. By inhibiting the production of prostaglandins, aspirin (and other cyclooxygenase inhibitors) interrupts the pathway that pyrogens utilize to raise the set-point temperature. When fever is treated with aspirin, the temperature sensors in the anterior hypothalamus now "see" body temperature as *too high* relative to the set-point temperature and set in motion the mechanisms for dissipating heat including vasodilation and sweating.

Disturbances of Temperature Regulation

Heat exhaustion can occur as a consequence of the body's responses to elevated environmental temperature. Normally, the response to increased temperature includes vasodilation and sweating in order to dissipate heat. However, if the sweating is excessive, it can result in decreased ECF volume, decreased blood volume, decreased arterial pressure, and fainting.

Heat stroke occurs when body temperature increases to the point of tissue damage. If the normal response to elevated environmental temperature is impaired (e.g., if sweating does not occur), then heat cannot be appropriately dissipated and core temperature increases to dangerous levels.

Malignant hyperthermia is characterized by a massive increase in metabolic rate, increased O_2 consumption, and increased heat production in skeletal muscle. The heat-dissipating mechanisms are unable to keep pace with the excessive heat production, and if the hyperthermia is not treated, body temperature may increase to dangerously high, or even fatal, levels. In susceptible individuals, malignant hyperthermia can be caused by **inhalation anesthetics.**

INTEGRATIVE FUNCTIONS OF THE CARDIOVASCULAR SYSTEM

The cardiovascular system *always* operates in an integrated manner. Thus, it is impossible to discuss a change *only* in cardiac function (e.g., a change in contractility) without then considering the effect such a change would have on arterial pressure, on hemodynamics, on the reflexes involving the sympathetic and parasympathetic nervous systems, on the renin–angiotensin II–aldosterone system, on filtration from capillaries and lymph flow, and on the distribution of blood flow among the organ systems.

The best and most enduring way to understand the integrative functions of the cardiovascular system is by describing its responses to exercise, to hemorrhage, and to changes in posture.

Responses to Exercise

The cardiovascular responses to exercise involve a combination of central nervous system (CNS) and local mechanisms. The CNS responses include a **central command** from the cerebral motor cortex, which directs changes in the autonomic nervous system. The **local responses** include effects of metabolites to increase blood flow and O_2 delivery to the exercising skeletal muscle. Changes in arterial P_{O_2}, P_{CO_2}, and pH apparently *play little role* in directing these responses because none of these parameters changes significantly during moderate exercise.

Central Command

The central command refers to a series of responses, directed by the cerebral motor cortex, which are initiated by the **anticipation of exercise.** These reflexes are triggered by muscle mechanoreceptors, and possibly muscle chemoreceptors, when exercise is anticipated or initiated. Details concerning the afferent limb of this reflex (i.e., information traveling from the muscles to the CNS) are lacking. It is clear, however, that the efferent limb of the reflex produces **increased sympathetic outflow to the heart and blood vessels** and **decreased parasympathetic outflow to the heart.**

One consequence of the central command is an increase in cardiac output. This increase is the result of two simultaneous effects on the heart. (1) The increase in sympathetic activity (β_1 receptors) and the decrease in parasympathetic activity cooperate to produce an **increase in heart rate.** (2) The increase in sympathetic activity (β_1 receptors) produces an **increase**

in contractility and a resulting **increase in stroke volume.**

Together, the increases in heart rate and stroke volume produce an **increase in cardiac output.** The increase in cardiac output is *essential* in the cardiovascular response to exercise. It ensures that more O_2 and nutrients are delivered to the exercising skeletal muscle. (If cardiac output did not increase, for example, the only way to increase blood flow to the skeletal muscle would be through redistribution of blood flow from other organs.)

Recall that cardiac output cannot increase without a concomitant increase in venous return (Frank-Starling relationship). In exercise, this concomitant **increase in venous return** is accomplished by two effects on the veins: The contraction of skeletal muscle around the veins has a mechanical (squeezing) action, and activation of the sympathetic nervous system produces venoconstriction. Together, these effects on the veins decrease the unstressed volume and increase venous return to the heart. Again, the increase in venous return makes the increase in cardiac output possible.

Another consequence of the increased sympathetic outflow in the central command is *selective* **arteriolar vasoconstriction.** (1) In the circulation of the skin, splanchnic regions, kidney, and inactive muscles, vasoconstriction occurs via α_1 receptors, which results in increased resistance and decreased blood flow to those organs. (2) In the exercising skeletal muscle, however, local metabolic effects override any sympathetic vasoconstricting effects, and **arteriolar vasodilation** occurs. (3) Other locations where vasoconstriction *does not* occur are in the coronary circulation (where blood flow increases to meet the increased level of myocardial O_2 consumption) and the cerebral circulation. (4) In the cutaneous circulation, there is a biphasic response. Initially, vasoconstriction occurs (due to increased sympathetic outflow); later, however, as body temperature increases, there is selective inhibition of sympathetic cutaneous vasoconstriction (see Temperature Regulation, pages 173–174), resulting in vasodilation and dissipation of heat through the skin.

In summary, there is vasoconstriction in some vascular beds so that blood flow can be redistributed to the exercising skeletal muscle and the heart, with blood flow being maintained in essential organs such as the brain.

Local Responses in Muscle

Local control of blood flow in the exercising skeletal muscle is orchestrated by **active hyperemia.** As the metabolic rate of the skeletal muscle increases, production of **vasodilator metabolites** such as lactate, potassium, and adenosine also increases. These metabolites act directly on the arterioles of the exercising muscle to produce local vasodilation. Vasodilation of the arterioles results in increased blood flow to meet the increased metabolic demand of the muscle. This vasodilation in the exercising muscle also produces an **overall decrease in TPR.** (If these local metabolic effects in the exercising muscle did not occur, TPR would increase because the central command directs an increase in sympathetic outflow to the blood vessels, which produces vasoconstriction.)

Overall Responses to Exercise

The two components of the cardiovascular response to exercise, the central command and the effects of local metabolites, now can be viewed together (Table 4-8 and Fig. 4-35). The central command directs an increase in sympathetic outflow and a decrease in parasympathetic outflow. This produces an **increase in cardiac output** and **vasoconstriction in several vascular beds** (excluding exercising skeletal muscle, coronary, and cerebral circulations). The increase in cardiac output has two components: increased heart rate and increased contractility. The increase in contractility results in increased stroke volume and is represented by an increased pulse pressure (increased volume is pumped into the low-compliance arteries). Increased cardiac output is possible because **venous return increases** (Frank-Starling relationship). Venous return increases because there is sympathetic constriction of the veins (which reduces unstressed volume) and because of the squeezing action of the exercising skeletal muscle on the veins.

A higher-than-normal percentage of this increased cardiac output will perfuse the exercising skeletal muscle because of local metabolic responses: Local metabolites produce **vasodilation.** Overall, **TPR decreases** because of this vasodilation in skeletal muscle, even though other vascular beds are vasoconstricted. There is an increase in systolic arterial pressure and

Table 4-8 Summary of Cardiovascular Responses to Exercise

Parameter	Response to Exercise
Heart rate	↑↑
Stroke volume	↑
Pulse pressure	↑ (increased stroke volume)
Cardiac output	↑↑
Venous return	↑
Mean arterial pressure	↑ (slight)
Total peripheral resistance (TPR)	↓↓ (vasodilation in skeletal muscle)
Arteriovenous O_2 difference	↑↑ (increased O_2 consumption by tissues)

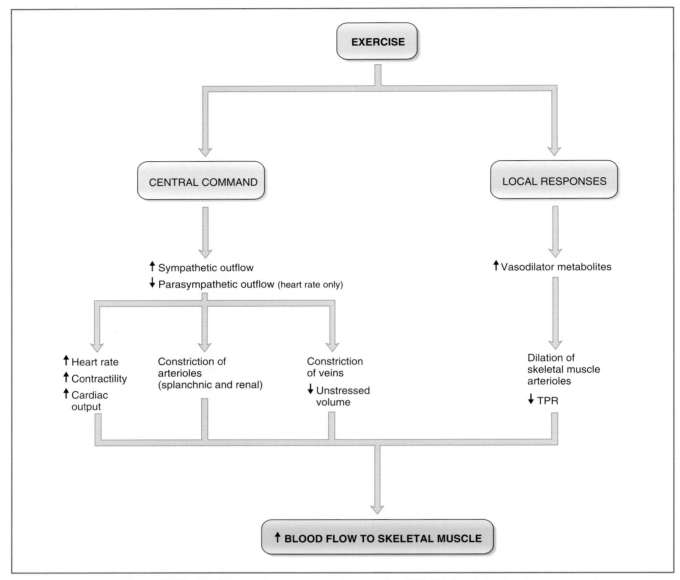

Figure 4–35 **Cardiovascular responses to exercise.** TPR, Total peripheral resistance.

pulse pressure because of the increase in stroke volume. However, diastolic arterial pressure remains the same or may even decrease secondary to the decrease in TPR.

Responses to Hemorrhage

When a person loses a large quantity of blood, arterial pressure decreases rapidly, followed by a series of compensatory cardiovascular responses that attempt to restore arterial pressure back to normal and to sustain life (Fig. 4-36 and Box 4-3).

Decreased Arterial Pressure—Initiating Event

The initiating event in **hemorrhage** is loss of blood and decreased blood volume. Recall, by referring to Figure

4-29B, how a decrease in blood volume leads to a **decrease in arterial pressure.** When blood volume decreases, mean systemic pressure decreases and the vascular function curve shifts to the left. In the new steady state, the cardiac and vascular function curves intersect at a new equilibrium point, where both cardiac output and right atrial pressure are decreased.

These events also can be understood without referring to the graphs. Consider that when hemorrhaging occurs, there is a decrease in total blood volume. The decrease in blood volume produces a decrease in venous return to the heart and a decrease in right atrial pressure. When venous return decreases, there is a corresponding decrease in cardiac output (Frank-Starling mechanism). The decrease in cardiac output then leads to a decrease in P_a because P_a is the product

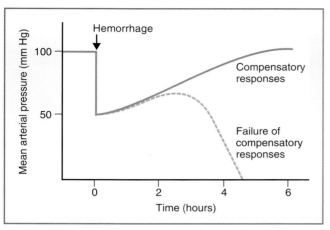

Figure 4–36 **Effect of hemorrhage on mean arterial pressure (P$_a$).** In some persons, compensatory responses to blood loss return P$_a$ to normal within a few hours; in other persons, the compensatory response fails and irreversible shock and death occur.

of cardiac output and TPR (P$_a$ = cardiac output × TPR). Hence, cardiac output and P$_a$ decrease almost immediately, but *thus far* there has been *no change in TPR* (although TPR will change as a later compensatory response).

Within the few hours immediately following hemorrhage, arterial pressure gradually begins to increase back toward the normal (prehemorrhagic) value. This increase in arterial pressure is the result of **compensatory responses** in the cardiovascular system (Fig. 4-37 and Table 4-9; see Fig. 4-36).

In some persons the compensatory responses fail, and after a brief upswing, mean arterial pressure falls irreversibly and death ensues (i.e., irreversible shock). There are multiple reasons for this irreversible process including severe vasoconstriction of essential vascular beds and cardiac failure.

BOX 4-3   Clinical Physiology: Hypovolemic Shock

DESCRIPTION OF CASE. Two teenagers, Adam and Ben, are involved in an automobile accident, and both suffer significant blood loss. They are taken to the nearest trauma center. Adam has a P$_a$ of 55 mm Hg, a pulse pressure of 20 mm Hg, and a heart rate of 120 beats/min. He is anxious but alert, has a slightly decreased urine output, and has cool, pale skin. Ben has a P$_a$ of 40 mm Hg, a barely measurable pulse pressure, and a heart rate of 160 beats/min. He is comatose, has no urine output, and is cold and cyanotic.

Adam is treated by stopping the bleeding and administering lactated Ringer solution intravenously and a blood transfusion. The physicians are prepared to administer a positive inotropic agent but find it unnecessary because Adam shows signs of improvement. During the next 5 hours, Adam's P$_a$ increases back to normal and his heart rate simultaneously decreases to a normal value of 75 beats/min. His skin gradually warms, and the normal pink color returns.

Ben is treated in the same way as Adam, but despite the efforts of the medical team, he dies.

EXPLANATION OF CASE. These teenagers illustrate two different responses to significant blood loss. In the first patient, Adam, the blood loss led to decreased P$_a$ (decreased blood volume → decreased mean systemic pressure → decreased venous return → decreased cardiac output → decreased P$_a$). The decreased P$_a$ triggered the baroreceptor reflex, resulting in increased sympathetic outflow to the heart and blood vessels. As a result of the reflex, the patient's heart rate increased in an attempt to increase cardiac output. There was vasoconstriction of several vascular beds (excluding the

heart and brain) and increased total peripheral resistance (TPR). Vasoconstriction of cutaneous blood vessels caused the skin to become cool and pale. Supportive therapy included intravenous infusion of buffered saline solution and transfusion, allowing the patient to fully recover. A positive inotropic agent might have been used to increase cardiac output; because the patient's own reflex mechanisms increased myocardial contractility, it was unnecessary.

In the second patient, Ben, the compensatory mechanisms failed. When compared with Adam, Ben's P$_a$ is lower, his stroke volume is *much* lower (he had no pulse pressure), his heart rate is much higher, and the vasoconstriction is more pronounced (his skin was cold). His kidneys are not producing urine, which may explain his deteriorating condition. Clearly, the baroreceptor reflex is strongly activated because his heart rate is high and there is intense peripheral vasoconstriction. Vasoconstriction reduces blood flow to *nonvital* organs, such as skin, in order to preserve blood flow to *vital* organs such as the brain, heart, and kidneys. In this patient, vasoconstriction unfortunately extended to the vital organs, and the ischemic damage in them proved fatal. In this patient, myocardial ischemia and renal ischemia were particularly devastating: Without oxygen, his heart could not adequately function as a pump; without blood flow, his kidney could not produce urine.

TREATMENT. Despite treatment, one patient dies. The other patient responds well to treatment, which includes stopping the bleeding and administering lactated Ringer solution and a blood transfusion.

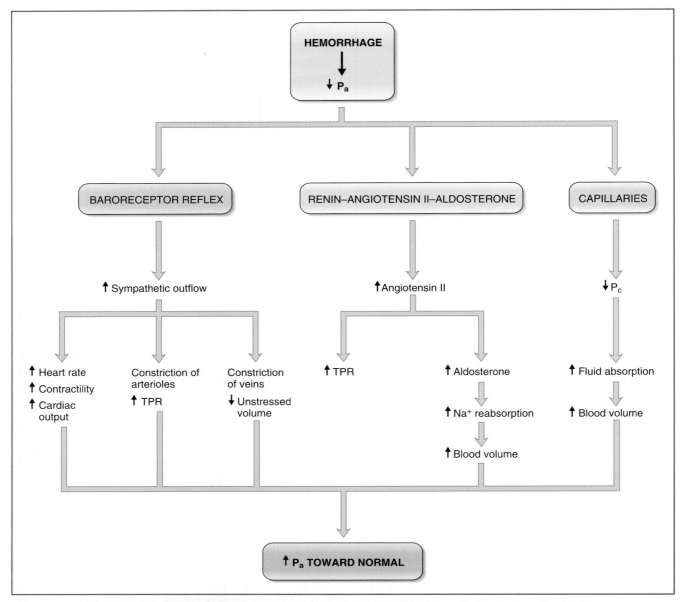

Figure 4–37 Cardiovascular responses to hemorrhage. P_a, Mean arterial pressure; P_c, capillary hydrostatic pressure; TPR, total peripheral resistance.

Responses of the Baroreceptor Reflex

Among the compensatory responses to a decrease in mean arterial pressure are those involved in the baroreceptor reflex. Baroreceptors in the carotid sinus detect the decrease in P_a and relay the information to the medulla via the carotid sinus nerve. The medulla coordinates an output that is intended to increase P_a back toward normal: Sympathetic outflow to the heart and blood vessels increases, and parasympathetic outflow to the heart decreases. The four consequences of these autonomic reflexes are (1) **increased heart rate,** (2) **increased contractility,** (3) **increased TPR** (due to arteriolar vasoconstriction in many vascular beds, but sparing of the coronary and cerebral vascular beds), and (4) **constriction of the veins,** which reduces unstressed volume, increases venous return, and increases stressed volume.

Notice that each of these four cardiovascular responses occurs in the direction of increasing P_a. Constriction of the veins (which decreases their compliance or capacitance) returns more blood to the heart, increases venous return and cardiac output, and shifts blood from the venous to the arterial side of the circulation. Increased heart rate and increased contractility result in increased cardiac output, which is possible because of the increased venous return. Finally, constriction of arterioles and increased TPR result in more

Table 4–9 Summary of Cardiovascular Responses to Hemorrhage

Parameter	Compensatory Response to Hemorrhage*
Carotid sinus nerve firing rate	↓
Heart rate	↑
Contractility	↑
Cardiac output	↑
Unstressed volume	↓ (produces an increase in venous return)
Total peripheral resistance (TPR)	↑
Renin	↑
Angiotensin II	↑
Aldosterone	↑
Circulating epinephrine	↑ (secreted from adrenal medulla)
Antidiuretic hormone (ADH)	↑ (stimulated by decreased blood volume)

*These compensatory responses should be compared with values immediately after the hemorrhage occurs, *not* with the prehemorrhagic values. For example, the compensatory increase in cardiac output does *not* mean that cardiac output is higher than it is in a normal person: It means that cardiac output is higher than just after the hemorrhage occurred.

blood being "held" on the arterial side (increased stressed volume and increased P_a).

Responses of the Renin–Angiotensin II–Aldosterone System

Another set of compensatory responses to the decrease in mean arterial pressure are those of the renin–angiotensin II–aldosterone system. When P_a decreases, renal perfusion pressure decreases, which stimulates the secretion of **renin** from the renal juxtaglomerular cells. Renin, in turn, increases the production of angiotensin I, which is then converted to angiotensin II. **Angiotensin II** has two major actions: (1) It causes arteriolar vasoconstriction, reinforcing and adding to the increase in TPR from the increased sympathetic outflow to the blood vessels. (2) It stimulates the secretion of **aldosterone,** which circulates to the kidney and causes increased reabsorption of Na^+. By increasing total body Na^+ content, aldosterone increases ECF volume, thereby raising blood volume and reinforcing the increase in stressed volume, which resulted from a shift of blood from the veins to the arteries.

Responses in the Capillaries

The compensatory responses to hemorrhage include changes in the Starling forces across capillary walls.

These compensatory changes favor **absorption** of fluid into capillaries as follows: Increased sympathetic outflow to blood vessels and increased angiotensin II both produce arteriolar vasoconstriction. As a result of this vasoconstriction, there is a **decrease in capillary hydrostatic pressure** (P_c), which opposes filtration out of the capillary and favors absorption.

Responses of Antidiuretic Hormone

Antidiuretic hormone (ADH) is secreted in response to decreases in blood volume, mediated by volume receptors in the atria. ADH has two actions: (1) It increases water reabsorption by the renal collecting ducts (V_2 receptors), which helps to restore blood volume. (2) It causes arteriolar vasoconstriction (V_1 receptors), which reinforces the vasoconstricting effects of sympathetic activity and angiotensin II.

Other Responses in Hemorrhage

If a person becomes hypoxemic (has decreased arterial P_{O_2}) following a hemorrhage, **chemoreceptors** in the **carotid and aortic bodies** sense the decrease in P_{O_2} and respond by increasing sympathetic outflow to the blood vessels. As a result, there is vasoconstriction, increased TPR, and increased P_a. This mechanism augments the baroreceptor reflex (which senses the decreased P_a rather than the decreased P_{O_2}).

If **cerebral ischemia** occurs following a hemorrhage, there will be a local increase in P_{CO_2} and a decrease in pH. These changes activate chemoreceptors in the medullary vasomotor center to increase sympathetic outflow to blood vessels, resulting in peripheral vasoconstriction, increased TPR, and increased P_a.

Responses to Changes in Posture

The cardiovascular responses to a change in posture (or gravity) are illustrated in a person who changes from a supine (lying) position to a standing position. A person who stands up too quickly may briefly experience **orthostatic hypotension** (i.e., a decrease in arterial blood pressure upon standing), light-headedness, and possibly fainting. Normally, a series of fast compensatory cardiovascular responses involving the baroreceptor reflex occurs to offset this brief, initial decrease in P_a (Fig. 4-38 and Table 4-10).

Pooling of Blood in the Extremities—Initiating Event

When a person moves from a supine to a standing position, **blood pools in the veins** of the lower extremities. The capacitance of the veins allows for large blood volumes to accumulate. When blood pools in the veins, venous return to the heart decreases and cardiac output decreases (Frank-Starling mechanism), which results in a **decrease in mean arterial pressure.**

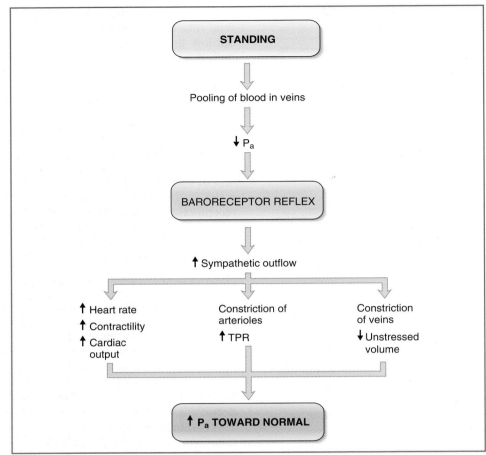

Figure 4–38 **Cardiovascular responses in a person moving from a supine to a standing position.** TPR, Total peripheral resistance.

Table 4–10 Summary of Cardiovascular Responses to Standing

Parameter	Initial Response to Standing	Compensatory Response
Mean arterial pressure	↓	↑ (toward normal)
Heart rate	—	↑
Stroke volume	↓ (decreased venous return)	↑ (toward normal)
Cardiac output	↓ (decreased stroke volume)	↑ (toward normal)
Total peripheral resistance (TPR)	—	↑
Central venous pressure	↓ (pooling of blood in lower extremities)	↑ (toward normal)

Venous pooling also causes increased capillary hydrostatic pressure in the veins of the legs, which results in **increased filtration** of fluid into the interstitial fluid with a loss of intravascular volume. For example, if a person stands for an extended period of time (e.g., a soldier who is standing at attention), filtration from capillaries can exceed the ability of the lymphatics to return fluid to the circulation, which results in **edema** formation in the lower extremities. Increased filtration of fluid out of the capillaries contributes further to the decreased venous return and decreased P_a. If the decrease in P_a is dramatic, then cerebral blood pressure may decrease and cause fainting.

Response of the Baroreceptor Reflex

The primary compensatory cardiovascular response to the decrease in mean arterial pressure involves the baroreceptor reflex. As blood pools in the veins of the lower extremities and is not returned to the heart, both cardiac output and P_a decrease. The baroreceptors in the carotid sinus detect this decrease in P_a and send this information to the medullary vasomotor center. The vasomotor center directs an **increase in**

BOX 4–4 Clinical Physiology: Heart Failure

DESCRIPTION OF CASE. A 60-year-old woman is admitted to the hospital after complaining of extreme fatigue and weakness, shortness of breath (dyspnea), and swelling of her ankles. Her clothes no longer fit around the waist, and she has gained 3 kg in the past month. She finds that breathing is particularly difficult when lying down (orthopnea). Sleeping propped on several pillows no longer brings her relief. She has a history of chest pain and shortness of breath upon exertion.

Her physical examination reveals cyanosis (blue skin tone), rapid respirations, rapid pulse, distended neck veins, ascites (fluid) in the abdomen, edema in the ankles, and cold clammy skin. Her ventricular ejection fraction is 0.30. Her systolic pressure is 100 mm Hg, with a reduced pulse pressure. She is treated with digoxin and a diuretic and placed on a low-sodium diet.

EXPLANATION OF CASE. The woman's signs and symptoms are a classic presentation of heart failure. The history of angina (chest pain) suggests that blockage of the coronary arteries has resulted in insufficient blood flow to the heart. With insufficient coronary blood flow, there is inadequate oxygen delivery to the working myocardial cells and the ventricles are unable to develop normal pressures for ejection of blood during systole. A negative inotropic state develops in the ventricles, resulting in decreased contractility and decreased stroke volume for a given end-diastolic volume (downward shift of the Frank-Starling relationship; see Figure 4-21). The decreased stroke volume is reflected both in the reduced pulse pressure and in the reduced ejection fraction of 0.30 (normal value is 0.55): A smaller-than-normal fraction of the end-diastolic volume is ejected during systole. Although not stated explicitly, cardiac output is also reduced. Cyanosis and easy fatigability are signs of inadequate blood flow to the tissues and inadequate oxygenation of blood.

The woman has edema (accumulation of interstitial fluid) in the lungs, as evidenced by shortness of breath, and in the peripheral tissues. Edema fluid accumulates when filtration out of capillaries exceeds the capacity of the lymphatics. In her case, there is increased filtration from capillaries because of a rise in venous pressure (note the distended neck veins). Venous pressure increases because blood "backs up" on the venous side of the circulation, as the ventricles are unable to efficiently eject blood during systole. Both left and right ventricles apparently have failed because edema has formed in the lungs (left heart failure) and in the periphery (right heart failure).

The baroreceptor reflex is activated in response to the decrease in P_a. (P_a is decreased because blood has shifted from the arterial to the venous side of the circulation, as the ventricles failed to pump adequately.) The woman's increased pulse rate and cold clammy skin result from the baroreceptor reflex: Decreased P_a activates the baroreceptors, causing an increased sympathetic outflow to the heart and blood vessels (increases heart rate and produces cutaneous vasoconstriction) and decreased parasympathetic outflow to the heart (also increases heart rate). TPR, if measured, would be increased as a result of sympathetic vasoconstriction of many vascular beds, in addition to that of the skin.

The renin–angiotensin II–aldosterone system also is activated by the low P_a, and the increased levels of angiotensin II contribute to peripheral vasoconstriction. The increased levels of aldosterone increase Na^+ reabsorption, total body Na^+ content, and ECF volume, perpetuating the cycle of edema formation.

TREATMENT. Treatment involves two strategies: (1) to increase contractility of the myocardial cells by administering a positive inotropic agent such as digoxin and (2) to reduce total body Na^+ content and the cycle of edema formation by administering a diuretic and by restricting sodium intake.

---

sympathetic outflow to the heart and blood vessels and a **decrease in parasympathetic outflow** to the heart, attempting to increase P_a back to normal. The results of these autonomic changes now are familiar: increased heart rate, increased contractility, constriction of arterioles (increased TPR), and constriction of the veins (decreased unstressed volume and increased venous return). Collectively, these changes increase cardiac output and increase TPR, attempting to restore P_a back to normal.

Box 4-4 describes heart failure and further illustrates the integrative nature of the cardiovascular system.

SUMMARY

- The cardiovascular system is composed of the heart and blood vessels. The heart, by contracting, pumps blood through the systemic and pulmonary vasculatures. Blood vessels act as conduits that deliver blood to the tissues. The thin-walled capillaries serve as the site of exchange of nutrients and waste products.

- Hemodynamics are the principles that govern blood flow: velocity of flow; flow, pressure, and resistance relationships; and compliance of blood vessels.

■ Velocity of blood flow is proportional to the rate of volume flow and inversely proportional to the cross-sectional area. Velocity is lowest in the capillaries, which have the largest cross-sectional area.

■ Blood flow is proportional to the size of the pressure gradient and inversely proportional to the resistance of the blood vessels.

■ Resistance to blood flow is proportional to the viscosity of blood and vessel length and inversely proportional to vessel radius to the fourth power. The arterioles are the site of highest resistance in the vasculature. Resistances can be arranged in series or in parallel.

■ Compliance is the relationship between volume and pressure: The higher the compliance of a blood vessel, the greater the volume contained at a given pressure. Veins have high compliance and hold large volumes of blood (the unstressed volume) at low pressure. Arteries have low compliance and hold small volumes of blood (the stressed volume) at high pressure.

■ The cardiac action potential is initiated in the SA node, which depolarizes spontaneously. The action potential spreads in a specific sequence throughout the myocardium via a specialized conducting system. Conduction is rapid, except through the AV node, where slow conduction ensures ample time for ventricular filling prior to contraction.

■ In atria and ventricles, the upstroke of the action potential is the result of an inward Na^+ current. The action potential in the atria and ventricles exhibits a plateau, which is the result of an inward Ca^{2+} current. This plateau accounts for the action potential's long duration and long refractory period.

■ In the SA node, the upstroke of the action potential is the result of an inward Ca^{2+} current. The SA node exhibits slow, spontaneous depolarization during phase 4, which brings the cells to threshold to fire action potentials. Slow depolarization is the result of an inward Na^+ current (I_f).

■ Excitation-contraction coupling in myocardial cells is similar to that in skeletal muscle. In myocardial cells, however, Ca^{2+} entering the cell during the plateau of the action potential serves as a trigger for the release of more Ca^{2+} from the sarcoplasmic reticulum. Ca^{2+} then binds to troponin C to allow cross-bridge formation.

■ Inotropism or contractility is the ability of the myocardial cell to develop tension at a given cell length: Intracellular $[Ca^{2+}]$ determines the degree of inotropism, with positive inotropic agents increasing intracellular $[Ca^{2+}]$ and contractility.

■ Myocardial cells and the myocardium exhibit a length-tension relationship based on the degree of overlap of contractile elements. The Frank-Starling law of the heart describes this relationship between cardiac output and end-diastolic volume. End-diastolic volume reflects venous return. Therefore, cardiac output is determined by venous return, and in the steady state, cardiac output and venous return are equal.

■ P_a is the product of cardiac output and TPR. P_a is carefully monitored and maintained at a normal value of 100 mm Hg. The baroreceptor reflex is a fast, neural mechanism that detects changes in P_a and orchestrates changes in sympathetic and parasympathetic outflow to the heart and blood vessels to restore P_a back to normal. The renin–angiotensin II–aldosterone system is a slower, hormonal mechanism that detects changes in P_a and, via aldosterone, restores P_a to normal through changes in blood volume.

■ The exchange of fluid across capillary walls is determined by the balance of Starling forces. The net Starling pressure determines whether there will be filtration out of the capillary or absorption into the capillary. If filtration of fluid exceeds the ability of the lymphatics to return it to the circulation, then edema occurs.

■ The blood flow to the organ systems is a variable percentage of the cardiac output. Blood flow is determined by arteriolar resistance, which can be altered by vasodilator metabolites or by sympathetic innervation.

Challenge Yourself

Answer each question with a word, phrase, sentence, or numerical solution. When a list of possible answers is supplied with the question, one, more than one, or none of the choices may be correct. Correct answers are provided at the end of the book.

1 *What are the units of hemodynamic resistance?*

2 *If heart rate is 75 beats/minute, what is the R-R interval in units of milliseconds?*

3 *What is the correct order of the following events: Ca^{2+} binding to troponin C, tension, Ca^{2+} release from sarcoplasmic reticulum, ventricular action potential, Ca^{2+} accumulation by sarcoplasmic reticulum?*

4 If heart rate is 85 beats/minute, end-diastolic volume is 150 mL, and stroke volume is 75 mL, what is the ejection fraction?

5 Which portion of the cardiac cycle has the lower ventricular volume: atrial systole or isovolumetric ventricular relaxation?

6 According to the cardiac and vascular function curves, an increase in blood volume leads to _____ right atrial pressure and _____ cardiac output.

7 If cardiac output is 5.2 L/min, heart rate is 76 beats/minute, and end-diastolic volume is 145 mL, what is the end-systolic volume?

8 In a capillary, if P_c is 35 mm Hg, π_c is 25 mm Hg, P_i is 2 mm Hg, and π_i is 1 mm Hg, is there net absorption or filtration, and what is the magnitude of the driving force?

9 When a person moves quickly from a lying to a standing position, which of the following decrease(s): venous return, cardiac output, arterial pressure (P_a)?

10 What is the name of the volume contained in the left ventricle immediately before it contracts?

11 Which of the following produce(s) an increase in contractility: decreased heart rate, increased phosphorylation of phospholamban, increased action potential duration?

12 During which phase of the ventricular action potential, phase 0 or phase 4, is inward current greater than outward current?

13 Which term best applies to the absolute refractory period of the ventricular action potential: automaticity, excitability, conduction velocity, maximum diastolic potential?

14 If, simultaneously, there is an increased rate of phase 4 depolarization and hyperpolarization of the threshold potential, will there be an increase, decrease, or no change in heart rate?

15 Among the responses that occur following hemorrhage, which of the following increase(s): unstressed volume, heart rate, resistance of cutaneous vascular beds, firing rate of carotid sinus nerves, angiotensin II levels?

16 In the myogenic mechanism of autoregulation, according to the law of Laplace, does an increase in pressure lead to an increase, decrease, or no change in the radius of the blood vessel?

17 Of the following, which circulation receives the highest percentage of the cardiac output: renal, pulmonary, coronary, skeletal muscle during intense exercise, skin during intense exercise?

18 Which of the following cause(s) an increase in stroke volume from the left ventricle: increased contractility, decrease in end-diastolic volume, increase in aortic pressure?

19 During which portion(s) of the cardiac cycle is the aortic valve open: atrial systole, rapid ventricular ejection, diastasis?

20 According to the cardiac and vascular function curves, an increase in TPR leads to _____ venous return and _____ cardiac output.

21 Which situation is associated with the higher efficiency of myocardial oxygen consumption: increased cardiac output secondary to increased heart rate or decreased cardiac output secondary to increased aortic pressure?

22 Three resistors, each with a value of 10, are arranged in parallel. How much does total resistance change if a fourth resistor with a value of 10 is added in parallel?

23 Blood vessel "A" has a cross-sectional area of 1 cm², and blood vessel "B" has a cross-sectional area of 10 cm². If blood flow through the two vessels is the same, in which vessel is velocity of blood flow higher?

24 Where am I? For each item in the following list, give its correct location in the cardiovascular system. The location may be anatomic, a graph or portion of a graph, an equation, or a concept.
Dicrotic notch
β_1 receptors
L_{max}
Radius to the fourth power
Phospholamban
Negative dromotropic effect
Pulse pressure
Normal automaticity
Ejection fraction

25 During which portions(s) of the cardiac cycle is the mitral valve closed? Atrial systole, rapid ventricular ejection, isovolumetric ventricular relaxation, diastasis.

26 During exercise, which of the following decrease(s)? Heart rate, venous return, stroke volume, diameter of splanchnic arterioles, TPR.

27 *According to the ventricular pressure-volume loop, an increase in afterload produces an increase in which of the following? End-diastolic volume, end-diastolic pressure, end-systolic volume, stroke volume.*

28 *Which of the following is/are mediated by an increase in I_{Ca}? Sympathetic effect to increase heart rate, parasympathetic effect to decrease heart rate, sympathetic effect to increase contractility, parasympathetic effect to decrease conduction velocity in AV node.*

SELECTED READINGS

Berne RM, Levy MN: Cardiovascular Physiology, 8th ed. St Louis, Mosby, 2001.

Guyton AC, Hall JE: Textbook of Medical Physiology, 9th ed. Philadelphia, WB Saunders, 1996.

Smith JJ, Kampine JP: Circulatory Physiology, 3rd ed. Baltimore, Williams & Wilkins, 1990.

Respiratory Physiology

The function of the respiratory system is the exchange of oxygen and carbon dioxide between the environment and the cells of the body. Fresh air is brought into the lungs during the inspiratory phase of the breathing cycle, oxygen and carbon dioxide are exchanged between inspired air and pulmonary capillary blood, and the air is then expired.

STRUCTURE OF THE RESPIRATORY SYSTEM

Airways

The respiratory system includes the lungs and a series of airways that connect the lungs to the external environment. The structures of the respiratory system are subdivided into a **conducting zone** (or conducting airways), which brings air into and out of the lungs, and a **respiratory zone** lined with alveoli, where gas exchange occurs. The functions of the conducting and respiratory zones differ, and the structures lining them also differ (Fig. 5-1).

Conducting Zone

The conducting zone includes the nose, nasopharynx, larynx, trachea, bronchi, bronchioles, and terminal bronchioles. These structures function to bring air into and out of the respiratory zone for gas exchange and to warm, humidify, and filter the air before it reaches the critical gas exchange region.

The trachea is the main conducting airway. The trachea divides into two bronchi, one leading into each lung, which divide into two smaller bronchi, which divide again. Ultimately, there are 23 such divisions into increasingly smaller airways.

The conducting airways are lined with mucus-secreting and ciliated cells that function to remove inhaled particles. Although large particles usually are filtered out in the nose, small particles may enter the airways, where they are captured by mucus, which is then swept upward by the rhythmic beating of the cilia.

The walls of the conducting airways contain **smooth muscle.** This smooth muscle has both sympathetic and parasympathetic innervation, which have opposite effects on airway diameter: (1) Sympathetic adrenergic neurons activate β_2 **receptors** on bronchial smooth muscle, which leads to relaxation and **dilation** of the airways. In addition, and what is more important, these β_2 receptors are activated by circulating epinephrine released from the adrenal medulla and by β_2-adrenergic agonists such as

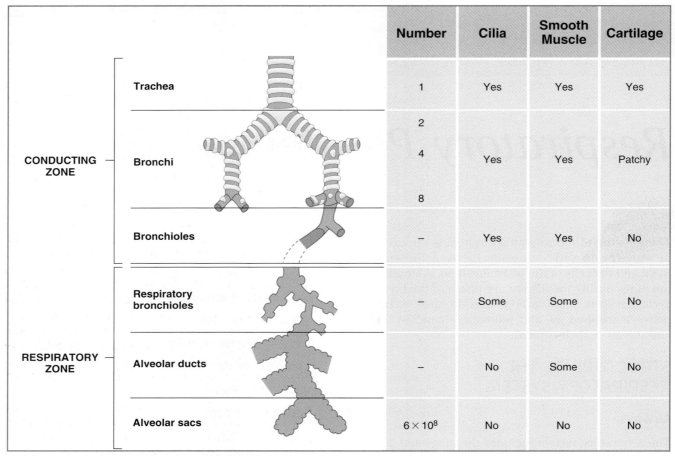

		Number	Cilia	Smooth Muscle	Cartilage
CONDUCTING ZONE	Trachea	1	Yes	Yes	Yes
	Bronchi	2 4 8	Yes	Yes	Patchy
	Bronchioles	–	Yes	Yes	No
RESPIRATORY ZONE	Respiratory bronchioles	–	Some	Some	No
	Alveolar ducts	–	No	Some	No
	Alveolar sacs	6×10^8	No	No	No

Figure 5–1 **Structure of the airways.** The number of the various structures is reported for two lungs.

isoproterenol. (2) Parasympathetic cholinergic neurons activate **muscarinic receptors,** which leads to contraction and **constriction** of the airways.

Changes in diameter of the conducting airways result in changes in their resistance, which produce changes in airflow. Thus, the effects of the autonomic nervous system on airway diameter have predictable effects on airway resistance and airflow. The most notable effects are those of β_2-adrenergic agonists (e.g., epinephrine, isoproterenol, albuterol), which are used to dilate the airways in the treatment of **asthma.**

Respiratory Zone

The respiratory zone includes the structures that are lined with alveoli and, therefore, participate in **gas exchange:** the respiratory bronchioles, alveolar ducts, and alveolar sacs. The **respiratory bronchioles** are transitional structures. Like the conducting airways, they have cilia and smooth muscle, but they also are considered part of the gas exchange region because alveoli occasionally bud off their walls. The **alveolar ducts** are completely lined with alveoli, but they contain no cilia and little smooth muscle. The alveolar

ducts terminate in **alveolar sacs,** which also are lined with alveoli.

The **alveoli** are pouchlike evaginations of the walls of the respiratory bronchioles, the alveolar ducts, and the alveolar sacs. Each lung has a total of approximately 300 million alveoli. The diameter of each alveolus is approximately 200 μm. Exchange of oxygen (O_2) and carbon dioxide (CO_2) between alveolar gas and pulmonary capillary blood can occur rapidly and efficiently across the alveoli because alveolar walls are thin and have a large **surface area** for diffusion.

The alveolar walls are rimmed with elastic fibers and lined with epithelial cells, called type I and type II pneumocytes (or alveolar cells). **Type II pneumocytes** synthesize **pulmonary surfactant** (necessary for reduction of surface tension of alveoli) and have regenerative capacity for the type I and type II pneumocytes.

The alveoli contain phagocytic cells called **alveolar macrophages.** Alveolar macrophages keep the alveoli free of dust and debris because the alveoli have no cilia to perform this function. Macrophages fill with debris and migrate to the bronchioles, where the beating cilia carry debris to the upper airways and the pharynx, where it can be swallowed or expectorated.

Pulmonary Blood Flow

Pulmonary blood flow is the cardiac output of the right heart. It is ejected from the right ventricle and delivered to the lungs via the pulmonary artery (see Chapter 4, Fig. 4-1). The pulmonary arteries branch into increasingly smaller arteries and travel with the bronchi toward the respiratory zones. The smallest arteries divide into arterioles and then into the pulmonary capillaries, which form dense networks around the alveoli.

Because of **gravitational effects,** pulmonary blood flow is not distributed evenly in the lungs. When a person is standing, blood flow is lowest at the apex (top) of the lungs and highest at the base (bottom) of the lungs. When the person is supine (lying down), these gravitational effects disappear. The physiologic significance of regional variations in blood flow is discussed later in the chapter.

As in other organs, **regulation of pulmonary blood flow** is accomplished by altering the resistance of the pulmonary arterioles. Changes in pulmonary arteriolar resistance are controlled by local factors, mainly O_2.

Bronchial circulation is the blood supply to the conducting airways (which do not participate in gas exchange) and is a very small fraction of the total pulmonary blood flow.

LUNG VOLUMES AND CAPACITIES

Lung Volumes

Static volumes of the lung are measured with a **spirometer** (Table 5-1). Typically, the subject is sitting and breathes into and out of the spirometer, displacing a bell. The volume displaced is recorded on calibrated paper (Fig. 5-2).

First, the subject is asked to breathe quietly. Normal, quiet breathing involves inspiration and expiration of a **tidal volume** (V_T). Normal tidal volume is approximately 500 mL and includes the volume of air that fills the alveoli *plus* the volume of air that fills the airways.

Next, the subject is asked to take a maximal inspiration, followed by a maximal expiration. With this maneuver, additional lung volumes are revealed. The additional volume that can be inspired *above* tidal volume is called the **inspiratory reserve volume,** which is approximately 3000 mL. The additional volume that can be expired *below* tidal volume is called the **expiratory reserve volume,** which is approximately 1200 mL.

The volume of gas remaining in the lungs after a maximal forced expiration is the **residual volume** (**RV**), which is approximately 1200 mL and cannot be measured by spirometry.

Lung Capacities

In addition to these lung volumes, there are several **lung capacities;** each lung capacity includes two or more lung volumes. The **inspiratory capacity** (**IC**) is composed of the tidal volume plus the inspiratory reserve volume and is approximately 3500 mL (500 mL + 3000 mL). The **functional residual capacity** (**FRC**) is composed of the expiratory reserve volume (ERV) plus the residual volume, or approximately 2400 mL (1200 mL + 1200 mL). FRC is the volume remaining in the lungs after a normal tidal volume is expired and can be thought of as the **equilibrium volume** of the lungs. The **vital capacity** (**VC**) is composed of the inspiratory capacity plus the expiratory reserve volume, or approximately 4700 mL (3500 mL + 1200 mL). Vital capacity is the volume that can be expired after maximal inspiration. Its value increases with body size, male gender, and physical conditioning and decreases with age. Finally, as the terminology suggests, the **total lung capacity** (**TLC**) includes all of the lung volumes: It is the vital capacity plus the residual volume, or 5900 mL (4700 mL + 1200 mL).

Because residual volume cannot be measured by spirometry, lung capacities that *include* the residual volume also cannot be measured by spirometry (i.e., FRC and TLC). Of the lung capacities *not* measurable by spirometry, the FRC (the volume remaining in the lungs after a normal expiration) is of greatest interest because it is the resting or equilibrium volume of the lungs.

Two methods are used to **measure FRC:** helium dilution and the body plethysmograph.

♦ In the **helium dilution** method, the subject breathes a known amount of helium, which has been added to the spirometer. Because helium is insoluble in blood, after a few breaths the helium concentration in the lungs becomes equal to that in the spirometer, which can be measured. The amount of helium that was added to the spirometer and its concentration in the lungs are used to "back-calculate" the lung volume. If this measurement is made after a normal tidal volume is expired, the lung volume being calculated is the FRC.

♦ The **body plethysmograph** employs a variant of Boyle's law, which states that for gases at constant temperature, gas pressure multiplied by gas volume is constant (P × V = constant). Therefore, if volume increases, pressure must decrease, and if volume decreases, pressure must increase. To measure FRC, the subject sits in a large airtight box called a plethysmograph. After expiring a normal

Table 5–1 Abbreviations and Normal Values Associated with Respiratory Physiology

Abbreviation	Meaning	Normal Value
P	Gas pressure or partial pressure	
$\dot{Q}$	Blood flow	
V	Gas volume	
$\dot{V}$	Gas flow rate	
F	Fractional concentration of gas	
A	Alveolar gas	
a	Arterial blood	
V	Venous blood	
E	Expired gas	
I	Inspired gas	
L	Transpulmonary	
TM	Transmural	
Arterial Blood		
Pa_{O_2}	Partial pressure of O_2 in arterial blood	100 mm Hg
Pa_{CO_2}	Partial pressure of CO_2 in arterial blood	40 mm Hg
Mixed Venous Blood		
$P\bar{v}_{O_2}$	Partial pressure of O_2 in venous blood	40 mm Hg
$P\bar{v}_{CO_2}$	Partial pressure of CO_2 in venous blood	46 mm Hg
Inspired Air		
PI_{O_2}	Partial pressure of O_2 in dry inspired air	160 mm Hg
PI_{CO_2}	Partial pressure of CO_2 in dry inspired air	0 mm Hg
Alveolar Air		
PA_{O_2}	Partial pressure of O_2 in alveolar air	100 mm Hg
PA_{CO_2}	Partial pressure of CO_2 in alveolar air	40 mm Hg
Respiratory Volumes and Rates		
TLC	Total lung capacity	6.0 L
FRC	Functional residual capacity	2.4 L
VC	Vital capacity	4.7 L
V_T	Tidal volume	0.5 L
$\dot{V}_A$	Alveolar ventilation	—
—	Breathing rate	15 breaths/min
V_D	Physiologic dead space	0.15 L
FVC	Forced vital capacity	4.7 L
FEV_1	Volume of forced vital capacity expired in 1 second	—
Constants		
P_{atm}, or P_B	Atmospheric (barometric) pressure	760 mm Hg (sea level)
P_{H_2O}	Water vapor pressure	47 mm Hg (37°C)
STPD	Standard temperature, pressure, dry	273 K, 760 mm Hg
BTPS	Body temperature, pressure, saturated	310 K, 760 mm Hg, 47 mm Hg
—	Solubility of O_2 in blood	0.003 mL O_2/100 mL blood/mm Hg
—	Solubility of CO_2 in blood	0.07 mL CO_2/100 mL blood/mm Hg
Other Values		
—	Hemoglobin concentration	15 g/100 mL blood
—	O_2-binding capacity of hemoglobin	1.34 mL O_2/g hemoglobin
$\dot{V}_{O_2}$	O_2 consumption	250 mL/min
$\dot{V}_{CO_2}$	CO_2 production	200 mL/min
R	Respiratory exchange quotient (CO_2 production/O_2 consumption)	0.8

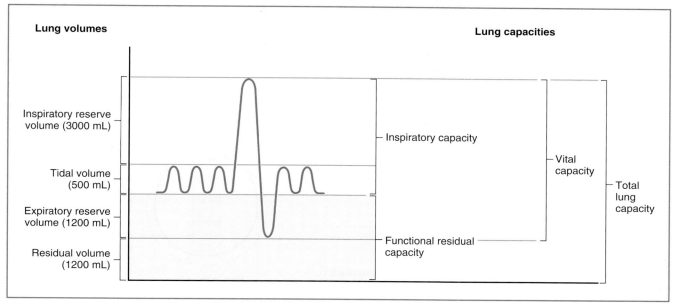

Figure 5–2 **Lung volumes and capacities.** Measurements of lung volumes and capacities are made by spirometry. Residual volume cannot be measured by spirometry.

tidal volume, the mouthpiece to the subject's airway is closed. The subject then attempts to breathe. As the subject tries to inspire, the volume in the subject's lungs increases and the pressure in his or her lungs decreases. Simultaneously, the volume in the box decreases, and the pressure in the box increases. The increase in pressure in the box can be measured and, from it, the preinspiratory volume in the lungs can be calculated, which is the FRC.

Dead Space

Dead space is the volume of the airways and lungs that **does not participate in gas exchange.** Dead space is a general term that refers to both the *anatomic* dead space of the conducting airways and a functional, or *physiologic,* dead space.

Anatomic Dead Space

The anatomic dead space is the **volume of the conducting airways** including the nose (and/or mouth), trachea, bronchi, and bronchioles. It does not include the respiratory bronchioles and alveoli. The volume of the conducting airways is approximately 150 mL. Thus, for example, when a tidal volume of 500 mL is inspired, the entire volume does not reach the alveoli for gas exchange. 150 mL fills the conducting airways (the anatomic dead space, where no gas exchange occurs), and 350 mL fills the alveoli. Figure 5-3 shows that at the end of expiration the conducting airways are filled with alveolar air; that is, they are filled with air that has already been in the alveoli and exchanged gases

with pulmonary capillary blood. With the inspiration of the next tidal volume, this alveolar air is first to enter the alveoli, although it will not undergo further gas exchange ("already been there, done that"). The next air to enter the alveoli is fresh air from the inspired tidal volume (350 mL), which will undergo gas exchange. The rest of the tidal volume (150 mL) does not make it to the alveoli but remains in the conducting airways; this air will not participate in gas exchange and will be the first air expired. (A related point arises from this discussion: The first air expired is dead space air that has not undergone gas exchange. To sample alveolar air, one must sample *end*-expiratory air.)

Physiologic Dead Space

The concept of physiologic dead space is more abstract than the concept of anatomic dead space. By definition, the physiologic dead space is the *total volume of the lungs that does not participate in gas exchange.* Physiologic dead space includes the *anatomic* dead space of the conducting airways plus a *functional* dead space in the alveoli.

The functional dead space can be thought of as ventilated alveoli that do not participate in gas exchange. The most important reason that alveoli do not participate in gas exchange is a mismatch of ventilation and perfusion, or so-called ventilation/perfusion defect, in which ventilated alveoli are not perfused by pulmonary capillary blood.

In normal persons, the physiologic dead space is nearly equal to the anatomic dead space. In other words, alveolar ventilation and perfusion (blood flow)

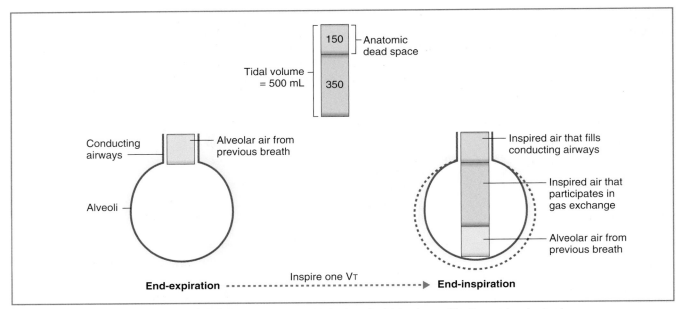

Figure 5–3 **Anatomic dead space.** One third of each tidal volume fills the anatomic dead space. V_T, Tidal volume.

are normally well matched and functional dead space is small. In certain pathologic situations, however, the physiologic dead space can become larger than the anatomic dead space, suggesting a ventilation/perfusion defect. The ratio of physiologic dead space to tidal volume provides an estimate of how much ventilation is "wasted" (either in the conducting airways or in nonperfused alveoli).

The **volume of the physiologic dead space** is estimated with the following method, which is based on the measurement of the partial pressure of CO_2 (P_{CO_2}) of mixed expired air (PE_{CO_2}) and the following three assumptions: (1) *All* of the CO_2 in expired air comes from exchange of CO_2 in functioning (ventilated and perfused) alveoli; (2) there is essentially no CO_2 in inspired air; and (3) the physiologic dead space (nonfunctioning alveoli and airways) neither exchanges nor contributes any CO_2. If physiologic dead space is zero, then PE_{CO_2} will be equal to alveolar P_{CO_2} (PA_{CO_2}). However, if a physiologic dead space is present, then PE_{CO_2} will be "diluted" by dead space air and PE_{CO_2} will be less than PA_{CO_2} by a dilution factor. Therefore, by comparing PE_{CO_2} with PA_{CO_2}, the dilution factor (i.e., volume of the physiologic dead space) can be measured. A potential problem in measuring physiologic dead space is that alveolar air cannot be sampled directly. This problem can be overcome, however, because alveolar air normally equilibrates with pulmonary capillary blood (which becomes systemic arterial blood). Thus, the P_{CO_2} of systemic arterial blood (Pa_{CO_2}) is equal to the P_{CO_2} of alveolar air (PA_{CO_2}). Using this assumption, the volume of physiologic dead space is calculated by the following equation:

$$V_D = V_T \times \frac{Pa_{CO_2} - PE_{CO_2}}{Pa_{CO_2}}$$

where

V_D = Physiologic dead space (mL)
V_T = Tidal volume (mL)
Pa_{CO_2} = P_{CO_2} of arterial blood (mm Hg)
PE_{CO_2} = P_{CO_2} of mixed expired air (mm Hg)

In words, the equation states that the volume of the physiologic dead space is the tidal volume (volume inspired with a single breath) multiplied by a fraction. The fraction represents the dilution of alveolar P_{CO_2} by dead space air (which contributes no CO_2).

To better appreciate the equation and its application, consider two extreme examples. In the first example, assume that physiologic dead space is *zero;* in the second example, assume that physiologic dead space is equal to the *entire* tidal volume. In the first example, in which dead space is zero, the P_{CO_2} of expired air (PE_{CO_2}) will be the same as the P_{CO_2} of alveolar gas (PA_{CO_2}) and arterial blood (Pa_{CO_2}) because there is no "wasted" ventilation: The fraction in the equation is equal to zero, and thus the calculated value of V_D is zero. In the second example, in which dead space is equal to the *entire* tidal volume, there is no gas exchange: Therefore, PE_{CO_2} will be zero, the fraction will be 1.0, and V_D will be equal to V_T.

Ventilation Rates

Ventilation rate is the volume of air moved into and out of the lungs per unit time. Ventilation rate can be expressed either as the *minute* ventilation, which is the total rate of air movement into and out of the lungs, or as *alveolar* ventilation, which corrects for the physiologic dead space. To calculate alveolar ventilation, the physiologic dead space first must be measured, which involves sampling systemic arterial blood, as described in the preceding section.

Minute ventilation is given by the following equation:

$$\text{Minute ventilation} = V_T \times \text{Breaths/min}$$

Alveolar ventilation is minute ventilation corrected for the physiologic dead space and is given by the following equation:

$$\dot{V}_A = (V_T - V_D) \times \text{Breaths/min}$$

where

$$\dot{V}_A = \text{Alveolar ventilation (mL/min)}$$
$$V_T = \text{Tidal volume (mL)}$$
$$V_D = \text{Physiologic dead space (mL)}$$

SAMPLE PROBLEM. A man who has a tidal volume of 550 mL is breathing at a rate of 14 breaths/min. The P_{CO_2} in his arterial blood is 40 mm Hg, and the P_{CO_2} in his expired air is 30 mm Hg. *What is his minute ventilation? What is his alveolar ventilation? What percentage of each tidal volume reaches functioning alveoli? What percentage of each tidal volume is dead space?*

SOLUTION. Minute ventilation is tidal volume times breaths per minute, or:

$$\text{Minute ventilation} = 550 \text{ mL} \times 14 \text{ breaths/min}$$
$$= 7700 \text{ mL/min}$$

Alveolar ventilation is minute ventilation corrected for the physiologic dead space, which must be calculated. This problem illustrates the usual method of assessing physiologic dead space, which represents structures that are ventilated but are not exchanging CO_2.

$$V_D = V_T \times \frac{Pa_{CO_2} - PE_{CO_2}}{Pa_{CO_2}}$$
$$= 550 \text{ mL} \times \frac{40 \text{ mm Hg} - 30 \text{ mm Hg}}{40 \text{ mm Hg}}$$
$$= 550 \text{ mL} \times 0.25$$
$$= 138 \text{ mL}$$

Thus, alveolar ventilation ($\dot{V}_A$) is

$$\dot{V}_A = (V_T - V_D) \times \text{Breaths/min}$$
$$= (550 \text{ mL} - 138 \text{ mL}) \times 14 \text{ breaths/min}$$
$$= 412 \text{ mL} \times 14 \text{ breaths/min}$$
$$= 5768 \text{ mL/min}$$

If tidal volume is 550 mL and physiologic dead space is 138 mL, then the volume of fresh air reaching functioning alveoli on each breath is 412 mL, or 75% of each tidal volume. Dead space is, accordingly, 25% of each tidal volume.

Alveolar Ventilation Equation

The alveolar ventilation equation is the *fundamental relationship of respiratory physiology* and describes the inverse relationship between alveolar ventilation and alveolar P_{CO_2} (PA_{CO_2}). The alveolar ventilation equation is expressed as follows:

$$\dot{V}_A = \frac{\dot{V}_{CO_2} \times K}{PA_{CO_2}}$$

or, rearranging,

$$PA_{CO_2} = \frac{\dot{V}_{CO_2} \times K}{\dot{V}_A}$$

where

$$\dot{V}_A = \text{Alveolar ventilation (mL/min)}$$
$$\dot{V}_{CO_2} = \text{Rate of } CO_2 \text{ production (mL/min)}$$
$$PA_{CO_2} = \text{Alveolar } P_{CO_2} \text{ (mm Hg)}$$
$$K = \text{Constant (863 mm Hg)}$$

The **constant, K,** equals 863 mm Hg for conditions of BTPS and when $\dot{V}_A$ and $\dot{V}_{CO_2}$ are expressed in the same units (e.g., mL/min). **BTPS** means body temperature (310 K), ambient pressure (760 mm Hg), and gas saturated with water vapor.

Using the rearranged form of the equation, alveolar P_{CO_2} can be predicted if two variables are known: (1) the rate of **CO_2 production** from aerobic metabolism of the tissues and (2) **alveolar ventilation,** which excretes this CO_2 in expired air.

A critical point to be understood from the alveolar ventilation equation is that *if CO_2 production is constant, then PA_{CO_2} is determined by alveolar ventilation.* For a constant level of CO_2 production, there is a hyperbolic relationship between PA_{CO_2} and $\dot{V}_A$ (Fig. 5-4). Increases in alveolar ventilation cause a decrease in PA_{CO_2}; conversely, decreases in alveolar ventilation cause an increase in PA_{CO_2}.

An additional critical point, which is not immediately evident from the equation, is that because CO_2 always equilibrates between pulmonary capillary blood and alveolar gas, the arterial P_{CO_2} (Pa_{CO_2}) always equals the alveolar P_{CO_2} (PA_{CO_2}). Consequently, Pa_{CO_2}, which can be measured, can be substituted for PA_{CO_2} in the earlier discussion.

So, *why does arterial (and alveolar) P_{CO_2} vary inversely with alveolar ventilation?* To understand the inverse relationship, first appreciate that alveolar ventilation is *pulling* CO_2 out of pulmonary capillary blood. With each breath, CO_2-free air is brought into the lungs, which creates a driving force for CO_2 diffusion from pulmonary capillary blood into the alveolar gas; the CO_2 pulled out of pulmonary capillary blood will then be expired. The higher the alveolar ventilation, the more CO_2 is pulled out of the blood and the lower the Pa_{CO_2} and the PA_{CO_2} (because alveolar P_{CO_2} always equilibrates with arterial P_{CO_2}). The lower the alveolar ventilation, the less CO_2 is pulled out of the blood and the higher the Pa_{CO_2} and PA_{CO_2}.

Another way to think about the alveolar ventilation equation is to consider how the relationship between PA_{CO_2} and $\dot{V}A$ would be altered by changes in CO_2 production. For example, if CO_2 production, or

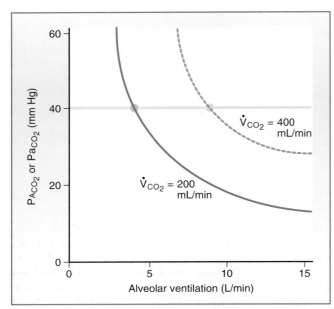

Figure 5–4   Alveolar or arterial P_{CO_2} as a function of alveolar ventilation. The relationship is described by the alveolar ventilation equation. When CO_2 production doubles from 200 mL/min to 400 mL/min, alveolar ventilation also must double to maintain the PA_{CO_2} and Pa_{CO_2} at 40 mm Hg.

$\dot{V}_{CO_2}$, doubles (e.g., during strenuous exercise), the hyperbolic relationship between PA_{CO_2} and $\dot{V}A$ shifts to the right (see Fig. 5-4). Under these conditions, the only way to maintain PA_{CO_2} at its normal value (i.e., 40 mm Hg) is for alveolar ventilation to also double. The graph confirms that if CO_2 production increases from 200 mL/min to 400 mL/min, PA_{CO_2} is maintained at 40 mm Hg if, simultaneously, $\dot{V}A$ increases from 5 L/min to 10 L/min.

Alveolar Gas Equation

The alveolar ventilation equation describes the dependence of alveolar and arterial P_{CO_2} on alveolar ventilation. A second equation, the **alveolar gas equation,** is used to predict the alveolar P_{O_2}, based on the alveolar P_{CO_2}, and is illustrated by the O_2-CO_2 diagram in Figure 5-5. The alveolar gas equation is expressed as

$$PA_{O_2} = PI_{O_2} - \frac{PA_{CO_2}}{R} + \text{Correction factor}$$

where

$$PA_{O_2} = \text{Alveolar } P_{O_2} \text{ (mm Hg)}$$
$$PI_{O_2} = P_{O_2} \text{ in inspired air (mm Hg)}$$
$$PA_{CO_2} = \text{Alveolar } P_{CO_2} \text{ (mm Hg)}$$
$$R = \text{Respiratory exchange ratio or}$$
$$\text{respiratory quotient (CO}_2$$
$$\text{production/O}_2 \text{ consumption)}$$

The correction factor is small and usually is ignored. In the steady state, R, the respiratory exchange ratio, equals the respiratory quotient. According to the earlier

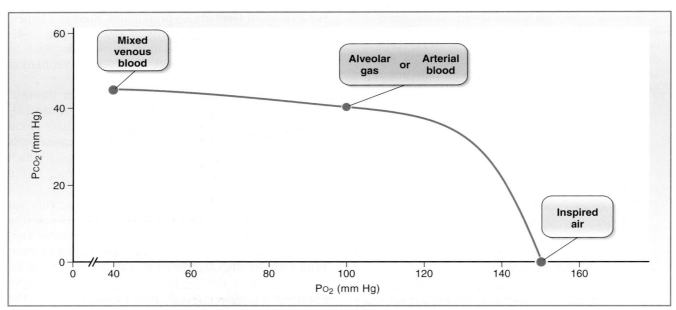

Figure 5–5 P_{CO_2} as a function of P_{O_2}. The relationship is described by the alveolar gas equation. The variations in P_{O_2} between inspired air and mixed venous blood are much greater than the variations in P_{CO_2}.

alveolar ventilation equation, when alveolar ventilation is halved, $P_{A_{CO_2}}$ doubles (because less CO_2 is removed from the alveoli). A second consequence of halving alveolar ventilation is that $P_{A_{O_2}}$ will decrease (a decrease in alveolar ventilation means that less O_2 is brought into the alveoli). The alveolar gas equation predicts the change in $P_{A_{O_2}}$ that will occur for a given change in $P_{A_{CO_2}}$. Because the normal value for the respiratory exchange ratio is 0.8, when alveolar ventilation is halved, the *decrease* in $P_{A_{O_2}}$ will be slightly greater than the *increase* in $P_{A_{CO_2}}$. To summarize, when $\dot{V}_A$ is halved, $P_{A_{CO_2}}$ is doubled and $P_{A_{O_2}}$ is slightly more than halved.

Further inspection of the alveolar gas equation reveals that if for some reason the respiratory exchange ratio changes, the relationship between $P_{A_{CO_2}}$ and $P_{A_{O_2}}$ also changes. As stated, the normal value of the respiratory exchange ratio is 0.8. However, if the rate of CO_2 production decreases relative to the rate of O_2 consumption (e.g., if the respiratory quotient and respiratory exchange ratio are 0.6 rather than 0.8), then $P_{A_{O_2}}$ would decrease relative to $P_{A_{CO_2}}$.

SAMPLE PROBLEM. A man has a rate of CO_2 production that is 80% the rate of O_2 consumption. If his arterial P_{CO_2} is 40 mm Hg and the P_{O_2} in humidified tracheal air is 150 mm Hg, what is his alveolar P_{O_2}?

SOLUTION. To solve this problem, a basic assumption is that CO_2 equilibrates between arterial blood and

---

alveolar air. Thus, $P_{A_{CO_2}}$ (needed for the alveolar gas equation) equals $P_{a_{CO_2}}$ (given in the problem). Using the alveolar gas equation, $P_{A_{O_2}}$ can be calculated from $P_{A_{CO_2}}$ if the respiratory quotient and the P_{O_2} of inspired air are known. It is stated that CO_2 production is 80% of O_2 consumption; thus, the respiratory quotient is 0.8, a normal value. $P_{A_{O_2}}$ is calculated as follows:

$$P_{A_{O_2}} = P_{I_{O_2}} - P_{A_{CO_2}}/R$$
$$= 150 \text{ mm Hg} - 40 \text{ mm Hg}/0.8$$
$$= 150 \text{ mm Hg} - 50 \text{ mm Hg}$$
$$= 100 \text{ mm Hg}$$

This calculated value for $P_{A_{O_2}}$ can be confirmed on the O_2-CO_2 diagram shown in Figure 5-4. The graph indicates that alveolar gas or arterial blood with a P_{CO_2} of 40 mm Hg will have a P_{O_2} of 100 mm Hg when the respiratory quotient is 0.8—exactly the value calculated by the alveolar gas equation!

Forced Expiratory Volumes

Vital capacity is the volume that can be expired following a maximal inspiration. ***Forced* vital capacity (FVC)** is the total volume of air that can be *forcibly* expired after a maximal inspiration, as shown in Figure 5-6. The volume of air that can be forcibly expired in the first second is called **FEV_1.** Likewise, the cumulative volume expired in 2 seconds is called **FEV_2,** and the cumulative volume expired in 3 seconds is called **FEV_3.** Normally, the entire vital capacity can be forcibly expired in 3 seconds, so there is no need for "FEV_4."

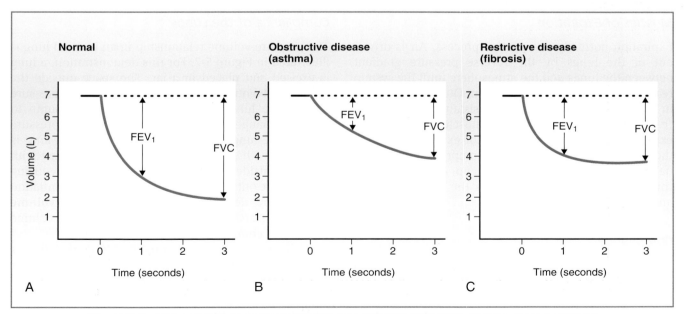

Figure 5–6 **FVC and FEV_1 in normal subjects and patients with lung disease.** Subjects inspired maximally and then expired forcibly. **A–C,** The graphs show the phase of forced expiration. The total volume that is forcibly expired is called the forced vital capacity (FVC). The volume expired in the first second is called FEV_1.

FVC and FEV$_1$ are useful indices of lung disease. Specifically, the fraction of the vital capacity that can be expired in the first second, FEV$_1$/FVC, can be used to differentiate among diseases. For example, in a **normal** person, FEV$_1$/FVC is approximately 0.8, meaning that 80% of the vital capacity can be expired in the first second of forced expiration (see Fig. 5-6*A*). In a patient with an obstructive lung disease such as **asthma,** both FVC and FEV$_1$ are decreased, but FEV$_1$ is decreased *more* than FVC is. Thus, FEV$_1$/FVC is also decreased, which is typical of airway obstruction with increased resistance to expiratory airflow (see Fig. 5-6*B*). In a patient with a restrictive lung disease such as **fibrosis,** both FVC and FEV$_1$ are decreased but FEV$_1$ is decreased *less* than FVC is. Thus, in fibrosis, FEV$_1$/FVC is actually increased (see Fig. 5-6*C*).

MECHANICS OF BREATHING

Muscles Used for Breathing

Muscles of Inspiration

The **diaphragm** is the most important muscle for inspiration. When the diaphragm contracts, the abdominal contents are pushed downward and the ribs are lifted upward and outward. These changes produce an increase in intrathoracic volume, which lowers intrathoracic pressure and initiates the flow of air into the lungs. During **exercise,** when breathing frequency and tidal volume increase, the **external intercostal muscles** and **accessory muscles** may also be used for more vigorous inspiration.

Muscles of Expiration

Expiration normally is a passive process. Air is driven out of the lungs by the reverse pressure gradient between the lungs and the atmosphere until the system reaches its equilibrium point again. During **exercise** or in diseases in which airway resistance is increased (e.g., **asthma**), the expiratory muscles may aid the expiratory process. The muscles of expiration include the **abdominal muscles,** which compress the abdominal cavity and push the diaphragm up, and the **internal intercostal muscles**, which pull the ribs downward and inward.

Compliance

The concept of compliance has the same meaning in the respiratory system as it has in the cardiovascular system: Compliance describes the **distensibility** of the system. In the respiratory system, the compliance of the lungs and the chest wall is of primary interest. Recall that compliance is a measure of how volume changes as a result of a pressure change. Thus, lung compliance describes the change in lung volume for a given change in pressure.

The compliance of the lungs and chest wall is *inversely* correlated with their elastic properties or **elastance.** To appreciate the inverse correlation between compliance and elastance, consider two rubber bands, one thin and one thick. The thin rubber band has the smaller amount of elastic "tissue"—it is easily stretched and is distensible and compliant. The thick rubber band has the larger amount of elastic "tissue"—it is difficult to stretch and is less distensible and compliant. Furthermore, when stretched, the thick rubber band, with its greater elastance, "snaps back" with more vigor than the thin rubber band does. So it is with the pulmonary structures: The greater the amount of elastic tissue, the greater the tendency to "snap back," and the greater the elastic recoil force, but the lower the compliance.

Measuring lung compliance requires simultaneous measurement of lung pressure and volume. The term for pressure can be ambiguous, however, because "pressure" can mean pressure *inside* the alveoli, pressure *outside* the alveoli, or even *transmural* pressure across the alveolar walls. **Transmural pressure** is the pressure across a structure. For example, transpulmonary pressure is the difference between intra-alveolar pressure and intrapleural pressure. (The intrapleural space lies between the lungs and the chest wall.) Finally, lung pressures are always *referred to atmospheric pressure,* which is called "zero." Pressures equal to atmospheric pressure are zero, pressures higher than atmospheric pressure are positive, and pressures lower than atmospheric pressure are negative.

Compliance of the Lungs

The pressure-volume relationship in an isolated lung is illustrated in Figure 5-7. For this demonstration, a lung is excised and placed in a jar. The space outside the lung is analogous to intrapleural pressure. The pressure outside the lung is varied with a vacuum pump to simulate changes in intrapleural pressures. As pressure outside the lung is varied, the volume of the lung is measured with a spirometer. The lung is inflated with negative outside pressure and then deflated by reducing the negative outside pressure. The sequence of inflation followed by deflation produces a **pressure-volume loop.** The slope of each limb of the pressure-volume loop is the **compliance** of the isolated lung.

In the experiment on the **air-filled** lung, the airways and the alveoli are open to the atmosphere and alveolar pressure equals atmospheric pressure. As the pressure outside the lung is made more negative with the vacuum pump, the lung inflates and its volume increases. This negative outside pressure that expands the lungs is, therefore, an **expanding pressure.** The lungs fill with air along the **inspiration** limb of the

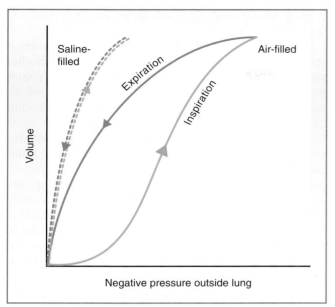

Figure 5–7 Compliance of the lung. The relationship between lung volume and lung pressure is obtained by inflating and deflating an isolated lung. The slope of each curve is the compliance. In the air-filled lung, inspiration (inflation) and expiration (deflation) follow different curves, which is known as hysteresis.

pressure-volume loop. At the highest expanding pressures, when the alveoli are filled to the limit, they become stiffer and less compliant and the curve flattens. Once the lungs are expanded maximally, the pressure outside the lungs is made gradually less negative, causing lung volume to decrease along the **expiration** limb of the pressure-volume loop.

An unusual feature of the pressure-volume loop for the air-filled lung is that the slopes of the relationships for inspiration and expiration are different, a phenomenon called **hysteresis.** Because the slope of the pressure-volume relationship is compliance, it follows that lung compliance also must differ for inspiration and for expiration. For a given outside pressure, the volume of the lung is greater during expiration than during inspiration (i.e., the compliance is higher during expiration than during inspiration). Usually, **compliance is measured on the expiration limb** of the pressure-volume loop because the inspiration limb is complicated by the decrease in compliance at maximal expanding pressures.

Why are the inspiration and expiration limbs of the lung compliance curve different? As compliance is an intrinsic property of the lung that depends on the amount of elastic tissue, one would think that the two curves would be the same. The explanation for the different curves (i.e., hysteresis) lies in **surface tension** at the liquid-air interface of the air-filled lung: The intermolecular attractive forces between liquid molecules lining the lung are much stronger than the forces between liquid and air molecules. Different curves are produced for inspiration and expiration in the air-filled lung as follows:

♦ On the **inspiration limb,** one begins at low lung volume where the liquid molecules are closest together and intermolecular forces are highest; to inflate the lung, one must first break up these intermolecular forces. Surfactant, which is discussed in a later section, plays a role in hysteresis. Briefly, surfactant is a phospholipid that is produced by type II alveolar cells and functions as a detergent to reduce surface tension and increase lung compliance. During inflation of the lung (inspiration limb), surfactant, which is newly produced by type II alveolar cells, enters the liquid layer lining the alveoli and breaks up these intermolecular forces to reduce surface tension. In the initial part of the inspiration curve, at lowest lung volumes, the lung surface area is increasing faster than surfactant can be added to the liquid layer; thus, surfactant density is low, surface tension is high, compliance is low, and the curve is flat. As inflation proceeds, the surfactant density increases, which decreases surface tension, increases compliance, and increases the slope of the curve.

♦ On the **expiration limb,** one begins at high lung volume, where intermolecular forces between liquid molecules are low; one does not need to break up intermolecular forces to deflate the lung. During deflation of the lung (expiration limb), lung surface area decreases faster than surfactant can be removed from the liquid lining and the density of surfactant molecules rapidly increases, which decreases surface tension and increases compliance; thus, the initial portion of the expiration limb is flat. As expiration proceeds, surfactant is removed from the liquid lining and the density of surfactant remains relatively constant, as does the compliance of the lung.

In summary, for the air-filled lung, the observed compliance curves are determined in part by the intrinsic compliance of the lung and in part by surface tension at the liquid-air interface. The role of surface tension is demonstrated by repeating the experiment in a **saline-filled lung.** The inspiration and expiration limbs are the same when the liquid-air interface, and thus surface tension, is eliminated.

Compliance of the Chest Wall

Figure 5-8 shows the relationship between the lungs and chest wall. The conducting airways are represented by a single tube, and the gas exchange region is represented by a single alveolus. The intrapleural space, between the lungs and chest wall, is shown much larger than its actual size. Like the lungs, the chest wall is compliant. Its compliance can be demonstrated by introducing air into the intrapleural space, which creates a pneumothorax.

To understand the consequences of a pneumothorax, it must first be recognized that, normally, the intrapleural space has a negative (less than atmospheric) pressure. This **negative intrapleural pressure** is created by two opposing elastic forces pulling on the intrapleural space: The lungs, with their elastic properties, tend to collapse, and the chest wall, with its elastic properties, tends to spring out (Fig. 5-9). When these two opposing forces pull on the intrapleural space, a negative pressure, or vacuum, is created. In turn, this negative intrapleural pressure opposes the natural tendency of the lungs to collapse and the chest wall to spring out (i.e.,

it prevents the lungs from collapsing and the chest wall from springing out).

When a sharp object punctures the intrapleural space, air is introduced into the space **(pneumothorax)**, and intrapleural pressure suddenly becomes equal to atmospheric pressure; thus, instead of its normal negative value, intrapleural pressure becomes zero. There are two important consequences of a pneumothorax (see Fig. 5-9). First, without the negative intrapleural pressure to hold the lungs open, the lungs collapse. Second, without the negative intrapleural pressure to keep the chest wall from expanding, the chest wall springs out. (If you have trouble picturing why the chest wall would want to spring out, think of the chest wall as a spring that you normally contain by compressing it between your fingers. Of course, the real chest wall is "contained" by the negative intrapleural pressure, rather than the force of your fingers. If you release your fingers, or eliminate the negative intrapleural pressure, the spring or the chest wall springs out.)

Pressure-Volume Curves for the Lungs, Chest Wall, and Combined Lung and Chest Wall

Pressure-volume curves can be obtained for the lungs alone (i.e., the isolated lung in a jar), for the chest wall alone, and for the combined lung and chest-wall system, as shown in Figure 5-10. The curve for the chest wall alone is obtained by subtraction of the lung curve from the curve for the combined lung and chest wall, described subsequently. The curve for the lung alone is similar to that shown in Figure 5-7, with the hysteresis eliminated for the sake of simplicity. The curve for the combined lung and chest-wall system is obtained

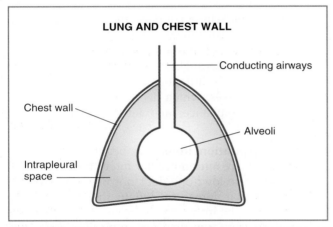

Figure 5–8 Schematic diagram of the lung and chest-wall system. The intrapleural space is exaggerated and lies between the lungs and the chest wall.

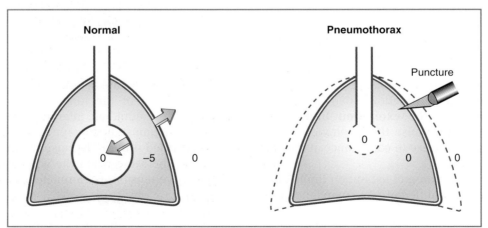

Figure 5–9 Intrapleural pressure in a normal person and in a person with a pneumothorax. The numbers are pressures in cm H_2O. Pressures are referred to atmospheric pressure; thus, zero pressure means equal to atmospheric pressure. The *arrows* show expanding or collapsing elastic forces. Normally, at rest, intrapleural pressure is –5 cm H_2O because of equal and opposite forces trying to collapse the lungs and expand the chest wall. With a pneumothorax, the intrapleural pressure becomes equal to atmospheric pressure, causing the lungs to collapse and the chest wall to expand.

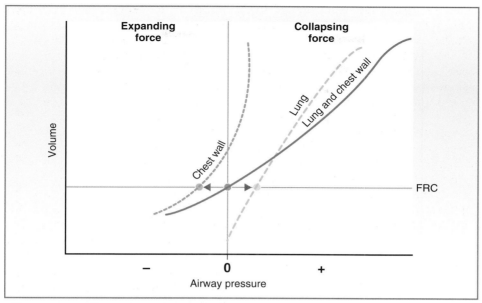

Figure 5–10 **Compliance of the lungs, chest wall, and combined lung and chest-wall system.** The equilibrium position is at functional residual capacity (FRC), where the expanding force on the chest wall is exactly equal to the collapsing force on the lungs.

by having a trained subject breathe in and out of a spirometer as follows: The subject inspires or expires to a given volume. The spirometer valve is closed, and as the subject relaxes his or her respiratory muscles, the subject's airway pressure is measured (called relaxation pressure). In this way, values for airway pressure are obtained at a series of static volumes of the combined lung and chest-wall system. When the volume is functional residual capacity (FRC), airway pressure is zero and equal to atmospheric pressure. At volumes lower than FRC, airway pressures are negative (less volume, less pressure). At volumes higher than FRC, airway pressures are positive (more volume, more pressure).

The slope of each of the curves in Figure 5-10 is **compliance.** The compliance of the chest wall alone is approximately equal to the compliance of the lungs alone. (Note that on the graph, the slopes are similar.) However, the compliance of the combined lung and chest-wall system is less than that of either structure alone (i.e., the curve for the combined lung and chest wall is "flatter"). Visualize one balloon (the lungs) inside another balloon (the chest wall). Each balloon is compliant by itself, but the combined system (the balloon within the balloon) is less compliant and harder to expand.

The easiest way to interpret the curves in Figure 5-10 is to begin at the volume called **FRC,** which is the resting, or equilibrium, volume of the combined lung and chest-wall system. FRC is the volume present in the lungs after a person has expired a normal tidal breath. When you understand the graphs at FRC, then compare the graphs at volumes less than FRC and greater than FRC.

♦ **Volume is FRC.** When the volume is FRC, the combined lung and chest-wall system is at equilibrium. Airway pressure is equal to atmospheric pressure, which is called zero. (Note that when the volume is FRC, the combined lung and chest-wall curve intersects the X-axis at an airway pressure of zero.) At FRC, because they are elastic structures, the lungs "want" to collapse and the chest wall "wants" to expand. If these elastic forces were unopposed, the structures would do exactly that! However, at FRC, the equilibrium position, the collapsing force on the lungs is exactly equal to the expanding force on the chest wall, as shown by the equidistant arrows; the *combined* lung and chest-wall system neither has a tendency to collapse nor to expand.

♦ **Volume is less than FRC.** When the volume in the system is less than FRC (i.e., the subject makes a forced expiration into the spirometer), there is less volume in the lungs and the collapsing (elastic) force of the lungs is smaller. The expanding force on the chest wall is greater, however, and the *combined* lung and chest-wall system "wants" to expand. (Notice on the graph that at volumes less than FRC, the collapsing force on the lungs is smaller than the expanding force on the chest wall and that airway pressure for the combined system is negative; thus, the combined system tends to expand, as air flows into the lungs down the pressure gradient.)

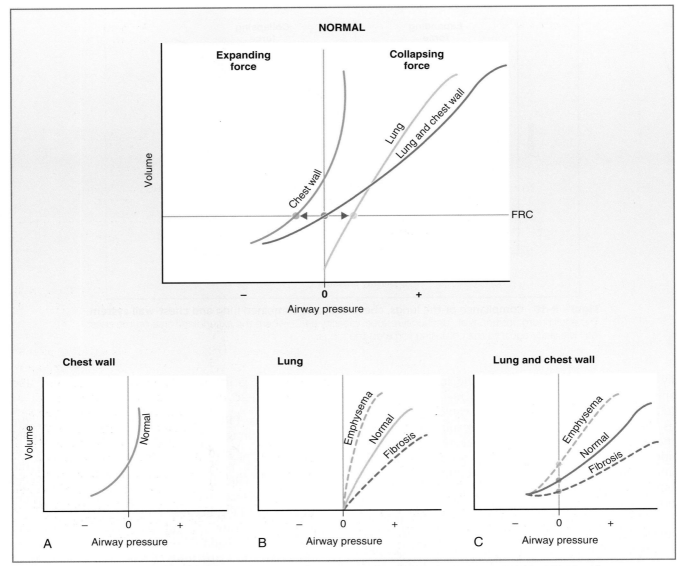

Figure 5–11 **Changes in compliance of the chest wall (A), lungs (B), and combined lung and chest-wall system (C) in emphysema and fibrosis.** The equilibrium point, functional residual capacity (FRC), is increased in emphysema and decreased in fibrosis.

♦ **Volume is greater than FRC.** When the volume in the system is greater than FRC (i.e., the subject inspires from the spirometer), there is more volume in the lungs and the collapsing (elastic) force of the lungs is greater. The expanding force on the chest wall is smaller, however, and the *combined* lung and chest-wall system "wants" to collapse. (Notice on the graph that at volumes greater than FRC, the collapsing force on the lungs is greater than the expanding force on the chest wall and that airway pressure for the combined system is positive; thus, the overall system tends to collapse, as air flows out of the lungs down the pressure gradient.) At highest lung volumes, *both* the lungs and the chest wall "want" to collapse [notice that the chest wall curve has

crossed the vertical axis at high volumes], and there is a large collapsing force on the combined system.)

Diseases of Lung Compliance

If the compliance of the lungs changes because of disease, the slopes of the relationships change, and as a result, the volume of the combined lung and chest-wall system also changes, as illustrated in Figure 5-11. As a reference, the normal relationships from Figure 5-10 are shown at the top of Figure 5-11. For convenience, each component of the system is shown on a separate graph (i.e., chest wall alone, lung alone, and combined lung and chest wall). The chest wall alone is included only for completeness because its compliance is not altered by these diseases. The solid

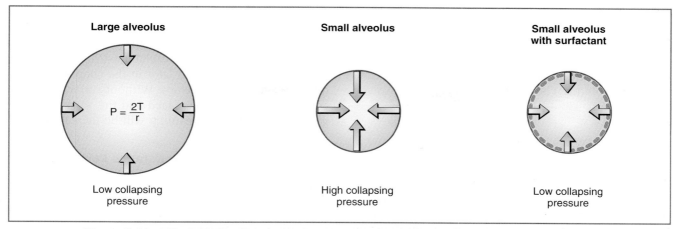

Figure 5–12 **Effect of alveolar size and surfactant on collapsing pressure.** The length of the *arrows* shows the relative magnitude of the collapsing pressure.

lines in each of the three graphs show the normal relationships from Figure 5-10. The dashed lines show the effects of disease.

♦ **Emphysema (increased lung compliance).** Emphysema, a component of chronic obstructive pulmonary disease (COPD), is associated with loss of elastic fibers in the lungs. As a result, the compliance of the lungs increases. (Recall again the inverse relationship between elastance and compliance.) An increase in compliance is associated with an increased (steeper) slope of the volume-versus-pressure curve for the lung (see Fig. 5-11*B*). As a result, at a given volume, the collapsing (elastic recoil) force on the lungs is decreased. At the original value for FRC, the tendency of the lungs to collapse is less than the tendency of the chest wall to expand, and these opposing forces will no longer be balanced. In order for the opposing forces to be balanced, volume must be added to the lungs to increase their collapsing force. Thus, the combined lung and chest-wall system seeks a new **higher FRC,** where the two opposing forces can be balanced (see Fig. 5-11*C*); the new intersection point, where airway pressure is zero, is increased. A patient with emphysema is said to breathe at higher lung volumes (in recognition of the higher FRC) and will have a **barrel-shaped chest.**

♦ **Fibrosis (decreased lung compliance).** Fibrosis, a so-called restrictive disease, is associated with stiffening of lung tissues and decreased compliance. A decrease in lung compliance is associated with a decreased slope of the volume-versus-pressure curve for the lung (see Fig. 5-11*B*). At the original FRC, the tendency of the lungs to collapse is greater than the tendency of the chest wall to expand and the opposing forces will no longer be balanced. To reestablish balance, the lung and chest-wall system will seek a

new **lower FRC** (see Fig. 5-11*C*); the new intersection point, where airway pressure is zero, is decreased.

Surface Tension of Alveoli

The small size of alveoli presents a special problem in keeping them open. This "problem" can be explained as follows: Alveoli are lined with a film of fluid. The attractive forces between adjacent molecules of the liquid are stronger than the attractive forces between molecules of liquid and molecules of gas in the alveoli, which creates a **surface tension.** As the molecules of liquid are drawn together by the attractive forces, the surface area becomes as small as possible, forming a sphere (like soap bubbles blown at the end of a tube). The surface tension generates a pressure that tends to collapse the sphere. The pressure generated by such a sphere is given by the **law of Laplace:**

$$P = \frac{2T}{r}$$

where

P = Collapsing pressure on alveolus (dynes/cm²)
or
Pressure required to keep alveolus open (dynes/cm²)
T = Surface tension (dynes/cm)
r = Radius of the alveolus (cm)

The law of Laplace states that the pressure tending to collapse an alveolus is directly proportional to the surface tension generated by the molecules of liquid lining the alveolus and inversely proportional to alveolar radius (Fig. 5-12). Because of the inverse relationship with radius, a **large alveolus** (one with a large radius) will have a low collapsing pressure and, therefore, will require only minimal pressure to keep it open. On the other hand, a **small alveolus** (one with a small radius) will have a high collapsing pressure and require more pressure to keep it open. Thus, small alveoli are not ideal because of their tendency to collapse. Yet from the standpoint of gas exchange, alveoli need to be as small as possible to increase their total surface area relative to volume. This fundamental conflict is solved by surfactant.

Surfactant

From the discussion of the effect of the radius on collapsing pressure, the question that arises is *How do small alveoli remain open under high collapsing pressures?* The answer to this question is found in **surfactant,** a mixture of phospholipids that line the alveoli and reduce their surface tension. By reducing surface tension, surfactant reduces the collapsing pressure for a given radius.

Figure 5-12 shows two small alveoli, one with surfactant and one without. *Without* surfactant, the law of Laplace predicts that the small alveolus will collapse **(atelectasis).** *With* surfactant present, the same small alveolus will remain open (inflated with air) because the collapsing pressure has been reduced.

Surfactant is synthesized from fatty acids by **type II alveolar cells.** The exact composition of surfactant remains unknown, but the most important constituent is **dipalmitoyl phosphatidylcholine (DPPC).** The mechanism by which DPPC reduces surface tension is based on the **amphipathic** nature of the phospholipid molecules (i.e., hydrophobic on one end and hydrophilic on the other). The DPPC molecules align themselves on the alveolar surface, with their hydrophobic portions attracted to each other and their hydrophilic portions repelled. Intermolecular forces between the DPPC molecules break up the attracting forces between liquid molecules lining the alveoli (which had been responsible for the high surface tension). Thus, when surfactant is present, surface tension and collapsing pressure are reduced and small alveoli are kept open.

Surfactant provides another advantage for pulmonary function: It **increases lung compliance,** which reduces the work of expanding the lungs during inspiration. (Recall from Figure 5-11 that increasing the compliance of the lungs reduces the collapsing force at any given volume so that it is easier for the lungs to expand.)

In **neonatal respiratory distress syndrome,** surfactant is lacking. In the developing fetus, surfactant synthesis begins as early as gestational week 24 and it is almost always present by week 35. The more prematurely the infant is born, the less it is likely that surfactant will be present. Infants born before gestational week 24 will *never* have surfactant, and infants born between weeks 24 and 35 will have *uncertain* surfactant status. The consequences of the lack of surfactant in the newborn should now be clear: Without surfactant, small alveoli have increased surface tension and increased pressures and will collapse **(atelectasis).** Collapsed alveoli are not ventilated and, therefore, cannot participate in gas exchange (this is called a shunt, which is discussed later in the chapter); consequently, hypoxemia develops. Without surfactant, **lung compliance will be decreased** and the work of inflating the lungs during breathing will be increased.

Airflow, Pressure, and Resistance Relationships

The relationship between airflow, pressure, and resistance in the lungs is analogous to the relationship in the cardiovascular system. Airflow is analogous to blood flow, gas pressures are analogous to fluid pressures, and resistance of the airways is analogous to resistance of the blood vessels. The following relationship is now familiar:

$$Q = \frac{\Delta P}{R}$$

where

$$Q = \text{Airflow (mL/min or L/min)}$$
$$\Delta P = \text{Pressure gradient (mm Hg or cm } H_2O)$$
$$R = \text{Airway resistance (cm } H_2O/L/sec)$$

In words, airflow (Q) is directly proportional to the pressure difference (ΔP) between the mouth or nose and the alveoli and it is inversely proportional to the resistance of the airways (R). It is important to understand that the *pressure difference is the driving force*—without a pressure difference, airflow will not occur. To illustrate this point, compare the pressures that exist in different phases of the breathing cycle, at rest (between breaths) and during inspiration. Between breaths, alveolar pressure equals atmospheric pressure; there is no pressure gradient, no driving force, and no airflow. On the other hand, during inspiration, the diaphragm contracts to increase lung volume, which decreases alveolar pressure and establishes a pressure gradient that drives airflow into the lungs.

Airway Resistance

In the respiratory system, as in the cardiovascular system, flow is inversely proportional to resistance ($Q = \Delta P/R$). Resistance is determined by **Poiseuille's law.** Thus,

$$R = \frac{8 \eta l}{\pi r^4}$$

where

$$R = \text{Resistance}$$
$$\eta = \text{Viscosity of inspired air}$$
$$l = \text{Length of the airway}$$
$$r = \text{Radius of the airway}$$

Notice the powerful relationship that exists between resistance (R) and radius (r) of the airways because of the fourth power dependence. For example, if the radius of an airway decreases by a factor of 2, resistance does not simply increase twofold, it increases by 2^4, or 16-fold. When resistance *increases* by 16-fold, airflow *decreases* by 16-fold, a dramatic effect.

The **medium-sized bronchi** are the sites of highest airway resistance. It would *seem* that the smallest airways would provide the highest resistance to airflow, based on the inverse fourth power relationship between resistance and radius. However, because of their parallel arrangement, the smallest airways *do not* have the highest collective resistance. Recall that when blood vessels are arranged in parallel, the total resistance is less than the individual resistances and that adding a blood vessel in parallel decreases total resistance (see Chapter 4). These same principles of parallel resistances apply to airways.

Changes in Airway Resistance

The relationship between airway resistance and airway diameter (radius) is a powerful one, based on the fourth power relationship. It is logical, therefore, that **changes in airway diameter** provide the major mechanism for altering resistance and airflow. The smooth muscle in the walls of the conducting airways is innervated by autonomic nerve fibers; when activated, these fibers produce constriction or dilation of the airways. Changes in lung volume and in the viscosity of inspired air also may change resistance to airflow.

♦ **Autonomic nervous system.** Bronchial smooth muscle is innervated by parasympathetic cholinergic nerve fibers and by sympathetic adrenergic nerve fibers. Activation of these fibers produces constriction or dilation of bronchial smooth muscle, which decreases or increases the diameter of the airway as follows: (1) **Parasympathetic stimulation** produces **constriction** of bronchial smooth muscle, decreasing airway diameter and increasing resistance to airflow. These effects can be simulated by muscarinic agonists (e.g., muscarine and carbachol) and can be blocked by muscarinic antagonists (e.g., atropine). Constriction of bronchial smooth muscle also occurs in asthma and in response to irritants. (2) **Sympathetic stimulation** produces **relaxation** of bronchial smooth muscle via stimulation of β_2 receptors. Relaxation of bronchial smooth muscle results in increases in airway diameter and decreases in resistance to airflow. Therefore, β_2 agonists such as epinephrine, isoproterenol, and albuterol produce relaxation of bronchial smooth muscle, which underlies their usefulness in the **treatment of asthma.**

♦ **Lung volume.** Changes in lung volume alter airway resistance because the surrounding lung parenchymal tissue exerts radial traction on the airways. High lung volumes are associated with greater traction, which decreases airway resistance. Low lung volumes are associated with less traction, which increases airway resistance, even to the point of airway collapse. Persons with asthma breathe at higher lung volumes and partially offset the high airway resistance of their disease (i.e., the volume mechanism helps to reduce airway resistance as a compensatory mechanism).

♦ **Viscosity of inspired air (η).** The effect of the viscosity of inspired air on resistance is clear from the Poiseuille relationship. Although not common, increases in gas viscosity (e.g., as occurs during deep sea diving) produce increases in resistance, and decreases in viscosity (e.g., breathing a low-density gas such as helium) produce decreases in resistance.

Breathing Cycle

The normal breathing cycle is illustrated in Figures 5-13 and 5-14. For purposes of discussion, the breathing cycle is divided into phases: **rest** (the period between breaths), **inspiration,** and **expiration.** In Figure 5-13,

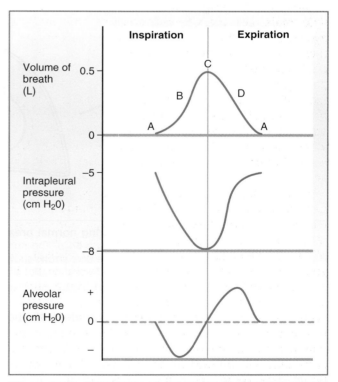

Figure 5–13 Volumes and pressures during the normal breathing cycle. Intrapleural pressure and alveolar pressure are referred to atmospheric pressure. Letters *A* to *D* correspond to phases of the breathing cycle in Figure 5-14.

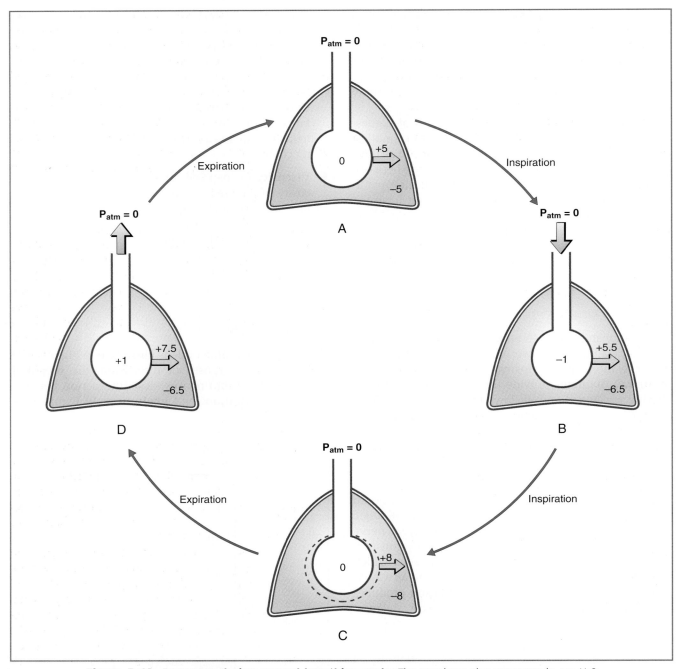

Figure 5–14 Pressures during normal breathing cycle. The numbers give pressures in cm H_2O relative to atmospheric pressure (P_{atm}). The numbers over the *yellow arrows* give the magnitude of transmural pressures. The *wide blue arrows* show airflow into and out of the lungs. **A,** Rest; **B,** halfway through inspiration; **C,** end of inspiration; **D,** halfway through expiration.

three parameters are shown graphically to describe the breathing cycle: volume of air moved in and out of the lungs, intrapleural pressure, and alveolar pressure.

Figure 5-14 shows the familiar picture of the lungs (represented by an alveolus), the chest wall, and the intrapleural space between the lung and chest wall. Pressures, in cm H_2O, are shown at different points in the breathing cycle. Atmospheric pressure is zero, and

values for alveolar and intrapleural pressure are given in the appropriate spaces. The *yellow arrows* show the direction and magnitude of the **transmural pressure** across the lungs. By convention, *transmural pressure is calculated as alveolar pressure **minus** intrapleural pressure*. If transmural pressure is positive, it is an expanding pressure on the lung and the yellow arrow points outward. For example, if alveolar pressure is zero and intrapleural pressure is −5 cm H_2O, there is an expanding pressure on the lungs of +5 cm H_2O (0 − [−5 cm H_2O] = +5 cm H_2O). If transmural pressure is negative, it is a collapsing pressure on the lung and the yellow arrow points inward (not illustrated in this figure). Note that for all phases of the normal breathing cycle, despite changes in alveolar and intrapleural pressures, transmural pressures across the lungs are such that they always remain open. The *wide blue arrows* show the direction of airflow into or out of the lungs.

Rest

Rest is the period between breathing cycles when the diaphragm is at its equilibrium position (see Figs. 5-13 and 5-14*A*). At rest, no air is moving into or out of the lungs. **Alveolar pressure equals atmospheric pressure,** and because lung pressures are always referred to atmospheric pressure, alveolar pressure is said to be zero. There is no airflow at rest because there is no pressure difference between the atmosphere (the mouth or nose) and the alveoli.

At rest, **intrapleural pressure is negative,** or approximately −5 cm H_2O. The reason that intrapleural pressure is negative has been explained previously: The opposing forces of the lungs trying to collapse and the chest wall trying to expand create a negative pressure in the intrapleural space between them. Recall from the experiment on the isolated lung in a jar that an outside negative pressure (i.e., negative intrapleural pressure) keeps the lungs inflated or expanded. The transmural pressure across the lungs at rest is +5 cm H_2O (alveolar pressure minus intrapleural pressure), which means that these structures will be open.

The volume present in the lungs at rest is the equilibrium volume or **FRC,** which, by definition, is the volume remaining in the lungs after a normal expiration.

Inspiration

During inspiration, the **diaphragm contracts,** causing the volume of the thorax to increase. As lung volume increases, the pressure in the lungs must decrease. (Boyle's law states that P × V is constant at a given temperature.) Halfway through inspiration (see Figs. 5-13 and 5-14*B*), alveolar pressure falls below atmospheric pressure (−1 cm H_2O). The pressure gradient between the atmosphere and the alveoli drives airflow into the lung. Air flows into the lungs until, at the end of inspiration (see Fig. 5-14*C*), alveolar pressure is once again equal to atmospheric pressure; the pressure gradient between the atmosphere and the alveoli has dissipated, and airflow into the lungs ceases. The volume of air inspired in one breath is the **tidal volume (V$_T$),** which is approximately 0.5 L. Thus, the volume present in the lungs at the end of normal inspiration is the functional residual capacity *plus* one tidal volume (FRC + V$_T$).

During inspiration, **intrapleural pressure becomes even *more negative*** than at rest. There are two explanations for this effect: (1) As lung volume increases, the elastic recoil of the lungs also increases and pulls more forcefully against the intrapleural space, and (2) airway and alveolar pressures become negative.

Together, these two effects cause the intrapleural pressure to become more negative, or approximately −8 cm H_2O at the end of inspiration. The extent to which intrapleural pressure changes during inspiration can be used to estimate the **dynamic compliance** of the lungs.

Expiration

Normally, expiration is a passive process. **Alveolar pressure becomes positive** (higher than atmospheric pressure) because the elastic forces of the lungs compress the greater volume of air in the alveoli. When alveolar pressure increases above atmospheric pressure (see Figs. 5-13 and 5-14*D*), air flows out of the lungs and the volume in the lungs returns to FRC. The volume expired is the tidal volume. At the end of expiration (see Figs. 5-13 and 5-14*A*), all volumes and pressures return to their values at rest and the system is ready to begin the next breathing cycle.

Forced Expiration

In a forced expiration, a person deliberately and forcibly breathes out. The expiratory muscles are used to make lung and airway pressures even more positive than those seen in a normal, passive expiration. Figure 5-15 shows an example of the pressures generated during a forced expiration; a person with normal lungs is compared with a person with chronic obstructive pulmonary disease (COPD).

In a person with **normal lungs,** the forced expiration makes the pressures in the lungs and airways very positive. Both airway and alveolar pressures are raised to much higher values than those occurring during passive expiration. Thus, during a normal passive expiration, alveolar pressure is +1 cm H_2O (see Fig. 5-14*D*); in this example of forced expiration, airway pressure is +25 cm H_2O and alveolar pressure is +35 cm H_2O (see Fig. 5-15).

During forced expiration, contraction of the expiratory muscles also raises intrapleural pressure, now to a positive value of, for example, +20 cm H_2O. An important question is *Will the lungs and airways collapse under these conditions of positive intrapleural pressure?* No, as long as the transmural pressure is positive, the airways and lungs will remain open. During a normal forced expiration, transmural pressure across the airways is airway pressure minus intrapleural pressure, or +5 cm H_2O (+25 − [+20] = +5 cm H_2O); transmural pressure across the lungs is alveolar pressure minus intrapleural pressure, or +15 cm H_2O

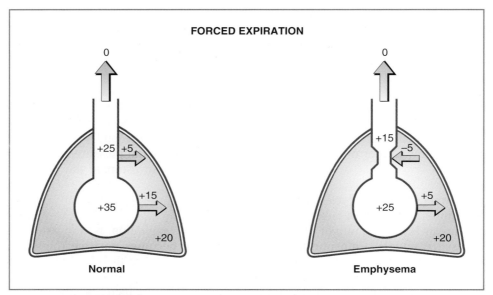

FORCED EXPIRATION

Normal

Emphysema

Figure 5–15 **Pressures across the alveoli and conducting airways during forced expiration in a normal person and a person with emphysema.** The numbers give pressure in cm H_2O and are expressed relative to atmospheric pressure. The numbers over the *yellow arrows* give the magnitude of the transmural pressure. The direction of the *yellow arrows* indicates whether the transmural pressure is expanding (*outward arrow*) or collapsing (*inward arrow*). The *blue arrows* show airflow into and out of the lungs.

(+35 − [+20] = +15 cm H_2O). Therefore, both the airways and the alveoli will remain open because transmural pressures are positive. Expiration will be rapid and forceful because the pressure gradient between the alveoli (+35 cm H_2O) and the atmosphere (0) is much greater than normal.

In a person with **emphysema,** however, forced expiration may cause the airways to collapse. In emphysema, lung compliance increases because of loss of elastic fibers. During forced expiration, intrapleural pressure is raised to the same value as in the normal person, +20 cm H_2O. However, because the structures have diminished elastic recoil, alveolar pressure and airway pressure are lower than in a normal person. The transmural pressure gradient across the lungs remains a positive expanding pressure, +5 cm H_2O, and the alveoli remain open. However, the large airways collapse because the transmural pressure gradient across them reverses, becoming a negative (collapsing) transmural pressure of −5 cm H_2O. Obviously, if the large airways collapse, resistance to airflow increases and expiration is more difficult. Persons with emphysema learn to **expire slowly** with **pursed lips,** which raises airway pressure, prevents the reversal of the transmural pressure gradient across the large airways, and, thus, prevents their collapse.

GAS EXCHANGE

Gas exchange in the respiratory system refers to diffusion of O_2 and CO_2 in the lungs and in the peripheral tissues. O_2 is transferred from alveolar gas into pulmonary capillary blood and, ultimately, delivered to the tissues, where it diffuses from systemic capillary blood into the cells. CO_2 is delivered from the tissues to venous blood, to pulmonary capillary blood, and is transferred to alveolar gas to be expired.

Gas Laws

The mechanisms of gas exchange are based on the fundamental properties of gases and include their behavior in solution. This section reviews those principles.

General Gas Law

The general gas law (familiar from chemistry courses) states that the product of pressure times volume of a gas is equal to the number of moles of the gas multiplied by the gas constant multiplied by the temperature. Thus,

$$PV = nRT$$

where

P = Pressure (mm Hg)
V = Volume (L)
n = Moles (mol)
R = Gas constant
T = Temperature (K)

The only "trick" in applying the general gas law to respiratory physiology is to know that in the gas phase BTPS is used, but in the liquid phase, STPD is used.

BTPS means body temperature (37°C, or 310 K), ambient pressure, and gas saturated with water vapor. For gases dissolved in blood, **STPD** is used, meaning standard temperature (0°C, or 273 K), standard pressure (760 mm Hg), and dry gas. Gas volume at BTPS can be converted to volume at STPD by multiplying the volume (at BTPS) by 273/310 × P$_B$- 47/760 (where P$_B$ is barometric pressure and 47 mm Hg is water vapor pressure at 37°C).

Boyle's Law

Boyle's law is a special case of the general gas law. It states that, at a given temperature, the product of pressure times volume for a gas is constant. Thus,

$$P_1 V_1 = P_2 V_2$$

The application of Boyle's law to the respiratory system has been discussed in a previous example. Recall the events occurring during inspiration when the diaphragm contracts to increase lung volume: To keep the product of pressure times volume constant, gas pressure in the lungs must decrease as lung volume increases. (It is this decrease in gas pressure that is the driving force for airflow into the lungs.)

Dalton's Law of Partial Pressures

Dalton's law of partial pressures is applied frequently in respiratory physiology. It states that the partial pressure of a gas in a mixture of gases is the pressure that gas would exert if it occupied the total volume of the mixture. Thus, partial pressure is the total pressure multiplied by the fractional concentration of *dry gas,* or

$$Px = P_B \times F$$

The relationship for *humidified gas* is determined by correcting the barometric pressure for the water vapor pressure. Thus,

$$Px = (P_B - P_{H_2O}) \times F$$

where

Px = Partial pressure of gas (mm Hg)
P$_B$ = Barometric pressure (mm Hg)
P$_{H_2O}$ = Water vapor pressure at 37°C (47 mm Hg)
F = Fractional concentration of gas (no units)

It follows, then, from Dalton's law of partial pressures, that the sum of partial pressures of all gases in a mixture equals the total pressure of the mixture. Thus, the barometric pressure (P$_B$) is the sum of the partial pressures of O_2, CO_2, N_2, and H_2O. The percentages of gases in dry air at a barometric pressure of 760 mm Hg (with the corresponding values for F in parentheses) are as follows: O_2, 21% (0.21); N_2, 79% (0.79); and CO_2, 0% (0). Because air is humidified in the airways, water vapor pressure is obligatory and equal to 47 mm Hg at 37°C.

SAMPLE PROBLEM. Calculate the partial pressure of O_2 (P$_{O_2}$) in dry inspired air, and compare that value to the P$_{O_2}$ in humidified tracheal air at 37°C. The fractional concentration of O_2 in inspired air is 0.21.

SOLUTION. The P$_{O_2}$ of dry inspired air is calculated by multiplying the pressure of the mixture of gases (i.e., the barometric pressure) by the fractional concentration of O_2, which is 0.21. Thus, in *dry inspired air,*

$$P_{I_{O_2}} = 760 \text{ mm Hg} \times 0.21$$
$$= 160 \text{ mm Hg}$$

The P$_{O_2}$ of humidified tracheal air is lower than the P$_{O_2}$ of dry inspired air because the total pressure must be corrected for water vapor pressure (or 47 mm Hg at 37°C). Thus, *in humidified tracheal air,*

$$P_{I_{O_2}} = (760 \text{ mm Hg} - 47 \text{ mm Hg}) \times 0.21$$
$$= 713 \text{ mm Hg} \times 0.21$$
$$= 150 \text{ mm Hg}$$

Henry's Law for Concentrations of Dissolved Gases

Henry's law deals with **gases dissolved in solution** (e.g., in blood). Both O_2 and CO_2 are dissolved in blood (a solution) en route to and from the lungs. To calculate a gas concentration in the liquid phase, the partial pressure in the gas phase first is converted to the partial pressure in the liquid phase; next, the partial pressure in liquid is converted to the concentration in liquid.

An important, but not necessarily self-evident, point is that at equilibrium, the *partial pressure of a gas in the liquid phase equals the partial pressure in the gas phase.* Thus, if alveolar air has a P$_{O_2}$ of 100 mm Hg, then the capillary blood that equilibrates with alveolar air also will have a P$_{O_2}$ of 100 mm Hg. Henry's law is used to convert the partial pressure of gas in the liquid phase to the concentration of gas in the liquid phase (e.g., in blood). The concentration of a gas in solution is expressed as volume percent (%), or volume of gas per 100 mL of blood (mL gas/100 mL blood).

Thus, for blood,

$$Cx = Px \times \text{Solubility}$$

where

Cx = Concentration of dissolved gas (mL gas/100 mL blood)
Px = Partial pressure of gas (mm Hg)
Solubility = Solubility of gas in blood (mL gas/100 mL blood/mm Hg)

Finally, it is important to understand that the concentration of a gas in solution applies *only to dissolved gas* that is free in solution (calculated with Henry's law), and it does not include any gas that is present in bound form (e.g., gas bound to hemoglobin or to plasma proteins).

SAMPLE PROBLEM. If the P_{O_2} of arterial blood is 100 mm Hg, what is the concentration of dissolved O_2 in blood, given that the solubility of O_2 is 0.003 mL O_2/100 mL blood/mm Hg?

SOLUTION. To calculate the concentration of dissolved O_2 in arterial blood, simply multiply the P_{O_2} by the solubility as follows:

$$[O_2] = P_{O_2} \times \text{Solubility}$$
$$= 100 \text{ mm Hg} \times 0.003 \text{ mL } O_2/100 \text{ mL blood/mm Hg}$$
$$= 0.3 \text{ mL}/100 \text{ mL blood}$$

Diffusion of Gases—Fick's Law

Transfer of gases across cell membranes or capillary walls occurs by **simple diffusion,** which is discussed in Chapter 1. For gases, the rate of transfer by diffusion ($\dot{V}x$) is directly proportional to the driving force, a diffusion coefficient, and the surface area available for diffusion; it is inversely proportional to the thickness of membrane barrier. Thus,

$$\dot{V}x = \frac{DA\Delta P}{\Delta x}$$

where

$\dot{V}x$ = Volume of gas transferred per unit time
D = Diffusion coefficient of the gas
A = Surface area
ΔP = Partial pressure difference of the gas
Δx = Thickness of the membrane

There are two special points regarding diffusion of gases. (1) The driving force for diffusion of a gas is the **partial pressure difference of the gas** (ΔP) across the membrane, *not* the concentration difference. Thus, if the P_{O_2} of alveolar air is 100 mm Hg and the P_{O_2} of mixed venous blood that enters the pulmonary capillary is 40 mm Hg, then the partial pressure difference, or driving force, for O_2 across the alveolar/pulmonary capillary barrier is 60 mm Hg (100 mm Hg − 40 mm Hg). (2) The **diffusion coefficient of a gas** (**D**) is a combination of the usual diffusion coefficient, which depends on molecular weight (see Chapter 1), and the solubility of the gas. The diffusion coefficient of the gas has enormous implications for its diffusion rate, as illustrated by differences in the diffusion rates of CO_2 and O_2. The diffusion coefficient for CO_2 is approximately 20 times higher than the diffusion coefficient for O_2; as a result, for a given partial pressure difference, CO_2 diffuses approximately 20 times faster than O_2.

Several of the terms in the previous equation for diffusion can be combined into a single term called the **lung diffusing capacity** (**DL**). DL combines the diffusion coefficient of the gas, the surface area of the membrane (A), and the thickness of the membrane

(Δx). DL also takes into account the time required for the gas to combine with proteins in pulmonary capillary blood (e.g., binding of O_2 to hemoglobin in red cells). DL can be measured with carbon monoxide (**CO**) because CO transfer across the alveolar/pulmonary capillary barrier is limited exclusively by the diffusion process. DL_{CO} is measured using the single breath method where the subject breathes a gas mixture containing a low concentration of CO; the rate of disappearance of CO from the gas mixture is proportional to DL. In various diseases, DL changes in a predictable way. In **emphysema,** for example, DL decreases because destruction of alveoli results in a decreased surface area for gas exchange. In **fibrosis** or **pulmonary edema,** DL decreases because the diffusion distance (membrane thickness or interstitial volume) increases. In **anemia,** DL decreases because the amount of hemoglobin in red blood cells is reduced (recall that DL includes the protein-binding component of O_2 exchange). During **exercise,** DL increases because additional capillaries are perfused with blood, which increases the surface area for gas exchange.

Forms of Gases in Solution

In alveolar air, there is one form of gas, which is expressed as a partial pressure. However, in solutions such as blood, gases are carried in additional forms. In solution, gas may be dissolved, it may be bound to proteins, or it may be chemically modified. It is important to understand that the *total gas concentration in solution is the sum of dissolved gas plus bound gas plus chemically modified gas.*

♦ **Dissolved gas.** All gases in solution are carried, to some extent, in the dissolved form. **Henry's law** gives the relationship between the partial pressure of a gas and its concentration in solution: For a given partial pressure, the higher the solubility of the gas, the higher the concentration of gas in solution. In solution, only *dissolved* gas molecules contribute to the partial pressure. In other words, bound gas and chemically modified gas do not contribute to the partial pressure.

Of the gases found in inspired air, nitrogen (N_2) is the only one that is carried *only* in dissolved form and it is never bound or chemically modified. Because of this simplifying characteristic, N_2 is used for certain measurements in respiratory physiology.

♦ **Bound gas.** O_2, CO_2, and carbon monoxide (CO) are bound to proteins in blood. O_2 and CO bind to hemoglobin inside red blood cells and are carried in this form. CO_2 binds to hemoglobin in red blood cells and to plasma proteins.

♦ **Chemically modified gas.** The most significant example of a chemically modified gas is the conversion

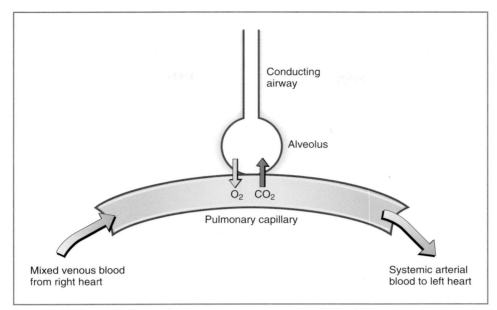

Figure 5–16 **Schematic diagram of an alveolus and a nearby pulmonary capillary.** Mixed venous blood enters the pulmonary capillary; O_2 is added to pulmonary capillary blood, and CO_2 is removed from it by transfer across the alveolar/capillary barrier. Systemic arterial blood leaves the pulmonary capillary.

of CO_2 to bicarbonate (HCO_3^-) in red blood cells by the action of carbonic anhydrase. In fact, most CO_2 is carried in blood as HCO_3^-, rather than as dissolved CO_2 or as bound CO_2.

Overview—Gas Transport in the Lungs

An alveolus and a nearby pulmonary capillary are shown in Figure 5-16. The diagram shows that the pulmonary capillaries are perfused with blood from the right heart (the equivalent of mixed venous blood). Gas exchange then occurs between alveolar gas and the pulmonary capillary: O_2 diffuses from alveolar gas into pulmonary capillary blood, and CO_2 diffuses from pulmonary capillary blood into alveolar gas. The blood leaving the pulmonary capillary is delivered to the left heart and becomes systemic arterial blood.

Figure 5-17 further elaborates on this scheme in which the values for P_{O_2} and P_{CO_2} have been included at various sites: dry inspired air, humidified tracheal air, alveolar air, mixed venous blood entering the pulmonary capillary, and systemic arterial blood leaving the pulmonary capillary.

◆ In **dry inspired air,** the P_{O_2} is approximately 160 mm Hg, which is computed by multiplying the barometric pressure times the fractional concentration of O_2, 21% (760 mm Hg $\times$ 0.21 = 160 mm Hg). For practical purposes, there is no CO_2 in dry inspired air and P_{CO_2} is zero.

◆ In **humidified tracheal air,** it is assumed that the air becomes fully saturated with water vapor. At

37°C, P_{H_2O} is 47 mm Hg. Thus, in comparison to dry inspired air, P_{O_2} is reduced because the O_2 is "diluted" by water vapor. Again, recall that partial pressures in humidified air are calculated by correcting the barometric pressure for water vapor pressure, then multiplying by the fractional concentration of the gas. Thus, the P_{O_2} of humidified tracheal air is 150 mm Hg ([760 mm Hg – 47 mm Hg] $\times$ 0.21 = 150 mm Hg). Because there is no CO_2 in inspired air, the P_{CO_2} of humidified tracheal air also is zero. The humidified air enters the alveoli, where gas exchange occurs.

◆ In **alveolar air,** the values for P_{O_2} and P_{CO_2} are changed substantially when compared with inspired air. (The notations for partial pressures in alveolar air use the modifier "A"; see Table 5-1.) $P_{A_{O_2}}$ is 100 mm Hg, which is less than in inspired air, and $P_{A_{CO_2}}$ is 40 mm Hg, which is greater than in inspired air. These changes occur because O_2 leaves alveolar air and is added to pulmonary capillary blood, and CO_2 leaves pulmonary capillary blood and enters alveolar air. Normally, the amounts of O_2 and CO_2 transferred between the alveoli and pulmonary capillary blood correspond to the needs of the body. Thus, on a daily basis, O_2 transfer *from* alveolar air equals O_2 consumption by the body, and CO_2 transfer *to* alveolar air equals CO_2 production.

◆ Blood entering the pulmonary capillaries is **mixed venous blood.** This blood has been returned from the tissues, via the veins, to the right heart. It is then pumped from the right ventricle into the

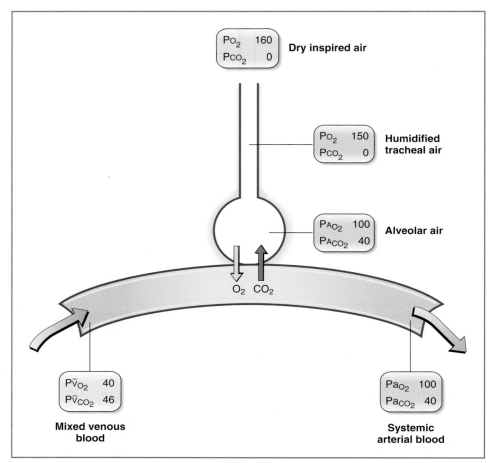

Figure 5–17 **Values for Po₂ and Pco₂ in dry inspired air, humidified tracheal air, alveolar air, and pulmonary capillary blood.** The numbers are partial pressures in mm Hg. Pa_{O_2} actually is slightly less than 100 mm Hg because of the physiologic shunt.

pulmonary artery, which delivers it to the pulmonary capillaries. The composition of this mixed venous blood reflects metabolic activity of the tissues: The Po₂ is relatively low, at 40 mm Hg, because the tissues have taken up and consumed O₂; the Pco₂ is relatively high, at 46 mm Hg, because the tissues have produced CO₂ and added it to venous blood.

♦ The blood that leaves the pulmonary capillaries has been *arterialized* (oxygenated) and will become **systemic arterial blood.** (The notations for systemic arterial blood use the modifier "a"; see Table 5-1.) The arterialization is effected by the exchange of O₂ and CO₂ between alveolar air and pulmonary capillary blood. Because diffusion of gases across the alveolar/capillary barrier is rapid, blood leaving the pulmonary capillaries normally has the same Po₂ and Pco₂ as alveolar air (i.e., there is complete equilibration). Hence, Pa_{O_2} is 100 mm Hg and Pa_{CO_2} is 40 mm Hg, just as PA_{O_2} is 100 mm Hg and PA_{CO_2} is 40 mm Hg. This arterialized blood will now be

returned to the left heart, pumped out of the left ventricle into the aorta, and begin the cycle again.

There is a small discrepancy between alveolar air and systemic arterial blood: Systemic arterial blood has a slightly lower Po₂ than alveolar air. This discrepancy is the result of a **physiologic shunt,** which describes the small fraction of pulmonary blood flow that bypasses the alveoli and, therefore, is not arterialized.

The physiologic shunt has two sources: bronchial blood flow and a small portion of coronary venous blood that drains directly into the left ventricle rather than going to the lungs to be oxygenated. The physiologic shunt is increased in several pathologic conditions (called a **ventilation/perfusion defect**). When the size of the shunt increases, equilibration between alveolar gas and pulmonary capillary blood cannot adequately occur and pulmonary capillary blood is not fully arterialized. The **A − a difference,** which is discussed later in this chapter, expresses the difference in Po₂ between alveolar gas ("A") and systemic arterial blood ("a"). If the shunt is small (i.e.,

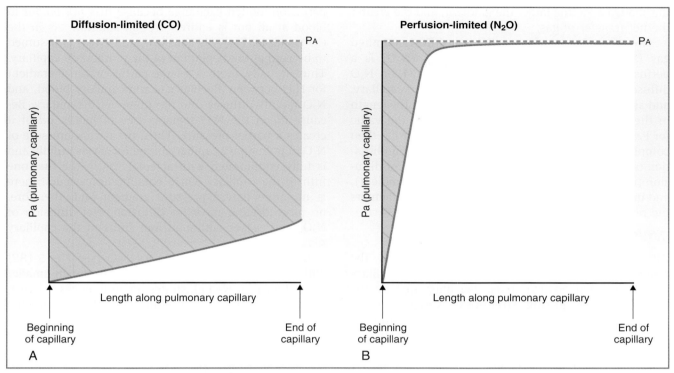

Figure 5–18 **Diffusion-limited (A) and perfusion-limited (B) gas exchange between alveolar air and pulmonary capillary blood.** The partial pressure of the gas in pulmonary capillary blood is shown as a function of capillary length by the *solid red line*. The *dashed green line* at the top of the figure shows the partial pressure of the gas in alveolar air (PA). The *shaded pink area* gives the size of the partial pressure difference between alveolar air and pulmonary capillary blood, which is the driving force for diffusion of the gas. CO, Carbon monoxide; N₂O, nitrous oxide.

physiologic), then the A − a difference is small or negligible; if the shunt is larger than normal, then the A − a difference increases to the extent that equilibration fails to occur.

The diagram in Figure 5-17 emphasizes the changes in PO₂ and PCO₂ that occur in the lungs. Not shown on the figure, but implied from the differences between systemic arterial blood and mixed venous blood, are the exchange processes that occur in the **systemic tissues.** Systemic arterial blood is delivered to the tissues, where O₂ diffuses from systemic capillaries into the tissues and is consumed, producing CO₂, which diffuses from the tissues into capillaries. This gas exchange in the tissues converts systemic arterial blood to mixed venous blood, which then leaves the capillaries, returns to the right heart, and is delivered to the lungs.

Diffusion-Limited and Perfusion-Limited Gas Exchange

Gas exchange across the alveolar/pulmonary capillary barrier is described as either diffusion-limited or perfusion-limited.

♦ **Diffusion-limited** gas exchange means that the total amount of gas transported across the alveolar-capillary barrier is limited by the *diffusion process.* In these cases, as long as the partial pressure gradient for the gas is maintained, diffusion will continue along the length of the capillary.

♦ **Perfusion-limited** gas exchange means that the total amount of gas transported across the alveolar/capillary barrier is limited by *blood flow* (i.e., perfusion) through the pulmonary capillaries. In perfusion-limited exchange, the *partial pressure gradient is not maintained,* and in this case, the only way to increase the amount of gas transported is by increasing blood flow.

Examples of gases transferred by diffusion-limited and perfusion-limited exchange are used to characterize these processes (Fig. 5-18). In the figure, the *solid red line* shows the partial pressure of a gas in pulmonary capillary blood (Pa) as a function of length along the capillary. The *dashed green line* across the top of each panel gives the partial pressure of the gas in alveolar air (PA), which is constant. The *shaded pink area* gives the **partial pressure gradient** between alveolar gas and pulmonary capillary blood along the length of the capillary. Because the partial pressure gradient is the driving force for diffusion of the gas, the larger the shaded area, the larger the gradient, and the greater the net transfer of gas.

Two examples are shown: CO is a diffusion-limited gas (see Fig. 5-18A), and nitrous oxide (N_2O) is a perfusion-limited gas (see Fig. 5-18B). CO or N_2O diffuse out of alveolar gas into the pulmonary capillary, and as a result, Pa for the gas increases along the length of the capillary and approaches or reaches the value for PA. If the value for Pa reaches the value of PA, then complete equilibration has occurred. Once equilibration occurs, there is no longer a driving force for diffusion (i.e., there is no longer a partial pressure gradient), and unless blood flow increases (i.e., more blood enters the pulmonary capillary), gas exchange will cease.

Diffusion-Limited Gas Exchange

Diffusion-limited gas exchange is illustrated by the transport of **CO** across the alveolar/pulmonary capillary barrier (see Fig. 5-18A). It is also illustrated by the transport of **O_2 during strenuous exercise** and in pathologic conditions such as **emphysema** and **fibrosis.**

The partial pressure of CO in alveolar air (PA_{CO}), shown as the dashed line, is constant along the length of the capillary. At the beginning of the pulmonary capillary, there is no CO in the blood because none has been transferred from alveolar air and the partial pressure of CO in capillary blood (Pa_{CO}) is zero. Thus, at the beginning of the capillary, there is the largest partial pressure gradient for CO and the largest driving force for diffusion of CO from alveolar air into the blood. Moving along the length of the pulmonary capillary, as CO diffuses into pulmonary capillary blood, Pa_{CO} begins to rise. As a result, the partial pressure gradient for diffusion decreases. Pa_{CO} rises only slightly along the capillary length, however, because in capillary blood, CO is avidly bound to hemoglobin inside the red blood cells. When CO is bound to hemoglobin, it is not free in solution, and therefore, it is not producing a partial pressure. (Recall that only free, dissolved gas causes a partial pressure.) Thus, the binding of CO to hemoglobin keeps the free CO concentration and the partial pressure low, thereby maintaining the gradient for diffusion along the *entire* length of the capillary.

In summary, net diffusion of CO into the pulmonary capillary depends on, or is "limited" by, the magnitude of the partial pressure gradient, which is maintained because CO is bound to hemoglobin in capillary blood. Thus, **CO does not equilibrate** by the end of the capillary. In fact, if the capillary were longer, net diffusion would continue indefinitely, or until equilibration occurred.

Perfusion-Limited Gas Exchange

Perfusion-limited gas exchange is illustrated by **N_2O** (see Fig. 5-18B), but also by **O_2 (under normal conditions)** and **CO_2.** N_2O is used as the classic example of

perfusion-limited exchange because it is *not bound* in blood at all but is entirely free in solution. As in the CO example, PA_{N_2O} is constant, and Pa_{N_2O} is assumed to be zero at the beginning of the pulmonary capillary. Thus, initially, there is a large partial pressure gradient for N_2O between alveolar gas and capillary blood, and N_2O rapidly diffuses into the pulmonary capillary. Because *all* of the N_2O remains free in blood, *all* of it creates a partial pressure. Thus, the partial pressure of N_2O in pulmonary capillary blood increases rapidly and is fully equilibrated with alveolar gas in the first one fifth of the capillary. Once equilibration occurs, there is no more partial pressure gradient and, therefore, no more driving force for diffusion. Net diffusion of N_2O then ceases, although four fifths of the capillary remains.

Compare the shaded area for N_2O (see Fig. 5-18B) with that for CO (see Fig. 5-18A). The much smaller shaded area for N_2O illustrates the differences between the two gases. Because equilibration of N_2O occurs, the only means for increasing net diffusion of N_2O is by increasing blood flow. If more "new" blood is supplied to the pulmonary capillary, then more *total* N_2O can be added to it. Thus, blood flow or perfusion determines, or "limits," the net transfer of N_2O, which is described as perfusion-limited.

O_2 Transport—Perfusion-Limited and Diffusion-Limited

Under normal conditions, O_2 transport into pulmonary capillaries is perfusion-limited, but under other conditions (e.g., fibrosis or strenuous exercise), it is diffusion-limited. Figure 5-19 illustrates both conditions.

◆ **Perfusion-limited O_2 transport.** In the lungs of a normal person at rest, O_2 transfer from alveolar air into pulmonary capillary blood is *perfusion-limited* (although not to the extreme that N_2O is perfusion-limited) (see Fig. 5-19A). PA_{O_2} is constant at 100 mm Hg. At the beginning of the capillary, Pa_{O_2} is 40 mm Hg, reflecting the composition of mixed venous blood. There is large partial pressure gradient for O_2 between alveolar air and capillary blood, which drives O_2 diffusion into the capillary. As O_2 is added to pulmonary capillary blood, Pa_{O_2} increases. The gradient for diffusion is maintained initially because O_2 binds to hemoglobin, which keeps the free O_2 concentration and the partial pressure low. Equilibration of O_2 occurs about one third of the distance along the capillary, at which point Pa_{O_2} becomes equal to PA_{O_2}, and unless blood flow increases, there can be no more net diffusion of O_2. Thus, under normal conditions, O_2 transport is perfusion-limited. Another way of describing perfusion-limited O_2 exchange is to say that pulmonary blood flow determines net O_2 transfer. Thus, increases in

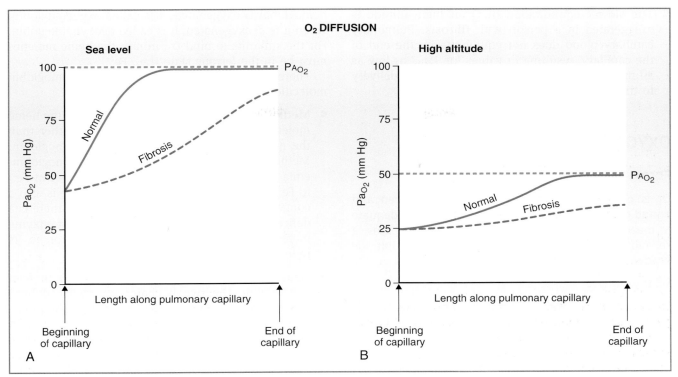

Figure 5–19 O$_2$ diffusion along the length of the pulmonary capillary in normal persons and persons with fibrosis. **A**, At sea level; **B**, at high altitude.

pulmonary blood flow (e.g., during exercise) will increase the total amount of O$_2$ transported, and decreases in pulmonary blood flow will decrease the total amount transported.

♦ **Diffusion-limited O$_2$ transport.** In certain pathologic conditions (e.g., **fibrosis**) and during **strenuous exercise**, O$_2$ transfer becomes *diffusion* limited. For example, in fibrosis the alveolar wall thickens, increasing the diffusion distance for gases and decreasing D$_L$ (see Fig. 5-19A). This increased diffusion distance slows the rate of diffusion of O$_2$ and prevents equilibration of O$_2$ between alveolar air and pulmonary capillary blood. In these cases, the partial pressure gradient for O$_2$ is maintained along the entire length of the capillary, converting it to a diffusion-limited process (although not as extreme as in the example of CO; see Fig. 5-18A). Because a partial pressure gradient is maintained along the entire length of the capillary, it may *seem* that the total amount of O$_2$ transferred would be greater in a person with fibrosis than in a person with normal lungs. Although it is true that the O$_2$ partial pressure gradient is maintained for a longer length of the capillary (because D$_L$ is markedly decreased in fibrosis), the total transfer of O$_2$ still is greatly decreased. At the end of the pulmonary capillary, equilibration has not occurred between alveolar air and pulmonary capillary blood (Pa$_{O_2}$ < PA$_{O_2}$), which

will be reflected in a decreased Pa$_{O_2}$ in systemic arterial blood and decreased P$\bar{v}_{O_2}$ in mixed venous blood.

♦ **O$_2$ transport at high altitude.** Ascent to high altitude alters some aspects of the O$_2$ equilibration process. At high altitude, barometric pressure is reduced, and with the same fraction of O$_2$ in inspired air, the partial pressure of O$_2$ in alveolar gas also will be reduced. In the example shown in Figure 5-19B, PA$_{O_2}$ is reduced to 50 mm Hg, compared with the normal value of 100 mm Hg. Mixed venous P$_{O_2}$ is 25 mm Hg (as opposed to the normal value of 40 mm Hg). Therefore, at high altitude, the partial pressure gradient for O$_2$ is greatly reduced compared with sea level (see Fig. 5-19A). Even at the beginning of the pulmonary capillary, the gradient is only 25 mm Hg (50 mm Hg − 25 mm Hg), instead of the normal gradient at sea level of 60 mm Hg (100 mm Hg − 40 mm Hg). This reduction of the partial pressure gradient means that diffusion of O$_2$ will be reduced, equilibration will occur more slowly along the capillary, and complete equilibration will be achieved at a later point along the capillary (two thirds of the capillary length at high altitude, compared with one third of the length at sea level). The final equilibrated value for Pa$_{O_2}$ is only 50 mm Hg because PA$_{O_2}$ is only 50 mm Hg (it is impossible for the equilibrated value to be higher than 50 mm Hg).

The slower equilibration of O_2 at high altitude is exaggerated in a person with **fibrosis.** Pulmonary capillary blood does not equilibrate by the end of the capillary, resulting in values for Pa_{O_2} as low as 30 mm Hg, which will seriously impair O_2 delivery to the tissues.

OXYGEN TRANSPORT IN BLOOD

Forms of O_2 in Blood

O_2 is carried in two forms in blood: dissolved and bound to hemoglobin. Dissolved O_2 alone is inadequate to meet the metabolic demands of the tissues; thus, a second form of O_2, combined with hemoglobin, is needed.

Dissolved O_2

Dissolved O_2 is free in solution and accounts for approximately **2% of the total O_2 content of blood.** Recall that dissolved O_2 is the *only form* of O_2 that produces a partial pressure, which, in turn, drives O_2 diffusion. (In contrast, O_2 bound to hemoglobin *does not* contribute to its partial pressure in blood.) As described by **Henry's law,** the concentration of dissolved O_2 is proportional to the partial pressure of O_2; the proportionality constant is simply the solubility of O_2 in blood, 0.003 mL O_2/100 mL blood/mm Hg. Thus, for a normal Pa_{O_2} of 100 mm Hg, the concentration of dissolved O_2 is 0.3 mL O_2/100 mL (100 mm Hg $\times$ 0.003 mL O_2/100 mL blood/mm Hg).

At this concentration, dissolved O_2 is grossly insufficient to meet the demands of the tissues. For example, in a person at rest, O_2 consumption is about 250 mL O_2/min. If O_2 delivery to the tissues were based strictly on the dissolved component, then 15 mL O_2/min would be delivered to the tissues (O_2 delivery = cardiac output $\times$ dissolved O_2 concentration, or 5 L/min $\times$ 0.3 mL O_2/100 mL = 15 mL O_2/min). Clearly, this amount is insufficient to meet the demand of 250 mL O_2/min. An additional mechanism for transporting large quantities of O_2 in blood is needed—that mechanism is O_2 bound to hemoglobin.

O_2 Bound to Hemoglobin

The remaining **98% of the total O_2 content of blood** is reversibly bound to hemoglobin inside the red blood cells. **Hemoglobin** is a globular protein consisting of **four subunits.** Each subunit contains a heme moiety, which is an iron-binding porphyrin, and a polypeptide chain, which is designated either α or β. **Adult hemoglobin** (hemoglobin A) is called $\alpha_2\beta_2$; two of the subunits have α chains and two have β chains. Each subunit can bind one molecule of O_2, for a total of four molecules of O_2 per molecule of hemoglobin. When

hemoglobin is oxygenated, it is called oxyhemoglobin; when it is deoxygenated, it is called deoxyhemoglobin. For the subunits to bind O_2, iron in the heme moieties must be in the ferrous state (i.e., **Fe^{2+}**).

There are several variants of the hemoglobin molecule:

♦ **Methemoglobin.** If the iron component of the heme moieties is in the ferric, or **Fe^{3+},** state (rather than the normal Fe^{2+} state), it is called methemoglobin. Methemoglobin *does not bind O_2.* Methemoglobinemia has several causes including oxidation of Fe^{2+} to Fe^{3+} by nitrites and sulfonamides. There is also a congenital variant of the disease in which there is a deficiency of methemoglobin reductase, an enzyme in red blood cells that normally keeps iron in its reduced state.

♦ **Fetal hemoglobin (hemoglobin F, HbF).** In fetal hemoglobin, the two β chains are replaced by γ chains, giving it the designation of $\alpha_2\gamma_2$. The physiologic consequence of this modification is that hemoglobin F has a **higher affinity for O_2** than hemoglobin A, facilitating O_2 movement from the mother to the fetus. Hemoglobin F is the normal variant present in the fetus and is replaced by hemoglobin A within the first year of life.

♦ **Hemoglobin S.** Hemoglobin S is an abnormal variant of hemoglobin that causes **sickle cell disease.** In hemoglobin S, the α subunits are normal and the β subunits are abnormal, giving it the designation $\alpha^A_2\beta^S_2$. In its deoxygenated form, hemoglobin S forms sickle-shaped rods in the red blood cells, distorting the shape of the red blood cells (i.e., sickling them). This deformation of the red blood cells can result in occlusion of small blood vessels. The O_2 affinity of hemoglobin S is less than the O_2 affinity of hemoglobin A.

O_2-Binding Capacity and O_2 Content

Because the majority of O_2 transported in blood is reversibly bound to hemoglobin, the O_2 content of blood is primarily determined by the hemoglobin concentration and by the O_2-binding capacity of that hemoglobin.

The **O_2-binding capacity** is the *maximum* amount of O_2 that can be bound to hemoglobin per volume of blood, assuming that hemoglobin is 100% saturated (i.e., all four heme groups on each molecule of hemoglobin are bound to O_2). The O_2-binding capacity is measured by exposing blood to air with a high P_{O_2} (so that hemoglobin will be 100% saturated) and by correcting for the small amount of O_2 that is present in the dissolved form. (To correct for dissolved O_2, remember that the solubility of O_2 in blood is 0.003 mL O_2/100 mL blood/mm Hg.) Other information needed to calculate the O_2-binding capacity is that 1 g of hemoglobin A can bind 1.34 mL O_2 and that the normal concentration of hemoglobin A in blood is 15 g/100 mL. The O_2-binding capacity of blood is therefore 20.1 mL O_2/100 mL blood (15 g/100 mL × 1.34 mL O_2/g hemoglobin = 20.1 mL O_2/100 mL blood).

The **O_2 content** is the actual amount of O_2 per volume of blood. The O_2 content can be calculated from the O_2-binding capacity of hemoglobin and the percent saturation of hemoglobin, plus any dissolved O_2. (Recall that O_2-binding capacity is determined at 100% saturation with all heme groups bound to O_2 on all hemoglobin molecules.)

$$O_2 \text{ content} = (O_2\text{-binding capacity} \times \% \text{ Saturation}) + \text{Dissolved } O_2$$

where

$$O_2 \text{ content} = \text{Amount of } O_2 \text{ in blood} \\ (\text{mL } O_2/100 \text{ mL blood})$$
$$O_2\text{-binding capacity} = \text{Amount of } O_2 \text{ bound} \\ \text{to hemoglobin} \\ (\text{mL } O_2/100 \text{ mL blood}) \\ \text{measured at } 100\% \\ \text{saturation}$$
$$\text{Percent saturation} = \% \text{ of heme groups bound} \\ \text{to } O_2$$
$$\text{Dissolved } O_2 = \text{Unbound } O_2 \text{ in blood} \\ (\text{mL } O_2/100 \text{ mL blood})$$

SAMPLE PROBLEM. A man who is anemic has a severely reduced hemoglobin concentration of 10 g/100 mL blood. Assuming that the patient has normal lungs and that the values of both PA_{O_2} and Pa_{O_2} are normal at 100 mm Hg, *what is the O_2 content of his blood, and how does that value compare with the normal value?* Assume that for a normal hemoglobin concentration of 15 g/100 mL, the O_2-binding capacity is 20.1 mL O_2/100 mL blood, and that hemoglobin is 98% saturated at a Pa_{O_2} of 100 mm Hg.

SOLUTION. (1) First, calculate the *O_2-binding capacity* (the maximum amount of O_2 that can be bound to hemoglobin) at a hemoglobin concentration of 10 g/100 mL blood. It is a given that at a normal hemoglobin concentration of 15 g/100 mL, O_2-binding capacity is 20.1 mL O_2/100 mL blood. Thus, at a hemoglobin concentration of 10 g/100 mL, O_2-binding capacity is 10/15 of normal. Thus,

$$O_2\text{-binding capacity} = 20.1 \text{ mL } O_2/100 \text{ mL blood} \\ \times \frac{10}{15} \\ = 13.4 \text{ mL } O_2/100 \text{ mL blood}$$

(2) Next, calculate the *actual amount of O_2 combined with hemoglobin* by multiplying the O_2-binding capacity by the % saturation. Thus,

$$O_2 \text{ bound to hemoglobin} = 13.4 \text{ mL } O_2/100 \text{ mL blood} \times 98\% \\ = 13.1 \text{ mL } O_2/100 \text{ mL blood}$$

(3) Finally, determine the *total O_2 content* by calculating the dissolved O_2 at Pa_{O_2} of 100 mm Hg and adding that amount to the O_2 bound to hemoglobin. The solubility of O_2 in blood is 0.003 mL O_2/100 mL/mm Hg. Thus,

$$\text{Dissolved } O_2 = 100 \text{ mm Hg} \times 0.003 \text{ mL } O_2/100 \text{ mL/mm Hg} \\ = 0.3 \text{ mL } O_2/100 \text{ mL blood}$$

$$\text{Total } O_2 \text{ content} = O_2 \text{ bound to hemoglobin} + \text{dissolved } O_2 \\ = 13.1 \text{ mL } O_2/100 \text{ mL blood} \\ + 0.3 \text{ mL } O_2/100 \text{ mL blood} \\ = 13.4 \text{ mL } O_2/100 \text{ mL blood}$$

An O_2 content of 13.4 mL O_2/100 mL blood is *severely* depressed. Compare this value with the O_2 content of 20.0 mL O_2/100 mL blood calculated at the normal hemoglobin concentration of 15 g/100 mL and 98% saturation. (Bound O_2 is 20.1 mL O_2/100 mL × 98% = 19.7 mL O_2/100 mL, and dissolved O_2 is 0.3 mL O_2/100 mL. Thus, normal total O_2 content is the sum, or 20.0 mL O_2/100 mL blood.)

O_2 Delivery to Tissues

The amount of O_2 delivered to tissues is determined by blood flow and the O_2 content of blood. In terms of the whole organism, blood flow is considered to be cardiac output. O_2 content of blood, as already described, is the sum of dissolved O_2 (2%) and O_2-hemoglobin (98%). Thus, O_2 delivery is described as follows:

$$O_2 \text{ delivery} = \text{Cardiac output} \times O_2 \text{ content of blood} \\ = \text{Cardiac output} \times (\text{Dissolved } O_2 \\ + O_2\text{-hemoglobin})$$

O_2-Hemoglobin Dissociation Curve

As a review, recall that O_2 combines reversibly and rapidly with hemoglobin, binding to heme groups on each of the four subunits of the hemoglobin molecule. Each hemoglobin molecule, therefore, has the capacity to bind **four molecules of O_2.** In this configuration, saturation is **100%.** If fewer than four molecules of O_2 are bound to heme groups, then saturation is less than 100%. For example, if, on average, each hemoglobin molecule has three molecules of O_2 bound, then saturation is **75%;** if, on average, each hemoglobin has two molecules of O_2 bound, then saturation is **50%;** and if only one molecule of O_2 is bound, saturation is **25%.**

Percent saturation of hemoglobin is a function of the P_{O_2} of blood, as described by the **O_2-hemoglobin dissociation curve** (Fig. 5-20). The most striking feature of this curve is its sigmoidal shape. In other words, the percent saturation of heme sites does not increase linearly as P_{O_2} increases. Rather, percent saturation increases steeply as P_{O_2} increases from zero to approximately 40 mm Hg, and it then levels off between

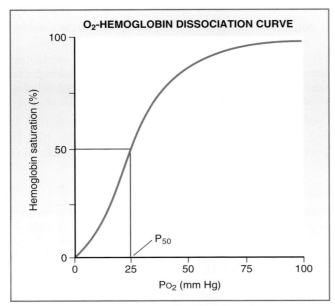

Figure 5–20 **O₂-hemoglobin dissociation curve.** P$_{50}$ is the partial pressure of O$_2$ at which hemoglobin is 50% saturated.

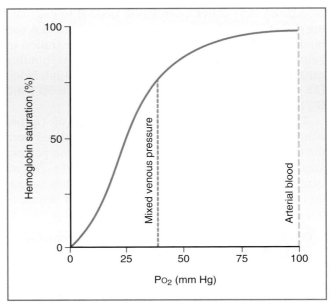

Figure 5–21 **Hemoglobin saturation as a function of P$_{O_2}$ in systemic arterial blood and mixed venous blood.**

Table 5–2 Values of P$_{O_2}$ and Corresponding Values of Percent Saturation of Hemoglobin

P$_{O_2}$ (mm Hg)	Saturation (%)
10	25
20	35
25	50
30	60
40	75
50	85
60	90
80	96
100	98

The P$_{O_2}$ that corresponds to 50% saturation of hemoglobin is called P$_{50}$.

50 mm Hg and 100 mm Hg. For convenience, Table 5-2 gives the values of percent saturation that correspond to various values of P$_{O_2}$.

Sigmoidal Shape

The shape of the steepest portion of the curve is the result of a **change in affinity** of the heme groups for O$_2$ as each successive O$_2$ molecule binds: Binding of the first molecule of O$_2$ to a heme group increases the affinity for the second O$_2$ molecule, binding of the second O$_2$ molecule increases the affinity for the third O$_2$ molecule, and so forth. Affinity for the fourth, and

last, molecule of O$_2$ is highest and occurs at values of P$_{O_2}$ between approximately 60 and 100 mm Hg (where saturation is nearly 100%, corresponding to four molecules of O$_2$ per one molecule of hemoglobin). This phenomenon is described as **positive cooperativity.**

P$_{50}$

A significant point on the O$_2$-hemoglobin dissociation curve is the P$_{50}$. By definition, P$_{50}$ is the **P$_{O_2}$ at which hemoglobin is 50% saturated** (i.e., where two of the four heme groups are bound to O$_2$). A change in the value of P$_{50}$ is used as an indicator for a change in affinity of hemoglobin for O$_2$. An increase in P$_{50}$ reflects a decrease in affinity, and a decrease in P$_{50}$ reflects an increase in affinity.

Loading and Unloading of O$_2$

The sigmoidal shape of the O$_2$-hemoglobin dissociation curve helps to explain why O$_2$ is *loaded into* pulmonary capillary blood from alveolar gas and *unloaded from* systemic capillaries into the tissues (Fig. 5-21). At the highest values of P$_{O_2}$ (i.e., in systemic arterial blood), the affinity of hemoglobin for O$_2$ is highest; at lower values of P$_{O_2}$ (i.e., in mixed venous blood), affinity for O$_2$ is lower.

Alveolar air, pulmonary capillary blood, and **systemic arterial blood** all have a P$_{O_2}$ of **100 mm Hg.** On the graph, a P$_{O_2}$ of 100 mm Hg corresponds to almost 100% saturation, with all heme groups bound to O$_2$, and affinity for O$_2$ at its highest value due to positive cooperativity. On the other hand, **mixed venous blood** has a P$_{O_2}$ of **40 mm Hg** (because O$_2$ has diffused from

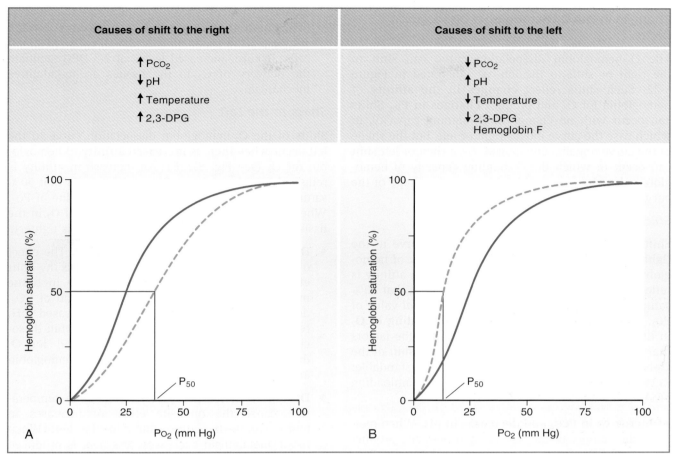

Figure 5–22 **Shifts of the O₂-hemoglobin dissociation curve. A,** Shifts to the right are associated with increased P_{50} and decreased affinity. **B,** Shifts to the left are associated with decreased P_{50} and increased affinity.

systemic capillaries into the tissues). On the graph, a P_{O_2} of 40 mm Hg corresponds to approximately 75% saturation and a lower affinity of hemoglobin for O_2. Thus, the sigmoidal shape of the curve reflects changes in the affinity of hemoglobin for O_2, and these changes in affinity facilitate loading of O_2 in the lungs (where P_{O_2} and affinity are highest) and unloading of O_2 in the tissues (where P_{O_2} and affinity are lower).

♦ In the **lungs,** Pa_{O_2} is 100 mm Hg. Hemoglobin is **nearly 100% saturated** (all heme groups are bound to O_2). Due to positive cooperativity, **affinity is highest** and O_2 is most tightly bound (the flat portion of the curve). The high affinity makes sense because it is important to have as much O_2 as possible loaded into arterial blood in the lungs. Also, because O_2 is so tightly bound to hemoglobin in this range, relatively less O_2 is in the dissolved form to produce a partial pressure; by keeping the P_{O_2} of pulmonary capillary blood lower than the P_{O_2} of alveolar gas, O_2 diffusion into the capillary will continue. The flat portion of the curve extends from 100 mm Hg to

60 mm Hg, which means that humans can tolerate substantial decreases in alveolar P_{O_2} to 60 mm Hg (e.g., caused by decreases in atmospheric pressure) without significantly compromising the amount of O_2 carried by hemoglobin.

♦ In the **tissues,** $P\bar{v}_{O_2}$ is approximately 40 mm Hg, much lower than it is in the lungs. At a P_{O_2} of 40 mm Hg, hemoglobin is only **75% saturated** and the **affinity for O_2** is decreased. O_2 is not as tightly bound in this part of the curve, which facilitates unloading of O_2 in the tissues.

The partial pressure gradient for O_2 diffusion into the tissues is maintained in two ways: First, the tissues consume O_2, keeping their P_{O_2} low. Second, the lower affinity for O_2 ensures that O_2 will be unloaded more readily from hemoglobin; unbound O_2 is free in blood, creates a partial pressure, and the P_{O_2} of blood is kept relatively high. Because the P_{O_2} of the tissue is kept relatively low, the partial pressure gradient that drives O_2 diffusion from blood to tissues is maintained.

Changes in the O₂-Hemoglobin Dissociation Curve

The O_2-hemoglobin dissociation curve can shift to the right or shift to the left, as illustrated in Figure 5-22. Such shifts reflect **changes in the affinity** of hemoglobin for O_2 and produce **changes in P_{50}.** Shifts can occur with no change in O_2-binding capacity, in which case the curve moves right or left, but the shape of the curve remains unchanged. Or, a right or left shift can occur in which the O_2-binding capacity of hemoglobin also changes and, in this case, the shape of the curve changes.

Shifts to the Right

Shifts of the O_2-hemoglobin dissociation curve to the right occur when there is **decreased affinity** of hemoglobin for O_2 (see Fig. 5-22A). A decrease in affinity is reflected in an **increase in P_{50},** which means that 50% saturation is achieved at a *higher-than-normal* value of Po_2. When the affinity is decreased, **unloading of O_2** in the tissues is facilitated. Physiologically, the factors that cause a decrease in affinity and a right shift of the O_2-hemoglobin dissociation curve are understandable: In each case, it is advantageous to facilitate unloading of O_2 in the tissues.

◆ **Increases in Pco_2 and decreases in pH.** When metabolic activity of the tissues increases, the production of CO_2 increases; the increase in tissue Pco_2 causes an increase in H^+ concentration and a decrease in pH. Together, these effects decrease the affinity of hemoglobin for O_2, shift the O_2-hemoglobin dissociation curve to the right, and increase the P_{50}, all of which facilitates unloading of O_2 from hemoglobin in the tissues. This mechanism helps to ensure that O_2 delivery can meet O_2 demand (e.g., in exercising skeletal muscle). The effect of Pco_2 and pH on the O_2-hemoglobin dissociation curve is called the **Bohr effect.**

◆ **Increases in temperature.** The increases in temperature also cause a right shift of the O_2-hemoglobin dissociation curve and an increase in P_{50}, facilitating unloading of O_2 in the tissues. Considering the example of exercising skeletal muscle, this effect also is logical. As heat is produced by the working muscle, the O_2-hemoglobin dissociation curve shifts to the right, providing more O_2 to the tissue.

◆ **Increases in 2,3-diphosphoglycerate (2,3-DPG) concentration.** 2,3-DPG is a byproduct of glycolysis in red blood cells. 2,3-DPG binds to the β chains of deoxyhemoglobin and reduces their affinity for O_2. This decrease in affinity causes the O_2-hemoglobin dissociation curve to shift to the right and facilitates unloading of O_2 in the tissues. 2,3-DPG production increases under hypoxic conditions. For example, living at **high altitude** causes hypoxemia, which stimulates the production of 2,3-DPG in red blood cells. In turn, increased levels of 2,3-DPG facilitate the delivery of O_2 to the tissues as an adaptive mechanism.

Shifts to the Left

Shifts of the O_2-hemoglobin dissociation curve to the left occur when there is **increased affinity** of hemoglobin for O_2 (see Fig. 5-22B). An increase in affinity is reflected in a **decrease in P_{50},** which means that 50% saturation occurs at a *lower-than-normal* value of Po_2. When the affinity is increased, **unloading of O_2** in the tissues is more difficult (i.e., binding of O_2 is tighter).

◆ **Decreases in Pco_2 and increases in pH.** The effect of decreases in Pco_2 and increases in pH is the Bohr effect again. When there is a decrease in tissue metabolism, there is decreased production of CO_2, decreased H^+ concentration, and increased pH, resulting in a left shift of the O_2-hemoglobin dissociation curve. Thus, when the demand for O_2 decreases, O_2 is more tightly bound to hemoglobin and less O_2 is unloaded to the tissues.

◆ **Decreases in temperature.** Decreases in temperature cause the opposite effect of increases in temperature—the curve shifts to the left. When tissue metabolism decreases, less heat is produced and less O_2 is unloaded in the tissues.

◆ **Decreases in 2,3-DPG concentration.** Decreases in 2,3-DPG concentration also reflect decreased tissue metabolism, causing a left shift of the curve and less O_2 to be unloaded in the tissues.

◆ **Hemoglobin F.** As previously described, hemoglobin F is the fetal variant of hemoglobin. The β chains of adult hemoglobin (hemoglobin A) are replaced by γ chains in hemoglobin F. This modification results in increased affinity of hemoglobin for O_2, a left shift of the O_2-hemoglobin dissociation curve, and decreased P_{50}.

The mechanism of the left shift is based on the binding of **2,3-DPG.** 2,3-DPG does not bind as avidly to the γ chains of hemoglobin F as it binds to the β chains of hemoglobin A. When less 2,3-DPG is bound, the affinity for O_2 increases. This increased affinity is beneficial to the fetus, whose Pa_{O_2} is low (approximately 40 mm Hg).

Carbon Monoxide

All the effects on the O_2-hemoglobin dissociation curve discussed thus far have involved right or left shifts. The effect of CO is different: It **decreases O_2 bound to hemoglobin** and also causes a **left shift** of the O_2-hemoglobin dissociation curve (Fig. 5-23).

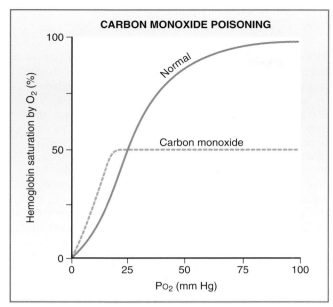

Figure 5–23 **Effect of carbon monoxide on the O₂-hemoglobin dissociation curve.** Carbon monoxide reduces the number of sites available for O_2 binding to hemoglobin and causes a shift of the O_2-hemoglobin dissociation curve to the left.

CO binds to hemoglobin with an affinity that is 250 times that of O_2 to form **carboxyhemoglobin**. In other words, when the partial pressure of CO is only 1/250 that of O_2, equal amounts of CO and O_2 will bind to hemoglobin! Because O_2 cannot bind to heme groups that are bound to CO, the presence of CO decreases the number of O_2-binding sites available on hemoglobin. In the example shown in Figure 5-23, hemoglobin bound to O_2 is reduced to 50%, which means that one half the binding sites would be bound to CO and one half the binding sites would be available for O_2. The implications for O_2 transport are obvious: This effect *alone* would reduce O_2 content of blood and O_2 delivery to tissues by 50%.

CO also causes a left shift of the O_2-hemoglobin dissociation curve: Those heme groups *not* bound to CO have an **increased affinity for O₂.** Thus, P_{50} is decreased, making it more difficult for O_2 to be unloaded in the tissues.

Together, these two effects of CO on O_2 binding to hemoglobin are catastrophic for O_2 delivery to tissues. Not only is there reduced O_2-binding capacity of hemoglobin, but the remaining heme sites bind O_2 more tightly (Box 5-1).

Erythropoietin

Erythropoietin (EPO) is a glycoprotein growth factor that is synthesized in the kidneys (and to a lesser extent in the liver) and serves as the major stimulus for erythropoiesis by promoting the differentiation of proerythroblasts into red blood cells.

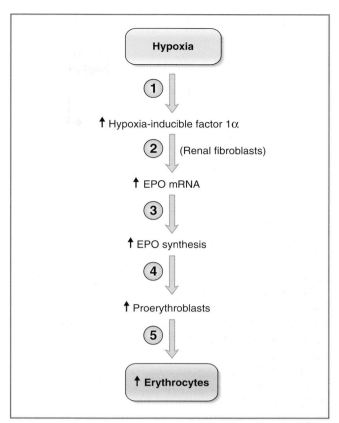

Figure 5–24 **Hypoxia induces synthesis of erythropoietin.** The circled numbers correspond to the numbered steps in the text. EPO, Erythropoietin; mRNA, messenger RNA.

EPO synthesis is induced in the kidney in response to **hypoxia** in the following steps (Fig. 5-24).

1. When there is decreased O_2 delivery to the kidneys (hypoxia), either due to decreased hemoglobin concentration or decreased Pa_{O_2}, there is increased production of the alpha subunit of hypoxia-inducible factor 1 (**hypoxia-inducible factor 1α**).
2. Hypoxia-inducible factor 1α acts on fibroblasts in the renal cortex and medulla to cause synthesis of the mRNA for EPO.
3. The mRNA directs increased synthesis of **EPO.**
4. EPO then acts to cause **differentiation of proerythroblasts.**
5. Proerythroblasts undergo further steps in development to form mature erythrocytes (red blood cells). These further maturation steps do not require EPO.

Interestingly, the kidneys are the ideal site for EPO synthesis because they can distinguish between decreased blood flow as a cause of decreased O_2 delivery and decreased O_2 content of arterial blood (e.g., due to decreased hemoglobin concentration or decreased Pa_{O_2}) as a cause of decreased O_2 delivery.

BOX 5–1   Clinical Physiology: Carbon Monoxide Poisoning

DESCRIPTION OF CASE. On a cold February morning in Boston, a 55-year-old man decides to warm his car in the garage. While the car is warming, he waits in a workshop adjoining the garage. About 30 minutes later, his wife finds him tinkering at his workbench, confused and breathing rapidly. He is taken to a nearby emergency department and given 100% O_2 to breathe. The following arterial blood values are measured:

Pa_{O_2}, 660 mm Hg

Pa_{CO_2}, 36 mm Hg

pH, 7.43

% O_2 saturation of hemoglobin, 60%

EXPLANATION OF CASE. The man inhaled the exhaust fumes from his automobile and is suffering from acute carbon monoxide (CO) poisoning. The arterial blood values obtained can be explained by the effects of CO-binding to hemoglobin.

CO binds avidly to hemoglobin, with an affinity that is 250 times that of O_2-binding to hemoglobin. Thus, heme groups that normally are bound to O_2 now are bound to CO. The percent saturation of hemoglobin with O_2 is measured as 60%, so 40% of the sites must be occupied by CO. Because O_2-hemoglobin is the major form of O_2 transport to the tissues, the first detrimental effect of CO poisoning is the decreased O_2-carrying capacity of blood. The second detrimental effect of CO poisoning is a shift of the O_2-hemoglobin dissociation curve to the left, which reduces P_{50} and increases the affinity of hemoglobin for what little O_2 is bound. As a result, it is more difficult to unload O_2 to the tissues. Together, these two effects of CO poisoning can result in death caused by a failure to deliver sufficient O_2 to critical tissues such as the brain.

TREATMENT. Treatment of this patient consists of having him breathe 100% O_2 in an effort to rapidly displace as much CO from hemoglobin as possible.

Notice the strikingly high value of Pa_{O_2} at 660 mm Hg. *Is this value plausible?* Assuming that there is no $\dot{V}/\dot{Q}$ defect, Pa_{O_2} should be equal to PA_{O_2} because there is equilibration of pulmonary capillary blood with alveolar gas. Therefore, a better question is *Why is PA_{O_2} 660 mm Hg?* The expected value for PA_{O_2} can be calculated from the alveolar gas equation, if values are known for the P_{O_2} of inspired air, PA_{CO_2}, and the respiratory quotient. PI_{O_2} can be calculated from the barometric pressure (corrected for water vapor) and the percent of O_2 in inspired air (100%). PA_{CO_2} is equal to Pa_{CO_2}, which is given. The respiratory quotient is assumed to be 0.8. Thus,

$$PI_{O_2} = (P_{atm} - PH_2O) \times FO_2$$
$$= (760 \text{ mm Hg} - 47 \text{ mm Hg}) \times 1.0$$
$$= 713 \text{ mm Hg}$$

$$PA_{O_2} = PI_{O_2} - \frac{PA_{CO_2}}{R}$$
$$= 713 \text{ mm Hg} - \frac{36 \text{ mm Hg}}{0.8}$$
$$= 668 \text{ mm Hg}$$

Again, assuming that systemic arterial blood has the same P_{O_2} as alveolar gas, and assuming that $\dot{V}/\dot{Q}$ ratios are normal, the *measured* value for Pa_{O_2} of 660 mm Hg is consistent with the *expected* PA_{O_2} value of 668 mm Hg, calculated with the alveolar gas equation. This extremely high Pa_{O_2} does little to improve O_2 delivery to the tissues because the solubility of O_2 in blood is so low (0.003 mL O_2/100 mL blood/mm Hg). Thus, at a Pa_{O_2} of 660 mm Hg, the dissolved O_2 content is only 1.98 mL O_2/100 mL blood.

This distinguishing ability is based on the fact that decreased renal blood flow causes decreased glomerular filtration, which leads to decreased filtration and reabsorption of Na^+. Because O_2 consumption in the kidneys is strongly linked to Na^+ reabsorption, decreased renal blood flow results in *both* decreased O_2 delivery *and* decreased O_2 consumption; thus, renal O_2 delivery and renal O_2 consumption remain matched in that scenario and, as is appropriate, the kidney *is not* alerted to a need for more erythrocytes. If there is decreased O_2 content of arterial blood, then the kidney *is* alerted to a need for more erythrocytes.

Anemia is a common finding in **chronic renal failure** because the decrease in functioning renal mass results in decreased synthesis of EPO and decreased production of erythrocytes and the accompanying decrease in hemoglobin concentration. The anemia of chronic renal failure can be treated with recombinant human EPO.

CARBON DIOXIDE TRANSPORT IN BLOOD

Forms of CO_2 in Blood

CO_2 is carried in the blood in three forms: as dissolved CO_2, as carbaminohemoglobin (CO_2 bound to hemoglobin), and as bicarbonate (HCO_3^-), which is a chemically modified form of CO_2. By far, *HCO_3^- is quantitatively the most important* of these forms.

Dissolved CO_2

As with O_2, a portion of the CO_2 in blood is in the dissolved form. The concentration of CO_2 in solution is given by **Henry's law,** which states that the concentration of CO_2 in blood is the partial pressure multiplied by the solubility of CO_2. The solubility of CO_2 is 0.07 mL CO_2/100 mL blood/mm Hg; thus, the concentration of dissolved CO_2 in arterial blood, as calculated by Henry's

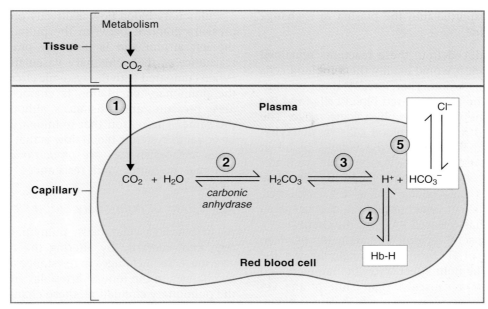

Figure 5–25 **Transport of carbon dioxide (CO₂) in the blood.** CO_2 and H_2O are converted to H^+ and HCO_3^- inside red blood cells. H^+ is buffered by hemoglobin (Hb-H) inside the red blood cells. HCO_3^- exchanges for Cl^- and is transported in plasma. The circled numbers correspond to the numbered steps discussed in the text.

law, is 2.8 mL CO_2/100 mL blood (40 mm Hg × 0.07 mL CO_2/100 mL blood/mm Hg), which is approximately **5% of the total CO_2 content of blood.** (Recall that because of the lower solubility of O_2, compared with CO_2, dissolved O_2 is only 2% of the total O_2 content of blood.)

Carbaminohemoglobin

CO_2 binds to terminal amino groups on proteins (e.g., hemoglobin and plasma proteins such as albumin). When CO_2 is bound to hemoglobin, it is called carbaminohemoglobin, which accounts for about **3% of the total CO_2.**

CO₂ binds to hemoglobin at a different site than O_2 binds to hemoglobin. As discussed previously, CO_2 binding to hemoglobin reduces its affinity for O_2 and causes a right-shift of the O_2-hemoglobin dissociation curve (Bohr effect). In turn, O_2 bound to hemoglobin changes its affinity for CO_2, such that when less O_2 is bound, the affinity of hemoglobin for CO_2 increases (the **Haldane effect**). These mutual effects of O_2 and CO_2 on each other's binding to hemoglobin makes sense—in the tissues, as CO_2 is produced and binds to hemoglobin, hemoglobin's affinity for O_2 is decreased and it releases O_2 to the tissues more readily; in turn, release of O_2 from hemoglobin increases its affinity for the CO_2 that is being produced in the tissues.

HCO₃⁻

Almost all of the CO_2 carried in blood is in a chemically modified form, HCO_3^-, which accounts for more than **90% of the total CO_2.** The reactions that produce

HCO_3^- from CO_2 involve the combination of CO_2 and H_2O to form the weak acid H_2CO_3. This reaction is catalyzed by the enzyme **carbonic anhydrase,** which is present in most cells. In turn, H_2CO_3 dissociates into H^+ and HCO_3^-. Both reactions are reversible, and carbonic anhydrase catalyzes both the hydration of CO_2 and the dehydration of H_2CO_3. Thus,

$$CO_2 + H_2O \underset{\textit{Carbonic anhydrase}}{\longleftrightarrow} H_2CO_3 \leftrightarrow H^+ + HCO_3^-$$

In the **tissues,** CO_2 generated from aerobic metabolism is added to systemic capillary blood, converted to HCO_3^- by the reactions described previously, and transported to the lungs. In the lungs, HCO_3^- is reconverted to CO_2 and expired. Figure 5-25 shows the steps that occur in systemic capillaries. The circled numbers shown in the figure correspond to the following steps:

1. In the tissues, **CO_2** is produced from aerobic metabolism. CO_2 then diffuses across the cell membranes and across the capillary wall, into the red blood cells. The transport of CO_2 across each of these membranes occurs by simple diffusion, driven by the partial pressure gradient for CO_2.

2. **Carbonic anhydrase** is found in high concentration in red blood cells. It catalyzes the hydration of CO_2 to form **H_2CO_3.** In red blood cells, the reactions are driven to the right by mass action because CO_2 is being supplied from the tissue.

3. In the red blood cells, H_2CO_3 dissociates into **H^+** and **HCO_3^-.** The H^+ remains in the red blood cells, where it will be buffered by deoxyhemoglobin, and the

HCO_3^- is transported into the plasma in exchange for Cl^- (chloride).

4. If the H^+ produced from these reactions remained free in solution, it would acidify the red blood cells and the venous blood. Therefore, H^+ must be buffered so that the pH of the red blood cells (and the blood) remains within the physiologic range. The **H^+ is buffered** in the red blood cells by **deoxyhemoglobin** and is carried in the venous blood in this form. Interestingly, deoxyhemoglobin is a better buffer for H^+ than oxyhemoglobin: By the time blood reaches the venous end of the capillaries, hemoglobin is conveniently in its deoxygenated form (i.e., it has released its O_2 to the tissues).

There is a useful reciprocal relationship between the buffering of H^+ by deoxyhemoglobin and the Bohr effect. The Bohr effect states that an increased H^+ concentration causes a right shift of the O_2-hemoglobin dissociation curve, which causes hemoglobin to unload O_2 more readily in the tissues; thus, the H^+ generated from tissue CO_2 causes hemoglobin to release O_2 more readily to the tissues. In turn, deoxygenation of hemoglobin makes it a better buffer for H^+.

5. The HCO_3^- produced from these reactions is exchanged for Cl^- across the red blood cell membrane (to maintain charge balance), and the HCO_3^- is carried to the lungs in the plasma of venous blood. **Cl^--HCO_3^- exchange,** or the Cl^- shift, is accomplished by an anion exchange protein called **band three protein** (so called because of its prominence in an electrophoretic profile of blood).

All of the reactions previously described occur in reverse in the **lungs** (not shown in Fig. 5-25). H^+ is released from its buffering sites on deoxyhemoglobin, HCO_3^- enters the red blood cells in exchange for Cl^-, H^+ and HCO_3^- combine to form H_2CO_3, and H_2CO_3 dissociates into CO_2 and H_2O. The regenerated CO_2 and H_2O are expired by the lungs.

VENTILATION/PERFUSION RELATIONSHIPS

Pulmonary Blood Flow

Pulmonary Blood Flow, Pressure, and Resistance Relationships

Pulmonary blood flow is the cardiac output of the right heart, which is equal to the cardiac output of the left heart. The difference is a result of a small amount of coronary venous blood that drains directly into the left ventricle through the thebesian vein (rather than going to the lungs via the pulmonary artery).

Pulmonary blood flow is directly proportional to the pressure gradient between the pulmonary artery and the left atrium and is inversely proportional to the resistance of the pulmonary vasculature ($Q = \Delta P/R$). When compared with the systemic circulation, however, the pulmonary circulation is characterized by *much lower* pressures and resistances, although blood flow is the same. The reason that pulmonary blood flow can be equal to systemic blood flow is that pulmonary pressures and resistances are *proportionately* lower than systemic pressures and resistances (see Chapter 4, Table 4-1).

Regulation of Pulmonary Blood Flow

As in other vascular beds, pulmonary blood flow is regulated primarily by altering the resistance of the arterioles. Such changes in resistance are accomplished by changes in the tone of arteriolar smooth muscle; in the pulmonary circulation, these changes are mediated by local vasoactive substances, especially O_2.

♦ **Hypoxic vasoconstriction.** By far, the major factor regulating pulmonary blood flow is the partial pressure of O_2 in alveolar gas, **$P_{A_{O_2}}$**. Decreases in $P_{A_{O_2}}$ produce pulmonary vasoconstriction (i.e., hypoxic vasoconstriction). Initially, this effect may seem counterintuitive because in several vascular beds decreases in P_{O_2} produce the exact opposite effect, vasodilation (to increase O_2 delivery to the tissue). In the lungs, however, hypoxic *vasoconstriction* occurs as an adaptive mechanism, reducing pulmonary blood flow to poorly ventilated areas where the blood flow would be "wasted." Thus, pulmonary blood flow is directed *away from* poorly ventilated regions of the lung, where gas exchange would be inadequate, and *toward* well-ventilated regions of the lung, where gas exchange will be better.

In certain types of lung disease, hypoxic vasoconstriction serves a protective role because, within limits, blood can be redirected to alveoli that are well oxygenated without changing overall pulmonary vascular resistance. The compensatory mechanism fails, however, if the lung disease is widespread (e.g., multilobar pneumonia); if there are insufficient areas of well-ventilated alveoli, hypoxemia will occur.

The **mechanism of hypoxic vasoconstriction** involves a *direct action of alveolar P_{O_2}* on the vascular smooth muscle of pulmonary arterioles. This action can be understood by recalling the proximity of the alveoli to the pulmonary microcirculation. The arterioles and their capillary beds densely surround the alveoli. O_2 is highly lipid soluble and, therefore, is quite permeable across cell membranes. When $P_{A_{O_2}}$ is normal (at 100 mm Hg), O_2 diffuses from the alveoli into the nearby arteriolar smooth muscle cells, keeping the arterioles relatively relaxed and dilated. If $P_{A_{O_2}}$ is reduced to values between 100 mm Hg and 70 mm Hg, vascular tone is minimally affected. However, if $P_{A_{O_2}}$ is reduced below 70 mm Hg, the vascular smooth muscle cells sense this hypoxia, vasoconstrict, and reduce pulmonary blood flow in that region. The mechanism whereby alveolar hypoxia causes contraction of nearby vascular smooth muscle is not precisely understood. It is believed that hypoxia causes depolarization of vascular smooth muscle cells; depolarization opens voltage-gated Ca^{2+} channels, leading to Ca^{2+} entry into the cell and contraction.

There is also evidence of a relationship between hypoxic vasoconstriction and **nitric oxide** (**NO**) synthesis in the endothelial cells of the pulmonary vasculature. Recall that NO is an endothelial-derived relaxing factor that is synthesized from L-arginine by the action of nitric oxide synthase. NO then activates guanylyl cyclase, leading to production of cyclic guanosine monophosphate (cGMP) and relaxation of vascular smooth muscle. Inhibition of nitric oxide synthase enhances hypoxic vasoconstriction, and inhaled NO reduces, or offsets, hypoxic vasoconstriction.

As described previously, hypoxic vasoconstriction can function locally to redirect blood flow to well-ventilated regions of the lung. It also can operate globally in an entire lung, in which case the vasoconstriction will produce an increase in pulmonary vascular resistance. For example, at **high altitude** or in persons breathing a low O_2 mixture, $P_{A_{O_2}}$ is reduced throughout the lungs, not just in one region. The low $P_{A_{O_2}}$ produces global vasoconstriction of pulmonary arterioles and an increase in pulmonary vascular resistance. In response to the increase in resistance, pulmonary arterial pressure increases. In chronic hypoxia, the increased pulmonary arterial pressure causes hypertrophy of the right ventricle, which must pump against an increased afterload.

Fetal circulation is another example of global hypoxic vasoconstriction. Because the fetus does not breathe, $P_{A_{O_2}}$ is much lower in the fetus than in the mother, producing vasoconstriction in the fetal lungs. This vasoconstriction increases pulmonary vascular resistance and, accordingly, decreases pulmonary blood flow to approximately 15% of the cardiac output. At birth, the neonate's first breath increases $P_{A_{O_2}}$ to 100 mm Hg, hypoxic vasoconstriction is reduced, pulmonary vascular resistance decreases, and pulmonary blood flow increases and eventually equals cardiac output of the left side of the heart (as in the adult).

♦ **Other vasoactive substances.** In addition to O_2, several other substances alter pulmonary vascular resistance. **Thromboxane A$_2$**, a product of arachidonic acid metabolism (via the cyclooxygenase pathway) in macrophages, leukocytes, and endothelial cells, is produced in response to certain types of lung injury. Thromboxane A$_2$ is a powerful local vasoconstrictor of both arterioles and veins. **Prostacyclin (prostaglandin I$_2$),** also a product of arachidonic acid metabolism via the cyclooxygenase pathway, is a potent local vasodilator. It is produced by lung endothelial cells. The **leukotrienes,** another product of arachidonic acid metabolism (via the lipoxygenase pathway), cause *airway* constriction.

Distribution of Pulmonary Blood Flow

The distribution of pulmonary blood flow within the lung is *uneven* and the distribution can be explained by the effects of **gravity.** When a person is supine, blood flow is nearly uniform because the entire lung is at the same gravitational level. However, when a person is upright, gravitational effects are not uniform and blood flow is lowest at the apex of the lung (zone 1) and highest at the base of the lung (zone 3). (Gravitational effects increase pulmonary arterial hydrostatic pressure more at the base of the lung than at the apex.)

In Figure 5-26, the pattern of blood flow in the three zones of the lungs is illustrated in a person who is standing. The pressures responsible for driving blood flow in each zone also are shown in the figure. For the following discussion, recall that pressures in the pulmonary vasculature are much lower than in the systemic vasculature.

♦ **Zone 1.** As a result of the gravitational effect, arterial pressure (Pa) at the apex of the lung may be lower than alveolar pressure (P$_A$), which is approximately equal to atmospheric pressure. If Pa is lower than P$_A$, the pulmonary capillaries will be compressed by the higher alveolar pressure outside of them. This compression will cause the capillaries to close, reducing regional blood flow. Normally, in zone 1, arterial pressure is *just high enough* to prevent this closure, and zone 1 is perfused, albeit at a low flow rate.

However, if arterial pressure is decreased (e.g., due to **hemorrhage**) or if alveolar pressure is increased (e.g., by **positive pressure breathing**), then P$_A$ will be greater than Pa and the blood vessels will be compressed and will close. Under these conditions, zone 1 will be ventilated but not perfused. There can be no gas exchange if there is no perfusion, and zone 1 will become part of the physiologic dead space.

♦ **Zone 2.** Because of the gravitational effect on hydrostatic pressure, Pa is higher in zone 2 than in zone 1 and higher than P$_A$. Alveolar pressure is still higher than pulmonary venous pressure (P$_V$),

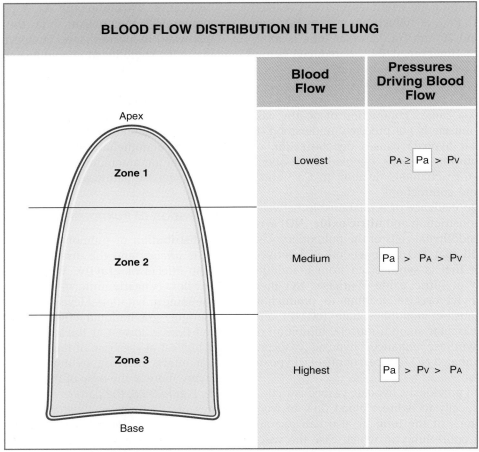

BLOOD FLOW DISTRIBUTION IN THE LUNG

	Blood Flow	Pressures Driving Blood Flow
Zone 1 (Apex)	Lowest	$P_A \geq P_a > P_v$
Zone 2	Medium	$P_a > P_A > P_v$
Zone 3 (Base)	Highest	$P_a > P_v > P_A$

Figure 5–26 **Variation of blood flow (perfusion) in the three zones of the lung.** P_A, Alveolar pressure; P_a, arterial pressure; P_v, venous pressure.

however. Although compression of the capillaries does not present a problem in zone 2, blood flow is driven by the difference between arterial and alveolar pressure, not by the difference between arterial and venous pressure (as it is in systemic vascular beds).

♦ **Zone 3.** In zone 3, the pattern is more familiar. The gravitational effect has increased arterial and venous pressures, and both are now higher than alveolar pressure. Blood flow in zone 3 is driven by the difference between arterial pressure and venous pressure, as it is in other vascular beds. In zone 3, the greatest number of capillaries is open and blood flow is highest.

Shunts

A shunt refers to a portion of the cardiac output or blood flow that is diverted or rerouted. For example, normally, a small fraction of the pulmonary blood flow bypasses the alveoli (e.g., bronchial blood flow), which is called a physiologic shunt. Several abnormal situations also may occur when there is shunting of blood between the right and left hearts through septal defects. Of these defects, left-to-right shunts are more common.

♦ **Physiologic shunt.** About 2% of the cardiac output normally bypasses the alveoli—there is a physiologic right-to-left shunt. Part of the physiologic shunt is the bronchial blood flow, which serves the metabolic functions of the bronchi. The other component of the shunt is the small amount of coronary blood flow that drains directly into the left ventricle through the thebesian veins and never perfuses the lungs. Small physiologic shunts are always present, and Pa_{O_2} will always be slightly less than PA_{O_2}.

♦ **Right-to-left shunts.** Shunting of blood from the right heart to the left heart can occur if there is a defect in the wall between the right and left ventricles. As much as 50% of the cardiac output can be routed from the right ventricle directly to the left ventricle and never be pumped to the lungs for arterialization. In a right-to-left shunt, **hypoxemia *always* occurs** because a significant fraction of the cardiac output is not delivered to the lungs for oxygenation. The portion of the cardiac output that is

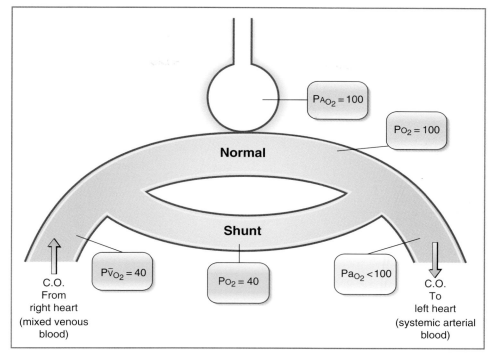

Figure 5–27 **Right-to-left shunt.** C.O., Cardiac output.

delivered to the lungs for oxygenation is "diluted" by the low O_2 shunted blood (Fig. 5-27).

A defining characteristic of the hypoxemia caused by a right-to-left shunt is that it *cannot be corrected by having the person breathe a high O_2 gas* (e.g., 100% O_2) because the shunted blood never goes to the lungs to be oxygenated. The shunted blood will continue to dilute the normally oxygenated blood, and no matter how high the alveolar Po_2, it cannot offset this dilutional effect. (Furthermore, because hemoglobin saturation is nearly 100% in this range, breathing 100% O_2 adds primarily dissolved O_2 to pulmonary capillary blood and adds little to the total O_2 content of blood.) However, having a person with a right-to-left shunt breathe 100% O_2 is a useful diagnostic tool; the magnitude of the shunt can be estimated from the extent of dilution of the oxygenated blood.

Usually, a right-to-left shunt does not cause an appreciable increase in Pa_{CO_2} (although it may seem that it should because of the high CO_2 content of the shunted blood). Pa_{CO_2} changes only minimally because the central chemoreceptors are sensitive to changes in Pa_{CO_2}. Thus, a small increase in Pa_{CO_2} produces an increase in ventilation rate, and the extra CO_2 is expired. Chemoreceptors for O_2 are not as sensitive as those for CO_2 and are not activated until the Pa_{O_2} decreases to less than 60 mm Hg.

The blood flow through a right-to-left shunt can be calculated with the shunt fraction equation, where flow through the shunt is expressed as a fraction of pulmonary blood flow, or cardiac output, as follows:

$$\frac{Q_s}{Q_T} = \frac{O_2 \text{ content ("normal" blood)} - O_2 \text{ content (arterial blood)}}{O_2 \text{ content ("normal" blood)} - O_2 \text{ content (mixed venous blood)}}$$

where

$$Q_s = \text{blood flow through}$$
$$\text{right-to-left shunt (L/min)}$$
$$Q_T = \text{cardiac output (L/min)}$$

$$\frac{O_2 \text{ content}}{\text{("normal" blood)}} = \frac{O_2 \text{ content of nonshunted}}{\text{blood}}$$

$$\frac{O_2 \text{ content}}{\text{(arterial blood)}} = \frac{O_2 \text{ content of systemic}}{\text{arterial blood}}$$

$$\frac{O_2 \text{ content (mixed}}{\text{venous blood)}} = \frac{O_2 \text{ content of mixed venous}}{\text{blood}}$$

♦ **Left-to-right shunts.** Left-to-right shunts are more common and *do not* **cause hypoxemia.** Among the causes of left-to-right shunts are **patent ductus arteriosus** and **traumatic injury.** If blood is shunted from the left side of the heart to the right side of the heart, pulmonary blood flow (right-heart cardiac output) becomes higher than systemic blood flow (left-heart cardiac output). In effect, oxygenated blood that has just returned from the lungs is added

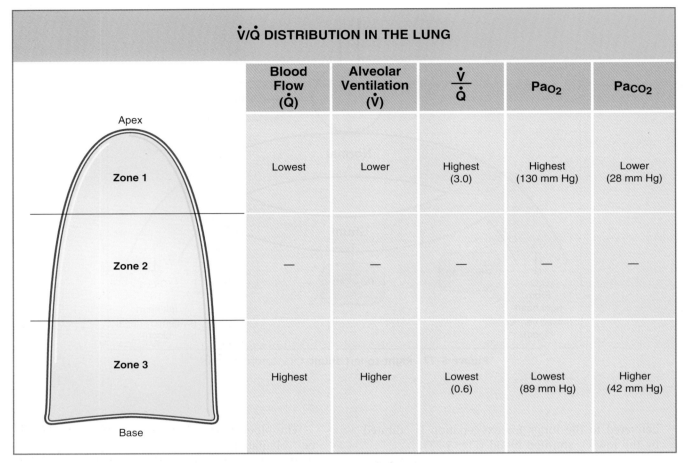

V̇/Q̇ DISTRIBUTION IN THE LUNG

	Blood Flow (Q̇)	Alveolar Ventilation (V̇)	$\frac{\dot{V}}{\dot{Q}}$	Pa$_{O_2}$	Pa$_{CO_2}$
Zone 1	Lowest	Lower	Highest (3.0)	Highest (130 mm Hg)	Lower (28 mm Hg)
Zone 2	—	—	—	—	—
Zone 3	Highest	Higher	Lowest (0.6)	Lowest (89 mm Hg)	Higher (42 mm Hg)

Figure 5–28 **Variation in ventilation/perfusion (V̇/Q̇) in the three zones of the lung.** The effects of regional differences in V̇/Q̇ on Pa$_{O_2}$ and Pa$_{CO_2}$ also are shown.

directly to the right heart without being delivered to the systemic tissues. Because the right side of the heart normally receives mixed venous blood, the P$_{O_2}$ in blood on the right side of the heart will be elevated.

Ventilation/Perfusion Ratios

The ventilation/perfusion ratio (V̇/Q̇) is the ratio of alveolar ventilation (V̇$_A$) to pulmonary blood flow (Q̇). Matching ventilation to perfusion is critically important for ideal gas exchange: It is useless for alveoli to be ventilated but not perfused, or for alveoli to be perfused but not ventilated.

Normal Value for (V̇/Q̇)

The **normal value** for V̇/Q̇ is **0.8.** This value means that alveolar ventilation (L/min) is 80% of the value for pulmonary blood flow (L/min). The term "normal" means that if breathing frequency, tidal volume, and cardiac output all are normal, V̇/Q̇ will be 0.8. In turn, if V̇/Q̇ is normal, then Pa$_{O_2}$ will be its normal value of 100 mm Hg and Pa$_{CO_2}$ will be its normal value of

40 mm Hg. If V̇/Q̇ changes due to an alteration of alveolar ventilation or an alteration of pulmonary blood flow, or both, then gas exchange will be less than ideal and the values for Pa$_{O_2}$ and Pa$_{CO_2}$ will change.

Distribution of V̇/Q̇ in the Lung

The value of 0.8 for V̇/Q̇ is an *average* for the entire lung. In fact, in the three zones of the lung, **V̇/Q̇ is uneven,** just as blood flow is uneven. These variations in V̇/Q̇ have consequences for Pa$_{O_2}$ and Pa$_{CO_2}$ in blood leaving those zones, as illustrated in Figure 5-28. As already described, regional variations in pulmonary blood flow are caused by gravitational effects: Zone 1 has the lowest blood flow, and zone 3 the highest. Alveolar ventilation also varies in the same direction among the zones of the lung. Ventilation is lower in zone 1 and higher in zone 3, again due to gravitational effects in the upright lung. To visualize how gravity produces differences in regional ventilation, imagine the lung as an accordion that is hung vertically. Between breaths (i.e., at FRC), the weight of the accordion

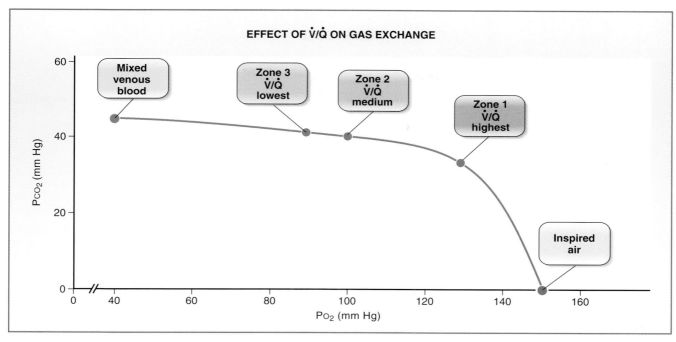

Figure 5-29 **Effect of regional differences in ventilation/perfusion ($\dot{V}/\dot{Q}$) on P_{CO_2} and P_{O_2}.** Regional differences in P_{O_2} are much greater than the regional differences in P_{CO_2}.

(lung) squeezes air out of the bellows at the base and most of the FRC fills the bellows at the apex. When the next breath is taken, most of the *potential* space to be ventilated is at the base of the lung, while the apex is already full. However, *regional variations in ventilation are not as great as regional variations in blood flow.* Therefore, the < $\dot{V}/\dot{Q}$ **ratio is highest in zone 1** and **lowest in zone 3,** with the average value for the entire lung being 0.8.

These regional differences in $\dot{V}/\dot{Q}$ produce regional differences in Pa_{O_2} and Pa_{CO_2}. The O_2-CO_2 diagram derived from the alveolar gas equation (see Fig. 5-5) is repeated in Figure 5-29. Notice that the regional differences in Pa_{O_2} are *much greater* than regional differences in Pa_{CO_2}. In zone 1, where $\dot{V}/\dot{Q}$ is highest, Pa_{O_2} is highest and Pa_{CO_2} is lowest. In zone 3, where $\dot{V}/\dot{Q}$ is lowest, Pa_{O_2} is lowest and Pa_{CO_2} is highest. These regional differences are present in healthy lungs, and the blood leaving the lungs via the pulmonary vein (representing the sum of blood from all zones) has an average Pa_{O_2} of 100 mm Hg and an average Pa_{CO_2} of 40 mm Hg.

Ventilation/Perfusion Defects

Normally, as previously described, there is ventilation/perfusion matching: Ventilated alveoli are close to perfused capillaries, and this arrangement provides for ideal gas exchange. Although there are regional variations in the $\dot{V}/\dot{Q}$ ratio, the average value for the lung is about 0.8.

A mismatch of ventilation and perfusion, called $\dot{V}/\dot{Q}$ **mismatch,** or $\dot{V}/\dot{Q}$ **defect,** results in abnormal gas exchange. A $\dot{V}/\dot{Q}$ defect can be caused by ventilation of lung regions that are not perfused (dead space), perfusion of lung regions that are not ventilated (shunt), and every possibility in between (Figs. 5-30 and 5-31). In some lung diseases, the entire range of possible $\dot{V}/\dot{Q}$ defects is exhibited.

♦ **Dead space ($\dot{V}/\dot{Q} = \infty$).** Dead space is ventilation of lung regions that are not perfused. This ventilation is wasted, or "dead." No gas exchange is possible in dead space because there is no blood flow to receive O_2 from alveolar gas or add CO_2 to alveolar gas. Dead space is illustrated by **pulmonary embolism,** in which blood flow to a portion of the lung (or even the entire lung) is occluded. In regions of dead space, because no gas exchange occurs, alveolar gas has the same composition as humidified inspired air: PA_{O_2} is 150 mm Hg and PA_{CO_2} is 0.

♦ **High $\dot{V}/\dot{Q}$.** Regions of high $\dot{V}/\dot{Q}$ have high ventilation relative to perfusion, usually because blood flow is decreased. Unlike dead space, which has *no* perfusion, high $\dot{V}/\dot{Q}$ regions have *some* blood flow. Because ventilation is high relative to perfusion, pulmonary capillary blood from these regions has a high P_{O_2} and a low P_{CO_2}.

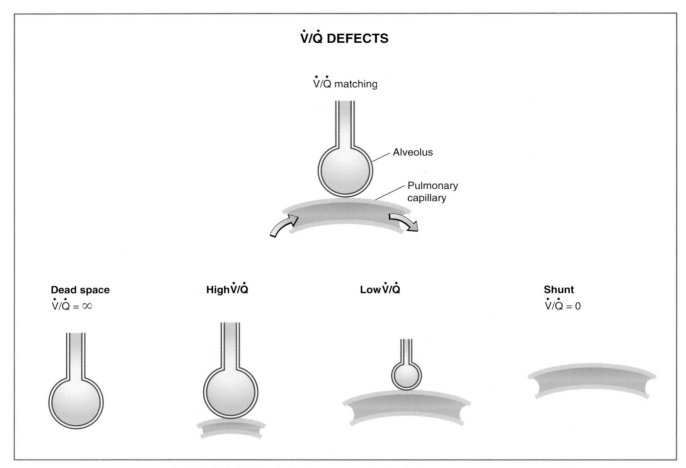

Figure 5–30   Ventilation-perfusion ($\dot{V}/\dot{Q}$) defects. $\dot{V}/\dot{Q}$ defects include dead space, high $\dot{V}/\dot{Q}$, low $\dot{V}/\dot{Q}$, and shunt.

♦ **Low $\dot{V}/\dot{Q}$.** Regions of low $\dot{V}/\dot{Q}$ have low ventilation relative to perfusion, usually because ventilation is decreased. Unlike shunt, which has *no* ventilation, low $\dot{V}/\dot{Q}$ regions have *some* ventilation. Because ventilation is low relative to perfusion, pulmonary capillary blood from these regions has a low P_{O_2} and high P_{CO_2}.

♦ **Shunt ($\dot{V}/\dot{Q} = 0$).** Right-to-left shunt is perfusion of lung regions that are not ventilated. No gas exchange is possible in regions of shunt because there is no ventilation to deliver O_2 to the blood or carry away CO_2 from the blood. Shunt is illustrated by **airway obstruction** and **right-to-left cardiac shunts.** Because no gas exchange can occur with a shunt, pulmonary capillary blood from these regions has the same composition as mixed venous blood: Pa_{O_2} is 40 mm Hg, and Pa_{CO_2} is 46 mm Hg.

CONTROL OF BREATHING

The volume of air inspired and expired per unit time is tightly controlled, both with respect to frequency of breaths and to tidal volume. Breathing is regulated so that the lungs can maintain the Pa_{O_2} and Pa_{CO_2} within the normal range, even under widely varying conditions such as exercise.

Breathing is controlled by centers in the brain stem. There are four components to this control system: (1) chemoreceptors for O_2 or CO_2; (2) mechanoreceptors in the lungs and joints; (3) control centers for breathing in the brain stem (medulla and pons); (4) respiratory muscles, whose activity is directed by the brain stem centers (Fig. 5-32). Voluntary control can also be exerted by commands from the cerebral cortex (e.g., breath-holding or voluntary hyperventilation), which can temporarily override the brain stem.

Brain Stem Control of Breathing

Breathing is an involuntary process that is controlled by the medulla and pons of the brain stem. The frequency of normal, involuntary breathing is controlled by three groups of neurons or **brain stem centers:** the medullary respiratory center, the apneustic center, and the pneumotaxic center.

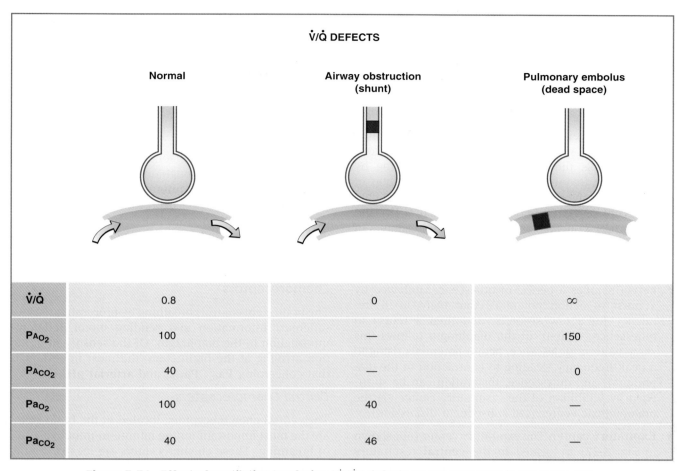

Figure 5–31 **Effect of ventilation/perfusion (V̇/Q̇) defects on gas exchange in the lungs.** With airway obstruction, the composition of systemic arterial blood approaches that of mixed venous blood. With pulmonary embolus, the composition of alveolar air approaches that of inspired air.

V̇/Q̇ DEFECTS

	Normal	Airway obstruction (shunt)	Pulmonary embolus (dead space)
V̇/Q̇	0.8	0	∞
$P_{A_{O_2}}$	100	—	150
$P_{A_{CO_2}}$	40	—	0
$P_{a_{O_2}}$	100	40	—
$P_{a_{CO_2}}$	40	46	—

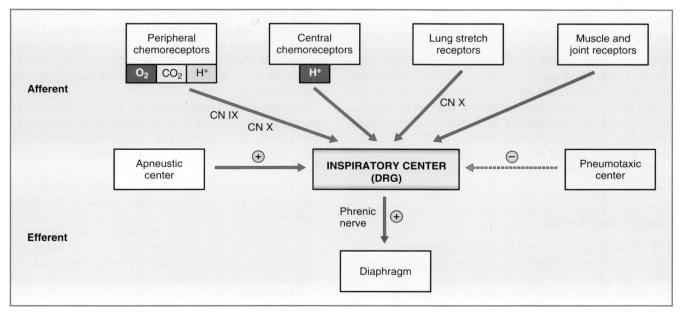

Figure 5–32 **Brain stem control of breathing.** Afferent (sensory) information reaches the medullary inspiratory center via central and peripheral chemoreceptors and mechanoreceptors. Efferent (motor) information is sent from the inspiratory center to the phrenic nerve, which innervates the diaphragm. CN, Cranial nerve; DRG, dorsal respiratory group.

Medullary Respiratory Center

The medullary respiratory center is located in the reticular formation and is composed of two groups of neurons that are distinguished by their anatomic location: the **inspiratory center** (dorsal respiratory group) and the **expiratory center** (ventral respiratory group).

♦ **Inspiratory center.** The inspiratory center is located in the **dorsal respiratory group** (**DRG**) of neurons and controls the **basic rhythm** for breathing by setting the frequency of inspiration. This group of neurons receives sensory input from peripheral chemoreceptors via the glossopharyngeal (CN IX) and vagus (CN X) nerves and from mechanoreceptors in the lung via the vagus nerve. The inspiratory center sends its motor output to the diaphragm via the **phrenic nerve.** The pattern of activity in the phrenic nerve includes a period of quiescence, followed by a burst of action potentials that increase in frequency for a few seconds, and then a return to quiescence. Activity in the diaphragm follows this same pattern: quiescence, action potentials rising to a peak frequency (leading to contraction of the diaphragm), and quiescence. Inspiration can be shortened by inhibition of the inspiratory center via the pneumotaxic center (see subsequent discussion).

♦ **Expiratory center.** The expiratory center (not shown in Fig. 5-32) is located in the **ventral** respiratory neurons and is responsible primarily for expiration. Because expiration is normally a passive process, these neurons are inactive during quiet breathing. However, during exercise when expiration becomes active, this center is activated.

Apneustic Center

Apneusis is an abnormal breathing pattern with prolonged **inspiratory gasps,** followed by brief expiratory movement. Stimulation of the apneustic center in the **lower pons** produces this breathing pattern in experimental subjects. Stimulation of these neurons apparently excites the inspiratory center in the medulla, prolonging the period of action potentials in the phrenic nerve, and thereby prolonging the contraction of the diaphragm.

Pneumotaxic Center

The pneumotaxic center **turns off inspiration,** limiting the burst of action potentials in the phrenic nerve. In effect, the pneumotaxic center, located in the **upper pons,** limits the size of the tidal volume, and secondarily, it regulates the respiratory rate. A normal breathing rhythm persists in the absence of this center.

Cerebral Cortex

Commands from the cerebral cortex can temporarily override the automatic brain stem centers. For example, a person can voluntarily **hyperventilate** (i.e., increase breathing frequency and volume). The consequence of hyperventilation is a decrease in Pa_{CO_2}, which causes arterial pH to increase. Hyperventilation is self-limiting, however, because the decrease in Pa_{CO_2} will produce unconsciousness and the person will revert to a normal breathing pattern. Although more difficult, a person may voluntarily **hypoventilate** (i.e., breath-holding). Hypoventilation causes a decrease in Pa_{O_2} and an increase in Pa_{CO_2}, both of which are strong drives for ventilation. A period of prior hyperventilation can prolong the duration of breath-holding.

Chemoreceptors

The brain stem controls breathing by processing sensory (afferent) information and sending motor (efferent) information to the diaphragm. Of the sensory information arriving at the brain stem, the most important is that concerning **Pa_{O_2}**, **Pa_{CO_2}**, and **arterial pH.**

Central Chemoreceptors

The central chemoreceptors, located in the brain stem, are the most important for the minute-to-minute control of breathing. These chemoreceptors are located on the ventral surface of the medulla, near the point of exit of the glossopharyngeal (CN IX) and vagus (CN X) nerves and only a short distance from the DRG in the medulla. Thus, central chemoreceptors *communicate directly* with the inspiratory center.

The brain stem chemoreceptors are exquisitely sensitive to **changes in the pH of cerebrospinal fluid (CSF).** Decreases in the pH of CSF produce increases in breathing rate (hyperventilation), and increases in the pH of CSF produce decreases in breathing rate (hypoventilation).

The medullary chemoreceptors respond directly to changes in the pH of CSF and indirectly to changes in arterial P_{CO_2} (Fig. 5-33). The circled numbers in the figure correspond with the following steps:

1. In the blood, CO_2 combines reversibly with H_2O to form H^+ and HCO_3^- by the familiar reactions. Because the blood-brain barrier is relatively *impermeable* to H^+ and HCO_3^-, these ions are trapped in the vascular compartment and do not enter the brain. CO_2, however, is quite *permeable* across the blood-brain barrier and enters the extracellular fluid of the brain.

2. CO_2 also is permeable across the brain-CSF barrier and enters the CSF.

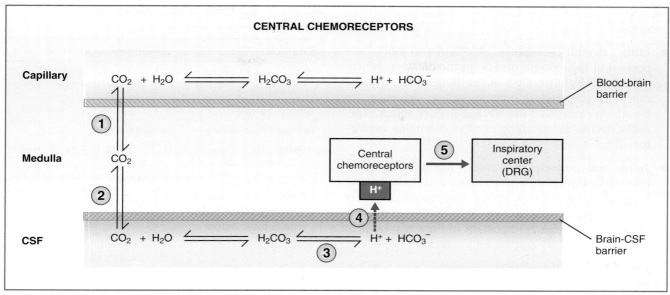

Figure 5–33 **Response of central chemoreceptors to pH.** The circled numbers correspond to the numbered steps discussed in the text. CSF, Cerebrospinal fluid; DRG, dorsal respiratory group.

3. In the CSF, CO_2 is converted to H^+ and HCO_3^-. Thus, increases in arterial P_{CO_2} produce increases in the P_{CO_2} of CSF, which results in an increase in H^+ concentration of CSF (decrease in pH).

4. and 5. The central chemoreceptors are in close proximity to CSF and detect the decrease in pH. A decrease in pH then signals the inspiratory center to increase the breathing rate (hyperventilation).

In summary, the goal of central chemoreceptors is to keep arterial P_{CO_2} within the normal range, if possible. Thus, increases in arterial P_{CO_2} produce increases in P_{CO_2} in the brain and the CSF, which decreases the pH of the CSF. A decrease in CSF pH is detected by central chemoreceptors for H^+, which instruct the DRG to increase the breathing rate. When the breathing rate increases, more CO_2 will be expired and the arterial P_{CO_2} will decrease toward normal.

Peripheral Chemoreceptors

There are peripheral chemoreceptors for **O_2, CO_2, and H^+** in the carotid bodies located at the bifurcation of the common carotid arteries and in the aortic bodies above and below the aortic arch (see Fig. 5-32). Information about arterial P_{O_2}, P_{CO_2}, and pH is relayed to the DRG via CN IX and CN X, which orchestrates an appropriate change in breathing rate.

Each of the following changes in arterial blood composition is detected by peripheral chemoreceptors and produces an **increase in breathing rate:**

♦ **Decreases in arterial P_{O_2}.** The most important responsibility of the peripheral chemoreceptors is to detect changes in arterial P_{O_2}. Surprisingly, however, the peripheral chemoreceptors are relatively insensitive to changes in P_{O_2}: They respond when P_{O_2} decreases to less than 60 mm Hg. Thus, if arterial P_{O_2} is between 100 mm Hg and 60 mm Hg, the breathing rate is virtually constant. However, if arterial P_{O_2} is **less than 60 mm Hg,** the breathing rate increases in a steep and linear fashion. In this range of P_{O_2}, chemoreceptors are exquisitely sensitive to O_2; in fact, they respond so rapidly that the firing rate of the sensory neurons may change during a single breathing cycle.

♦ **Increases in arterial P_{CO_2}.** The peripheral chemoreceptors also detect increases in P_{CO_2}, but the effect is less important than their response to decreases in P_{O_2}. Detection of changes in P_{CO_2} by the peripheral chemoreceptors also is less important than detection of changes in P_{CO_2} by the central chemoreceptors.

♦ **Decreases in arterial pH.** Decreases in arterial pH cause an increase in ventilation, mediated by peripheral chemoreceptors for H^+. This effect is independent of changes in the arterial P_{CO_2} and is mediated *only* by chemoreceptors in the carotid bodies (not by those in the aortic bodies). Thus, in metabolic acidosis, in which there is decreased arterial pH, the peripheral chemoreceptors are stimulated directly to increase the ventilation rate (the respiratory compensation for metabolic acidosis; see Chapter 7).

Other Receptors

In addition to chemoreceptors, several other types of receptors are involved in the control of breathing including lung stretch receptors, joint and muscle receptors, irritant receptors, and juxtacapillary (J) receptors.

◆ **Lung stretch receptors.** Mechanoreceptors are present in the smooth muscle of the airways. When stimulated by distention of the lungs and airways, mechanoreceptors initiate a reflex decrease in breathing rate called the **Hering-Breuer reflex.** The reflex decreases breathing rate by prolonging expiratory time.

◆ **Joint and muscle receptors.** Mechanoreceptors located in the joints and muscles detect the movement of limbs and instruct the inspiratory center to increase the breathing rate. Information from the joints and muscles is important in the early (anticipatory) ventilatory response to exercise.

◆ **Irritant receptors.** Irritant receptors for noxious chemicals and particles are located between epithelial cells lining the airways. Information from these receptors travels to the medulla via CN X and causes a reflex constriction of bronchial smooth muscle and an increase in breathing rate.

◆ **J receptors.** Juxtacapillary (J) receptors are located in the alveolar walls and, therefore, are *near the capillaries.* Engorgement of pulmonary capillaries with blood and increases in interstitial fluid volume may activate these receptors and produce an increase in the breathing rate. For example, in **left-sided heart failure,** blood "backs up" in the pulmonary circulation and J receptors mediate a change in breathing pattern, including rapid shallow breathing and dyspnea (difficulty in breathing).

INTEGRATIVE FUNCTIONS

As in the cardiovascular system, the coordinated functions of the respiratory system are best appreciated through examples. Two examples that illustrate many of the principles presented in this chapter are the responses to exercise and the adaptation to high altitude. A third example, chronic obstructive pulmonary disease, is discussed in Box 5-2.

Responses to Exercise

The response of the respiratory system to exercise is remarkable. As the body's demand for O_2 increases, more O_2 is supplied by increasing the ventilation rate: Excellent matching occurs between O_2 consumption, CO_2 production, and the ventilation rate.

For example, when a trained athlete is exercising, his O_2 consumption may increase from its resting value of 250 mL/min to 4000 mL/min and his ventilation rate may increase from 7.5 L/min to 120 L/min. Both

Table 5–3 Summary of Respiratory Responses to Exercise

Parameter	Response to Exercise
O_2 consumption	↑
CO_2 production	↑
Ventilation rate	↑
Arterial P_{O_2} and P_{CO_2}	No change
Arterial pH	No change during moderate exercise ↓ During strenuous exercise
Venous P_{CO_2}	↑
Pulmonary blood flow and cardiac output	↑
$\dot{V}/\dot{Q}$ ratio	More evenly distributed throughout the lung
Physiologic dead space	↓
O_2-hemoglobin dissociation curve	Shifts to the right; ↑P_{50}; decreased affinity

O_2 consumption and ventilation rate increase more than 15 times the resting level! An interesting question is *What factors ensure that the ventilation rate will match the need for O_2?* At this time, there is no completely satisfactory answer to this question. The responses of the respiratory system to exercise are summarized in Table 5-3 and Figure 5-34.

Arterial P_{O_2} and P_{CO_2}

Remarkably, **mean values for arterial P_{O_2} and P_{CO_2} do not change during exercise.** An increased ventilation rate and increased efficiency of gas exchange ensure that there is neither a decrease in arterial P_{O_2} nor an increase in arterial P_{CO_2}. (The arterial pH may decrease, however, during strenuous exercise because the exercising muscle produces lactic acid.) Recalling that the peripheral and central chemoreceptors respond, respectively, to changes in Pa_{O_2} and Pa_{CO_2}, it is a mystery, therefore, how the ventilation rate can be altered so precisely to meet the increased demand when these parameters seem to remain constant. One hypothesis states that although *mean* values of arterial P_{O_2} and P_{CO_2} do not change, oscillations in their values do occur during the breathing cycle. These oscillatory changes may, via the chemoreceptors, produce such immediate adjustments in ventilation that mean values in arterial blood remain constant.

Venous P_{CO_2}

The P_{CO_2} of mixed venous blood *must* increase during exercise because skeletal muscle is adding more CO_2 than usual to venous blood. However, because mean

BOX 5–2   Clinical Physiology: Chronic Obstructive Pulmonary Disease (COPD)

DESCRIPTION OF CASE. A 65-year-old man has smoked two packs of cigarettes a day for more than 40 years. He has a long history of producing morning sputum, cough, and progressive shortness of breath on exertion (dyspnea). For the past decade, each fall and winter he has had bouts of bronchitis with dyspnea and wheezing, which have gradually worsened over the years. When admitted to the hospital, he is short of breath and cyanotic. He is barrel-chested. His breathing rate is 25 breaths/min, and his tidal volume is 400 mL. His vital capacity is 80% of the normal value for a man his age and size, and FEV_1 is 60% of normal. The following arterial blood values were measured (normal values are in parentheses):

pH, 7.47 (normal, 7.4)

Pa_{O_2}, 60 mm Hg (normal, 100 mm Hg)

Pa_{CO_2}, 30 mm Hg (normal, 40 mm Hg)

Hemoglobin saturation, 90%

Hemoglobin concentration, 14 g/L (normal, 15 g/L)

EXPLANATION OF CASE. The man's history of smoking and bronchitis suggests severe lung disease. Of the arterial blood values, the one most notably abnormal is the Pa_{O_2} of 60 mm Hg. Hemoglobin concentration (14 g/L) is normal, and the percent saturation of hemoglobin of 90% is in the expected range for a Pa_{O_2} of 60 mm Hg (see Fig. 5-20).

The low value for Pa_{O_2} at 60 mm Hg can be explained in terms of a gas exchange defect in the lungs. This defect is best understood by comparing Pa_{O_2} (measured as 60 mm Hg) with PA_{O_2} (calculated with the alveolar gas equation). If the two are equal, then gas exchange is normal and there is no defect. If Pa_{O_2} is less than PA_{O_2} (i.e., there is an A − a difference), then there is a $\dot{V}/\dot{Q}$ defect, with insufficient amounts of O_2 being added to pulmonary capillary blood.

The alveolar gas equation can be used to calculate PA_{O_2}, if the PI_{O_2}, PA_{CO_2}, and respiratory quotient are known. PI_{O_2} is calculated from the barometric pressure (corrected for water vapor pressure) and the percent O_2 in inspired air (21%). PA_{CO_2} is equal to Pa_{CO_2}, which is given. The respiratory quotient is assumed to be 0.8. Thus,

$$
\begin{aligned}
PI_{O_2} &= (P_{atm} - PH_2O) \times FI_{O_2} \\
&= (760 \text{ mm Hg} - 47 \text{ mm Hg}) \times 0.21 \\
&= 150 \text{ mm Hg}
\end{aligned}
$$

$$
\begin{aligned}
PA_{O_2} &= PI_{O_2} - \frac{PA_{CO_2}}{R} \\
&= 150 \text{ mm Hg} - \frac{30 \text{ mm Hg}}{0.8} \\
&= 113 \text{ mm Hg}
\end{aligned}
$$

Because the measured Pa_{O_2} (60 mm Hg) is much less than the calculated PA_{O_2} (113 mm Hg), there must be a mismatch of ventilation and perfusion. Some blood is perfusing alveoli that are not ventilated, thereby diluting the oxygenated blood and reducing arterial P_{O_2}.

The man's Pa_{CO_2} is lower than normal because he is hyperventilating and blowing off more CO_2 than his body is producing. He is hyperventilating because he is hypoxemic. His Pa_{O_2} is just low enough to stimulate peripheral chemoreceptors, which drive the medullary inspiratory center to increase the ventilation rate. His arterial pH is slightly alkaline because his hyperventilation has produced a mild respiratory alkalosis.

The man's FEV_1 is reduced more than his vital capacity; thus, FEV_1/FVC is decreased, which is consistent with an obstructive lung disease in which airway resistance is increased. His barrel-shaped chest is a compensatory mechanism for the increased airway resistance: High lung volumes exert positive traction on the airways and decrease airway resistance; by breathing at a higher lung volume, he can partially offset the increased airway resistance from his disease.

TREATMENT. The man is advised to stop smoking immediately. He is given an antibiotic to treat a suspected infection and an inhalant form of albuterol (a β_2 agonist) to dilate his airways.

---

arterial PCO_2 does not increase, the ventilation rate must increase sufficiently to rid the body of this excess CO_2 (i.e., the "extra" CO_2 is expired by the lungs and never reaches systemic arterial blood).

Muscle and Joint Receptors

Muscle and joint receptors send information to the medullary inspiratory center and participate in the coordinated response to exercise. These receptors are activated early in exercise, and the inspiratory center is commanded to increase the ventilation rate.

Cardiac Output and Pulmonary Blood Flow

Cardiac output increases during exercise to meet the tissues' demand for O_2, as discussed in Chapter 4. Because pulmonary blood flow is the cardiac output of the right heart, **pulmonary blood flow increases.** There is a decrease in pulmonary resistance associated with perfusion of more pulmonary capillary beds, which also improves gas exchange. As a result, pulmonary blood flow becomes more evenly distributed throughout the lungs, and the $\dot{V}/\dot{Q}$ ratio becomes

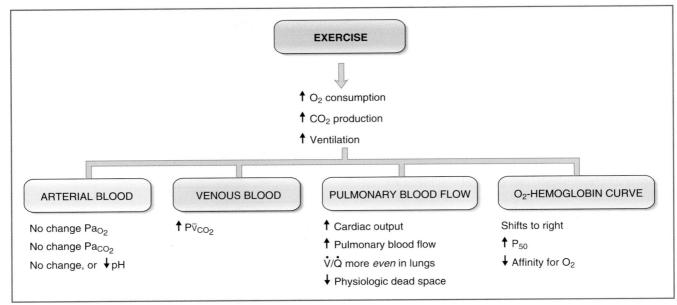

Figure 5-34 **Responses of the respiratory system to exercise.**

more "even," producing a **decrease in the physiologic dead space.**

O₂-Hemoglobin Dissociation Curve

During exercise, the O_2-hemoglobin dissociation curve **shifts to the right** (see Fig. 5-22). There are multiple reasons for this shift including increased tissue P_{CO_2}, decreased tissue pH, and increased temperature. The shift to the right is advantageous, of course, because it is associated with an increase in P_{50} and **decreased affinity** of hemoglobin for O_2, making it easier to unload O_2 in the exercising skeletal muscle.

Adaptation to High Altitude

Ascent to high altitude is one of several causes of **hypoxemia.** The respiratory responses to high altitude are the adaptive adjustments a person must make to the decreased P_{O_2} in inspired and alveolar air.

The decrease in P_{O_2} at high altitudes is explained as follows: At sea level, the barometric pressure is 760 mm Hg; at 18,000 feet above sea level, the barometric pressure is one-half that value, or 380 mm Hg. To calculate the P_{O_2} of humidified inspired air at 18,000 feet above sea level, correct the barometric pressure of dry air by the water vapor pressure of 47 mm Hg, then multiply by the fractional concentration of O_2, which is 21%. Thus, at 18,000 feet, $P_{O_2} = 70$ mm Hg ([380 mm Hg − 47 mm Hg] × 0.21 = 70 mm Hg). A similar calculation for pressures at the peak of Mount Everest yields a P_{O_2} of inspired air of only 47 mm Hg!

Despite severe reductions in the P_{O_2} of both inspired and alveolar air, it is possible to live at high altitudes

Table 5-4 Summary of Adaptive Respiratory Responses to High Altitude

Parameter	Response to High Altitude
Alveolar P_{O_2}	↓ (due to decreased barometric pressure)
Arterial P_{O_2}	↓ (hypoxemia)
Ventilation rate	↑ (hyperventilation due to hypoxemia)
Arterial pH	↑ (respiratory alkalosis due to hyperventilation)
Hemoglobin concentration	↑ (increased red blood cell concentration)
2,3-DPG concentration	↑
O_2-hemoglobin dissociation curve	Shifts to right; increased P_{50}; decreased affinity
Pulmonary vascular resistance	↑ (due to hypoxic vasoconstriction)
Pulmonary arterial pressure	↑ (secondary to increased pulmonary resistance)

if the following adaptive responses occur (Table 5-4 and Fig. 5-35).

Hyperventilation

The most significant response to high altitude is hyperventilation, an increase in ventilation rate. For example, if the alveolar P_{O_2} is 70 mm Hg, then arterial blood,

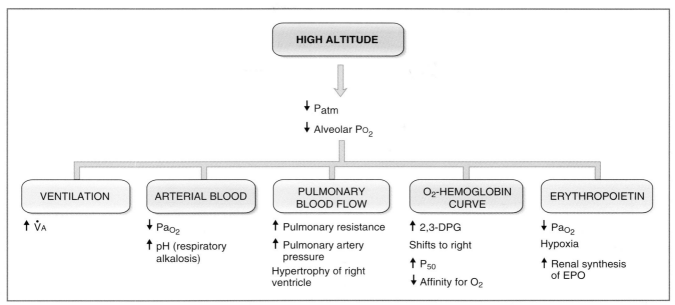

Figure 5-35 **Responses of the respiratory system to high altitude.** EPO, Erythropoietin.

which is almost perfectly equilibrated, also will have a P_{O_2} of 70 mm Hg, which will not stimulate peripheral chemoreceptors. However, if alveolar P_{O_2} is 60 mm Hg, then arterial blood will have a P_{O_2} of 60 mm Hg, in which case the **hypoxemia** is severe enough to stimulate **peripheral chemoreceptors** in the carotid and aortic bodies. In turn, the chemoreceptors instruct the medullary inspiratory center to increase the breathing rate.

A consequence of the hyperventilation is that "extra" CO_2 is expired by the lungs and arterial P_{CO_2} decreases, producing **respiratory alkalosis.** However, the decrease in P_{CO_2} and the resulting increase in pH will inhibit central and peripheral chemoreceptors and offset the increase in ventilation rate. These offsetting effects of CO_2 and pH occur initially, but within several days HCO_3^- excretion increases, HCO_3^- leaves the CSF, and the pH of the CSF decreases toward normal. Thus, within a few days, the offsetting effects are reduced and hyperventilation resumes.

The respiratory alkalosis that occurs as a result of ascent to high altitude can be treated with **carbonic anhydrase inhibitors** (e.g., acetazolamide). These drugs increase HCO_3^- excretion, creating a mild compensatory metabolic acidosis.

Polycythemia

Ascent to high altitude produces an increase in red blood cell concentration (polycythemia) and, as a consequence, an increase in hemoglobin concentration. The increase in hemoglobin concentration means that the O_2-carrying capacity is increased, which increases the total O_2 content of blood in spite of arterial P_{O_2}

being decreased. Polycythemia is advantageous in terms of O_2 transport to the tissues, but it is disadvantageous in terms of blood viscosity. The increased concentration of red blood cells increases blood viscosity, which increases resistance to blood flow (see Chapter 4, the Poiseuille equation).

The stimulus for polycythemia is hypoxia, which increases the synthesis of **erythropoietin (EPO)** in the kidney. Erythropoietin acts on bone marrow to stimulate red blood cell production.

2,3-DPG and O_2-Hemoglobin Dissociation Curve

One of the most interesting features of the body's adaptation to high altitude is an **increased synthesis of 2,3-DPG** by red blood cells. The increased concentration of 2,3-DPG causes the O_2-hemoglobin dissociation curve to **shift to the right.** This right shift is advantageous in the tissues because it is associated with increased P_{50}, decreased affinity, and increased unloading of O_2. However, the right shift is disadvantageous in the lungs because it becomes more difficult to load the pulmonary capillary blood with O_2.

Pulmonary Vasoconstriction

At high altitude, alveolar gas has a low P_{O_2}, which has a direct vasoconstricting effect on the pulmonary vasculature (i.e., **hypoxic vasoconstriction**). As pulmonary vascular resistance increases, pulmonary arterial pressure also must increase to maintain a constant blood flow. The right ventricle must pump against this higher pulmonary arterial pressure and may hypertrophy in response to the increased afterload.

Table 5-5   Causes of Hypoxemia

Cause	Pa_{O_2}	A – a Gradient	Supplemental O_2 Helpful?
High altitude ($\downarrow P_B$; $\downarrow P_{I_{O_2}}$)	Decreased	Normal	Yes
Hypoventilation ($\downarrow PA_{O_2}$)	Decreased	Normal	Yes
Diffusion defect (e.g., fibrosis)	Decreased	Increased	Yes
$\dot{V}/\dot{Q}$ defect	Decreased	Increased	Yes
Right-to-left shunt	Decreased	Increased	Limited

Acute Altitude Sickness

The initial phase of ascent to high altitude is associated with a constellation of complaints including headache, fatigue, dizziness, nausea, palpitations, and insomnia. The symptoms are attributable to the initial hypoxia and respiratory alkalosis, which abate when the adaptive responses are established.

HYPOXEMIA AND HYPOXIA

Hypoxemia is defined as a decrease in arterial P_{O_2}. Hypoxia is defined as a decrease in O_2 delivery to, or utilization by, the tissues. Hypoxemia is one cause of tissue hypoxia, although it is not the only cause.

Hypoxemia

Hypoxemia, a **decrease in arterial P_{O_2},** has multiple causes, which are summarized in Table 5-5.

One useful tool for comparing the various causes of hypoxemia is the A – a gradient, or A – a difference. The **A – a gradient** is the difference between the P_{O_2} of alveolar gas (PA_{O_2}) and the P_{O_2} of systemic arterial blood (Pa_{O_2}). As explained earlier in this chapter, in this context, "A" stands for alveolar P_{O_2} and "a" stands for systemic arterial P_{O_2}.

$$A - a \text{ gradient} = PA_{O_2} - Pa_{O_2}$$

PA_{O_2} is calculated with the alveolar gas equation and substituted as follows:

$$A - a \text{ gradient} = \left(P_{I_{O_2}} - \frac{PA_{CO_2}}{R} \right) - Pa_{O_2}$$

Briefly, the A – a gradient describes whether there has been equilibration of O_2 between alveolar gas and pulmonary capillary blood (which becomes systemic arterial blood). Normally, O_2 equilibrates across the alveolar-pulmonary capillary barrier and the A – a gradient is close to zero. In some but not all causes of hypoxemia, the A – a gradient is increased, or widened, signifying a defect in O_2 equilibration.

♦ **High altitude** causes hypoxemia because barometric pressure (P_B) is decreased, which decreases the P_{O_2} of inspired air ($P_{I_{O_2}}$) and of alveolar air (PA_{O_2}). Equilibration of O_2 across the alveolar/pulmonary capillary barrier is normal, and systemic arterial blood achieves the same (lower) P_{O_2} as alveolar air. Because PA_{O_2} and Pa_{O_2} are nearly equal, the A – a gradient is normal. At high altitude, breathing supplemental O_2 raises arterial P_{O_2} by raising inspired and alveolar P_{O_2}.

♦ **Hypoventilation** causes hypoxemia by decreasing alveolar P_{O_2} (less fresh inspired air is brought into alveoli). Equilibration of O_2 is normal, and systemic arterial blood achieves the same (lower) P_{O_2} as alveolar air. PA_{O_2} and Pa_{O_2} are nearly equal, and the A – a gradient is normal. In hypoventilation, breathing supplemental O_2 raises arterial P_{O_2} by raising the alveolar P_{O_2}.

♦ **Diffusion defects** (e.g., fibrosis, pulmonary edema) cause hypoxemia by increasing diffusion distance or decreasing surface area for diffusion. Equilibration of O_2 is impaired, Pa_{O_2} is less than PA_{O_2}, and the A – a gradient is increased, or widened. With diffusion defects, breathing supplemental O_2 raises arterial P_{O_2} by raising alveolar P_{O_2} and increasing the driving force for O_2 diffusion.

♦ **$\dot{V}/\dot{Q}$ defects** always cause hypoxemia and increased A – a gradient. Recall that $\dot{V}/\dot{Q}$ defects usually present as a constellation of abnormalities that may include regions of dead space, high $\dot{V}/\dot{Q}$, low $\dot{V}/\dot{Q}$ and shunt. Recall also that high $\dot{V}/\dot{Q}$ regions have a high P_{O_2} and low $\dot{V}/\dot{Q}$ regions have a low P_{O_2}. The question may then arise: *In $\dot{V}/\dot{Q}$ defects, why don't regions of high $\dot{V}/\dot{Q}$ compensate for regions of low $\dot{V}/\dot{Q}$ so that the P_{O_2} of blood leaving the lungs is normal?* The answer is that while high $\dot{V}/\dot{Q}$ regions have blood with a high P_{O_2}, blood flow to those regions is low (i.e., high $\dot{V}/\dot{Q}$ ratio) and contributes little to total blood flow. Low $\dot{V}/\dot{Q}$ regions, where P_{O_2} is low, have the highest blood flow and the greatest overall effect on P_{O_2} of blood leaving the lungs. In $\dot{V}/\dot{Q}$ defects, supplemental O_2 can be helpful, primarily because it raises the P_{O_2} of low $\dot{V}/\dot{Q}$ regions where blood flow is highest.

♦ **Right-to-left shunts** (right-to-left cardiac shunts, intrapulmonary shunts) always cause hypoxemia and increased A – a gradient. Shunted blood completely bypasses ventilated alveoli and cannot be oxygenated (see Fig. 5-27). Because shunted blood mixes with, and dilutes, normally oxygenated blood (nonshunted blood), the P_{O_2} of blood leaving the lungs must be lower than normal. Supplemental O_2 has a limited effect in raising the P_{O_2} of systemic arterial blood because it can only raise the P_{O_2} of normal nonshunted blood; the shunted blood continues to have a dilutional effect. Therefore, the ability of supplemental O_2 to raise the P_{O_2} of systemic arterial blood will depend on the size of the shunt: The larger the shunt, the less effective is supplemental O_2.

Another feature of treating right-to-left shunts with supplemental O_2 is that it never corrects the increased A – a gradient; in fact, as supplemental O_2 is administered, the A – a increases or widens because $P_{A_{O_2}}$ increases faster than $P_{a_{O_2}}$ increases.

Hypoxia

Hypoxia is decreased O_2 delivery to the tissues. Because O_2 delivery is the product of cardiac output and O_2 content of blood, hypoxia is caused by decreased cardiac output (blood flow) or decreased O_2 content of blood. Recall that O_2 content of blood is determined primarily by the amount of O_2-hemoglobin. Causes of hypoxia are summarized in Table 5-6.

Table 5–6 Causes of Hypoxia

Cause	Mechanism	Pa_{O_2}
↓ Cardiac output	↓ Blood flow	—
Hypoxemia	↓ Pa_{O_2} ↓ O_2 saturation of hemoglobin ↓ O_2 content of blood	↓
Anemia	↓ Hemoglobin concentration ↓ O_2 content of blood	—
Carbon monoxide poisoning	↓ O_2 content of blood Left shift of O_2-hemoglobin curve	—
Cyanide poisoning	↓ O_2 utilization by tissues	—

A **decrease in cardiac output** and a decrease in regional (local) blood flow are self-evident causes of hypoxia. **Hypoxemia** (due to any cause; see Table 5-5) is a major cause of hypoxia. The reason that hypoxemia causes hypoxia is that a decreased Pa_{O_2} reduces the percent saturation of hemoglobin (see Fig. 5-20). O_2-hemoglobin is the major form of O_2 in blood; thus, a decrease in the amount of O_2-hemoglobin means a decrease in total O_2 content. **Anemia,** or decreased hemoglobin concentration, also decreases the amount of O_2-hemoglobin in blood. **Carbon monoxide (CO) poisoning** causes hypoxia because CO occupies binding sites on hemoglobin that normally are occupied by O_2; thus, CO decreases the O_2 content of blood. **Cyanide poisoning** interferes with O_2 utilization of tissue; it is one cause of hypoxia that does not involve decreased blood flow or decreased O_2 content of blood.

SUMMARY

■ Lung volumes and capacities are measured with a spirometer (except for those volumes and capacities that include the residual volume).

■ Dead space is the volume of the airways and lungs that does not participate in gas exchange. Anatomic dead space is the volume of conducting airways. Physiologic dead space includes the anatomic dead space plus those regions of the respiratory zone that do not participate in gas exchange.

■ The alveolar ventilation equation expresses the inverse relationship between $P_{A_{CO_2}}$ and alveolar ventilation. The alveolar gas equation extends this relationship to predict $P_{A_{O_2}}$.

■ In quiet breathing, respiratory muscles (diaphragm) are used only for inspiration; expiration is passive.

■ Compliance of the lungs and the chest wall is measured as the slope of the pressure-volume relationship. As a result of their elastic forces, the chest wall tends to spring out and the lungs tend to collapse. At FRC, these two forces are exactly balanced and intrapleural pressure is negative. Compliance of the lungs increases in emphysema and with aging. Compliance decreases in fibrosis and when pulmonary surfactant is absent.

■ Surfactant, a mixture of phospholipids produced by type II alveolar cells, reduces surface tension so that the alveoli can remain inflated despite their small radii. Neonatal respiratory distress syndrome occurs when surfactant is absent.

■ Airflow into and out of the lungs is driven by the pressure gradient between the atmosphere and the alveoli and is inversely proportional to the resistance of the airways. Stimulation of β_2-adrenergic receptors dilates the airways, and stimulation of cholinergic muscarinic receptors constricts the airways.

■ Diffusion of O_2 and CO_2 across the alveolar/pulmonary capillary barrier is governed by Fick's law and driven by the partial pressure difference of the gas. Mixed venous blood enters the pulmonary capillaries and is "arterialized" as O_2 is added to it and CO_2 is removed from it. Blood leaving the pulmonary capillaries will become systemic arterial blood.

■ Diffusion-limited gas exchange is illustrated by CO and by O_2 in fibrosis or strenuous exercise. Perfusion-limited gas exchange is illustrated by N_2O, CO_2, and O_2 under normal conditions.

■ O_2 is transported in blood in dissolved form and bound to hemoglobin. One molecule of hemoglobin can bind four molecules of O_2. The sigmoidal shape of the O_2-hemoglobin dissociation curve reflects increased affinity for each successive molecule of O_2 that is bound. Shifts to the right of the O_2-hemoglobin dissociation curve are associated with decreased affinity, increased P_{50}, and increased unloading of O_2 in the tissues. Shifts to the left are associated with increased affinity, decreased P_{50}, and decreased unloading of O_2 in the tissues. CO decreases the O_2-binding capacity of hemoglobin and causes a shift to the left.

■ CO_2 is transported in blood in dissolved form, as carbaminohemoglobin, and as HCO_3^-. HCO_3^- is produced in red blood cells from CO_2 and H_2O, catalyzed by carbonic anhydrase. HCO_3^- is transported in the plasma to the lungs where the reactions occur in reverse to regenerate CO_2, which then is expired.

■ Pulmonary blood flow is the cardiac output of the right heart, and it is equal to the cardiac output of the left heart. Pulmonary blood flow is regulated primarily by PA_{O_2}, with alveolar hypoxia producing vasoconstriction.

■ Pulmonary blood flow is unevenly distributed in the lungs of a person who is standing: Blood flow is lowest at the apex of the lung and highest at the base. Ventilation is similarly distributed, although regional variations in ventilatory rates are not as great as for blood flow. Thus, $\dot{V}/\dot{Q}$ is highest at the apex of the lung and lowest at the base, with an average value of 0.8. Where $\dot{V}/\dot{Q}$ is highest, Pa_{O_2} is highest and Pa_{CO_2} is lowest.

■ $\dot{V}/\dot{Q}$ defects impair gas exchange. If ventilation is decreased relative to perfusion, then Pa_{O_2} and Pa_{CO_2} will approach their values in mixed venous blood. If perfusion is decreased relative to ventilation, then PA_{O_2} and PA_{CO_2} will approach their values in inspired air.

■ Breathing is controlled by the medullary respiratory center, which receives sensory information from central chemoreceptors in the brain stem, from peripheral chemoreceptors in the carotid and aortic bodies, and from mechanoreceptors in the lungs and joints. Central chemoreceptors are sensitive primarily to changes in the pH of CSF, with decreases in pH causing hyperventilation. Peripheral chemoreceptors are sensitive primarily to O_2, with hypoxemia causing hyperventilation.

■ During exercise, the ventilation rate and cardiac output increase to match the body's needs for O_2 so that mean values for Pa_{O_2} and Pa_{CO_2} do not change. The O_2-hemoglobin dissociation curve shifts to the right as a result of increased tissue P_{CO_2}, increased temperature, and decreased tissue pH.

■ At high altitude, hypoxemia results from the decreased P_{O_2} of inspired air. Adaptive responses to hypoxemia include hyperventilation, respiratory alkalosis, pulmonary vasoconstriction, polycythemia, increased 2,3-DPG production, and a right shift of the O_2-hemoglobin dissociation curve.

■ Hypoxemia, or decreased Pa_{O_2}, is caused by high altitude, hypoventilation, diffusion defects, $\dot{V}/\dot{Q}$ defects, and right-to-left shunts. Hypoxia, or decreased O_2 delivery to tissues, is caused by decreased cardiac output or decreased O_2 content of blood.

Challenge Yourself

Answer each question with a word, phrase, sentence, or numerical solution. When a list of possible answers is supplied with the question, one, more than one, or none of the choices may be correct. Correct answers are provided at the end of the book.

1 If tidal volume is 500 mL, inspiratory reserve volume is 3 L, and vital capacity is 5 L, what is expiratory reserve volume?

2 What are the units of FEV_1?

3 Room air is a mixture of O_2 and N_2 saturated with H_2O vapor. If barometric pressure is 740 mm Hg and the fractional concentration of O_2 is 21%, what is the partial pressure of N_2?

4 A person at sea level breathes a mixture containing 0.1% carbon monoxide (CO). The uptake of CO was measured using the single breath method as 28 mL/minute. What is the lung diffusing capacity for CO (DL_{CO})?

5 Which of the following increase(s) hemoglobin P_{50}: increased H^+ concentration, increased pH, increased P_{CO_2}, increased 2,3-diphosphoglycerate (DPG) concentration?

6 Which of the following decrease(s) the O_2-binding capacity of hemoglobin: decreasing hemoglobin concentration, decreasing Pa_{O_2} to 60 mm Hg, increasing arterial P_{O_2} to 120 mm Hg, left-shift of the O_2-hemoglobin dissociation curve?

7 If the ventilation/perfusion ($\dot{V}/\dot{Q}$) ratio of a lung region decreases, how will the P_{O_2} and P_{CO_2} in the blood in that region change?

8 In perfusion-limited O_2 exchange, is the P_{O_2} at the end of the pulmonary capillary closer to PA_{O_2} or $P\bar{V}_{O_2}$?

9 Which of the following is/are higher at the base of the lung than at the apex: blood flow, $\dot{V}/\dot{Q}$, ventilation, P_{O_2}, P_{CO_2}?

10 Which cause(s) of hypoxemia is/are associated with increased A − a gradient: high altitude, hypoventilation, breathing 10% O_2, $\dot{V}/\dot{Q}$ defects, fibrosis, right-to-left shunt?

11 What is the largest lung volume or capacity that can be inspired above FRC?

12 Which of the following is/are decreased in both restrictive and obstructive lung diseases: vital capacity, FEV_1, FEV_1/FVC?

13 If tidal volume = 450 mL, breaths/minute = 14/minute, Pa_{CO_2} = 45 mm Hg, Pa_{O_2} = 55 mm Hg, PA_{O_2} = 100 mm Hg, $P_{E_{CO_2}}$ = 25 mm Hg, and cardiac output = 5 L/minute, what is alveolar ventilation?

14 In persons with emphysema, to balance the collapsing force on the lungs with the expanding force on the chest wall, does functional residual capacity (FRC) increase, decrease, or remain unchanged?

15 Which of the following pairs of pressures would cause the structure to collapse: alveolar pressure = +5 cm H_2O and intrapleural pressure = −5 cm H_2O; airway pressure = 0 and intrapleural pressure = −5 cm H_2O; airway pressure = +15 cm H_2O and intrapleural pressure = +20 cm H_2O?

16 Which cause of hypoxia is corrected best with supplemental O_2: anemia, decreased cardiac output, high altitude, right-to-left shunt?

17 Upon ascent to high altitude, what is the correct sequence of these events: hyperventilation, decreased PA_{O_2}, decreased Pa_{CO_2}, decreased Pa_{O_2}, decreased PI_{O_2}, increased pH?

18 Where am I? For each item in the following list, give its correct location in the respiratory system. (The location may be anatomic, a graph or portion of a graph, an equation, or a concept.)

FEV_1

$\dot{V}/\dot{Q}$ = 0

$PA > P_a$

Afterload of right ventricle

γ chains

P_{50}

Slope of pressure-volume curve

Normally, pressure lower than P_B

DL

P_{O_2} <60 mm Hg stimulates breathing

19 In perfusion-limited gas exchange, P_{O_2} at the end of the pulmonary capillary is: equal to mixed venous P_{O_2}, greater than alveolar P_{O_2}, less than alveolar P_{O_2}, or equal to systemic arterial P_{O_2}?

20 In persons with restrictive lung disease, to balance the collapsing force on the lungs with the expanding force on the chest wall, does functional residual capacity (FRC) increase, decrease, or remain unchanged?

SELECTED READINGS

Slonim NB, Hamilton LH: Respiratory Physiology, 5th ed. St Louis, Mosby, 1987.

West JB: Pulmonary Pathophysiology, 5th ed. Baltimore, Lippincott, Williams & Wilkins, 1998.

West JB: Respiratory Physiology—the Essentials, 6th ed. Baltimore, Williams & Wilkins, 2000.

Renal Physiology

The kidneys function in several capacities. As excretory organs, the kidneys ensure that those substances in excess or that are harmful are excreted in urine in appropriate amounts. As regulatory organs, the kidneys maintain a constant volume and composition of the body fluids by varying the excretion of solutes and water. Finally, as endocrine organs, the kidneys synthesize and secrete three hormones: renin, erythropoietin, and 1,25-dihydroxycholecalciferol.

ANATOMY AND BLOOD SUPPLY

Gross Anatomic Features of the Kidney

The kidneys are bean-shaped organs that lie in the retroperitoneal cavity of the body. In sagittal section, the kidneys have three main regions (Fig. 6-1): (1) The **cortex** is the outer region, located just under the kidney capsule. (2) The **medulla** is a central region, divided into an outer medulla and an inner medulla. The outer medulla has an outer stripe and an inner stripe. (3) The **papilla** is the innermost tip of the inner medulla and empties into pouches called minor and major calyces, which are extensions of the ureter. The urine from each kidney drains into a ureter and is transported to the bladder for storage and subsequent elimination.

Structure of the Nephron

The functional units of the kidney are nephrons. Each kidney contains approximately 1 million nephrons (Fig. 6-2). A nephron consists of a glomerulus and a renal tubule. The glomerulus is a **glomerular capillary network,** which emerges from an afferent arteriole. Glomerular capillaries are surrounded by **Bowman's capsule** (or **Bowman's space**), which is continuous with the first portion of the nephron. Blood is ultrafiltered across the glomerular capillaries into Bowman's space, which is the first step in urine formation. The remainder of the nephron is a tubular structure lined with epithelial cells, which serve the functions of reabsorption and secretion.

The nephron or renal tubule comprises the following segments (beginning with Bowman's space): the proximal convoluted tubule, the proximal straight tubule, the loop of Henle (which contains a thin descending limb, a thin ascending limb, and a thick ascending limb), the distal convoluted tubule, and the collecting ducts. Each segment

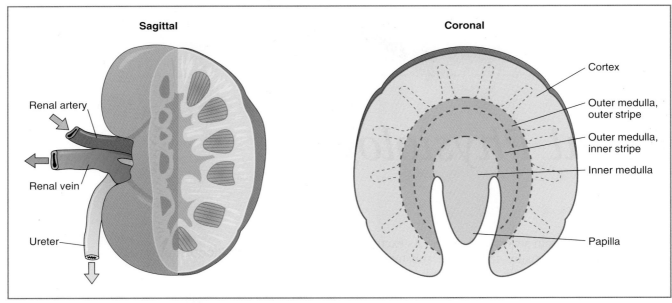

Figure 6–1 Sagittal and coronal sections of the kidney.

of the nephron is functionally distinct, and the epithelial cells lining each segment have a different ultrastructure (Fig. 6-3). For example, the cells of the proximal convoluted tubule are unique in having an extensive development of microvilli, called a brush border, on their luminal side. The brush border provides a large surface area for the major reabsorptive function of the proximal convoluted tubule. Other correlations between cell ultrastructure and function will be emphasized throughout the chapter.

There are two types of nephrons, superficial cortical nephrons and juxtamedullary nephrons, which are distinguished by the location of their glomeruli. The **superficial cortical nephrons** have their glomeruli in the outer cortex. These nephrons have relatively short loops of Henle, which descend only into the outer medulla. The **juxtamedullary nephrons** have their glomeruli near the corticomedullary border. The glomeruli of the juxtamedullary nephrons are larger than those of the superficial cortical nephrons and, accordingly, have higher glomerular filtration rates. The juxtamedullary nephrons are characterized by long loops of Henle that descend deep into the inner medulla and papilla and are essential for the concentration of urine.

Renal Vasculature

Blood enters each kidney via a renal artery, which branches into interlobar arteries, arcuate arteries, and then cortical radial arteries. The smallest arteries subdivide into the *first* set of arterioles, the **afferent arterioles.** The afferent arterioles deliver blood to the *first* capillary network, the **glomerular capillaries,** across

which ultrafiltration occurs. Blood leaves the glomerular capillaries via a *second* set of arterioles, the **efferent arterioles,** which deliver blood to a *second* capillary network, the **peritubular capillaries.** The peritubular capillaries surround the nephrons. Solutes and water are reabsorbed into the peritubular capillaries, and a few solutes are secreted from the peritubular capillaries. Blood from the peritubular capillaries flows into small veins and then into the renal vein.

The blood supply of superficial cortical nephrons differs from that of juxtamedullary nephrons. In the **superficial nephrons,** peritubular capillaries branch off the efferent arterioles and deliver nutrients to the epithelial cells. These capillaries also serve as the blood supply for reabsorption and secretion. In the **juxtamedullary nephrons,** the peritubular capillaries have a specialization called the **vasa recta,** which are long, hairpin-shaped blood vessels that follow the same course as the loop of Henle. The vasa recta serve as osmotic exchangers for the production of concentrated urine.

BODY FLUIDS

Water is the medium of the internal environment and constitutes a large percentage of the body weight. Discussion in this section includes the distribution of water in various compartments of the body; the methods of measuring volumes of the body fluid compartments; the differences in concentrations of major cations and anions among the compartments; and the shifts of water that occur between the body fluid compartments when a physiologic disturbance occurs.

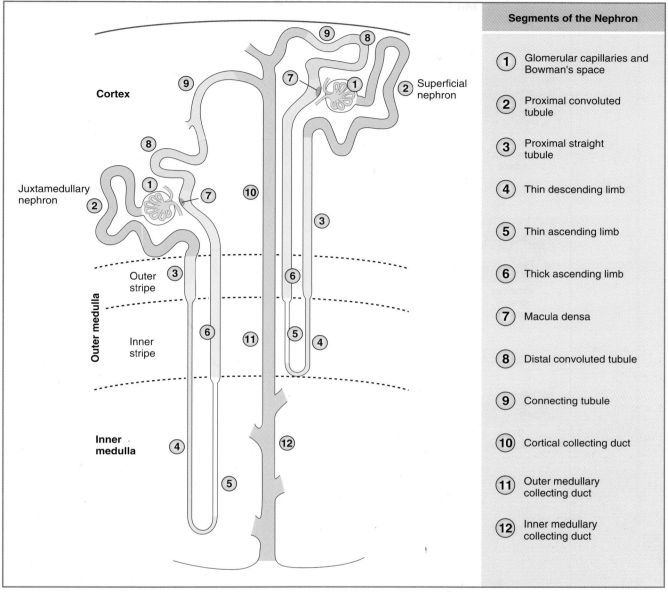

Figure 6–2 **Segments of a superficial and a juxtamedullary nephron.**

Segments of the Nephron

1. Glomerular capillaries and Bowman's space
2. Proximal convoluted tubule
3. Proximal straight tubule
4. Thin descending limb
5. Thin ascending limb
6. Thick ascending limb
7. Macula densa
8. Distal convoluted tubule
9. Connecting tubule
10. Cortical collecting duct
11. Outer medullary collecting duct
12. Inner medullary collecting duct

Distribution of Water among the Body Fluids

Total Body Water

Water accounts for **50% to 70% of body weight,** with an average value of 60% (Fig. 6-4). The percentage of total body water varies, depending on gender and the amount of adipose tissue in the body. Water content of the body correlates inversely with fat content. Women have lower percentages of water than men (because women have the higher percentage of adipose tissue). For these reasons, thin men have the highest percentage of body weight as water ($\approx$70%) and obese women have the lowest percentage ($\approx$50%).

The relationship between water content and body weight is clinically important because changes in body weight can be used to estimate changes in body water content. For example, in the absence of other explanations, a sudden weight loss of 3 kg reflects a loss of 3 kg ($\approx$3 L) of total body water.

The distribution of water among the body fluid compartments is shown in Figure 6-4. Total body water is distributed between two major compartments: **intracellular fluid (ICF)** and **extracellular fluid (ECF).** Approximately two thirds of total body water is in the ICF, and about one third is in the ECF. When expressed as percentage of body weight, 40% of body weight is in ICF (two thirds of 60%), and 20% of body weight is in ECF (one third of 60%). (The **60-40-20 rule** is useful to know: 60% of body weight is water, 40% is ICF, and 20% is ECF.) ECF is further divided among

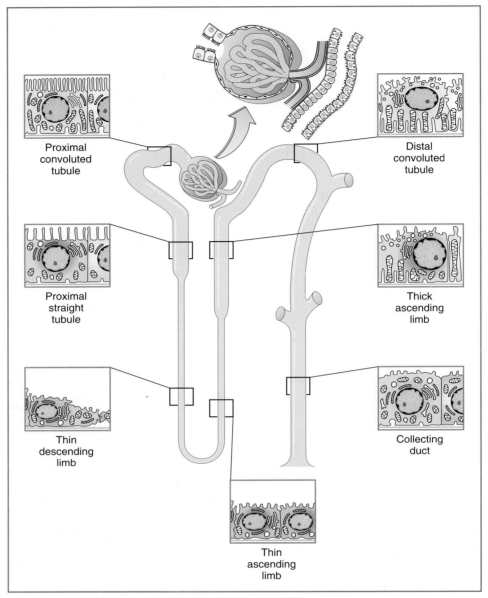

Figure 6–3 Schematic diagram of a nephron. Ultrastructural features are shown for major segments of the nephron.

two minor compartments: the interstitial fluid and the plasma. Approximately three fourths of the ECF is found in the interstitial compartment, and the remaining one fourth is found in the plasma. A third body fluid compartment, the **transcellular compartment** (not shown in Fig. 6-4), is quantitatively small and includes the cerebrospinal, pleural, peritoneal, and digestive fluids.

Intracellular Fluid

ICF is the water inside the cells in which all intracellular solutes are dissolved. It constitutes **two thirds of total body water** or 40% of body weight. The composition of ICF is discussed in Chapter 1. Briefly, the major cations are potassium (K^+) and magnesium (Mg^{2+}), and the major anions are **proteins** and **organic phosphates** such as adenosine triphosphate (ATP), adenosine diphosphate (ADP), and adenosine monophosphate (AMP).

Extracellular Fluid

ECF is the water outside the cells. It constitutes **one third of total body water** or 20% of body weight. ECF is divided among two subcompartments: plasma and interstitial fluid. Plasma is the fluid that circulates in the blood vessels, and interstitial fluid bathes the cells. The composition of ECF differs substantially from ICF: The major cation of ECF is sodium (Na^+), and the major anions are chloride (Cl^-) and bicarbonate (HCO_3^-).

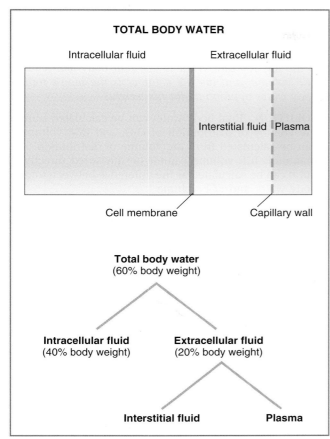

Figure 6–4 **Body fluid compartments**. Total body water is distributed between intracellular fluid and extracellular fluid. Water as a percentage of body weight is indicated for the major compartments.

Plasma is the aqueous component of blood. It is the fluid in which the blood cells are suspended. On a volume basis, plasma constitutes 55% of blood volume and blood cells (i.e., red blood cells, white blood cells, and platelets) constitute the remaining 45% of blood volume. The percent of blood volume occupied by red blood cells is called the **hematocrit,** which averages 0.45 or 45% and is higher in males (0.48) than in females (0.42). **Plasma proteins** constitute about 7% of plasma by volume; thus, only 93% of plasma volume is **plasma water,** a correction that usually is ignored.

Interstitial fluid is an **ultrafiltrate** of plasma: It has nearly the same composition as plasma, excluding plasma proteins and blood cells. To understand why interstitial fluid contains little protein and no blood cells, simply remember that it is formed by filtration across capillary walls (see Chapter 4). Pores in the capillary wall permit free passage of water and small solutes, but these pores are not large enough to permit passage of large protein molecules or cells. There are also small differences in the concentrations of small

cations and anions between interstitial fluid and plasma, explained by the **Gibbs-Donnan effect** of the negatively charged plasma proteins (see Chapter 1). The Gibbs-Donnan effect predicts that plasma will have a slightly higher concentration of small cations (e.g., Na^+) than interstitial fluid and a slightly lower concentration of small anions (e.g., Cl^-).

Measuring Volumes of Body Fluid Compartments

In humans, the volumes of the body fluid compartments are measured by the **dilution method**. The basic principle underlying this method is that a marker substance will be distributed in the body fluid compartments according to its physical characteristics. For example, a large molecular weight sugar such as **mannitol** cannot cross cell membranes and it will be distributed in ECF but not in ICF. Thus, mannitol is a marker for ECF volume. In contrast, **isotopic water** (e.g., D_2O) will be distributed everywhere that water is distributed and it is used as a marker for total body water.

The following steps are used to measure volumes of body fluid compartments by the dilution method:

1. **Identification of an appropriate marker substance.** The markers are selected according to their physical characteristics (Table 6-1). The markers for **total body water** are substances that are distributed wherever water is found. These substances include isotopic water (e.g., D_2O and tritiated water [THO]) and antipyrine, a substance that is lipid soluble. The markers for **ECF volume** are substances that distribute throughout the ECF but do not cross cell membranes. These substances include large molecular weight sugars such as mannitol and inulin and large molecular weight anions such as sulfate. Markers for **plasma volume** are substances that distribute in plasma but not in interstitial fluid, because they are too large to cross capillary walls. These substances include radioactive albumin and Evans blue, a dye that binds to albumin.

   ICF and interstitial fluid volumes cannot be measured directly because there are no unique markers for these compartments. Hence, ICF volume and interstitial fluid volume are determined indirectly. **ICF volume** is the difference between total body water and ECF volume. **Interstitial fluid volume** is the difference between ECF volume and plasma volume.

2. **Injection of a known amount of the marker substance.** The amount of marker substance injected into the blood is measured in milligrams (mg), millimoles (mmol), or units of radioactivity (e.g., millicuries [mCi]).

Table 6–1 Summary of Body Fluid Compartments

Body Fluid Compartment	Percent of Body Weight	Fraction of TBW	Marker
TBW	60%*	1.0	D_2O; THO; antipyrine
ECF	20%	⅓	Sulfate; mannitol; inulin
ICF	40%	⅔	TBW–ECF
Plasma	4%	¹⁄₁₂ (¼ of ECF)	Radioiodinated serum albumin (RISA); Evan's blue
Interstitial fluid	16%	¼ (¾ of ECF)	ECF–plasma

D_2O, Deuterium oxide; ECF, extracellular fluid; ICF, intracellular fluid; TBW, total body water; THO, tritiated water.
*Range of normal values for total body water is 50% to 70% of body weight.

3. **Equilibration and measurement of plasma concentration.** The marker is allowed to equilibrate in the body fluids, correction is made for any urinary losses during the equilibration period, and the concentration of the marker is then measured in plasma.

4. **Calculation of the volume of the body fluid compartment.** Because the *amount* of marker present in the body is known (i.e., the difference between the amount originally injected and the amount excreted in urine) and the *concentration* is measured, the volume of distribution of the marker substance can be calculated as follows:

$$\text{Volume} = \frac{\text{Amount}}{\text{Concentration}}$$

where

Volume = Volume of distribution (L)
or
Volume of body fluid compartment (L)

Amount = Amount of marker injected – Amount excreted (mg)

Concentration = Concentration in plasma (mg/L)

SAMPLE PROBLEM. A 65-kg man is participating in a research study for which it is necessary to know the volumes of his body fluid compartments. To measure these volumes, the man is injected with 100 mCi of D_2O and 500 mg of mannitol. During a 2-hour equilibration period, he excretes 10% of the D_2O and 10% of the mannitol in his urine. Following equilibration, the concentration of D_2O in plasma is 0.213 mCi/100 mL and the concentration of mannitol is 3.2 mg/100 mL. *What is his total body water, his ECF volume, and his ICF volume? Is the man's total body water appropriate for his weight?*

SOLUTION. Total body water can be calculated from the volume of distribution of D_2O, and ECF volume can be calculated from the volume of distribution of mannitol. ICF volume cannot be measured directly, but it can be calculated as the difference between total body water and ECF volume.

$$\text{Total body water} = \frac{\substack{\text{Amount of} \\ D_2O \text{ injected}} - \substack{\text{Amount of} \\ D_2O \text{ excreted}}}{\text{Concentration of } D_2O}$$

$$= \frac{100 \text{ mCi} - (10\% \text{ of } 100 \text{ mCi})}{0.213 \text{ mCi}/100 \text{ mL}}$$

$$= \frac{90 \text{ mCi}}{0.213 \text{ mCi}/100 \text{ mL}}$$

$$= \frac{90 \text{ mCi}}{2.13 \text{ mCi/L}}$$

$$= 42.3 \text{ L}$$

$$\text{ECF volume} = \frac{\substack{\text{Amount of} \\ \text{mannitol} \\ \text{injected}} - \substack{\text{Amount of} \\ \text{mannitol} \\ \text{excreted}}}{\text{Concentration of mannitol}}$$

$$= \frac{500 \text{ mg} - (10\% \text{ of } 500 \text{ mg})}{3.2 \text{ mg}/100 \text{ mL}}$$

$$= \frac{450 \text{ mg}}{3.2 \text{ mg}/100 \text{ mL}}$$

$$= \frac{450 \text{ mg}}{32 \text{ mg/L}}$$

$$= 14.1 \text{ L}$$

$$\text{ICF volume} = \text{Total body water} - \text{ECF volume}$$

$$= 42.3 \text{ L} - 14.1 \text{ L}$$

$$= 28.2 \text{ L}$$

The man's total body water is 42.3 L, which is 65.1% of his body weight (42.3 L is approximately 42.3 kg; 42.3 kg/65 kg = 65.1%). This percentage falls within the normal range of 50% to 70% of body weight.

Shifts of Water between Body Fluid Compartments

The normal distribution of total body water is described earlier in this chapter and in Chapter 1. There are, however, a number of disturbances that, by altering solute or water balance, cause a shift of water *between* the body fluid compartments. Among the disturbances to be considered are diarrhea, severe dehydration, adrenal insufficiency, infusion of isotonic saline, high sodium chloride (NaCl) intake, and syndrome of inappropriate antidiuretic hormone (SIADH). This section provides a systematic approach to understanding common disturbances of fluid balance.

The following key principles are necessary to understand fluid shifts between the body fluid compartments. Learn and understand these principles!

1. The **volume** of a body fluid compartment depends on the amount of solute it contains. For example, the volume of the ECF is determined by its total solute content. Because the major cation of ECF is Na^+ (and its accompanying anions Cl^- and HCO_3^-), ECF volume is determined by the *amount* of NaCl and sodium bicarbonate ($NaHCO_3$) it contains.

2. **Osmolarity** is the concentration of osmotically active particles, expressed as milliosmoles per liter (mOsm/L). In practice, osmolarity is the same as osmolality (mOsm/kgH$_2$O) because 1 L of water is equivalent to 1 kg of water. The normal value for osmolarity of the body fluids is **290 mOsm/L,** or, for simplicity, 300 mOsm/L.

   Plasma osmolarity can be estimated from the plasma Na^+ concentration, plasma glucose concentration, and blood urea nitrogen (BUN), as these are the major solutes of ECF and plasma.

$$\text{Plasma osmolarity} = 2 \times \text{Plasma Na}^+ + \frac{\text{Glucose}}{18} + \frac{\text{BUN}}{2.8}$$

where

Plasma osmolarity = Plasma osmolarity (total osmolar concentration) in mOsm/L
Na^+ = Plasma Na^+ concentration in mEq/L
Glucose = Plasma glucose concentration in mg/dL
BUN = Blood urea nitrogen concentration in mg/dL

The Na^+ concentration is multiplied by 2 because Na^+ must be balanced by an equal concentration of anions. (In plasma, these anions are Cl^- and HCO_3^-.) The glucose concentration in mg/dL is converted to mOsm/L when it is divided by 18. The BUN in mg/dL is converted to mOsm/L when it is divided by 2.8.

3. In the steady state, **intracellular osmolarity is equal to extracellular osmolarity.** In other words, osmolarity is the same throughout the body fluids. To maintain this equality, **water shifts** freely across cell membranes. Thus, if a disturbance occurs to change the ECF osmolarity, water will shift across cell membranes to make the ICF osmolarity equal to the new ECF osmolarity. After a brief period of equilibration (while the shift of water occurs), a new steady state will be achieved and the osmolarities again will be equal.

4. Solutes such as **NaCl** and **NaHCO$_3$** and large sugars such as **mannitol** are assumed to be confined to the ECF compartment because they do not readily cross cell membranes. For example, if a person ingests a large quantity of NaCl, that NaCl will be added only to the ECF compartment and the total solute content of the ECF will be increased.

Six disturbances of body fluids are summarized in Table 6-2 and are illustrated in Figure 6-5. The disturbances are grouped and named according to whether they involve volume contraction or volume expansion and whether they involve an increase or a decrease in body fluid osmolarity.

Volume contraction means a *decrease* in ECF volume. **Volume expansion** means an *increase* in ECF volume. The terms isosmotic, hyperosmotic, and hyposmotic refer to the osmolarity of the ECF. Thus, an **isosmotic** disturbance means that there is no change in ECF osmolarity; a **hyperosmotic** disturbance means that there has been an increase in ECF osmolarity; and a **hyposmotic** disturbance means that there has been a decrease in ECF osmolarity.

Table 6–2 Disturbances of Body Fluids

Type	Example	ECF Volume	ICF Volume	Osmolarity	Hematocrit	Plasma [protein]
Isosmotic volume contraction	Diarrhea; burn	↓	N.C.	N.C.	↑	↑
Hyperosmotic volume contraction	Sweating; fever; diabetes insipidus	↓	↓	↑	N.C.	↑
Hyposmotic volume contraction	Adrenal insufficiency	↓	↑	↓	↑	↑
Isosmotic volume expansion	Infusion of isotonic NaCl	↑	N.C.	N.C.	↓	↓
Hyperosmotic volume expansion	High NaCl intake	↑	↓	↑	↓	↓
Hyposmotic volume expansion	SIADH	↑	↑	↓	N.C.	↓

ECF, Extracellular fluid; ICF, intracellular fluid; NaCl, sodium chloride; N.C., no change; SIADH, syndrome of inappropriate antidiuretic hormone.

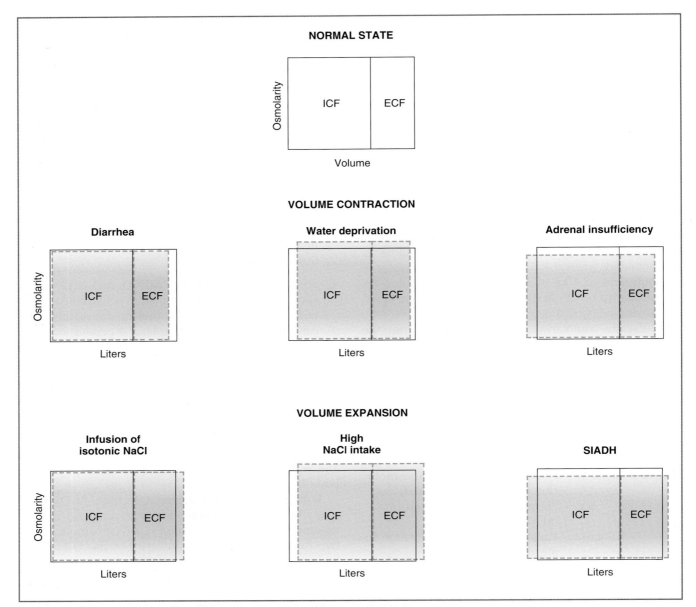

Figure 6–5 **Shifts of water between body fluid compartments.** Normal extracellular fluid (ECF) and intracellular fluid (ICF) osmolarity are shown by *solid lines*. Changes in volume and osmolarity in response to various disturbances are shown by *dashed lines*. SIADH, Syndrome of inappropriate antidiuretic hormone.

To understand the events that occur in these disturbances, a three-step approach should be used. First, identify any change occurring in the ECF (e.g., Was solute added to the ECF? Was water lost from the ECF?). Second, decide whether that change will produce an increase, a decrease, or no change in ECF osmolarity. Third, if there is a change in ECF osmolarity, determine whether water will shift into or out of the cells to reestablish equality between ECF osmolarity and ICF osmolarity. If there is no change in ECF osmolarity, no water shift will occur. If there is a change in ECF osmolarity, then a water shift must occur.

Isosmotic Volume Contraction—Diarrhea

A person with diarrhea loses a large volume of fluid from the gastrointestinal tract. The osmolarity of the fluid lost is approximately equal to that of the ECF—it is isosmotic. Thus, the disturbance in diarrhea is **loss of isosmotic fluid** from ECF. As a result, ECF volume decreases, but there is no accompanying change in ECF osmolarity (because the fluid that was lost is isosmotic). Because there is no change in ECF osmolarity, there is no need for a fluid shift across cell membranes and ICF volume remains unchanged. In the new steady state, ECF volume decreases and the osmolarities of ECF and ICF are unchanged. The decrease in ECF volume means that blood volume (a component of ECF) also is reduced, which produces a decrease in arterial pressure.

Other consequences of diarrhea include increased hematocrit and increased plasma protein concentration, which are explained by the loss of isosmotic fluid from the ECF compartment. The red blood cells and proteins that remain behind in the vascular component of the ECF are concentrated by this fluid loss.

Hyperosmotic Volume Contraction— Water Deprivation

A person who is lost in the desert without adequate drinking water loses both NaCl and water in sweat. A key piece of information, not immediately obvious, is that *sweat is hyposmotic* relative to ECF; that is, compared with the body fluids, sweat contains relatively more water than solute. Because **hyposmotic fluid is lost** from the ECF, ECF volume decreases and ECF osmolarity increases. ECF osmolarity is transiently higher than ICF osmolarity, and this difference in osmolarity causes water to shift from ICF into ECF. Water will flow until ICF osmolarity increases and becomes equal to ECF osmolarity. This shift of water out of cells decreases ICF volume. In the new steady state, both ECF and ICF volumes will be decreased and ECF and ICF osmolarities will be increased and equal to each other.

In hyperosmotic volume contraction, the plasma protein concentration is increased but the hematocrit is unchanged. The explanation for the increase in plasma protein concentration is straightforward: Fluid is lost from ECF, and the plasma protein remaining behind becomes concentrated. It is less obvious, however, why the hematocrit is unchanged. Loss of fluid from ECF alone would cause an increase in the concentration of red blood cells and an increase in hematocrit. However, there also is a fluid shift in this disturbance: Water moves from ICF to ECF. Because red blood cells are *cells*, water shifts out of them, decreasing their volume. Thus, the concentration of red blood cells increases, but red blood cell volume decreases. The two effects offset each other, and hematocrit is unchanged.

What is the final state of the ECF volume? Is it decreased (because of the loss of ECF volume in sweat), increased (because of the water shift from ICF to ECF), or unchanged (because both occur)? Figure 6-5 shows that ECF volume is lower than normal, but why? Determining the ECF volume in the new steady state is complicated because, although volume is lost from ECF in sweat, water also shifts from ICF to ECF. The following sample problem shows how to determine the new ECF volume to answer the questions posed:

SAMPLE PROBLEM. A woman runs a marathon on a hot September day and drinks no fluids to replace the volumes lost in sweat. It is determined that she lost 3 L of sweat, which had an osmolarity of 150 mOsm/L. Before the marathon, her total body water was 36 L, her ECF volume was 12 L, her ICF volume was 24 L, and her body fluid osmolarity was 300 mOsm/L. Assume that a new steady state is achieved and that all of the solute (i.e., NaCl) lost from her body came from the ECF. *What is her ECF volume and osmolarity after the marathon?*

SOLUTION. Values before the marathon will be called *old*, and values after the marathon will be called *new*. To solve this problem, first calculate the new osmolarity because osmolarity will be the same throughout the body fluids in the new steady state. Then calculate the new ECF volume using the new osmolarity.

To calculate the *new* **osmolarity,** calculate the total number of osmoles in the body after the fluid is lost in sweat (New osmoles = Old osmoles − Osmoles lost in sweat). Then divide the new osmoles by the new total body water to obtain the new osmolarity. (Remember that the new total body water is 36 L *minus* the 3 L lost in sweat.)

$$Old \text{ osmoles} = \text{Osmolarity} \times \text{Total body water}$$
$$= 300 \text{ mOsm/L} \times 36 \text{ L}$$
$$= 10{,}800 \text{ mOsm}$$

$$\text{Osmoles lost in sweat} = 150 \text{ mOsm/L} \times 3 \text{ L}$$
$$= 450 \text{ mOsm}$$

$$New \text{ osmoles} = 10{,}800 \text{ mOsm} - 450 \text{ mOsm}$$
$$= 10{,}350 \text{ mOsm}$$

$$New \text{ osmolarity} = \frac{\text{New osmoles}}{\text{New total body water}}$$
$$= \frac{10{,}350 \text{ mOsm}}{36 \text{ L} - 3 \text{ L}}$$
$$= 313.6 \text{ mOsm/L}$$

To calculate the *new* **ECF volume,** assume that all of the solute (NaCl) lost in sweat comes from the ECF. Calculate the new ECF osmoles after this loss, then divide by the new osmolarity (previously calculated) to obtain the new ECF volume.

$$Old \text{ ECF osmoles} = 300 \text{ mOsm/L} \times 12 \text{ L}$$
$$= 3600 \text{ mOsm}$$

$$New \text{ ECF osmoles} = \text{Old ECF osmoles} - \text{Osmoles lost in sweat}$$
$$= 3600 \text{ mOsm} - 450 \text{ mOsm}$$
$$= 3150 \text{ mOsm}$$

$$New \text{ ECF volume} = \frac{\text{New ECF osmoles}}{\text{New osmolarity}}$$
$$= \frac{3150 \text{ mOsm}}{313.6 \text{ mOsm/}L}$$
$$= 10.0 \text{ L}$$

To summarize the calculations in this example, after the marathon the ECF osmolarity increases to

313.6 mOsm/L because a hyposmotic solution is lost from the body (i.e., relatively more water than solute was lost in sweat). After the marathon, the ECF volume decreases to 10 L (from the original 12 L). Therefore, some, but not all, of the ECF volume lost in sweat was replaced by the shift of water from ICF to ECF. Had there been no shift of water, then the new ECF volume would have been even lower (i.e., 9 L).

Hyposmotic Volume Contraction—Adrenal Insufficiency

A person with adrenal insufficiency has a deficiency of several hormones including aldosterone, a hormone that normally promotes Na$^+$ reabsorption in the distal tubule and collecting ducts. As a result of **aldosterone deficiency,** excess NaCl is excreted in the urine. Because NaCl is an ECF solute, ECF osmolarity decreases. Transiently, ECF osmolarity is less than ICF osmolarity, which causes water to shift from ECF to ICF until ICF osmolarity decreases to the same level as ECF osmolarity. In the new steady state, both ECF and ICF osmolarities will be lower than normal and equal to each other. Because of the shift of water, ECF volume will be decreased and ICF volume will be increased.

In hyposmotic volume contraction, both plasma protein concentration and hematocrit will be increased because of the decrease in ECF volume. Hematocrit increases *also* because of the shift of water into red blood cells, increasing cell volume.

Isosmotic Volume Expansion—Infusion of NaCl

A person who receives an infusion of isotonic NaCl presents the opposite clinical picture of the person who has lost isotonic fluid through diarrhea. Because NaCl is an extracellular solute, all of the **isotonic NaCl solution is added to the ECF,** causing an increase in ECF volume but no change in ECF osmolarity. There will be no shift of water between ICF and ECF because there is no difference in osmolarity between the two compartments. Both plasma protein concentration and hematocrit will decrease (i.e., be diluted) because of the increase in ECF volume.

Hyperosmotic Volume Expansion—High NaCl Intake

Ingesting dry NaCl (e.g., eating a bag of potato chips) will increase the total amount of solute in the ECF. As a result, ECF osmolarity increases. Transiently, ECF osmolarity is higher than ICF osmolarity, which causes water to shift from ICF to ECF, decreasing ICF volume and increasing ECF volume. In the new steady state,

both ECF and ICF osmolarities will be higher than normal and equal to each other. Because of the shift of water out of cells, ICF volume will decrease and ECF volume will increase.

In hyperosmotic volume expansion, both plasma protein concentration and hematocrit will decrease due to the increase in ECF volume. Hematocrit *also* will be decreased because of the water shift out of the red blood cells.

Hyposmotic Volume Expansion—SIADH

A person with **syndrome of inappropriate antidiuretic hormone** (**SIADH**) secretes inappropriately high levels of antidiuretic hormone (ADH), which promotes water reabsorption in the collecting ducts. When ADH levels are abnormally high, too much water is reabsorbed and the excess water is retained and distributed throughout the total body water. The volume of water that is added to ECF and ICF is in direct proportion to their original volumes. For example, if an extra 3 L of water is reabsorbed by the collecting ducts, 1 L will be added to the ECF and 2 L will be added to the ICF (because ECF constitutes one third and ICF constitutes two thirds of the total body water). When compared with the normal state, ECF and ICF volumes will be increased and ECF and ICF osmolarities will be decreased.

In hyposmotic volume expansion, plasma protein concentration is decreased by dilution. However, the hematocrit is unchanged as a result of two offsetting effects: The concentration of red blood cells decreases because of dilution, but red blood cell volume increases because water shifts into the cells.

RENAL CLEARANCE

Clearance is a general concept that describes the rate at which substances are removed (or cleared) from plasma. Thus, whole-body clearance means the total rate of removal of a substance by all organs, hepatic clearance means the rate of removal by the liver, and renal clearance means the rate of removal by the kidneys. The concept of renal clearance is being introduced at this point because it is employed in several basic concepts of renal physiology discussed throughout the chapter. For reference, see the tables of commonly used abbreviations (Table 6-3) and commonly used equations (Table 6-4).

By definition, **renal clearance** is the volume of plasma completely cleared of a substance by the kidneys per unit time. The higher the renal clearance, the more plasma that is cleared of the substance. Substances with the highest renal clearances may be completely removed on a single pass of blood through the kidneys; substances with the lowest renal clearances are not removed at all.

Table 6-3 Commonly Used Abbreviations in Renal Physiology

Structure	Abbreviation	Meaning	Units and/or Normal Value
Whole Kidney	C	Clearance	mL/min
	[U]	Concentration in urine	mg/mL
	[P]	Concentration in plasma	mg/mL
	$\dot{V}$	Urine flow rate	mL/min
	GFR	Glomerular filtration rate	120 mL/min
	RPF	Renal plasma flow	660 mL/min
	RBF	Renal blood flow	1200 mL/min
Single Nephron	[TF]	Concentration in tubular fluid	mg/mL
	$[TF/P]_x$	Concentration of x in tubular fluid relative to concentration of x in plasma	None
	$[TF/P]_{inulin}$	Concentration of inulin in tubular fluid relative to concentration of inulin in plasma	None
	$[TF/P]_x/[TF/P]_{inulin}$	Fraction of the filtered load remaining in tubular fluid or fractional excretion	None

Table 6-4 Commonly Used Equations in Renal Physiology

Name	Equation	Units	Comments
Clearance	$C_x = \dfrac{[U]_x \dot{V}}{[P]_x}$	mL/min	x is any substance
Clearance ratio	$\text{Clearance ratio} = \dfrac{C_x}{C_{inulin}}$	None	Also means fractional excretion of x
Renal plasma flow	$RPF = \dfrac{[U]_{PAH} \dot{V}}{[RA]_{PAH} - [RV]_{PAH}}$	mL/min	
Effective renal plasma flow	$\text{Effective } RPF = \dfrac{[U]_{PAH} \dot{V}}{[P]_{PAH}}$	mL/min	Underestimates RPF by 10%; equals C_{PAH}
Renal blood flow	$RBF = \dfrac{RPF}{1 - Hct}$	mL/min	1 minus Hct is fraction of blood volume that is plasma
Glomerular filtration rate	$GFR = \dfrac{[U]_{inulin} \dot{V}}{[P]_{inulin}}$	mL/min	Equals C_{inulin}
Filtration fraction	$FF = \dfrac{GFR}{RPF}$	None	
Filtered load	$\text{Filtered load} = GFR \times [P]_x$	mg/min	
Excretion rate	$\text{Excretion} = \dot{V} \times [U]_x$	mg/min	
Reabsorption or secretion rate	$\text{Reabsorption or secretion} = \text{Filtered load} - \text{Excretion}$	mg/min	If *positive*, net reabsorption. If *negative*, net secretion
Free-water clearance	$C_{H_2O} = \dot{V} - C_{osm}$	mL/min	If *positive*, free water is excreted. If *negative*, free water is reabsorbed

The equation for renal clearance is as follows:

$$C = \frac{[U]_x \times \dot{V}}{[P]_x}$$

where

C = Clearance (mL/min)
$[U]_x$ = Urine concentration of substance X (mg/mL)
$\dot{V}$ = Urine flow rate per minute (mL/min)
$[P]_x$ = Plasma concentration of substance X (mg/mL)

Thus, renal clearance is the ratio of urinary excretion ($[U]_x \times \dot{V}$) to plasma concentration. For a given plasma concentration, renal clearance of a substance increases as the urinary excretion increases. Again, the units of clearance are volume per unit time (e.g., mL/min;

L/hour; L/day), which means the volume of plasma cleared of the substance per unit time.

Clearance of Various Substances

Renal clearance can be calculated for any substance. Depending on the characteristics of the substance and its renal handling, renal clearance can vary from zero to greater than 600 mL/min. For example, renal clearance of **albumin** is approximately zero because, normally, albumin is not filtered across the glomerular capillaries. The renal clearance of **glucose** is also zero, although for a different reason: Glucose is filtered and then completely reabsorbed back into the bloodstream. Other substances such as Na^+, urea, phosphate, and Cl^- have clearances that are higher than zero because they are filtered and partially reabsorbed. **Inulin,** a fructose polymer, is a special case. Inulin is freely filtered across the glomerular capillaries, but it is neither reabsorbed nor secreted; therefore, its clearance measures the glomerular filtration rate. Organic acids such as *para*-aminohippuric acid (**PAH**) have the highest clearances of all substances because they are both filtered and secreted.

Clearance Ratios

Inulin has unique properties that make it the only substance whose clearance is exactly equal to the glomerular filtration rate (GFR). Inulin is freely filtered across the glomerular capillaries, but once filtered, it is neither reabsorbed nor secreted. Thus, the amount of inulin filtered will be exactly equal to the amount of inulin excreted. For these reasons, inulin is a reference substance called a **glomerular marker.**

The clearance of any substance (x) can be compared with the clearance of inulin and is expressed as the **clearance ratio.** Thus,

$$\text{Clearance ratio} = \frac{C_x}{C_{inulin}}$$

The meanings of various values of the clearance ratio are as follows:

♦ $C_x/C_{inulin} = 1.0$. The clearance of x equals the clearance of inulin. The substance also must be a glomerular marker (filtered, but neither reabsorbed nor secreted).

♦ $C_x/C_{inulin} < 1.0$. The clearance of x is lower than the clearance of inulin. *Either* the substance is not filtered, *or* it is filtered and subsequently reabsorbed. For example, albumin is not filtered, and the clearance of albumin is less than the clearance of inulin. The clearances of Na^+, Cl^-, HCO_3^-, phosphate, urea, glucose, and amino acids also are less than the

clearance of inulin because these substances are filtered and then reabsorbed.

♦ $C_x/C_{inulin} > 1.0$. The clearance of x is higher than the clearance of inulin. The substance is filtered and secreted. Examples of substances whose clearances are higher than that of inulin are organic acids and bases and, under some conditions, K^+.

SAMPLE PROBLEM. In a 24-hour period, 1.44 L of urine is collected from a man receiving an infusion of inulin. In his urine, the [inulin] is 150 mg/mL and the $[Na^+]$ is 200 mEq/L. In his plasma, the [inulin] is 1 mg/mL and the $[Na^+]$ is 140 mEq/L. *What is the clearance ratio for Na^+, and what is the significance of its value?*

SOLUTION. The clearance ratio for Na^+ is the clearance of Na^+ relative to the clearance of inulin. The clearance equation for any substance is $C = [U] \times \dot{V}/[P]$. All of the values needed are provided in the description, although urine flow rate ($\dot{V}$) must be calculated.

$$\dot{V} = \text{Urine volume/time}$$
$$= 1.44 \text{ L/24 hr}$$
$$= 1440 \text{ mL/1440 min}$$
$$= 1.0 \text{ mL/min}$$

$$C_{Na^+} = \frac{[U]_{Na^+} \times \dot{V}}{[P]_{Na^+}}$$

$$= \frac{200 \text{ mEq/L} \times 1 \text{ mL/min}}{140 \text{ mEq/L}}$$

$$= 1.43 \text{ mL/min}$$

$$C_{inulin} = \frac{[U]_{inulin} \times \dot{V}}{[P]_{inulin}}$$

$$= \frac{150 \text{ mg/mL} \times 1 \text{ mL/min}}{1 \text{ mg/mL}}$$

$$= 150 \text{ mL/min}$$

$$\frac{C_{Na^+}}{C_{inulin}} = \frac{1.43 \text{ mL/min}}{150 \text{ mL/min}}$$

$$= 0.01 \text{ or } 1\%$$

The calculated clearance ratio for Na^+ of 0.01 (or 1%) provides a great deal of information about the renal handling of Na^+. Because Na^+ is freely filtered across the glomerular capillaries, it also must be extensively reabsorbed by the renal tubule, making its clearance much less than the clearance of inulin. The clearance ratio of 0.01 means that only 1% of the filtered Na^+ is excreted. Stated differently, 99% of the filtered Na^+ must have been reabsorbed.

RENAL BLOOD FLOW

The kidneys receive about 25% of the cardiac output, which is among the highest of all the organ systems.

Thus, in a person whose cardiac output is 5 L/min, renal blood flow (RBF) is 1.25 L/min or 1800 L/day! Such high rates of RBF are not surprising in light of the central role the kidneys play in maintaining the volume and composition of the body fluids.

Regulation of Renal Blood Flow

As with blood flow in any organ, RBF (Q) is directly proportional to the **pressure gradient** (ΔP) between the renal artery and the renal vein, and it is inversely proportional to the **resistance** (R) of the renal vasculature. (Recall from Chapter 4 that $Q = \Delta P/R$. Recall, also, that resistance is provided mainly by the arterioles.) The kidneys are unusual, however, in that there are *two sets of arterioles,* the afferent and the efferent. The major mechanism for changing blood flow is by changing arteriolar resistance. In the kidney, this can be accomplished by changing afferent arteriolar resistance and/ or efferent arteriolar resistance (Table 6-5).

♦ **Sympathetic nervous system and circulating catecholamines.** Both afferent and efferent arterioles are innervated by sympathetic nerve fibers that produce **vasoconstriction** by activating α_1 **receptors.** However, because there are far more α_1 receptors on afferent arterioles, increased sympathetic nerve activity causes a decrease in both RBF and GFR. The effects of the sympathetic nervous system on renal vascular resistance can be appreciated by considering the responses to hemorrhage. Recall from Chapter 4 that blood loss and the resulting decrease in arterial pressure causes, via the baroreceptor mechanism, an increase in sympathetic outflow to the heart and blood vessels. When renal α_1 receptors are activated by this increase in sympathetic activity, there is vasoconstriction of afferent arterioles that leads to a decrease in RBF and GFR. Thus, the cardiovascular system will attempt to raise arterial pressure even at the expense of blood flow to the kidneys.

♦ **Angiotensin II.** Angiotensin II is a potent vasoconstrictor of both afferent and efferent arterioles. The effect of angiotensin on RBF is clear: It constricts both sets of arterioles, increases resistance, and decreases blood flow. However, **efferent arterioles** are more sensitive to angiotensin II than afferent arterioles, and this difference in sensitivity has consequences for its effect on GFR (see the discussion on regulation of GFR). Briefly, low levels of angiotensin II produce an *increase in GFR* by constricting efferent arterioles, while high levels of angiotensin II produce a *decrease in GFR* by constricting both afferent and efferent arterioles. In **hemorrhage,** blood loss leads to decreased arterial pressure, which activates the renin-angiotensin-aldosterone

Table 6-5 Renal Vasoconstrictors and Vasodilators

Vasoconstrictors	Vasodilators
Sympathetic nerves (catecholamines)	PGE_2
	PGI_2
Angiotensin II	Nitric oxide
Endothelin	Bradykinin
	Dopamine
	Atrial natriuretic peptide

PG, Prostaglandin.

system. The high level of angiotensin II, together with increased sympathetic nerve activity, constricts afferent and efferent arterioles and causes a decrease in RBF and GFR.

♦ **Atrial natriuretic peptide (ANP).** ANP and related substances such as brain natriuretic peptide (BNP) cause dilation of afferent arterioles and constriction of efferent arterioles. Because the dilatory effect of ANP on afferent arterioles is greater than the constrictor effect on efferent arterioles, there is an overall decrease in renal vascular resistance and resulting increase in RBF. Dilation of afferent arterioles and constriction of efferent arterioles both lead to increased GFR (see discussion on regulation of GFR).

♦ **Prostaglandins.** Several prostaglandins (e.g., prostaglandin E_2 and prostaglandin I_2) are produced locally in the kidneys and cause **vasodilation** of both afferent and efferent arterioles. The same stimuli that activate the sympathetic nervous system and increase angiotensin II levels in hemorrhage also activate local renal prostaglandin production. Although these actions may seem contradictory, the vasodilatory effects of prostaglandins are clearly protective for RBF. Thus, prostaglandins modulate the vasoconstriction produced by the sympathetic nervous system and angiotensin II. Unopposed, this vasoconstriction can cause a profound reduction in RBF, resulting in renal failure. **Nonsteroidal antiinflammatory drugs** (**NSAIDs**) inhibit synthesis of prostaglandins and, therefore, interfere with the protective effects of prostaglandins on renal function following a hemorrhage.

♦ **Dopamine.** Dopamine, a precursor of norepinephrine, has selective actions on arterioles in several vascular beds. At low levels, dopamine *dilates* cerebral, cardiac, splanchnic, and renal arterioles, and it *constricts* skeletal muscle and cutaneous arterioles. Thus, a low dosage of dopamine can be administered in the treatment of **hemorrhage** because of its protective (vasodilatory) effect on blood flow in several critical organs including the kidneys.

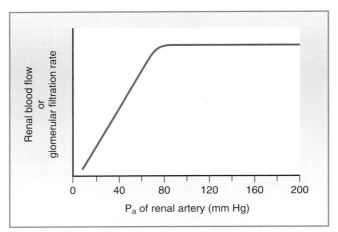

Figure 6-6 Autoregulation of renal blood flow and glomerular filtration rate. P_a, Renal artery pressure.

Autoregulation of Renal Blood Flow

RBF is autoregulated over a wide range of mean arterial pressures (P_a) (Fig. 6-6). Renal arterial pressure can vary from 80 to 200 mm Hg, yet RBF will be kept constant. Only when renal arterial pressure decreases to less than 80 mm Hg does RBF also decrease. The only way to maintain this constancy of blood flow in the face of changing arterial pressure is by varying the resistance of the arterioles. Thus, as renal arterial pressure increases or decreases, renal resistance must increase or decrease proportionately (recall that $Q = \Delta P/R$).

For renal autoregulation, it is believed that resistance is controlled primarily at the level of the afferent arteriole, rather than the efferent arteriole. The **mechanism of autoregulation** is not completely understood. Clearly, the autonomic nervous system is *not* involved because a denervated (e.g., transplanted) kidney autoregulates as well as an intact kidney. The major theories explaining renal autoregulation are a myogenic mechanism and tubuloglomerular feedback.

♦ **Myogenic hypothesis.** The myogenic hypothesis states that increased arterial pressure stretches the blood vessels, which causes reflex contraction of smooth muscle in the blood vessel walls and consequently increased resistance to blood flow (see Chapter 4). The mechanism of stretch-induced contraction involves the opening of **stretch-activated calcium (Ca^{2+}) channels** in the smooth muscle cell membranes. When these channels are open, more Ca^{2+} enters vascular smooth muscle cells, leading to more tension in the blood vessel wall. The myogenic hypothesis explains autoregulation of RBF as follows: Increases in renal arterial pressure stretch the walls of the afferent arterioles, which respond by contracting. Afferent arteriolar contraction leads to increased

afferent arteriolar resistance. The increase in resistance then balances the increase in arterial pressure, and RBF is kept constant.

♦ **Tubuloglomerular feedback.** Tubuloglomerular feedback is also a mechanism for autoregulation (Fig. 6-7), explained as follows: When renal arterial pressure increases, both RBF and GFR increase. The increase in GFR results in increased delivery of solute and water to the **macula densa** region of the early distal tubule, which senses some component of the increased delivered load. The macula densa, which is a part of the **juxtaglomerular apparatus,** responds to the increased delivered load by secreting a vasoactive substance that constricts afferent arterioles via a paracrine mechanism. Local vasoconstriction of afferent arterioles then reduces RBF and GFR back to normal; that is, there is autoregulation.

There are two major unanswered questions concerning the mechanism of tubuloglomerular feedback: (1) *What component of tubular fluid is sensed at the macula densa?* The major candidates are luminal Na^+ and Cl^-. (2) *What vasoactive substance is secreted by the juxtaglomerular apparatus to act locally on afferent arterioles?* Here, the candidates are adenosine, ATP, and thromboxane.

Measurement of Renal Plasma Flow and Renal Blood Flow

Renal *plasma* flow (RPF) can be estimated from the clearance of an organic acid **para-aminohippuric acid (PAH)**. Renal *blood* flow (RBF) is calculated from the RPF and the hematocrit.

Measuring True Renal Plasma Flow— Fick Principle

The **Fick principle** states that the amount of a substance entering an organ equals the amount of the substance leaving the organ (assuming that the substance is that the amount of degraded by the organ). Applied to the kidney, the Fick principle states that the amount of a substance entering the kidney via the renal artery equals the amount of the substance leaving the kidney via the renal vein *plus* the amount excreted in the urine (Fig. 6-8).

PAH is the substance used to measure RPF with the Fick principle, and the derivation is as follows:

$$\text{Amount of PAH entering kidney} = \text{Amount of PAH leaving kidney}$$

$$\text{Amount of PAH entering kidney} = [RA]_{PAH} \times RPF$$

$$\text{Amount of PAH leaving kidney} = [RV]_{PAH} \times RPF + [U]_{PAH} \times \dot{V}$$

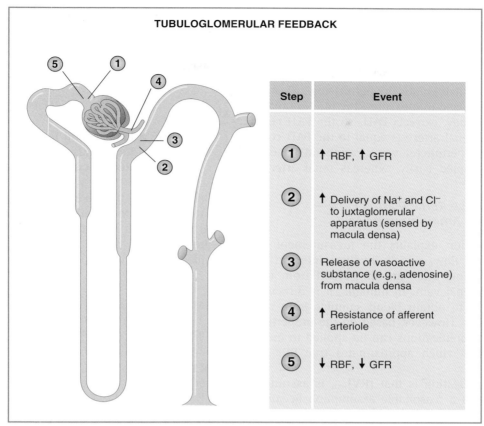

TUBULOGLOMERULAR FEEDBACK

Step	Event
1	↑ RBF, ↑ GFR
2	↑ Delivery of Na⁺ and Cl⁻ to juxtaglomerular apparatus (sensed by macula densa)
3	Release of vasoactive substance (e.g., adenosine) from macula densa
4	↑ Resistance of afferent arteriole
5	↓ RBF, ↓ GFR

Figure 6–7 **Mechanism of tubuloglomerular feedback.** GFR, Glomerular filtration rate; RBF, renal blood flow.

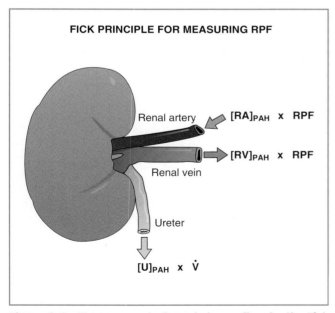

FICK PRINCIPLE FOR MEASURING RPF

Renal artery — $[RA]_{PAH} \times RPF$

Renal vein — $[RV]_{PAH} \times RPF$

Ureter

$[U]_{PAH} \times \dot{V}$

Figure 6–8 **Measurement of renal plasma flow by the Fick principle.** PAH, *Para*-aminohippuric acid; [RA], concentration in renal artery; RPF, renal plasma flow; [RV], concentration in renal vein; [U], concentration in urine.

Substituting,

$$[RA]_{PAH} \times RPF = [RV]_{PAH} \times RPF + [U]_{PAH} \times \dot{V}$$

Solving for RPF,

$$RPF = \frac{[U]_{PAH} \times \dot{V}}{[RA]_{PAH} - [RV]_{PAH}}$$

where

$$RPF = \text{Renal plasma flow}$$
$$[U]_{PAH} = [PAH] \text{ in urine}$$
$$\dot{V} = \text{Urine flow rate}$$
$$[RA]_{PAH} = [PAH] \text{ in renal artery}$$
$$[RV]_{PAH} = [PAH] \text{ in renal vein}$$

PAH has the following characteristics that make it the ideal substance for measuring RPF: (1) PAH is neither metabolized nor synthesized by the kidney. (2) PAH does not alter RPF. (3) The kidneys extract (remove) most of the PAH from renal arterial blood by a combination of filtration and secretion. As a result, almost all of the PAH entering the kidney via the renal artery is excreted in urine, leaving little in the renal vein. Because the renal vein concentration of PAH is nearly zero, the denominator of the previous equation ($[RA]_{PAH} - [RV]_{PAH}$) is large and, therefore, can be measured accurately. To elaborate this point, compare a substance such as glucose, which is *not* removed from renal arterial blood at all. Renal vein blood will have the same glucose concentration as renal artery blood, and the denominator of the equation will be zero, which is not mathematically permissible. Clearly, glucose cannot be used to measure RPF. (4) No organ, other than the kidney, extracts PAH, so the PAH concentration in the renal artery is equal to the PAH concentration in any peripheral vein. Peripheral venous blood can be sampled easily, whereas renal arterial blood cannot.

Measuring Effective Renal Plasma Flow— Clearance of Para-Aminohippuric Acid

The previous section explains the measurement of *true* renal plasma flow, which involves infusion of PAH, sampling urine, and sampling blood from the renal artery and renal vein. In humans, it is difficult, if not impossible, to obtain blood samples from the renal blood vessels. However, based on the properties of PAH, certain simplifications can be applied to measure *effective* RPF, which approximates *true* RPF to within 10%.

The first simplification is that **[RV]$_{PAH}$ is assumed to be zero.** This is a reasonable assumption because most of the PAH entering the kidney via the renal artery is excreted in the urine by the combined processes of filtration and secretion. The second simplification is that **[RA]$_{PAH}$ equals the PAH concentration in any peripheral vein,** which can be easily sampled. With these modifications, the equation for RPF becomes

$$\text{Effective RPF} = \frac{[U]_{PAH} \times \dot{V}}{[P]_{PAH}} = C_{PAH}$$

where

$$\begin{aligned}
\text{Effective RPF} &= \text{Effective renal plasma flow} \\
&\quad \text{(mL/min)} \\
[U]_{PAH} &= \text{Urine concentration of PAH} \\
&\quad \text{(mg/mL)} \\
\dot{V} &= \text{Urine flow rate (mL/min)} \\
[P]_{PAH} &= \text{Plasma concentration of PAH} \\
&\quad \text{(mg/mL)} \\
C_{PAH} &= \text{Clearance of PAH (mL/min)}
\end{aligned}$$

Thus, in the simplified form, *effective* RPF equals the clearance of PAH. Effective RPF underestimates *true* RPF by approximately 10% because [RV]$_{PAH}$ is not zero—it is *nearly zero*. [RV]$_{PAH}$ is not zero because a small fraction of the RPF serves kidney tissue that is not involved in filtration and secretion of PAH (e.g., renal adipose tissue, renal capsule). PAH will not be extracted from this portion of the RPF, and the PAH contained in that blood is returned to the renal vein.

Measuring Renal Blood Flow

RBF is calculated from RPF and the hematocrit (Hct). The formula used to calculate RBF is as follows:

$$\text{RBF} = \frac{\text{RPF}}{1 - \text{Hct}}$$

where

$$\begin{aligned}
\text{RBF} &= \text{Renal blood flow (mL/min)} \\
\text{RPF} &= \text{Renal plasma flow (mL/min)} \\
\text{Hct} &= \text{Hematocrit}
\end{aligned}$$

Thus, RBF is the RPF divided by 1 minus the hematocrit, where **hematocrit** is the fraction of blood volume that is occupied by red blood cells, and **1 − hematocrit** is the fraction of blood volume that is occupied by plasma.

SAMPLE PROBLEM. A man with a urine flow rate of 1 mL/min has a plasma concentration of PAH of 1 mg%, a urine concentration of PAH of 600 mg%, and a hematocrit of 0.45. *What is his RBF?*

SOLUTION. Because values are not given for renal artery and renal vein concentrations of PAH, *true* RPF (and true RBF) cannot be calculated. However, *effective* RPF can be calculated from the clearance of PAH. Effective RBF can then be calculated by using the hematocrit. Remember, *mg%* means mg/100 mL.

$$\begin{aligned}
\text{Effective RPF} &= C_{PAH} \\
&= \frac{[U]_{PAH} \times \dot{V}}{[P]_{PAH}} \\
&= \frac{600 \text{ mg/100 mL} \times 1 \text{ mL/min}}{1 \text{ mg/100 mL}} \\
&= 600 \text{ mL/min}
\end{aligned}$$

$$\begin{aligned}
\text{Effective RBF} &= \frac{\text{Effective RPF}}{1 - \text{Hct}} \\
&= \frac{600 \text{ mL/min}}{1 - 0.45} \\
&= \frac{600 \text{ mL/min}}{0.55} \\
&= 1091 \text{ mL/min}
\end{aligned}$$

GLOMERULAR FILTRATION

Glomerular filtration is the first step in the formation of urine. As the renal blood flow enters the glomerular capillaries, a portion of that blood is filtered into Bowman's space, the first part of the nephron. The fluid that is filtered is similar to interstitial fluid and is called an **ultrafiltrate.** The ultrafiltrate contains water and all of the small solutes of blood, but it does not contain proteins and blood cells. The forces responsible for glomerular filtration are similar to the forces that

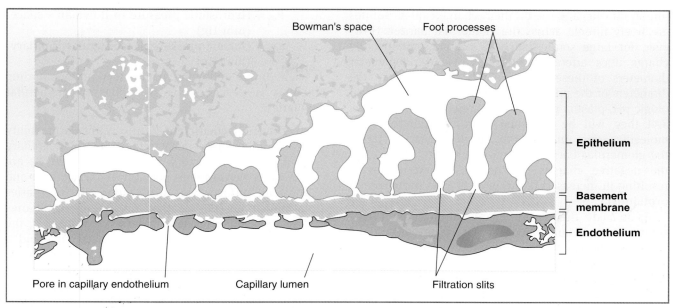

Bowman's space   Foot processes

Epithelium

Basement membrane

Endothelium

Pore in capillary endothelium   Capillary lumen   Filtration slits

Figure 6–9   **Structure of the glomerular capillary wall.**

operate in systemic capillaries—the Starling forces (see Chapter 4). There are differences, however, in the characteristics and surface area of the glomerular capillary barrier, making the glomerular filtration rates much higher than the filtration rates across systemic capillaries.

Characteristics of the Glomerular Filtration Barrier

The physical characteristics of the glomerular capillary wall determine both the rate of glomerular filtration and the characteristics of the glomerular filtrate. These characteristics determine *what* is filtered and *how much* is filtered into Bowman's space.

Layers of the Glomerular Capillary

Figure 6-9 shows the key features of a glomerular capillary at approximately 30,000 times magnification. Beginning with the capillary lumen and moving toward Bowman's space, the three layers, discussed in the following sections, constitute the glomerular capillary wall.

ENDOTHELIUM

The endothelial cell layer has pores 70 to 100 nanometers (nm) in diameter. Because these pores are relatively large, fluid, dissolved solutes, and plasma proteins all are filtered across this layer of the glomerular capillary barrier. On the other hand, the pores are not so large that blood cells can be filtered.

BASEMENT MEMBRANE

The basement membrane has three layers. The **lamina rara interna** is fused to the endothelium; the **lamina**

densa is located in the middle of the basement membrane; and the **lamina rara externa** is fused to the epithelial cell layer. The multilayered basement membrane does not permit filtration of plasma proteins and, therefore, constitutes the most significant barrier of the glomerular capillary.

EPITHELIUM

The epithelial cell layer consists of specialized cells called **podocytes,** which are attached to the basement membrane by **foot processes.** Between the foot processes are **filtration slits,** 25 to 60 nm in diameter, which are bridged by thin diaphragms. Because of the relatively small size of the filtration slits, the epithelial layer (in addition to the basement membrane) also is considered an important barrier to filtration.

Negative Charge on the Glomerular Capillary Barrier

In addition to the size barriers to filtration imposed by the various pores and slits, another feature of the glomerular barrier is the presence of **negatively charged glycoproteins.** These fixed negative charges are present on the endothelium, on the lamina rara interna and externa of the basement membrane, on the podocytes and foot processes, and on the filtration slits of the epithelium. A consequence of these fixed negative charges is that they add an electrostatic component to filtration. Positively charged solutes will be attracted to the negative charges on the barrier and be more readily filtered; negatively charged solutes will be repelled from the negative charges on the barrier and be less readily filtered.

For small solutes such as Na^+, K^+, Cl^-, or HCO_3^-, the effect of charge on filtration of the solute is not important. Regardless of their charge, small solutes are freely filtered across the glomerular barrier. However, for large solutes such as plasma proteins, the charge does affect filtration because the molecular diameters of these larger solutes are similar to the diameters of the pores and slits. For example, at physiologic pH, plasma proteins have a net negative charge, and they will be restricted from filtration by their molecular size *and* by the negative charges lining the glomerular barrier. In certain glomerular diseases, the negative charges on the barrier are removed, resulting in increased filtration of plasma proteins and **proteinuria.**

As an aside, the effect of charge on filtration of large solutes was demonstrated in rats by measuring the filtration rate of a series of dextran molecules of different sizes (molecular radii) and with different net charges. For a given molecular radius, there was a neutral dextran, a negatively charged (anionic) dextran, and a positively charged (cationic) dextran. At any molecular radius, cationic dextran was most filterable, anionic dextran was least filterable, and neutral dextran was in the middle. The cations were attracted to the negative charges on the pores, the anions were repelled, and the neutral molecules were unaffected.

Starling Forces Across Glomerular Capillaries

As in systemic capillaries, the pressures that drive fluid movement across the glomerular capillary wall are the Starling pressures, or Starling forces. Theoretically, there are four Starling pressures: two hydrostatic pressures (one in capillary blood and one in interstitial fluid) and two oncotic pressures (one in capillary blood and one in interstitial fluid). When applying these pressures to glomerular capillaries, there is one small modification: The oncotic pressure of Bowman's space, which is analogous to interstitial fluid, is considered to be zero because filtration of protein is negligible.

Starling Equation

Fluid movement across the glomerular capillary wall is glomerular filtration. It is driven by the Starling pressures across the wall and, with the assumption that the oncotic pressure of Bowman's space is zero, is described by the **Starling equation:**

$$GFR = K_f[(P_{GC} - P_{BS}) - \pi_{GC}]$$

where

    GFR = Glomerular filtration rate (mL/min)
    K_f = Hydraulic conductance (mL/min • mm Hg)
             or
       Filtration coefficient (mL/min • mm Hg)
    P_{GC} = Hydrostatic pressure in glomerular
           capillary (mm Hg)

    P_{BS} = Hydrostatic pressure in Bowman's space
          (mm Hg)
    π_{GC} = Oncotic pressure in glomerular capillary
          (mm Hg)

Each of the following parameters in the Starling equation is described as it applies to glomerular capillaries:

♦ **K_f, filtration coefficient,** is the water permeability or hydraulic conductance of the glomerular capillary wall. The two factors that contribute to K_f are the water permeability per unit of surface area and the total surface area. K_f for glomerular capillaries is more than 100-fold that for systemic capillaries (e.g., skeletal muscle capillaries) because of the combination of a higher total surface area and a higher intrinsic water permeability of the barrier. The consequence of this extremely high K_f is that much more fluid is filtered from glomerular capillaries than from other capillaries (i.e., GFR is 180 L/day).

♦ **P_{GC}, hydrostatic pressure in glomerular capillaries,** is a force favoring filtration. When compared with systemic capillaries, P_{GC} is relatively high (45 mm Hg). In systemic capillaries, hydrostatic pressure falls along the length of the capillary; in glomerular capillaries, it remains constant along the entire length.

♦ **P_{BS}, hydrostatic pressure in Bowman's space,** is a force opposing filtration. The origin of this pressure (10 mm Hg) is the fluid present in the lumen of the nephron.

♦ **π_{GC}, oncotic pressure in glomerular capillaries,** is another force opposing filtration. π_{GC} is determined by the protein concentration of glomerular capillary blood. π_{GC} *does not remain constant* along the capillary length; rather, it progressively increases as fluid is filtered out of the capillary. π_{GC} eventually increases to the point where net ultrafiltration pressure becomes zero and glomerular filtration stops (called filtration equilibrium).

In words, glomerular filtration rate is the product of K_f and the net ultrafiltration pressure. The **net ultrafiltration pressure,** the driving force, is the algebraic sum of the three Starling pressures (omitting the oncotic pressure in Bowman's space). For glomerular capillaries, the net ultrafiltration pressure **always favors filtration,** so the direction of fluid movement is always *out* of the capillaries. The greater the net pressure, the higher the rate of glomerular filtration.

Figure 6-10 is a pictorial presentation of the three Starling pressures, each of which is represented by an arrow. The *direction* of the arrow indicates whether the pressure favors filtration out of the capillary or

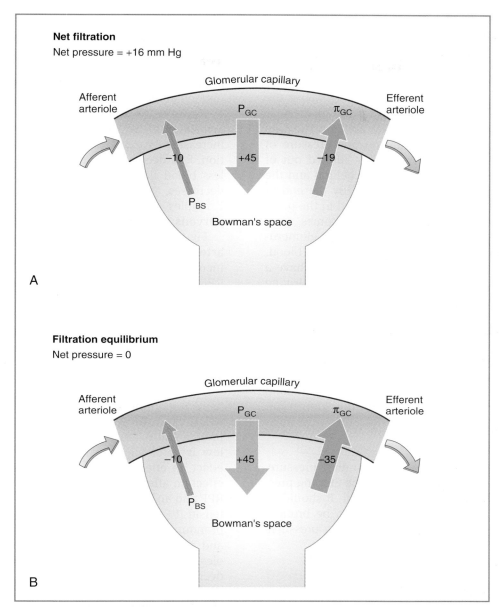

Figure 6–10 **Starling forces across the glomerular capillaries. A,** Net filtration; **B,** filtration equilibrium. *Arrows* show the direction of the Starling pressures; *numbers* are the magnitude of the pressure (mm Hg); *+ signs* show pressures that favor filtration; *– signs* show pressures that oppose filtration. P_{GC}, Hydrostatic pressure in the glomerular capillary; P_{BS}, hydrostatic pressure in Bowman's space; π_{GC}, oncotic pressure in the glomerular capillary.

absorption into the capillary. The *size* of the arrow indicates the relative magnitude of the pressure. The numerical value of the pressure (in mm Hg) has a *plus sign* if the pressure favors filtration and a *minus sign* if the pressure favors absorption. The net ultrafiltration pressure, which is the driving force, is the algebraic sum of the three pressures.

Figure 6-10*A* shows the profile of the Starling pressures at the **beginning of the glomerular capillary.** At the beginning of the glomerular capillary, blood has just come from the afferent arteriole and no filtration

has yet occurred. The sum of the three Starling pressures, or the net ultrafiltration pressure, is +16 mm Hg; thus, the net ultrafiltration pressure strongly favors filtration.

Figure 6-10*B* shows the three Starling pressures at the **end of the glomerular capillary.** At this point, the blood has been extensively filtered and is about to leave the glomerular capillary to enter the efferent arteriole. The sum of the three Starling pressures now is zero. Because net ultrafiltration is zero, no filtration can occur, a point called **filtration equilibrium.**

Conveniently, filtration equilibrium normally occurs at the end of the glomerular capillary.

An important question to ask is *What causes filtration equilibrium to occur?* Stated differently, *Which Starling pressure has changed to make the net ultrafiltration pressure zero?* To answer this question, compare the Starling pressures at the beginning of the glomerular capillary with those at the end of the capillary. The only pressure that changes is π_{GC}, the oncotic pressure of glomerular capillary blood. As fluid is filtered out of the glomerular capillary, protein is left behind and the protein concentration and π_{GC} increase. By the end of the glomerular capillary, π_{GC} has increased to the point where the net ultrafiltration pressure becomes zero. (A related point is that this blood leaving the glomerular capillaries will become peritubular capillary blood. The peritubular capillary blood will, therefore, have a high oncotic pressure $[\pi_c]$, which becomes a driving force for reabsorption in the proximal tubule of the nephron.) There is no decrease in P_{GC} along the length of the glomerular capillaries, as occurs in systemic capillaries. The difference for glomerular capillaries is the presence of a second set of arterioles, the efferent arterioles. Constriction of efferent arterioles prevents the decline in P_{GC} that would otherwise occur as fluid is filtered out along the length of the glomerular capillaries.

Changes in Starling Pressures

The GFR depends on the net ultrafiltration pressure, which in turn depends on the sum of the Starling pressures across the glomerular capillary wall. It should be clear, therefore, that changes in GFR can be brought about by changes in any one of the Starling pressures (Table 6-6).

Table 6–6 Effect of Changes in Starling Forces on Renal Plasma Flow, Glomerular Filtration Rate, and the Filtration Fraction

Effect	RPF	GFR	Filtration Fraction (GFR/RPF)
Constriction of afferent arteriole	↓	↓	N.C.
Constriction of efferent arteriole	↓	↑	↑
Increased plasma protein concentration	N.C.	↓	↓
Decreased plasma protein concentration	N.C.	↑	↑
Constriction of the ureter	N.C.	↓	↓

GFR, Glomerular filtration rate; N.C., no change; RPF, renal plasma flow.

♦ **Changes in P_{GC}** are produced by changes in the resistance of the afferent and efferent arterioles. For reasons that will be apparent, changes in GFR occur in opposite directions, depending on which arteriole is affected. The mechanism underlying this phenomenon is shown in Figure 6-11.

Figure 6-11A shows **constriction of the afferent arteriole,** in which afferent arteriolar resistance increases. As expected with any arteriolar constriction, RPF decreases. GFR also decreases because, as less blood flows into the glomerular capillary, P_{GC} decreases, reducing net ultrafiltration pressure. Examples include the effects of the **sympathetic nervous system** and *high* levels of angiotensin II.

Figure 6-11B shows **constriction of the efferent arteriole,** in which efferent arteriolar resistance increases. The effect of arteriolar constriction on RPF is the same as with constriction of the afferent arteriole (decreases), yet the effect on GFR is opposite (increases). GFR increases because blood is restricted from leaving the glomerular capillary, causing P_{GC} and net ultrafiltration pressure to increase. An example is the effect of *low* levels of **angiotensin II.**

The effects of **angiotensin II** on RPF and GFR have important implications. Angiotensin II constricts both afferent and efferent arterioles, but it preferentially constricts efferent arterioles. Thus, a low level of angiotensin II has a large constrictor effect on efferent arterioles and a small constrictor effect on afferent arterioles, leading to a decrease in RPF and an increase in GFR. A higher level of angiotensin II (as seen in response to hemorrhage) has a pronounced constrictor effect on efferent arterioles and a medium constrictor effect on afferent arterioles, leading to a decrease in RPF and a smaller decrease in GFR. Thus, with both low and high levels of angiotensin II, because of its preferential effect on efferent arterioles, the GFR is "protected" or "preserved" in the setting of vasoconstriction. **Angiotensin-converting enzyme** (ACE) **inhibitors** block the production of angiotensin II and offset or eliminate its protective effect on GFR.

♦ **Changes in π_{GC}** are produced by changes in plasma protein concentration. Thus, increases in plasma protein concentration produce **increases in π_{GC},** which decrease both the net ultrafiltration pressure and GFR. On the other hand, decreases in plasma protein concentration (e.g., nephrotic syndrome, in which large amounts of protein are lost in urine) produce **decreases in π_{GC},** which increase both net ultrafiltration pressure and GFR.

♦ **Changes in P_{BS}** can be produced by obstructing urine flow (e.g., ureteral stone or constriction of a ureter). For example, if the **ureter is constricted,** urine cannot flow through that ureter to the bladder,

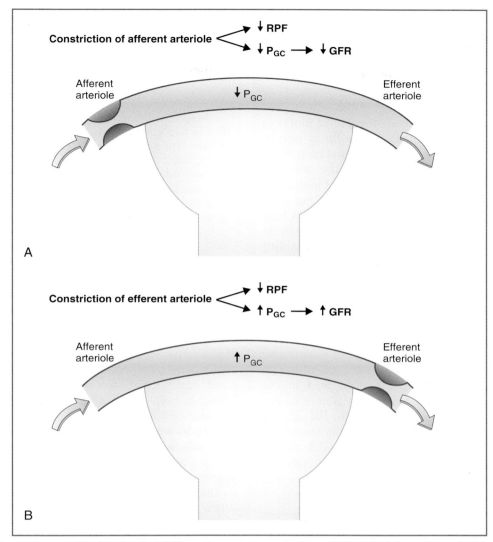

Figure 6–11 **Effects of constricting afferent (A) and efferent (B) arterioles on renal plasma flow (RPF) and glomerular filtration rate (GFR).** P_{GC}, Hydrostatic pressure in the glomerular capillary.

causing urine to back up in the kidney. Consequently, hydrostatic pressure in the nephrons will increase as far back as Bowman's space, producing an increase in P_{BS}. An increase in P_{BS} decreases the net ultrafiltration pressure, thereby decreasing GFR.

Measurement of Glomerular Filtration Rate

GFR is measured by the clearance of a glomerular marker. A **glomerular marker** has the following three characteristics: (1) It must be freely filtered across the glomerular capillaries, with no size or charge restrictions; (2) it cannot be reabsorbed or secreted by the renal tubule; and (3) when infused, it cannot alter the GFR. Thus, the properties of the ideal glomerular marker differ from those of a marker substance used to measure RPF (i.e., PAH).

Clearance of Inulin

The ideal glomerular marker is **inulin,** a fructose polymer with a molecular weight of approximately 5000 daltons. Inulin is not bound to plasma proteins, nor is it charged, and its molecular size is such that it is **freely filtered** across the glomerular capillary wall. Once filtered, inulin is completely inert in the renal tubule: It is **neither reabsorbed nor secreted** by the renal tubular cells. Thus, the amount of inulin filtered across the glomerular capillaries is exactly equal to the amount of inulin that is excreted in the urine.

The clearance of inulin equals the GFR, as expressed in the following equation:

$$GFR = \frac{[U]_{inulin} \times \dot{V}}{[P]_{inulin}} = C_{inulin}$$

where

$$\text{GFR} = \text{Glomerular filtration rate (mL/min)}$$
$$[\text{U}]_{\text{inulin}} = \text{Urine concentration of inulin (mg/mL)}$$
$$[\text{P}]_{\text{inulin}} = \text{Plasma concentration of inulin (mg/mL)}$$
$$\dot{\text{V}} = \text{Urine flow rate (mL/min)}$$
$$\text{C}_{\text{inulin}} = \text{Clearance of inulin (mL/min)}$$

Several additional points about the use of inulin to measure GFR should be noted: (1) Inulin is not an endogenous substance and, therefore, must be infused intravenously. (2) The numerator of the fraction, $[\text{U}]_{\text{inulin}} \times \dot{\text{V}}$, is equal to the excretion rate of inulin. (3) Changes in plasma inulin concentration *do not alter GFR*, although examination of the equation might lead to the opposite conclusion. For example, an increase in plasma inulin concentration (by infusing more inulin) *does not* decrease GFR, according to the following logic: When the plasma inulin concentration increases, the amount of inulin filtered also increases, which increases the amount of inulin excreted (i.e., $[\text{U}]_{\text{inulin}} \times \dot{\text{V}}$). Thus, both the numerator and the denominator increase proportionately, and the calculated value of GFR is unaffected. (4) GFR (or the clearance of inulin) also is unaffected by changes in urine flow rate, although inspection of the equation might again lead to the opposite conclusion. When urine flow rate ($\dot{\text{V}}$) increases, the urine concentration of inulin, $[\text{U}]_{\text{inulin}}$, decreases proportionately by dilution. Thus, the numerator ($[\text{U}]_{\text{inulin}} \times \dot{\text{V}}$) and the calculated value of GFR will be unaffected by such a change in urine flow rate, as illustrated in the following sample problem:

SAMPLE PROBLEM. A woman who consents to renal studies in the Clinical Research Center is infused with inulin to measure her GFR. Over the course of the measurement, her urine flow rate is intentionally varied by having her drink large amounts of water. The $[\text{P}]_{\text{inulin}}$ is kept constant at 1 mg/mL with an infusion. The urine flow rate and $[\text{U}]_{\text{inulin}}$ before and after she drinks water are as follows:

Before drinking water	After drinking water
$[\text{U}]_{\text{inulin}} = 100$ mg/mL	$[\text{U}]_{\text{inulin}} = 20$ mg/mL
$\dot{\text{V}} = 1$ mL/min	$\dot{\text{V}} = 5$ mL/min

What is the effect of the increase in urine flow (produced by drinking water) on the woman's GFR?

SOLUTION. Calculate the GFR from the clearance of inulin before and after the woman drank water.

$$\text{GFR before drinking water} = \frac{[\text{U}]_{\text{inulin}} \times \dot{\text{V}}}{[\text{P}]_{\text{inulin}}}$$
$$= \frac{100 \text{ mg/mL} \times 1 \text{ mL/min}}{1 \text{ mg/mL}}$$
$$= 100 \text{ mL/min}$$

$$\text{GFR after drinking water} = \frac{[\text{U}]_{\text{inulin}} \times \dot{\text{V}}}{[\text{P}]_{\text{inulin}}}$$
$$= \frac{20 \text{ mg/mL} \times 5 \text{ mL/min}}{1 \text{ mg/mL}}$$
$$= 100 \text{ mL/min}$$

Despite urine flow rate being markedly different in the two conditions, GFR was absolutely constant. As the urine flow rate increased from 1 mL/min to 5 mL/min, $[\text{U}]_{\text{inulin}}$ decreased (by dilution) from 100 mg/mL to 20 mg/mL (a proportional change).

Other Markers for Glomerular Filtration Rate

Inulin is the only perfect glomerular marker; no other marker is perfect. The closest substance is **creatinine,** which is freely filtered across the glomerular capillaries but also secreted to a small extent. Thus, the clearance of creatinine slightly overestimates the GFR. The convenience of using creatinine, however, outweighs this small error: Creatinine is an endogenous substance (inulin is not), and it need not be infused in order to measure GFR.

Both **blood urea nitrogen** (**BUN**) and **serum creatinine concentration** can be used to estimate GFR because both urea and creatinine are filtered across the glomerular capillaries. Thus, each substance depends on the filtration step in order to be excreted in urine. When there is a decrease in GFR (e.g., in renal failure), BUN and serum creatinine increase because they are not adequately filtered.

Volume contraction (hypovolemia) results in decreased renal perfusion and, as a consequence, decreased GFR (**prerenal azotemia**). In prerenal azotemia, both BUN and serum creatinine are increased due to the decrease in GFR. However, because urea is reabsorbed and creatinine is not, BUN increases more than serum creatinine; in volume contraction, there is increased proximal reabsorption of all solutes, including urea, which is responsible for the greater increase in BUN. One indicator, therefore, of volume contraction (*prerenal* azotemia) is an **increased ratio of BUN/creatinine** to more than 20. In contrast, renal failure due to *renal* causes (e.g., chronic renal failure) produces an increase in both BUN and serum creatinine, but it does not produce an increase in the ratio of BUN/creatinine.

Filtration Fraction

The filtration fraction expresses the relationship between the glomerular filtration rate (GFR) and renal plasma flow (RPF). The filtration fraction is given by the following equation:

$$\text{Filtration fraction} = \frac{\text{GFR}}{\text{RPF}}$$

In other words, the filtration fraction is that fraction of the RPF that is filtered across the glomerular capillaries. The value for the filtration fraction is normally about **0.20, or 20%.** That is, 20% of the RPF is filtered and 80% is not filtered. The 80% of RPF that is not filtered leaves the glomerular capillaries via the efferent arterioles and becomes the peritubular capillary blood flow.

As an exercise, think about the effect of changes in filtration fraction on the protein concentration and oncotic pressure (π_c) of peritubular capillary blood. If the filtration fraction were to increase (see Table 6-6), relatively more fluid would be filtered out of glomerular capillary blood, resulting in a greater than usual increase in the protein concentration of the capillary blood. Thus, increases in the filtration fraction produce increases in the protein concentration and π_c of peritubular capillary blood (which has consequences for the reabsorptive mechanism in the proximal tubule that is discussed later in this chapter).

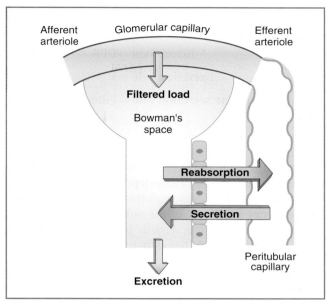

Figure 6–12 **Processes of filtration, reabsorption, and secretion in a nephron.** The sum of the three processes is excretion.

REABSORPTION AND SECRETION

Glomerular filtration results in the production of large quantities (180 L/day) of an ultrafiltrate of plasma. If this ultrafiltrate were excreted unmodified, the following quantities would be lost in the urine each day: 180 L of water; 25,200 mEq of Na^+; 19,800 mEq of Cl^-; 4320 mEq of HCO_3^-; and 14,400 mg of glucose. Each of these losses represents more than 10-fold the amount present in the *entire* ECF. Fortunately, reabsorptive mechanisms in the epithelial cells lining the renal tubule return these substances to the circulation and to the ECF. In addition, secretion mechanisms in the epithelial cells remove certain substances from the peritubular capillary blood and add it to urine.

Measurement of Reabsorption and Secretion

The processes of filtration, reabsorption, and secretion are illustrated in Figure 6-12. A glomerular capillary is shown with its afferent and efferent arterioles. The initial part of the nephron (Bowman's space and the beginning of the proximal convoluted tubule) is shown, lined with epithelial cells. Nearby is a peritubular capillary, which emerges from the efferent arteriole and supplies blood to the nephron.

♦ **Filtration.** An interstitial-type fluid is filtered across the glomerular capillary into Bowman's space. The

amount of a substance filtered into Bowman's space per unit time is called the **filtered load.** The fluid in Bowman's space and in the lumen of the nephron is called tubular fluid or luminal fluid.

♦ **Reabsorption.** Water and many solutes (e.g., Na^+, Cl^-, HCO_3^-, glucose, amino acids, urea, Ca^{2+}, Mg^{2+}, phosphate, lactate, and citrate) are reabsorbed from the glomerular filtrate into the peritubular capillary blood. The mechanisms for reabsorption involve transporters in the membranes of the renal epithelial cells. As emphasized, if reabsorption did not occur, most of these constituents of ECF would be rapidly lost in the urine.

♦ **Secretion.** A few substances (e.g., organic acids, organic bases, K^+) are secreted from peritubular capillary blood into tubular fluid. Thus, in addition to filtration, secretion provides a mechanism for excreting substances in the urine. As with reabsorption, the secretion mechanisms involve transporters in the membranes of the epithelial cells lining the nephron.

♦ **Excretion.** Excretion or excretion rate refers to the amount of a substance excreted per unit time. Excretion is the net result, or sum, of the processes of filtration, reabsorption, and secretion. The excretion rate can be compared with the filtered load to determine whether a substance has been reabsorbed or secreted.

The following equations are used to calculate filtered load, excretion rate, and reabsorption or secretion rate:

$$\text{Filtered load} = \text{GFR} \times [P]_x$$

$$\text{Excretion rate} = \dot{V} \times [U]_x$$

$$\text{Reabsorption or secretion rate} = \text{Filtered load} - \text{Excretion rate}$$

In words, the difference between the filtered load and the excretion rate is the rate of net reabsorption or net secretion. If the filtered load is greater than the excretion rate, there has been **net reabsorption** of the substance. If the filtered load is less than the excretion rate, there has been **net secretion** of the substance. This type of calculation is shown in Figure 6-13; one example is given for a substance that is reabsorbed, and another example is given for a substance that is secreted.

Figure 6-13*A* illustrates the renal handling of Na^+, a solute that is freely filtered and subsequently reabsorbed. In this example, the filtered load of Na^+ is 25,200 mEq/day (GFR × $[P]_{Na^+}$), and the excretion rate of Na^+ is 100 mEq/day ($\dot{V} \times [U]_{Na^+}$). Because the filtered load of Na^+ is higher than the excretion rate, there must have been **net reabsorption of Na^+.** The kidney reabsorbs 25,100 mEq/day, which is 99.4% of the filtered load (25,100 mEq/25,200 mEq).

Figure 6-13*B* illustrates the renal handling of PAH, a solute that is filtered and subsequently secreted. In this example, the filtered load of PAH is 18 g/day (GFR × $[P]_{PAH}$), and the excretion rate of PAH is 54 g/day ($\dot{V} \times [U]_{PAH}$). Because the filtered load of PAH is less than the excretion rate, there must have been **net secretion of PAH,** amounting to 36 g/day (excretion rate − filtered load). In this example, the secretion rate of PAH is twice that of the original filtered load.

Glucose—Example of Reabsorption

Glucose is filtered across glomerular capillaries and reabsorbed by the epithelial cells of the proximal convoluted tubule. Glucose reabsorption is a two-step process involving **Na^+-glucose cotransport** across the luminal membrane and **facilitated glucose transport** across the peritubular membrane. Because there are a limited number of glucose transporters, the mechanism is saturable; that is, it has a **transport maximum,** or **T_m.**

Cellular Mechanism for Glucose Reabsorption

Figure 6-14 shows the cellular mechanism for glucose reabsorption in the early proximal tubule. The luminal membrane of the epithelial cells faces the tubular fluid (lumen) and contains the Na^+-glucose cotransporter. The peritubular membrane or basolateral membrane of the cells faces the peritubular capillary blood and contains the Na^+-K^+ ATPase and the facilitated glucose transporter. The following steps are involved in reabsorbing glucose from tubular fluid into peritubular capillary blood:

1. Glucose moves from tubular fluid into the cell on the **Na^+-glucose cotransporter** (called **SGLT**) in the luminal membrane. Two Na^+ ions and one glucose bind to the cotransport protein, the protein rotates in the membrane, and Na^+ and glucose are released into the ICF. In this step, glucose is transported against an electrochemical gradient; the energy for this *uphill* transport of glucose comes from the *downhill* movement of Na^+.

2. The Na^+ gradient is maintained by the Na^+-K^+ ATPase in the peritubular membrane. Because ATP is used *directly* to energize the Na^+-K^+ ATPase and *indirectly* to maintain the Na^+ gradient, Na^+-glucose cotransport is called **secondary active transport.**

3. Glucose is transported from the cell into peritubular capillary blood by **facilitated diffusion.** In this step, glucose is moving down its electrochemical gradient and no energy is required. The proteins involved in facilitated diffusion of glucose are called **GLUT 1** and **GLUT 2,** which belong to a larger family of glucose carriers.

Glucose Titration Curve and T_m

A **glucose titration curve** depicts the relationship between plasma glucose concentration and glucose reabsorption (Fig. 6-15). For comparison, the filtered load of glucose and the excretion rate of glucose are plotted on the same graph. The glucose titration curve is obtained experimentally by infusing glucose and measuring its rate of reabsorption as the plasma concentration is increased. The titration curve is best understood by examining each relationship separately and then by considering all three relationships together.

♦ **Filtered load.** Glucose is freely filtered across glomerular capillaries, and the filtered load is the product of GFR and plasma glucose concentration (filtered load = GFR × $[P]_x$). Thus, as the plasma glucose concentration is increased, the filtered load increases linearly.

♦ **Reabsorption.** At plasma glucose concentrations less than 200 mg/dL, all of the filtered glucose can be reabsorbed because Na^+-glucose cotransporters are plentiful. In this range, the curve for reabsorption is identical to that for filtration; that is, reabsorption equals filtration. The number of carriers is limited, however. At plasma concentrations above 200 mg/dL, the reabsorption curve *bends* because some of the filtered glucose is not reabsorbed. At plasma concentrations above 350 mg/dL, the carriers are completely **saturated** and reabsorption levels off at its maximal value, **T_m.**

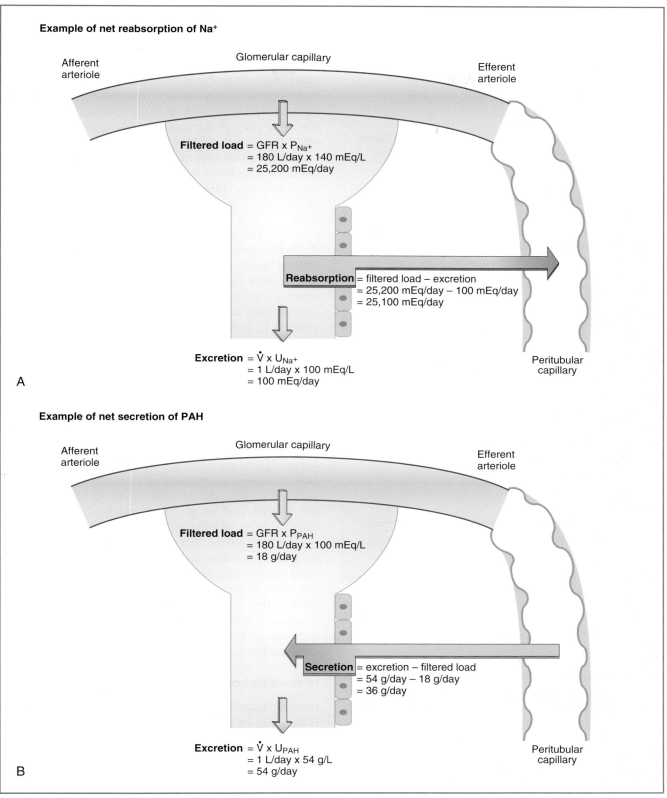

Figure 6–13 **Examples of substances that are reabsorbed or secreted. A,** Example of net reabsorption of Na⁺. Na⁺ is filtered and reabsorbed by the renal epithelial cells; Na⁺ excretion is the difference between filtered load and reabsorption rate. **B,** Example of net secretion of PAH (*Para*-aminohippuric acid). PAH is filtered and secreted by renal epithelial cells; PAH excretion is the sum of filtered load plus secretion rate. Calculations are shown for filtered load, reabsorption or secretion rate, and excretion rate (mEq/day). GFR, Glomerular filtration rate; P_{Na^+}, plasma concentration of Na⁺; P_{PAH}, plasma concentration of PAH; U_{Na^+}, urine concentration of Na⁺; U_{PAH}, urine concentration of PAH.

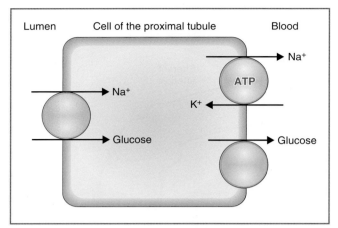

Figure 6–14 **Cellular mechanism of glucose reabsorption in the early proximal tubule.**

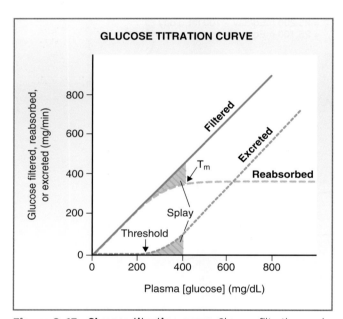

Figure 6–15 **Glucose titration curve.** Glucose filtration, reabsorption, and excretion are shown as a function of plasma glucose concentration. *Hatched areas* are the splay. T_m, Tubular transport maximum.

♦ **Excretion.** To understand the curve for excretion, compare those for filtration and reabsorption. Below plasma glucose concentrations of 200 mg/dL, all of the filtered glucose is reabsorbed and none is excreted. At plasma glucose concentrations above 200 mg/dL, the carriers are nearing the saturation point. Most of the filtered glucose is reabsorbed, but some is not; the glucose that is not reabsorbed is excreted. The plasma concentration at which glucose is first excreted in the urine is called **threshold,** which occurs at a lower plasma concentration than does T_m. Above 350 mg/dL, T_m is reached and the carriers are fully saturated. The curve for excretion now increases linearly as a function

of plasma glucose concentration, paralleling that for filtration.

The T_m for glucose is approached gradually, rather than sharply (see Fig. 6-15), a phenomenon called **splay.** Splay is that portion of the titration curve where reabsorption is *approaching* saturation, but it is not *fully* saturated. Because of splay, glucose is excreted in the urine (i.e., at threshold) before reabsorption levels off at the T_m value.

There are two explanations for splay. The first explanation is based on a **low affinity** of the Na⁺-glucose cotransporter. Thus, near T_m, if glucose detaches from its carrier, it will be excreted into the urine because there are few remaining binding sites where it may reattach. The second explanation for splay is based on the **heterogeneity** of nephrons. T_m for the whole kidney reflects the *average* T_m of all nephrons, yet all nephrons do not have exactly the same T_m. Some nephrons will reach T_m at lower plasma concentration than others, and glucose will be excreted in the urine before the average T_m is reached.

Glucosuria

At normal plasma glucose concentrations (70 to 100 mg/dL), all of the filtered glucose is reabsorbed and none is excreted. Under some circumstances, however, **glucosuria** (excretion or spilling of glucose in the urine) occurs. The causes of glucosuria can be understood by referring again to the glucose titration curve. (1) In uncontrolled **diabetes mellitus,** lack of insulin causes the plasma concentration of glucose to increase to abnormally high levels. In this condition, the filtered load of glucose exceeds the reabsorptive capacity (i.e., plasma glucose concentration is above the T_m), and glucose is excreted in the urine. (2) During **pregnancy,** GFR is increased, which increases the filtered load of glucose to the extent that it may exceed the reabsorptive capacity. (3) Several congenital **abnormalities of the Na⁺-glucose cotransporter** are associated with decreases in T_m, causing glucose to be excreted in the urine at lower than normal plasma concentrations (Box 6-1).

Urea—Example of Passive Reabsorption

Urea is transported in most segments of the nephron (Fig. 6-16). In contrast to glucose, which is reabsorbed by carrier-mediated mechanisms, urea is reabsorbed or secreted by diffusion (simple diffusion and facilitated diffusion). The rate of reabsorption or secretion is determined by the concentration difference for urea between tubular fluid and blood and by the permeability of the epithelial cells to urea. When there is a large concentration difference and the permeability is high, urea reabsorption is high; when there is a small concentration difference and/or the permeability is low, urea reabsorption is low.

BOX 6–1   Clinical Physiology: Glucosuria

DESCRIPTION OF CASE. A woman sees her physician because of excessive thirst and urination. During the previous week, she urinated hourly during the day and four or five times each night. Her physician tests her urine using a dipstick and detects glucose. She is asked to fast overnight and to report the following morning for a glucose tolerance test. After drinking a glucose solution, her blood glucose concentration increases from 200 to 800 mg/dL. Urine is collected at timed intervals throughout the test to measure urine volume and glucose concentration. The woman's glomerular filtration rate (GFR) is estimated to be 120 mL/min from her endogenous creatinine clearance. When the reabsorption rate of glucose is calculated (filtered load of glucose – excretion rate of glucose), it is found to be constant, at 375 mg/min. The physician concludes that the cause of the woman's glucosuria is type I diabetes mellitus (rather than a defect in the renal glucose transport mechanism).

EXPLANATION OF CASE. There are two possible explanations for this woman's glucosuria: (1) a defect in the renal transport mechanism for glucose or (2) an increased filtered load of glucose that exceeds the reabsorptive capacity of the proximal tubule. To determine which explanation is correct, the maximal reabsorption rate for glucose (T_m) is determined by measuring the reabsorption rate as the plasma glucose concentration is increased. A value of T_m of 375 mg/min is found, which is considered normal. Thus, the physician concludes that the basis for the woman's glucosuria is an abnormally elevated blood glucose concentration due to insufficient secretion of insulin from the pancreas. If the glucosuria had been caused by a renal defect, the T_m would be lower than normal.

Excessive urination is caused by the presence of nonreabsorbed glucose in tubular fluid. The glucose acts as an osmotic diuretic, holds water, and increases urine production. The woman's excessive thirst is partially explained by the excessive urine production. In addition, the high blood glucose concentration increases her blood osmolarity and stimulates the thirst center.

TREATMENT. The woman is treated with regular injections of insulin.

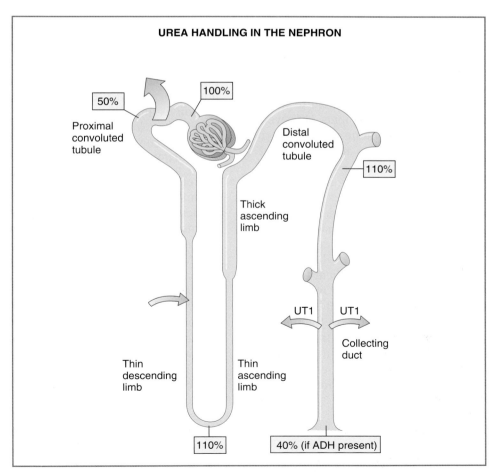

Figure 6–16   Urea handling in the nephron. *Arrows* show locations of urea reabsorption or secretion; numbers are percentages of the filtered load remaining at various points along the nephron. UT1, urea transporter 1. ADH, Antidiuretic hormone.

Urea is freely filtered across the glomerular capillaries, and the concentration in the initial filtrate is identical to that in blood (i.e., initially, there is no concentration difference or driving force for urea reabsorption). However, as water is reabsorbed along the nephron, the urea concentration in tubular fluid increases, creating a driving force for passive urea reabsorption. Therefore, urea reabsorption generally follows the same pattern as water reabsorption—the greater the water reabsorption, the greater the urea reabsorption and the lower the urea excretion.

In the **proximal tubule,** 50% of the filtered urea is reabsorbed by simple diffusion. As water is reabsorbed in the proximal tubule, urea lags slightly behind, causing the urea concentration in the tubular lumen to become slightly higher than the urea concentration in blood; this concentration difference then drives passive urea reabsorption. At the end of the proximal tubule, 50% of the filtered urea has been reabsorbed; thus, 50% remains in the lumen. In the **thin descending limb of Henle's loop,** urea is secreted. By mechanisms that will be described later, there is a high concentration of urea in the interstitial fluid of the inner medulla. The thin descending limb of Henle's loop passes through the inner medulla, and urea diffuses from high concentration in the interstitial fluid into the lumen of the nephron. More urea is secreted into the thin descending limbs than was reabsorbed in the proximal tubule; thus, at the bend of the loop of Henle, 110% of the filtered load of urea is present. The **thick ascending limb of Henle, distal tubule, and cortical and outer medullary collecting ducts** are impermeable to urea, so no urea transport occurs in these segments. However, in the presence of antidiuretic hormone (ADH), water is reabsorbed in the late distal tubule and the cortical and outer medullary collecting ducts—consequently, in these segments, urea is "left behind" and the urea concentration of the tubular fluid becomes quite high. In the **inner medullary collecting ducts,** there is a specific transporter for the facilitated diffusion of urea (urea transporter 1, **UT1**), which is activated by ADH. Thus, in the presence of ADH, urea is reabsorbed by UT1, moving down its concentration gradient from the lumen into the interstitial fluid of the inner medulla. In the presence of ADH, approximately 70% of the filtered urea is reabsorbed by UT1, leaving 40% of the filtered urea to be excreted in the urine. The urea that is reabsorbed into the inner medulla contributes to the corticopapillary osmotic gradient in a process called **urea recycling,** which is discussed in later sections.

Para-Aminohippuric Acid—Example of Secretion

PAH has been introduced as the substance used to measure RPF. PAH is an **organic acid** that is both

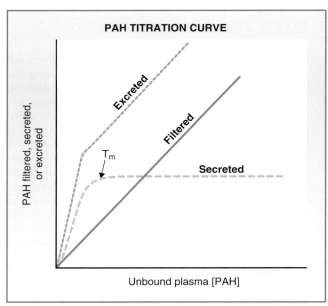

Figure 6-17 **PAH titration curve.** PAH (*para*-aminohippuric acid) filtration, secretion, and excretion are shown as a function of plasma PAH concentration. T_m, Tubular transport maximum.

filtered across glomerular capillaries and secreted from peritubular capillary blood into tubular fluid. As with glucose, PAH filtration, secretion, and excretion can be plotted simultaneously (Fig. 6-17). (For PAH, secretion is plotted instead of reabsorption.)

♦ **Filtered load.** Ten percent of the PAH in blood is bound to plasma proteins, and only the *unbound* portion is filterable across glomerular capillaries. The filtered load of PAH increases linearly as the *unbound* concentration of PAH increases (filtered load = GFR × [P]$_x$).

♦ **Secretion.** The transporters for PAH (and other organic anions) are located in the peritubular membranes of proximal tubule cells. These carriers have a finite capacity to bind and transport PAH across the cell, from blood to lumen. At low concentrations of PAH, many carriers are available and secretion increases linearly as the plasma concentration increases. When the PAH concentration increases to a level where the carriers are saturated, T_m is reached. After this point, no matter how much the PAH concentration increases, there can be no further increase in the secretion rate. The PAH transporter also is responsible for secretion of drugs such as **penicillin** and is inhibited by **probenecid.**

Incidentally, just as there is secretion of organic acids such as PAH, there are parallel secretory mechanisms for **organic bases** (e.g., quinine, morphine) in the proximal tubule. These secretory mechanisms for organic acids and bases are relevant in the discussion of non-ionic diffusion that follows.

♦ **Excretion.** For a secreted substance such as PAH, excretion is the sum of filtration and secretion. At low PAH concentrations (below T_m), excretion increases steeply with increases in plasma PAH concentration because both filtration and secretion are increasing. At PAH concentrations above T_m, excretion increases less steeply (and parallels the curve for filtration) because only the filtration component increases as concentration increases; secretion is already saturated.

Weak Acids and Bases—Non-Ionic Diffusion

Many of the substances secreted by the proximal tubule are weak acids (e.g., PAH, salicylic acid) or weak bases (e.g., quinine, morphine). Weak acids and bases exist in two forms, charged and uncharged, and the relative amount of each form depends on pH (see Chapter 7). **Weak acids** exist in an acid form, HA, and a conjugate base form, A^-. At low pH, the HA form, which is *uncharged,* predominates. At high pH, the A^- form, which is *charged,* predominates. For **weak bases,** the base form is B and the conjugate acid is BH^+. At low pH, the BH^+ form, which is *charged,* predominates. At high pH, the B form, which is *uncharged,* predominates. With respect to the renal excretion of weak acids and bases, the relevant points are (1) the relative amounts of the charged and uncharged species depend on urine pH, and (2) only the uncharged (i.e., "non-ionic") species can diffuse across the cells.

To illustrate the role of **non-ionic diffusion** in the renal excretion of weak acids and bases, consider the excretion of a **weak acid,** salicylic acid (HA) and its conjugate base, salicylate (A^-). For the remainder of this discussion, both forms are called "salicylate." Like PAH, salicylate is filtered across the glomerular capillaries and secreted by an organic acid secretory mechanism in the proximal tubule. As a result of these two processes, the urinary concentration of salicylate becomes much higher than the blood concentration and a concentration gradient across the cells is established. In the urine, salicylate exists in both HA and A^- forms. The HA form, being uncharged, can diffuse across the cells, from urine to blood, down this concentration gradient; the A^- form, being charged, cannot diffuse. At **acidic urine pH,** HA predominates, there is more "back-diffusion" from urine into blood, and the excretion (and clearance) of salicylate is decreased. At **alkaline urine pH,** A^- predominates, there is less "back-diffusion" from urine to blood, and the excretion (and clearance) of salicylate is increased. This relationship is illustrated in Figure 6-18, which shows that the clearance of a weak acid is highest at alkaline urine pH and lowest at acidic urine pH. The principle of non-ionic diffusion is the basis for treating aspirin (salicylate) overdose by alkalinizing the urine—at

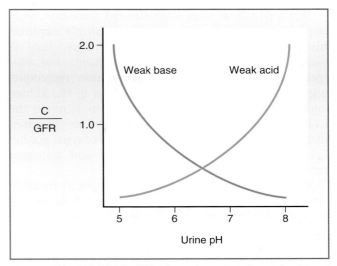

Figure 6–18 **Nonionic diffusion.** Clearance of a weak acid and a weak base as a function of urine pH. C, Clearance of weak acid or base; GFR, glomerular filtration rate.

alkaline urine pH, relatively more salicylate is in the A^- form, which does not diffuse back into blood and is excreted in the urine.

The effect of nonionic diffusion on the excretion of weak bases is the mirror image of its effect on weak acids (see Fig. 6-18). The **weak base** is both filtered and secreted, which results in a urine concentration that is higher than the blood concentration. In the urine, the weak base exists in both BH^+ and B forms. The B form, being uncharged, can diffuse across the cells, from urine to blood, down this concentration gradient; the BH^+ form, being charged, cannot diffuse. At **alkaline urine pH,** B predominates, there is more "back-diffusion" from urine into blood, and the excretion (and clearance) of the weak base is decreased. At **acidic urine pH,** BH^+ predominates, there is less "back-diffusion" from urine to blood, and the excretion (and clearance) of the weak base is increased.

TERMINOLOGY ASSOCIATED WITH THE SINGLE NEPHRON

The remainder of the chapter is concerned with the renal handling of specific substances such as Na^+, Cl^-, HCO_3^-, K^+, and H_2O. One level of understanding can be achieved at the level of whole kidney function. For example, Na^+ is freely filtered across the glomerular capillaries, almost completely reabsorbed, and only a small fraction of the filtered load is excreted. However, *What are the details of the reabsorption process? Is Na^+ reabsorbed throughout the nephron or only in certain segments, and what cellular transport mechanisms are involved?*

To answer these more sophisticated questions, techniques have been developed to study **single nephron function.** In the micropuncture technique, fluid is sampled directly from individual nephrons and analyzed. In the isolated perfused nephron technique, segments of nephrons are dissected out of the kidney and perfused with artificial solutions in vitro. In the isolated membrane technique, vesicles are prepared from luminal or basolateral membranes of renal epithelial cells to study their biochemical and transport properties.

The terms associated with single nephron function are parallel to those used to describe whole kidney function. For example, "U" represents urine in whole kidney terminology and the parallel term for the single nephron, "TF," represents tubular fluid. "GFR" represents whole kidney glomerular filtration rate, and "SNGFR" is the filtration rate of a single nephron. A summary of terms, abbreviations, and meanings is provided in Table 6-3.

[TF/P]$_x$ Ratio

The [TF/P]$_x$ ratio compares the concentration of a substance in tubular fluid with its concentration in systemic plasma. Using the micropuncture technique, the [TF/P]$_x$ ratio can be measured at various points along the nephron, beginning in Bowman's space. *Plasma concentrations are assumed to be constant,* and any changes in the [TF/P]$_x$, therefore, reflect changes in tubular fluid concentration.

To understand how the [TF/P]$_x$ ratio is applied, consider a simple example. Assume that the [TF/P]$_{Na^+}$ ratio was measured in Bowman's space and found to be 1.0. A value of 1.0 means that the tubular fluid Na^+ concentration is equal to the plasma Na^+ concentration. This value makes perfect sense, based on knowledge of glomerular filtration: Na^+ is freely filtered across the glomerular capillaries into Bowman's space, and the Na^+ concentration of the filtrate should be identical to the plasma concentration (with a small Gibbs-Donnan correction). No reabsorption or secretion has yet taken place. The generalization can be made that *for any freely filtered substance, [TF/P]$_x$ is 1.0 in Bowman's space* (before any reabsorption or secretion has taken place to modify it).

The following interpretations can be given for values of [TF/P]$_x$, where x is any solute. Again, the plasma concentration of x is assumed to be constant.

♦ **[TF/P]$_x$ = 1.0.** A value of 1.0 can have two meanings. The *first* meaning is illustrated in the preceding example: In Bowman's space, [TF/P]$_x$ for a freely filtered substance is 1.0 because no reabsorption or secretion has yet occurred. The *second* meaning is more complicated. Suppose that tubular fluid is sampled at the end of the proximal tubule, and [TF/P]$_x$ is found to be 1.0. *Does that mean that no reabsorption or secretion of the solute has occurred in the proximal tubule?* Not necessarily. It is also possible that reabsorption of the solute has occurred, but reabsorption of water has occurred in exactly the same proportion. If the solute and water are proportionally reabsorbed, the concentration of the solute in tubular fluid does not change. In fact, this is precisely what happens in the case of Na^+ in the proximal tubule: Na^+ is reabsorbed, but [TF/P]$_{Na^+}$ remains 1.0 along the entire proximal tubule because there is proportionality of Na^+ and water reabsorption.

♦ **[TF/P]$_x$ < 1.0.** A value less than 1.0 has only one meaning. Reabsorption of the solute must have been greater than reabsorption of water, causing the concentration of solute in tubular fluid to decrease below that in plasma.

♦ **[TF/P]$_x$ > 1.0.** A value greater than 1.0 has two possible meanings. The *first* meaning is that there has been net reabsorption of the solute, but solute reabsorption has been less than water reabsorption. When solute reabsorption lags behind water reabsorption, the tubular fluid concentration of the solute increases. The *second* meaning is that there has been net secretion of the solute into tubular fluid, causing its concentration to increase above that in plasma.

[TF/P]$_{Inulin}$

The previous discussion about values of [TF/P]$_x$ emphasizes how their interpretation requires a simultaneous knowledge of water reabsorption. Recall one of the questions asked: *Does [TF/P]$_x$ equal 1.0 because there has been filtration but no reabsorption or secretion? Or, does [TF/P]$_x$ equal 1.0 because there has been proportional reabsorption of the solute and water?* These two very different possibilities can be distinguished only if water reabsorption is measured simultaneously.

Inulin, the substance used to measure GFR, can also be used to **measure water reabsorption** in the single nephron. Recall that once inulin is filtered across glomerular capillaries, it is inert—that is, it is neither reabsorbed nor secreted. Thus, the concentration of inulin in tubular fluid is not affected by its own reabsorption or secretion, and it is only affected by the volume of water present. For example, in Bowman's space, the tubular fluid inulin concentration is identical to the plasma inulin concentration (because inulin is freely filtered). As water is reabsorbed along the nephron, the inulin concentration of tubular fluid steadily increases and becomes higher than the plasma concentration.

Water reabsorption can be calculated from the value of $[TF/P]_{inulin}$. Consider an example in which tubular fluid is sampled and the measured **$[TF/P]_{inulin}$ = 2.0.** In words, this means that the tubular fluid inulin concentration is twice the plasma inulin concentration. Water must have been reabsorbed in earlier portions of the nephron to cause the tubular fluid inulin concentration to double. *How much water was reabsorbed to achieve this value of [TF/P]$_{inulin}$?* This simple example can be analyzed intuitively: If the tubular fluid inulin concentration doubles, then 50% of the water must have been removed (i.e., reabsorbed).

Other values of $[TF/P]_{inulin}$ can be used to measure water reabsorption by the following equation:

$$\text{Fraction of filtered water reabsorbed} = 1 - \frac{1}{[TF/P]_{inulin}}$$

The equation can be understood by comparing it with the intuitive solution for **$[TF/P]_{inulin}$ = 2.0.** In that example, the fraction of the filtered water reabsorbed = 1 − 1/2 = 0.5 or 50%. The mathematical solution provides exactly the same answer as the intuitive approach, which also concluded that 50% of the water was reabsorbed.

Other values of $[TF/P]_{inulin}$ are not as easy to solve intuitively, and it may be necessary to use the equation. For example, if **$[TF/P]_{inulin}$ = 100,** the fraction of the filtered water reabsorbed = 1 − 1/100 = 1 − 0.01 = 0.99 or 99%. Incidentally, this is the value of $[TF/P]_{inulin}$ that could occur at the end of the collecting ducts, at which point 99% of the filtered water has been reabsorbed back into blood.

$[TF/P]_X/[TF/P]_{Inulin}$

The $[TF/P]_{inulin}$ ratio provides a tool for correcting $[TF/P]_x$ for water reabsorption. With this correction, it can be known with certainty whether a substance has been reabsorbed, secreted, or not transported at all. $[TF/P]_x/[TF/P]_{inulin}$ is a **double ratio** that makes this correction. The exact meaning of the double ratio is this: **fraction of the filtered load of substance x remaining** at any point along the nephron. For example, if $[TF/P]_x/[TF/P]_{inulin}$ = 0.3, then 30% of the filtered load of the solute remains in the tubular fluid at that point in the nephron, or 70% has been reabsorbed. This is approximately the situation for Na$^+$ at the end of the proximal tubule: $[TF/P]_{Na^+}/[TF/P]_{inulin}$ = 0.3, which means that 30% of the filtered Na$^+$ remains at that point and 70% has been reabsorbed. From the earlier discussion, recall that at the end of the proximal tubule $[TF/P]_{Na^+}$ = 1.0, which led to confusion about whether Na$^+$ was reabsorbed in the proximal tubule. Now, using the double ratio to correct for water reabsorption, the answer is clear: A large fraction of the filtered Na$^+$ *has been* reabsorbed, but because water is reabsorbed along with it, $[TF/P]_{Na^+}$ does not change from its value in Bowman's space.

SODIUM BALANCE

Of all functions of the kidney, reabsorption of sodium (Na$^+$) is the most important. Consider that Na$^+$ is the major cation of the ECF compartment, which consists of plasma and interstitial fluid. The amount of Na$^+$ in ECF determines the ECF volume, which in turn determines plasma volume, blood volume, and blood pressure (see Chapter 4). The renal mechanisms involved in reabsorption of Na$^+$ (i.e., returning Na$^+$ to ECF after filtration), therefore, are critically important for the maintenance of normal ECF volume, normal blood volume, and normal blood pressure.

The kidneys are responsible for maintaining a normal body Na$^+$ content. On a daily basis, the kidneys must ensure that Na$^+$ excretion exactly equals Na$^+$ intake, a matching process called **Na$^+$ balance.** For example, to remain in Na$^+$ balance, a person who ingests 150 mEq of Na$^+$ daily must excrete exactly 150 mEq of Na$^+$ daily.

If Na$^+$ excretion is less than Na$^+$ intake, then the person is in **positive Na$^+$ balance.** In this case, extra Na$^+$ is retained in the body, primarily in the ECF. When the Na$^+$ content of ECF is increased, there is increased ECF volume or **ECF volume expansion;** blood volume and arterial pressure also increase, and there may be **edema.**

Conversely, if Na$^+$ excretion is greater than Na$^+$ intake, then a person is in **negative Na$^+$ balance.** When excess Na$^+$ is lost from the body, there is a decreased Na$^+$ content of ECF, decreased ECF volume or **ECF volume contraction,** and decreased blood volume and arterial pressure.

An important distinction should be made between *Na$^+$ content* of the body (which determines ECF volume) and *Na$^+$ concentration.* Na$^+$ concentration is determined not only by the amount of Na$^+$ present but also by the volume of water. For example, a person can have an *increased* Na$^+$ content but a *normal* Na$^+$ concentration (if water content is increased proportionately). Or, a person can have an *increased* Na$^+$ concentration with a *normal* Na$^+$ content (if water content is decreased). In nearly all cases, changes in Na$^+$ *concentration* are caused by changes in body *water* content rather than Na$^+$ content. The kidney has separate mechanisms for regulating Na and water reabsorption.

Overall Handling of Na$^+$

Figure 6-19 shows the renal handling of Na$^+$ in the nephron. Na$^+$ is freely filtered across glomerular capillaries and subsequently reabsorbed throughout the

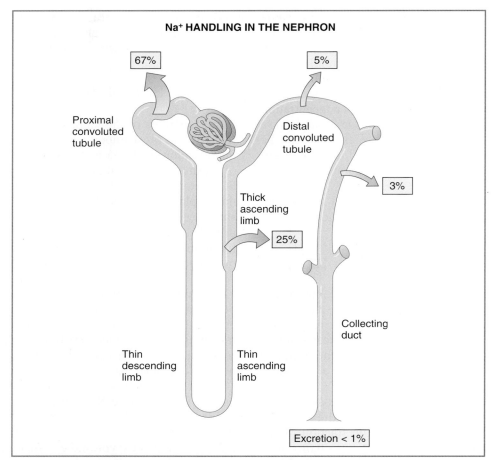

Figure 6–19 **Na⁺ handling in the nephron.** *Arrows* show locations of Na⁺ reabsorption; *numbers* are percentages of the filtered load reabsorbed or excreted.

nephron. The *arrows* show reabsorption in the various segments of the nephron, and the numbers give the approximate percentage of the filtered load reabsorbed in each segment. Excretion of Na⁺ is less than 1% of the filtered load, corresponding to net reabsorption of more than 99% of the filtered load.

By far, the bulk of the Na⁺ reabsorption occurs in the **proximal convoluted tubule,** where two thirds (or 67%) of the filtered load is reabsorbed. In the proximal tubule, water reabsorption is always linked to Na⁺ reabsorption and the mechanism is described as isosmotic.

The **thick ascending limb of the loop of Henle** reabsorbs 25% of the filtered load of Na⁺. In contrast to the proximal tubule, where water reabsorption is linked to Na⁺ reabsorption, the thick ascending limb is impermeable to water.

The terminal portions of the nephron (the distal tubule and the collecting ducts) reabsorb approximately 8% of the filtered load. The **early distal convoluted tubule** reabsorbs approximately 5% of the filtered load, and, like the thick ascending limb, it is impermeable to water. The **late distal convoluted tubule and**

collecting ducts reabsorb the final 3% of the filtered load and are responsible for the fine-tuning of Na⁺ reabsorption, which ultimately ensures Na⁺ balance. Not surprisingly, then, the late distal convoluted tubule and collecting duct are the sites of action of the Na⁺-regulating hormone **aldosterone.**

As emphasized, for a person to remain in **Na⁺ balance,** the amount of Na⁺ excreted in the urine (e.g., mEq/day) must be exactly equal to daily Na⁺ intake. With an average Na⁺ intake of 150 mEq/day, to maintain Na⁺ balance, excretion should be 150 mEq/day, which is less than 1% of the filtered load. (If GFR is 180 L/day and plasma Na⁺ concentration is 140 mEq/L, then the filtered load of Na⁺ is 25,200 mEq/day. Excretion of 150 mEq/day, therefore, is 0.6% of the filtered load [150 mEq/day divided by 25,200 mEq/day], as shown in Fig. 6-19.)

In terms of maintaining overall Na⁺ balance, each nephron segment plays a different role. Therefore, the segments will be discussed individually with regard to the quantity of the filtered Na⁺ reabsorbed and the cellular transport mechanisms. For a summary of the functions of each nephron segment, see Table 6-7.

Table 6–7 Summary of the Functions of the Major Nephron Segments

Segment/Cell Type	Major Functions	Cellular Mechanisms	Hormone Actions	Diuretic Actions
Early Proximal Tubule	Isosmotic reabsorption of solute and water	Na^+-glucose, Na^+-amino acid, Na^+-phosphate cotransport Na^+-H^+ exchange	PTH inhibits Na^+-phosphate cotransport Angiotensin II stimulates Na^+-H^+ exchange	Osmotic diuretics Carbonic anhydrase inhibitors
Late Proximal Tubule	Isosmotic reabsorption of solute and water	NaCl reabsorption driven by Cl^- gradient	—	Osmotic diuretics
Thick Ascending Limb of the Loop of Henle	Reabsorption of NaCl without water Dilution of tubular fluid Single effect of countercurrent multiplication Reabsorption of Ca^{2+} and Mg^{2+} driven by lumen-positive potential	Na^+-K^+-$2Cl^-$ cotransport	ADH stimulates Na^+-K^+-$2Cl^-$ cotransport	Loop diuretics
Early Distal Tubule	Reabsorption of NaCl without water Dilution of tubular fluid	Na^+-Cl^- cotransport	PTH stimulates Ca^{2+} reabsorption	Thiazide diuretics
Late Distal Tubule and Collecting Ducts (principal cells)	Reabsorption of NaCl K^+ secretion Variable water reabsorption	Na^+ channels (ENaC) K^+ channels AQP2 water channels	Aldosterone stimulates Na^+ reabsorption Aldosterone stimulates K^+ secretion ADH stimulates water reabsorption	K^+-sparing diuretics
Late Distal Tubule and Collecting Ducts (α-intercalated cells)	Reabsorption of K^+ Secretion of H^+	H^+-K^+ ATPase H^+ ATPase	— Aldosterone simulates H^+ secretion	— K^+-sparing diuretics

ADH, Antidiuretic hormone; PTH, parathyroid hormone; ENaC, epithelial Na^+ channel; AQP2, aquaporin 2.

Proximal Convoluted Tubule

The proximal convoluted tubule consists of an early proximal convoluted tubule and a late proximal convoluted tubule. The mechanisms for Na^+ reabsorption in the early and late proximal tubules are different, as reflected in the anions and other solutes that accompany Na^+. In the early proximal tubule, Na^+ is reabsorbed primarily with HCO_3^- and organic solutes such as glucose and amino acids. In the late proximal tubule, Na^+ is reabsorbed primarily with Cl^-, but without organic solutes.

Despite these differences, several statements can be made that describe the proximal tubule as a whole. (1) The entire proximal tubule reabsorbs **67%** of the filtered Na^+. (2) The entire proximal tubule also reabsorbs 67% of the filtered water. The tight coupling between Na^+ and water reabsorption is called **isosmotic reabsorption.** (3) This bulk reabsorption of Na^+ and water

(the major constituents of ECF) is critically important for maintaining ECF volume. (4) The proximal tubule is the site of **glomerulotubular balance,** a mechanism for coupling reabsorption to the GFR.

The features of the early and late proximal tubule are described first, followed by a discussion of those general properties of the proximal tubule.

Early Proximal Convoluted Tubule

The first half of the proximal convoluted tubule is called the early proximal tubule. In this segment, the most essential solutes are reabsorbed along with Na^+: glucose, amino acids, and HCO_3^-. Because of the critical metabolic roles of glucose and amino acids and the critical buffering role of HCO_3^-, the early proximal tubule can be thought of as performing the "highest priority" reabsorptive work.

The cellular mechanisms for reabsorption in the early proximal tubule are shown in Figure 6-20. The

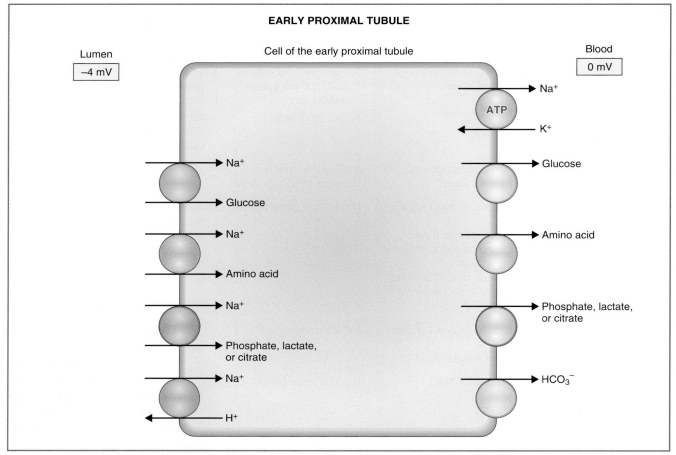

EARLY PROXIMAL TUBULE

Lumen −4 mV

Cell of the early proximal tubule

Blood 0 mV

Figure 6–20 **Cellular mechanisms of Na⁺ reabsorption in the early proximal tubule.** The transepithelial potential difference is the difference between the potential in the lumen and the potential in blood, −4 mV. ATP, Adenosine triphosphate.

luminal membrane contains multiple secondary active transport mechanisms, which derive their energy from the transmembrane Na⁺ gradient. Recall from Chapter 1 that secondary active transport can be cotransport, where all solutes move in the same direction across the cell membrane, or countertransport or exchange, where solutes move in opposite directions across the cell membrane.

The **cotransport** mechanisms in the luminal membrane of the early proximal tubule are Na⁺-glucose (SGLT), Na⁺-amino acid, Na⁺-phosphate, Na⁺-lactate, and Na⁺-citrate. In each case, Na⁺ moves into the cell and down its electrochemical gradient coupled to glucose, amino acid, phosphate, lactate, or citrate, which move into the cell against their electrochemical gradients. Na⁺ then is extruded from the cell into blood by the Na⁺-K⁺ ATPase; glucose and the other solutes are extruded by facilitated diffusion.

There is one **countertransport** or **exchange** mechanism in the luminal membrane of the early proximal tubule, Na⁺-H⁺ exchange. The details of this mechanism are discussed in relation to acid-base physiology in Chapter 7. Briefly, hydrogen (H^+) is transported into the lumen in exchange for Na⁺. The H⁺ combines with filtered HCO_3^-, converting it to carbon dioxide (CO_2) and water, which then move from the lumen into the cell. Inside the cell, CO_2 and water are reconverted to H⁺ and HCO_3^-. The H⁺ is transported again by the Na⁺-H⁺ exchanger, and HCO_3^- is reabsorbed into the blood by facilitated diffusion. The net result of the cycle is the **reabsorption of filtered HCO_3^-**. Thus, in the early proximal tubule, HCO_3^-, not Cl^-, is the anion that is reabsorbed with Na⁺.

There is a **lumen-negative** potential difference across the cells of the early proximal tubule, which is created by Na⁺-glucose and Na⁺-amino acid cotransport. These transporters bring net positive charge into the cell and leave negative charge in the lumen. The other transporters are electroneutral (e.g., Na⁺-H⁺ exchange) and, therefore, do not contribute to the transepithelial potential difference.

As a result of these secondary active transport processes, the following modifications are made to the glomerular filtrate by the time it reaches the midpoint

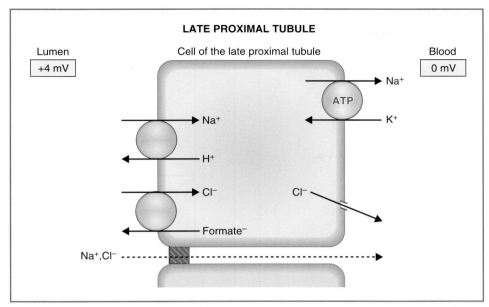

Figure 6–21 **Cellular mechanisms of Na⁺ reabsorption in the late proximal tubule.** The transepithelial potential difference is +4 mV. ATP, Adenosine triphosphate.

of the proximal tubule: (1) 100% of the filtered glucose and amino acids have been reabsorbed; (2) 85% of the filtered HCO_3^- has been reabsorbed; (3) most of the filtered phosphate, lactate, and citrate have been reabsorbed; and (4) because Na⁺ reabsorption is coupled to each of these transport processes, it, too, has been extensively reabsorbed.

Late Proximal Convoluted Tubule

As noted, the tubular fluid that leaves the early proximal tubule differs significantly from the original glomerular filtrate. All of the filtered glucose and amino acids and most of the filtered HCO_3^- have been reabsorbed. Therefore, the fluid entering the late proximal tubule has no glucose or amino acids and little HCO_3^-. Furthermore, this fluid has a **high Cl⁻ concentration**, although it may not be immediately evident why this is so. The Cl⁻ concentration is high because HCO_3^- has been preferentially reabsorbed in the early proximal tubule, leaving Cl⁻ behind in the tubular fluid. As water is reabsorbed isosmotically along with solute, the tubular fluid Cl⁻ concentration increases and becomes higher than the Cl⁻ concentration of the glomerular filtrate and of blood.

In contrast to the early proximal tubule, the late proximal tubule reabsorbs primarily NaCl (Fig. 6-21). The high tubular fluid Cl⁻ concentration is the driving force for this reabsorption, for which there are both cellular and paracellular (between cells) components.

The *cellular* component of **NaCl reabsorption** is explained as follows: The luminal membrane of late proximal cells contains two exchange mechanisms, including the familiar Na⁺-H⁺ exchanger and a

Cl⁻-formate⁻ anion exchanger, which is driven by the high tubular fluid Cl⁻ concentration. The combined function of the two exchangers is to transport NaCl from the lumen into the cell. Na⁺ then is extruded into blood by the Na⁺-K⁺ ATPase, and Cl⁻ moves into blood by diffusion.

The *paracellular* component also depends on the high tubular fluid Cl⁻ concentration. The tight junctions between cells of the proximal tubule are, in fact, not tight: They are quite permeable to small solutes, such as NaCl, and to water. Thus, the Cl⁻ concentration gradient drives Cl⁻ diffusion between the cells, from lumen to blood. This Cl⁻ diffusion establishes a **Cl⁻ diffusion potential**, making the **lumen positive** with respect to blood. Na⁺ reabsorption follows, driven by the lumen-positive potential difference. Like the cellular route, the net result of the paracellular route is reabsorption of NaCl.

Isosmotic Reabsorption

Isosmotic reabsorption is a hallmark of proximal tubular function: Solute and water reabsorption are coupled and are proportional to each other. Thus, if 67% of the filtered solute is reabsorbed by the proximal tubule, then 67% of the filtered water also will be reabsorbed.

What solutes are included in the general term "solute"? The major cation is Na⁺, with its accompanying anions HCO_3^- (early proximal tubule) and Cl⁻ (late proximal tubule). Minor anions are phosphate, lactate, and citrate. Other solutes are glucose and amino acids. Quantitatively, however, most of the solute reabsorbed by the proximal tubule is NaCl and $NaHCO_3$.

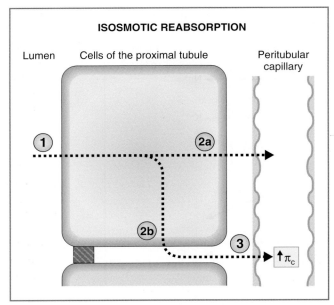

Figure 6–22 Mechanism of isosmotic reabsorption in the proximal tubule. *Dashed arrows* show the pathways for reabsorption. See the text for an explanation of the *circled numbers.* π_c, Peritubular capillary oncotic pressure.

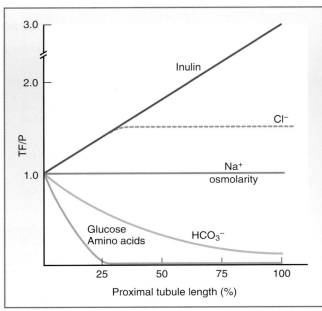

Figure 6-23 Changes in TF/P concentration ratios for various solutes along the proximal convoluted tubule.

One of the consequences of isosmotic reabsorption has already been mentioned: The values for $[TF/P]_{Na^+}$ and $[TF/P]_{osmolarity} = 1.0$ along the entire proximal tubule. This is remarkable because there is extensive reabsorption of both Na^+ and solute (osmoles) along the proximal tubule. The reason that these ratios remain at a value of 1.0 is that water reabsorption is coupled directly to both Na^+ reabsorption and total solute reabsorption.

Figure 6-22 is a schematic diagram of the **mechanism of isosmotic reabsorption.** A fundamental question to be asked is *Does solute follow water reabsorption, or does water follow solute reabsorption?* The answer is that solute reabsorption is the primary event, and water follows passively, as explained in Figure 6-22. The routes of solute and water reabsorption are shown by the dashed lines, and the circled numbers in the figure correlate with the following steps:

1. Na^+ enters the cell across the luminal membrane by any one of the mechanisms described in the preceding sections. Because the luminal membrane is permeable to water, water follows the solute to maintain isosmolarity.

2. Na^+ is pumped out of the cell by the Na^+-K^+ ATPase, which is located in the peritubular or basolateral membranes. ("Basal" refers to the cell membranes facing the peritubular capillary [2a], and "lateral" refers to the cell membranes facing the lateral intercellular spaces between cells [2b].) As Na^+ is pumped out of the cell, water again follows passively.

3. The **lateral intercellular space** is an important route for reabsorption of solute and water. Isosmotic fluid accumulates in these spaces between the proximal tubule cells, as described in step 2. (Electron micrographs show the spaces actually widening when there is increased proximal tubule reabsorption.) This isosmotic fluid in the spaces is then acted upon by Starling forces in the peritubular capillary.

The major Starling force driving reabsorption is the **high oncotic pressure** (π_c) of peritubular capillary blood. Recall that glomerular filtration elevates the protein concentration (and π_c) of the glomerular capillary blood; this blood leaves glomerular capillaries to become the peritubular capillary blood. The high π_c is then a pressure favoring reabsorption of isosmotic fluid.

TF/P Ratios Along the Proximal Tubule

Functions of the proximal tubule can be envisioned graphically by plotting the TF/P concentration ratios for various substances as a function of length along the proximal tubule (Fig. 6-23). At the beginning of the proximal tubule (i.e., Bowman's space), the TF/P ratio for all freely filtered substances is 1.0; because no reabsorption or secretion has yet occurred, the solute concentrations in tubular fluid equal their concentrations in plasma. Moving along the proximal tubule, because both Na^+ and total solute are reabsorbed in proportion to water (i.e., isosmotic reabsorption), the values for $[TF/P]_{Na}$ and $[TF/P]_{osmolarity}$ both remain at 1.0. Because reabsorption of glucose, amino acids, and HCO_3^- is proportionately greater than water reabsorption in the early proximal tubule, $[TF/P]_{glucose}$, $[TF/P]_{amino\ acids}$, and $[TF/P]_{HCO_3^-}$ fall below 1.0. Cl^- reabsorption is less than water reabsorption in the early proximal tubule (i.e., HCO_3^- is preferred over Cl^-); thus, $[TF/P]_{Cl}$ rises above 1.0. Finally, $[TF/P]_{inulin}$ rises steadily along the proximal tubule because inulin, once filtered, is not reabsorbed; $[TF/P]_{inulin}$ rises because as water is reabsorbed and inulin is left behind in the lumen, the tubular fluid inulin concentration increases. (Two thirds of the filtered water is reabsorbed along the entire proximal tubule; thus, the $[TF/P]_{inulin}$ ratio is approximately 3.0 at the end of the proximal tubule.)

Glomerulotubular Balance

Glomerulotubular balance is the major regulatory mechanism of the proximal tubule. It describes the balance between filtration (the glomerulus) and reabsorption (the proximal tubule), which is illustrated in the following example: If GFR were to spontaneously increase by 1%, the filtered load of Na^+ also would increase by 1% (filtered load = GFR $\times$ $[P]_x$). Thus, if GFR is 180 L/day and $[P]_{Na^+}$ is 140 mEq/L, the filtered load of Na^+ is 25,200 mEq/day. An increase of 1% in the filtered load of Na^+ corresponds to an increase of 252 mEq/day. If there was no accompanying increase in reabsorption, then an *extra* 252 mEq/day of Na^+ would be excreted in the urine. Because the total amount of Na^+ in ECF is only 1960 mEq (14 L $\times$ 140 mEq/L), a loss of 252 mEq/day is significant.

This loss of Na^+ does not occur, however, because of the protective mechanism of glomerulotubular balance. Glomerulotubular balance ensures that a **constant fraction of the filtered load is reabsorbed** by the proximal tubule, even if the filtered load increases or decreases. This constant fraction (or percentage) is normally maintained at 67% of the filtered load (by now, a familiar number).

How does the glomerulus "communicate" with the proximal tubule to maintain constant fractional reabsorption? The mechanism of glomerulotubular balance involves the filtration fraction and the Starling forces in peritubular capillary blood (see Fig. 6-22). In the previous example, GFR was said to increase spontaneously by 1%, with no change in RPF. As a result, the **filtration fraction** (GFR/RPF) increased, meaning that a greater than usual fraction of fluid was filtered out of glomerular capillary blood. Consequently, the protein concentration and oncotic pressure of the glomerular capillary blood increased more than usual. This blood becomes the peritubular capillary blood, but now with a **higher π_c** than usual. Because π_c is the most important driving force for reabsorption of isosmotic fluid in the proximal tubule, reabsorption is increased.

In summary, increases in GFR produce increases in the filtration fraction, which leads to increased π_c and increased reabsorption in the proximal tubule; decreases in GFR produce decreases in the filtration fraction, which leads to decreased π_c and decreased reabsorption. The proportionality of filtration and proximal tubule reabsorption is thereby maintained (i.e., there is glomerulotubular balance).

Changes in Extracellular Fluid Volume

Glomerulotubular balance ensures that normally 67% of the filtered Na^+ and water is reabsorbed in the proximal tubule. This balance is maintained because the glomerulus communicates with the proximal tubule via changes in the π_c of peritubular capillary blood. However, *glomerulotubular balance can be altered* by changes in ECF volume. The mechanisms underlying these changes can be explained by the Starling forces in the peritubular capillaries (Fig. 6-24).

♦ **ECF volume expansion** produces a decrease in fractional reabsorption in the proximal tubule (see Fig. 6-24*A*). When ECF volume is increased (e.g., by infusion of isotonic NaCl), the plasma protein concentration is decreased by dilution and the capillary hydrostatic pressure (P_c) is increased. For the peritubular capillaries, these changes result in a decrease in π_c and an increase in P_c. Both of these changes in Starling forces in the peritubular capillary produce a **decrease in fractional reabsorption** of isosmotic fluid in the proximal tubule. A portion of the fluid that would have been reabsorbed instead leaks back into the lumen of the tubule (across the tight junction) and is excreted. This alteration of glomerulotubular balance is one of several mechanisms that aids in the excretion of excess NaCl and water when there is ECF volume expansion.

♦ **ECF volume contraction** produces an increase in fractional reabsorption in the proximal tubule (see Fig. 6-24*B*). When ECF volume is decreased (e.g., diarrhea or vomiting), the plasma protein concentration increases (is concentrated) and the capillary hydrostatic pressure decreases. As a result, there is an increase in π_c and a decrease in P_c of peritubular capillary blood. These changes in Starling forces in the peritubular capillaries produce an **increase in fractional reabsorption** of isosmotic fluid. This alteration of glomerulotubular balance is a logical protective mechanism, as the kidneys are trying to restore ECF volume by reabsorbing more solute and water than usual.

In addition to the Starling forces, a second mechanism contributes to the increased proximal tubule reabsorption that occurs in ECF volume contraction. A decrease in ECF volume causes a decrease in blood volume and arterial pressure that activates the

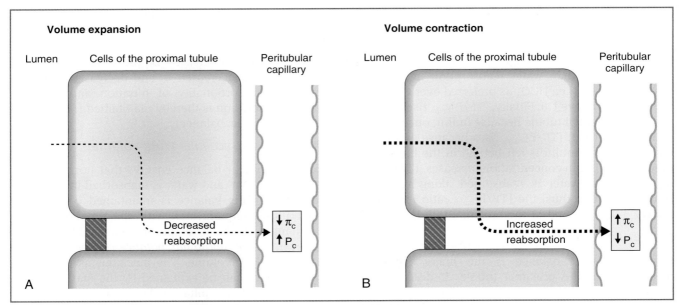

Figure 6–24 **Effects of ECF volume expansion (A) and ECF volume contraction (B) on isosmotic fluid reabsorption in the proximal tubule.** Changes in Starling forces in the peritubular capillary blood are responsible for the effects. π_c, Peritubular capillary oncotic pressure; P_c, peritubular capillary hydrostatic pressure.

renin-angiotensin-aldosterone system. **Angiotensin II** stimulates **Na$^+$-H$^+$ exchange** in the proximal tubule, and thereby stimulates reabsorption of Na$^+$, HCO$_3^-$, and water. Because the angiotensin II mechanism specifically stimulates HCO$_3^-$ reabsorption (along with Na$^+$ and water), ECF volume contraction causes **contraction alkalosis** (metabolic alkalosis secondary to volume contraction), which is discussed in Chapter 7.

Loop of Henle

The loop of Henle comprises three segments: the thin descending limb, the thin ascending limb, and the thick ascending limb. Together, the three segments are responsible for countercurrent multiplication, which is essential for the concentration and dilution of urine. Countercurrent multiplication is discussed later in the chapter.

Thin Descending Limb and Thin Ascending Limb

The thin descending limb and the thin ascending limb of the loop of Henle are characterized primarily by their high permeability to small solutes and water. The **thin descending limb** is permeable to water and small solutes such as NaCl and urea. In countercurrent multiplication, water moves out of the thin descending limb, solutes move into the thin descending limb, and the tubular fluid becomes progressively hyperosmotic as it flows down the descending limb. The **thin ascending limb** also is permeable to NaCl, but it is impermeable to water. During countercurrent multiplication, solute moves out of the thin ascending limb without water and the tubular fluid becomes progressively hyposmotic as it flows up the ascending limb.

Thick Ascending Limb

Unlike the thin limbs, which have only passive permeability properties, the thick ascending limb reabsorbs a significant amount of Na$^+$ by an active mechanism. Normally, the thick ascending limb reabsorbs about **25%** of the filtered Na$^+$.

The reabsorption mechanism is **load-dependent** (a property shared by the distal tubule). Load-dependent means that the more Na$^+$ delivered to the thick ascending limb, the more it reabsorbs. This property of load-dependency explains the observation that inhibition of Na$^+$ reabsorption in the proximal tubule produces smaller than expected increases in Na$^+$ excretion. For example, a diuretic that acts in the proximal tubule typically produces only mild diuresis. Although the diuretic does indeed inhibit proximal Na$^+$ reabsorption, some of the "extra" Na$^+$ then delivered to the loop of Henle is reabsorbed by the load-dependent mechanism. Thus, the loop of Henle (and the distal tubule) partially offsets the proximal diuretic effect.

The cellular mechanism in the thick ascending limb is shown in Figure 6-25. As the figure shows, the luminal membrane contains a **Na$^+$-K$^+$-2Cl$^-$ cotransporter** (a three-ion cotransporter). The energy for the cotransporter is derived from the familiar Na$^+$ gradient, which

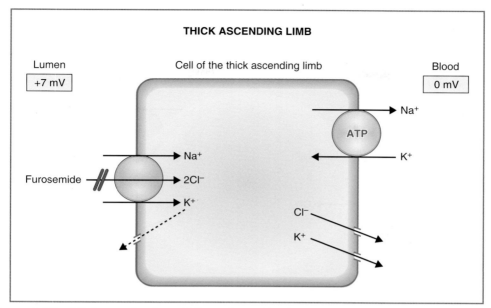

Figure 6–25 **Cellular mechanism of Na⁺ reabsorption in the thick ascending limb of the loop of Henle.** The transepithelial potential difference is +7 mV. ATP, Adenosine triphosphate.

is maintained by the Na⁺-K⁺ ATPase in the basolateral membranes. There is net reabsorption of Na⁺, K⁺, and Cl⁻ in the thick ascending limb, as follows: All three ions are transported into the cell on the cotransporter; Na⁺ is extruded from the cell by the Na⁺-K⁺ ATPase, and Cl⁻ and K⁺ diffuse through channels in the basolateral membrane, down their respective electrochemical gradients. As shown in the figure, most, but not all, of the K⁺ that enters the cell on the three-ion cotransporter leaves the cell across the basolateral membrane. A portion of the K⁺, however, diffuses back into the lumen. One consequence of this recycling of K⁺ across the luminal membrane is that the cotransporter is **electrogenic:** It brings slightly more negative than positive charge into the cell. The electrogenic property of the Na⁺-K⁺-2Cl⁻ cotransporter results in a **lumen-positive potential difference** across the cells of the thick ascending limb. (The role of the lumen-positive potential in driving the reabsorption of divalent cations such as Ca²⁺ and Mg²⁺ is discussed later in the chapter.)

The thick ascending limb is the site of action of the most potent diuretics, the **loop diuretics** (e.g., furosemide, bumetanide, ethacrynic acid). The loop diuretics are organic acids that are related to PAH. At physiologic pH, the loop diuretics are anions that attach to the Cl⁻-binding site of the Na⁺-K⁺-2Cl⁻ cotransporter. When diuretic is bound to the Cl⁻-binding site, the three-ion cotransporter is unable to cycle and transport stops. At maximal dosages, loop diuretics completely inhibit NaCl reabsorption in the thick ascending limb and, theoretically, can cause excretion of as much as 25% of the filtered Na⁺.

The cells of the thick ascending limb are **impermeable to water,** clearly an unusual characteristic because virtually all other cell membranes are highly permeable to water. As a consequence of the water impermeability, NaCl is reabsorbed by the thick ascending limb, but water is not reabsorbed along with it. For this reason, the thick ascending limb also is called the **diluting segment:** Solute is reabsorbed, but water remains behind, *diluting* the tubular fluid. Proof of this diluting function is seen in the values for tubular fluid Na⁺ concentration and tubular fluid osmolarity. The tubular fluid that leaves the thick ascending limb has a lower Na⁺ concentration and a lower osmolarity than blood and, accordingly, **[TF/P]ₙₐ⁺ and [TF/P]osmolarity < 1.0.**

Distal Tubule and Collecting Duct

The distal tubule and collecting duct constitute the **terminal nephron,** and together they reabsorb about 8% of the filtered Na⁺. Like the thick ascending limb, reabsorption in the terminal nephron is **load-dependent,** with considerable capacity to reabsorb extra Na⁺ that may be delivered from the proximal tubule. The mechanism of Na⁺ transport in the early distal tubule differs from that of the late distal tubule and collecting duct, and each segment is discussed separately.

Early Distal Tubule

The early distal tubule reabsorbs **5%** of the filtered Na⁺. At the cellular level, the mechanism is an **Na⁺-Cl⁻ cotransporter** in the luminal membrane, the energy for which derives from the Na⁺ gradient (Fig. 6-26). There is net reabsorption of Na⁺ and Cl⁻ in the early distal

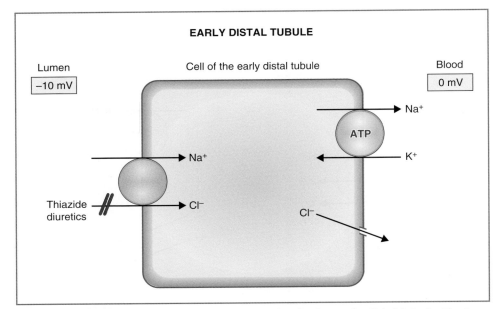

EARLY DISTAL TUBULE

Lumen
−10 mV

Cell of the early distal tubule

Blood
0 mV

ATP

Na⁺

K⁺

Na⁺

Cl⁻

Thiazide diuretics

Cl⁻

Figure 6–26 Cellular mechanism of Na⁺ reabsorption in the early distal tubule. The transepithelial potential difference is −10 mV. ATP, Adenosine triphosphate.

tubule, which is explained as follows: Both ions enter the cell on the Na⁺-Cl⁻ cotransporter; Na⁺ then is extruded from the cell into the blood by the Na⁺-K⁺ ATPase, and Cl⁻ diffuses out of the cell through Cl⁻ channels in the basolateral membrane.

The Na⁺-Cl⁻ cotransporter of the early distal tubule differs from the Na⁺-K⁺-2Cl⁻ cotransporter of the thick ascending limb in the following respects: It transports two ions (not three), it is electroneutral (not electrogenic), and it is inhibited by a different class of diuretics, the **thiazide diuretics** (e.g., chlorothiazide, hydrochlorothiazide, metolazone). Like the loop diuretics, the thiazides are organic acids, which are anions at physiologic pH. Thiazide diuretics bind to the Cl⁻ site of the Na⁺-Cl⁻ cotransporter and prevent it from cycling, thus inhibiting NaCl reabsorption in the early distal tubule.

Like the thick ascending limb, the early distal tubule is **impermeable to water.** Thus, it reabsorbs solute but leaves water behind, which then dilutes the tubular fluid. For this reason, the early distal tubule is called the *cortical* **diluting segment** ("cortical" because distal tubules are in the kidney cortex). Recall that the tubular fluid entering the early distal tubule is *already* dilute (compared with blood) because of the function of the thick ascending limb; the early distal tubule *further* dilutes it.

Late Distal Tubule and Collecting Duct

Anatomically and functionally, the late distal tubule and collecting duct are similar and can be discussed together. There are two major cell types interspersed along these segments: the **principal cells** and the

α-intercalated cells. The principal cells are involved in Na⁺ reabsorption, K⁺ secretion, and water reabsorption; the α-intercalated cells are involved in K⁺ reabsorption and H⁺ secretion. Discussion in this section focuses on Na⁺ reabsorption by the principal cells. (Water reabsorption, K⁺ reabsorption, and K⁺ secretion are discussed later in this chapter, and H⁺ secretion is discussed in Chapter 7.)

The late distal tubule and collecting duct reabsorb only **3%** of the filtered Na⁺. Quantitatively, this amount is small when compared with the amounts reabsorbed in the proximal tubule, the thick ascending limb, and even the early distal tubule. The late distal tubule and collecting duct, however, are the last segments of the nephron to influence the amount of Na⁺ that is to be excreted (i.e., they make the fine adjustments of Na⁺ reabsorption).

The mechanism for Na⁺ reabsorption in the **principal cells** of the late distal tubule and collecting duct is shown in Figure 6-27. Rather than the coupled transport mechanisms seen in other nephron segments, the luminal membrane of the principal cells contains **Na⁺ channels** (epithelial Na⁺ channels, or **ENaC**). Na⁺ diffuses through these channels down its electrochemical gradient, from the lumen into the cell. Na⁺ then is extruded from the cell via the Na⁺-K⁺ ATPase in the basolateral membrane. The anion that accompanies Na⁺ is mainly Cl⁻, although the transport mechanism for Cl⁻ has not been elucidated.

Given the critical role of the late distal tubule and collecting duct in the fine adjustments to Na⁺ excretion, it should not be surprising that Na⁺ reabsorption in these segments is hormonally regulated. **Aldosterone**

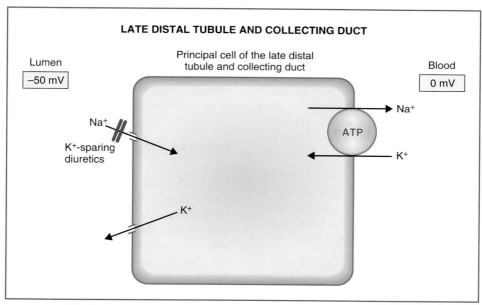

Figure 6–27 **Cellular mechanism of Na⁺ reabsorption in the principal cells of the late distal tubule and collecting duct.** The transepithelial potential difference is –50 mV. ATP, Adenosine triphosphate.

is a steroid hormone that acts directly on the principal cells to **increase Na⁺ reabsorption.** Aldosterone is secreted by the zona glomerulosa of the adrenal cortex, is delivered to the principal cells via the circulation, and diffuses into the cells across the basolateral cell membrane. In the cell, the hormone is transferred to the nucleus, where it directs the synthesis of specific messenger RNAs (mRNAs). These mRNAs then direct the synthesis of new proteins that are involved in Na⁺ reabsorption by the principal cells. The aldosterone-induced proteins include the luminal membrane **Na⁺ channel** itself, the Na⁺-K⁺ ATPase, and enzymes of the citric acid cycle (e.g., citrate synthase).

Na⁺ reabsorption by the principal cells is inhibited by the **K⁺-sparing diuretics** (e.g., amiloride, triamterene, spironolactone). **Spironolactone,** a steroid and aldosterone-antagonist, prevents aldosterone from entering the nucleus of the principal cells and therefore blocks the synthesis of mRNAs and new proteins. **Amiloride** and **triamterene** bind to the luminal membrane Na⁺ channels and inhibit the aldosterone-induced increase in Na⁺ reabsorption. The K⁺-sparing diuretics produce only mild diuresis because they inhibit such a small percentage of the total Na⁺ reabsorption. However, as the name suggests, their main use is in combination with other diuretics to inhibit K⁺ secretion by the principal cells, as discussed in the section on K⁺ handling.

Water reabsorption by the late distal tubule and collecting duct is variable, as described later in this chapter. Water permeability of the principal cells is controlled by **ADH,** which is secreted by the posterior lobe of the pituitary gland according to the body's need for water. When ADH levels are low or absent, the water permeability of the principal cells is low, and little, if any, water is reabsorbed along with NaCl. When ADH levels are high, aquaporin 2 (AQP2) channels are inserted in the luminal membranes of the principal cells, turning on their water permeability; thus, in the presence of ADH water is reabsorbed along with NaCl.

Regulation of Na⁺ Balance

Na⁺ and its associated anions Cl⁻ and HCO₃⁻ are the major solutes of ECF. In turn, the amount of Na⁺ in the ECF determines the ECF volume. Consequently, an increase in the amount of Na⁺ in the body leads to an increase in ECF volume, blood volume, and blood pressure; a decrease in the amount of Na⁺ leads to a decrease in ECF volume, blood volume, and blood pressure.

A useful concept for understanding the regulation of Na⁺ balance is that of **effective arterial blood volume (EABV).** EABV is that portion of the ECF volume contained in the arteries and is the volume "effectively" perfusing the tissues. In general, changes in ECF volume lead to changes in EABV in the same direction. For example, increases in ECF volume are associated with increases in EABV and decreases in ECF volume are associated with decreases in EABV. There are exceptions, however, such as edema, in which an *increase* in ECF volume is associated with a *decrease* in EABV (due to excessive filtration of fluid out of the capillaries into the interstitial fluid). The kidneys detect changes in EABV and, through a variety of mechanisms, direct changes in Na^+ excretion that attempt to restore EABV toward normal.

The renal mechanisms that regulate Na^+ excretion include sympathetic nerve activity, atriopeptin (atrial natriuretic peptide [ANP]), Starling forces in peritubular capillaries, and the renin-angiotensin-aldosterone system, as follows:

1. **Sympathetic nerve activity.** Sympathetic activity is activated by the baroreceptor mechanism in response to a decrease in arterial pressure and causes vasoconstriction of afferent arterioles and increased proximal tubule Na^+ reabsorption.

2. **Atriopeptin (ANP).** ANP is secreted by the atria in response to an increase in ECF volume and causes vasodilation of afferent arterioles, vasoconstriction of efferent arterioles, increased GFR, and decreased Na^+ reabsorption in the late distal tubule and collecting ducts. Other peptides in the ANP family have similar effects to increase GFR and decrease renal Na^+ reabsorption. These include **urodilatin,** which is secreted by the kidney, and **brain natriuretic peptide (BNP),** which is secreted by cardiac atrial cells and the brain.

3. **Starling forces in peritubular capillaries.** The role of Starling forces has been discussed previously in the context of glomerulotubular balance. Briefly, increases in ECF volume dilute π_c and inhibit proximal tubule Na^+ reabsorption; decreases in ECF volume concentrate π_c and stimulate proximal tubule Na^+ reabsorption.

4. **Renin-angiotensin-aldosterone system.** The renin-angiotensin-aldosterone system is activated in response to decreased arterial pressure (i.e., decreased renal perfusion pressure). As previously described, angiotensin II stimulates Na^+ reabsorption in the proximal tubule (Na^+-H^+ exchange), and aldosterone stimulates Na^+ reabsorption in the late distal tubule and the collecting duct.

Two examples will be considered in which these mechanisms are employed to restore Na^+ balance: the response of the kidneys to increased Na^+ intake and the response of the kidneys to decreased Na^+ intake.

Response to Increased Na⁺ Intake

When a person eats a high Na^+ diet, because Na^+ is primarily distributed in the ECF, there is an increase in ECF volume and EABV. The increase in EABV is detected, and the kidneys orchestrate an increase in Na^+ excretion that attempts to return ECF volume and EABV to normal (Fig. 6-28).

Response to Decreased Na⁺ Intake

When a person eats a low Na^+ diet, there is a decrease in ECF volume and EABV. The decrease in EABV is detected, and the kidneys orchestrate a decrease in Na^+ excretion that attempts to return ECF volume and EABV to normal (Fig. 6-29).

POTASSIUM BALANCE

The maintenance of potassium (K^+) balance is essential for the normal function of excitable tissues (e.g., nerve, skeletal muscle, cardiac muscle). Recall from Chapters 1 and 4 that the K^+ concentration gradient across excitable cell membranes sets the resting membrane potential. Recall, also, that changes in resting membrane potential alter excitability by opening or closing gates on the Na^+ channels, which are responsible for the upstroke of the action potential. Changes in either intracellular or extracellular K^+ concentration alter the resting membrane potential and, as a consequence, alter the excitability of these tissues.

Most of the **total body K^+** is located in the ICF: 98% of the total K^+ content is in the intracellular compartment and 2% is in the extracellular compartment. A consequence of this distribution is that the intracellular K^+ concentration (150 mEq/L) is much higher than the extracellular concentration (4.5 mEq/L). This large concentration gradient for K^+ is maintained by the Na^+-K^+ ATPase that is present in all cell membranes.

One challenge to maintaining the low extracellular K^+ concentration is the large amount of K^+ present in the intracellular compartment. A small shift of K^+ into or out of the cells can produce a large change in the extracellular K^+ concentration. The distribution of K^+ across cell membranes is called **internal K^+ balance.** Hormones, drugs, and various pathologic states alter this distribution and, as a consequence, can alter the extracellular K^+ concentration.

Another challenge to maintaining the low extracellular K^+ concentration is the variation in dietary K^+ intake in humans: Dietary K^+ can vary from as low as 50 mEq/day to as high as 150 mEq/day. To maintain K^+ balance, urinary excretion of K^+ must be equal to K^+ intake. Thus, on a daily basis, urinary excretion of K^+ must be capable of varying from 50 to 150 mEq/day. The renal mechanisms that allow for this variability are called **external K^+ balance.**

Internal K⁺ Balance

Internal K^+ balance is the distribution of K^+ across cell membranes. To reemphasize, most K^+ is present inside the cells and even small K^+ shifts across cell membranes can cause large changes in K^+ concentrations in ECF

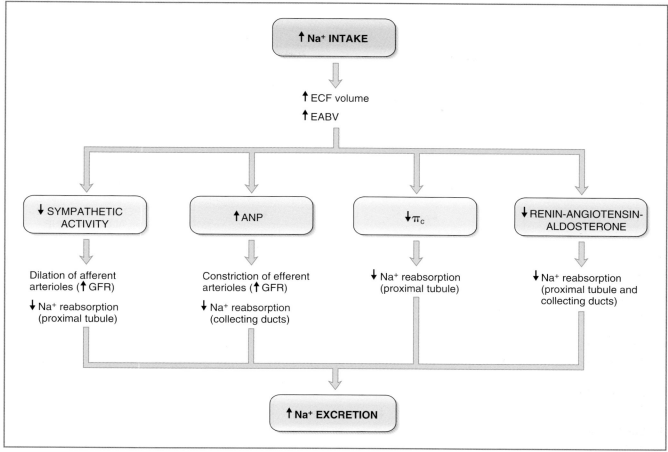

Figure 6–28 **Responses to increased Na⁺ intake.** ANP, Atriopeptin; EABV, effective arterial blood volume; ECF, extracellular fluid; GFR, glomerular filtration rate; π_c, peritubular capillary oncotic pressure.

and blood. The effects of hormones, drugs, and pathologic states that alter this distribution of K⁺ are summarized in Figure 6-30 and in Table 6-8. A shift of K⁺ out of cells produces an increase in the blood K⁺ concentration called **hyperkalemia.** A shift of K⁺ into cells produces a decrease in the blood K⁺ concentration called **hypokalemia.**

Insulin

Insulin stimulates K⁺ uptake into cells by increasing the activity of Na⁺-K⁺ ATPase. Physiologically, this effect of insulin is responsible for the uptake of dietary K⁺ into the cells following a meal. Thus, in response to food ingestion, insulin is secreted by the endocrine pancreas. One effect of this insulin (in addition to stimulation of glucose uptake into cells) is to stimulate K⁺ uptake into cells. This action ensures that ingested K⁺ does not remain in the ECF and produce hyperkalemia.

Deficiency of insulin, as occurs in **type I diabetes mellitus,** produces the opposite effect: decreased uptake of K⁺ into cells and **hyperkalemia.** When a

Table 6–8 Internal K⁺ Balance—Shifts across Cell Membranes

Causes of K⁺ Shift Out of Cells → Hyperkalemia	Causes of K⁺ Shift into Cells → Hypokalemia
Insulin deficiency	Insulin
β_2-Adrenergic antagonists	β_2-Adrenergic agonists
α-Adrenergic agonists	α-Adrenergic antagonists
Acidosis	Alkalosis
Hyperosmolarity	Hyposmolarity
Cell lysis	
Exercise	

person with untreated type I diabetes mellitus ingests a meal containing K⁺, the K⁺ remains in the ECF because insulin is not available to promote its uptake into cells. (Conversely, high levels of insulin can produce hypokalemia.)

Acid-Base Abnormalities

Acid-base abnormalities often are associated with K⁺ disturbances. One of the mechanisms underlying

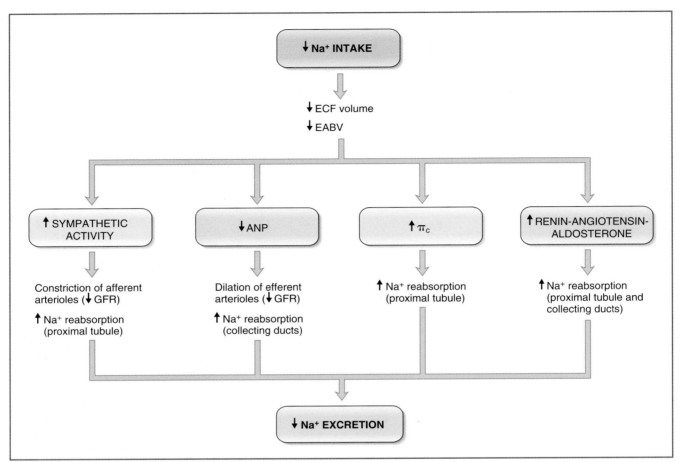

Figure 6–29 Responses to decreased Na⁺ intake. ANP, Atriopeptin; EABV, effective arterial blood volume; ECF, extracellular fluid; GFR, glomerular filtration rate; π_c, peritubular capillary oncotic pressure.

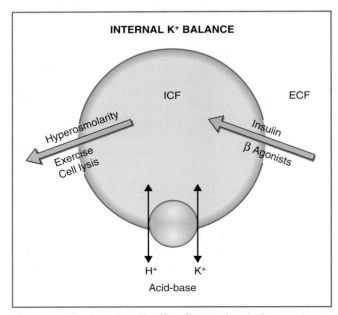

Figure 6–30 Agents affecting internal K⁺ balance. *Arrows* show directions of K⁺ movement into and out of cells. ECF, Extracellular fluid; ICF, intracellular fluid.

internal K⁺ balance involves **H⁺-K⁺ exchange** across cell membranes. This exchange is useful because ICF has considerable buffering capacity for H⁺. In order to take advantage of these buffers, H⁺ must enter or leave the cells. To preserve electroneutrality, however, H⁺ cannot enter or leave cells by itself; either it must be accompanied by an anion, or it must be exchanged for another cation. When H⁺ is exchanged for another cation, that cation is K⁺.

In **alkalemia**, the H⁺ concentration in blood is decreased: H⁺ leaves the cells and K⁺ enters the cells, producing **hypokalemia.** On the other hand, in **acidemia,** the H⁺ concentration in blood is increased: H⁺ enters the cells and K⁺ leaves the cells, producing **hyperkalemia.**

Acid-base disturbances *do not always* produce a K⁺ shift across cell membranes, however, and it is important to note the following exceptions: First, respiratory acidosis and respiratory alkalosis typically *do not* cause a K⁺ shift because these conditions are caused by a primary disturbance in CO_2. Because CO_2 is lipid soluble, it freely crosses cell membranes and needs no exchange with K^+ to preserve electroneutrality. Second, several forms of metabolic acidosis are caused by an excess of an organic acid (e.g., lactic acid, ketoacids, salicylic acid), which does not require a K^+ shift. When an organic anion such as lactate is available to enter the cell with H^+, electroneutrality is preserved. (Chapter 7 discusses the conditions under which an acid-base disturbance causes a K^+ shift and when it does not.)

Adrenergic Agonists and Antagonists

Catecholamines alter the distribution of K^+ across cell membranes by two separate receptors and mechanisms. Activation of β_2-**adrenergic receptors** by β_2 agonists (e.g., albuterol), by increasing the activity of the Na^+-K^+ ATPase, causes a shift of K^+ into cells and may produce hypokalemia. On the other hand, activation of α-**adrenergic receptors** causes a shift of K^+ out of cells and may produce hyperkalemia. The effects of adrenergic antagonists on the blood K^+ concentration also are predictable: β_2-adrenergic antagonists (e.g., propranolol) cause a shift of K^+ out of cells, and α-adrenergic antagonists cause a shift of K^+ into cells.

Osmolarity

Hyperosmolarity (increased osmolarity of ECF) causes a shift of K^+ out of cells. The mechanism involves water flow across cell membranes, which occurs in response to a change in ECF osmolarity. For example, if the osmolarity of ECF is increased, water will flow from ICF to ECF because of the osmotic gradient. As water leaves the cells, the intracellular K^+ concentration increases, which then drives the diffusion of K^+ from ICF to ECF. (A simpler way of visualizing the mechanism is to think of water flow from ICF to ECF as "dragging" K^+ with it.)

Cell Lysis

Cell lysis (breakdown of cell membranes) releases a large amount of K^+ from the ICF and produces hyperkalemia. Examples of cell lysis include burn, rhabdomyolysis (breakdown of skeletal muscle), and malignant cells being destroyed during cancer chemotherapy.

Exercise

Exercise causes a K^+ shift out of cells; the depletion of cellular ATP stores opens K^+ channels in the muscle cell membranes and K^+ moves out of the cells down its electrochemical gradient. Usually, the shift is small and produces only a slight increase in blood K^+ concentration, which is reversed during a subsequent period of rest. However, in a person treated with a β_2-adrenergic antagonist (which independently produces a K^+ shift out of cells), or in those with impaired renal function (in which K^+ cannot be adequately excreted), strenuous exercise can result in hyperkalemia.

As an aside, a K^+ shift out of cells assists in the local control of blood flow to exercising skeletal muscle. Recall that blood flow in exercising muscle is controlled by vasodilator metabolites, one of which is K^+. As K^+ is released from cells during exercise, it acts directly on skeletal muscle arterioles, dilating them and increasing local blood flow.

External K+ Balance—Renal Mechanisms

On a daily basis, the urinary excretion of K^+ is exactly equal to the dietary K^+ (minus small amounts of K^+ lost from the body via extrarenal routes such as the gastrointestinal tract or sweat). The physiologic concept of balance is now familiar. A person is in **K^+ balance** when excretion of K^+ equals intake of K^+. If excretion of K^+ is less than intake, then a person is in **positive K^+ balance** and hyperkalemia can occur. If excretion of K^+ is greater than intake, then a person is in **negative K^+ balance** and hypokalemia can occur.

Maintaining K^+ balance is a particular challenge because dietary K^+ intake is so variable (50 to 150 mEq/day), both from one person to another and from day-to-day in the same person. Thus, the renal mechanisms responsible for external K^+ balance must be flexible enough to ensure that K^+ excretion matches K^+ intake over a wide range. To accomplish this, K^+ is handled in the kidneys by a combination of **filtration, reabsorption,** and **secretion** mechanisms (Fig. 6-31).

♦ **Filtration.** K^+ is not bound to plasma proteins and is freely filtered across the glomerular capillaries.

♦ The **proximal convoluted tubule** reabsorbs about 67% of the filtered load of K^+ as part of the isosmotic fluid reabsorption.

♦ The **thick ascending limb** reabsorbs an additional 20% of the filtered load of K^+. Recall from the discussion of Na^+ reabsorption that K^+ enters the cells of the thick ascending limb via the Na^+-K^+-$2Cl^-$ cotransporter and then leaves the cell along either of two possible routes: K^+ may diffuse across the basolateral membrane through K^+ channels, to be reabsorbed, and K^+ may diffuse back into the lumen, which does not result in reabsorption (but creates the lumen-positive potential difference across the thick ascending limb cells).

♦ The **distal tubule and collecting ducts** are responsible for the adjustments in K^+ excretion that occur when dietary K^+ varies. These segments either reabsorb K^+ or secrete K^+, as dictated by the need to remain in K^+ balance.

In the case of a person on a low K^+ diet, there is further reabsorption of K^+ by the α-**intercalated cells** of the late distal tubule and collecting ducts.

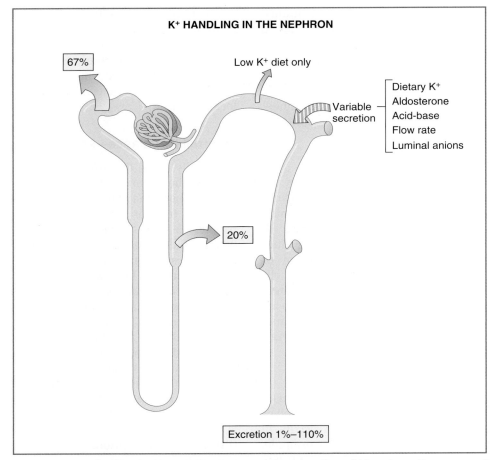

Figure 6–31 K⁺ handling in the nephron. *Arrows* show location of K⁺ reabsorption or secretion; numbers are percentages of the filtered load reabsorbed, secreted, or excreted.

On a low K⁺ diet, urinary excretion can be as low as 1% of the filtered load.

More commonly, though, in persons on a normal or high K⁺ diet, K⁺ is secreted by the **principal cells** of the late distal tubule and collecting duct. The magnitude of this K⁺ secretion is variable, depending on the amount of K⁺ ingested in the diet and several other factors including mineralocorticoids, acid-base status, and flow rate. Urinary K⁺ excretion can be as high as 110% of the filtered load.

The greatest attention should be paid to the handling of K⁺ by the late distal tubule and collecting ducts because these segments perform the fine-tuning of K⁺ excretion to maintain K⁺ balance. (Reabsorption of K⁺ in the proximal convoluted tubule and in the thick ascending limb is constant under most conditions.)

K⁺ Reabsorption by α-Intercalated Cells

When a person is on a low K⁺ diet, K⁺ can be reabsorbed in the terminal nephron segments by the α-intercalated cells (Fig. 6-32A). Briefly, the luminal membrane of these cells contains an **H⁺-K⁺ ATPase,** similar to the H⁺-K⁺ ATPase of the gastric parietal cells. The H⁺-K⁺ ATPase is a **primary active transport** mechanism that pumps H⁺ from the cell to the lumen and simultaneously pumps K⁺ from the lumen into the cell. K⁺ then diffuses from the cell into blood (is reabsorbed) via K⁺ channels. (In Figure 6-32A, another ATPase, the H⁺ ATPase, also is shown in the luminal membrane for completeness. It does not relate to the K⁺ reabsorptive function of the α-intercalated cells, but it will be discussed with acid-base balance in Chapter 7.)

K⁺ Secretion by Principal Cells

The function of the principal cells is to secrete, rather than to reabsorb, K⁺. Thus, the cellular mechanisms in the principal cells differ from those in the α-intercalated cells. The diagram of the principal cell in Figure 6-32B should be familiar because this cell type has been discussed previously in relation to Na⁺ reabsorption (see Fig. 6-27).

K⁺ secretion is net transfer of K⁺ from blood into the lumen. K⁺ is brought into the cell from the blood by the Na⁺-K⁺ ATPase, which is responsible for maintaining the high intracellular K⁺ concentration. Both the

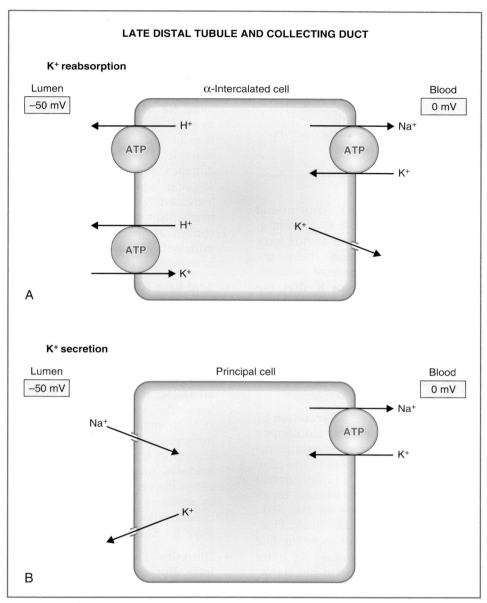

Figure 6–32 Cellular mechanisms of K⁺ reabsorption in α-intercalated cells (A) and K⁺ secretion in principal cells (B) of the late distal tubule and collecting duct. ATP, Adenosine triphosphate.

luminal and basolateral membranes have K⁺ channels, so, theoretically, K⁺ can diffuse into the lumen (secretion) or back into the blood. The K⁺ permeability and the size of the electrochemical gradient for K⁺ are higher in the luminal membrane; therefore, most of the K⁺ diffuses across the luminal membrane rather than being recycled across the basolateral membrane into the blood. (For simplicity, the basolateral K⁺ channels are omitted from the figure.)

The single most important principle for understanding the **factors that alter K⁺ secretion** is that *the magnitude of K⁺ secretion is determined by the size of the electrochemical gradient for K⁺ across the luminal membrane.* By employing this principle, it is then

easy to predict the effects of aldosterone, acid-base disturbances, dietary K⁺, and flow rate (diuretics). Any factor that increases the magnitude of the electrochemical gradient for K⁺ across the luminal membrane will increase K⁺ secretion; conversely, any factor that decreases the size of the electrochemical gradient will decrease K⁺ secretion (Table 6-9).

♦ **Dietary K⁺.** It has been emphasized that the fundamental mechanism for maintaining external K⁺ balance involves changes in K⁺ secretion by the principal cells. Knowing this, it is easy to understand the body's response to a **high K⁺ diet:** The ingested K⁺ enters the cells (aided by the insulin response to

Table 6–9 Regulation of K⁺ Secretion by the Principal Cells

Causes of Increased K⁺ Secretion	Causes of Decreased K⁺ Secretion
High K⁺ diet	Low K⁺ diet
Hyperaldosteronism	Hypoaldosteronism
Alkalosis	Acidosis
Thiazide diuretics	K⁺-sparing diuretics
Loop diuretics	
Luminal anions	

a meal) and raises the intracellular K⁺ content and concentration. When the intracellular K⁺ concentration of the principal cells increases, the driving force for K⁺ secretion across the luminal membrane increases and the ingested K⁺ is excreted in urine. Conversely, when a person eats a **low K⁺ diet,** the principal cells are relatively depleted of K⁺; the intracellular K⁺ concentration decreases, which decreases the driving force for K⁺ secretion. On a low K⁺ diet, in addition to the decrease in K⁺ secretion by the principal cells, there is an increase in K⁺ reabsorption by the α-intercalated cells. Together, the two effects account for low rates of K⁺ excretion.

♦ **Aldosterone.** Aldosterone **increases K⁺ secretion** by the principal cells. Recall the effect of aldosterone on Na⁺ reabsorption that was discussed previously: Aldosterone increases Na⁺ reabsorption in the principal cells by inducing synthesis of the luminal membrane Na⁺ channels and the basolateral membrane Na⁺-K⁺ ATPase. These actions on Na⁺ reabsorption are related to K⁺ secretion as follows: First, aldosterone induces the synthesis of more luminal membrane Na⁺ channels, which increases Na⁺ entry into the cell and provides more Na⁺ to the Na⁺-K⁺ ATPase. As more Na⁺ is pumped out of the cell, more K⁺ must be simultaneously pumped into the cell. Second, aldosterone increases the quantity of Na⁺-K⁺ ATPase, further increasing the amount of K⁺ pumped into the cell. Together, the two effects raise the intracellular K⁺ concentration, which increases the driving force for K⁺ secretion from the cell into the lumen. Finally, as a separate effect, aldosterone increases the number of K⁺ channels in the luminal membrane, which coordinates with the increased driving force to increase K⁺ secretion.

This discussion of the effects of aldosterone on Na⁺ reabsorption emphasizes the close relationship between Na⁺ reabsorption and K⁺ secretion in the principal cells. As described, much of the effect of aldosterone on K⁺ secretion is secondary to the effect of aldosterone on Na⁺ reabsorption. Other situations also demonstrate this relationship, and two examples are included here. The first example is of a person eating a **high Na⁺ diet.** This person will have increased Na⁺ excretion, as expected, to maintain Na⁺ balance, and *also* increased K⁺ excretion. The explanation for the increased K⁺ excretion is increased delivery of Na⁺ to the principal cells. As more Na⁺ is delivered to the principal cells, more Na⁺ enters the cells across the luminal membrane, more Na⁺ is extruded by the Na⁺-K⁺ ATPase, and more K⁺ is pumped into the cell, which increases the driving force for K⁺ secretion. The second example is a person treated with **diuretics.** Loop diuretics and thiazide diuretics inhibit Na⁺ reabsorption "upstream" to the principal cells, causing increased Na⁺ delivery to the principal cells. The mechanism discussed for a high Na⁺ diet can be applied again here: More Na⁺ is delivered to the principal cells, more Na⁺ is reabsorbed, and more K⁺ is secreted (Box 6-2).

♦ **Acid-base disturbances.** Acid-base disturbances can have profound effects on the blood K⁺ concentration, attributable to alterations in K⁺ secretion by the principal cells. Usually, alkalosis increases K⁺ secretion, and acidosis decreases K⁺ secretion. The exchange of H⁺ and K⁺ ions across *basolateral* cell membranes underlies these effects as follows: In **alkalosis,** there is a deficit of H⁺ in the ECF. H⁺ leaves the cells to aid in buffering, and K⁺ enters the cells to maintain electroneutrality. The increased intracellular K⁺ concentration increases the driving force for K⁺ secretion, causing hypokalemia. In **acidosis,** there is an excess of H⁺ in the ECF. H⁺ enters the cells for buffering, and K⁺ leaves the cells to maintain electroneutrality. The intracellular K⁺ concentration decreases, which decreases the driving force for K⁺ secretion, causing hyperkalemia.

♦ **Diuretics.** The most commonly used diuretics, the **loop diuretics** and the **thiazide diuretics,** cause increased K⁺ excretion or kaliuresis. Therefore, an important side effect of diuretic therapy is **hypokalemia.** The basis for the diuretic-induced increase in K⁺ excretion is **increased K⁺ secretion** by the principal cells, by the mechanism explained in the previous section. Loop diuretics and thiazide diuretics inhibit Na⁺ reabsorption "upstream" to the site of K⁺ secretion (in the thick ascending limb and in the early distal tubule, respectively), thereby delivering more Na⁺ to the principal cells. When more Na⁺ is delivered to the principal cells, more Na⁺ enters the cells across the luminal membrane and more Na⁺ is extruded from the cells by the Na⁺-K⁺ ATPase. Simultaneously, more K⁺ is pumped into the cells, which increases the intracellular K⁺ concentration and increases the driving force for K⁺ secretion.

A second factor contributing to the increased K⁺ secretion is the **increased flow rate** produced by these diuretics. When the flow rate through the late distal tubule and collecting duct increases, the

BOX 6–2 Clinical Physiology: Primary Hyperaldosteronism

DESCRIPTION OF CASE. A 50-year-old man is referred to his physician for evaluation of weakness and hypertension. On physical examination, his systolic and diastolic blood pressures are elevated (160/110) in the supine position. The following blood and urine values are obtained:

Venous blood	Urine
[Na$^+$], 142 mEq/L	[Na$^+$], 60 mEq/L (normal)
[K$^+$], 2.1 mEq/L	[K$^+$], 55 mEq/L (high)
[Cl$^-$], 98 mEq/L	Osmolarity, 520 mOsm/L
Osmolarity, 289 mOsm/L	

EXPLANATION OF CASE. The man's physical examination was notable for hypertension, which suggests ECF volume expansion. Increased ECF volume and increased blood volume explain his increased systolic and diastolic pressures. Because plasma [Na$^+$] and osmolarity are normal, it can be concluded that the water content of his body is normal relative to solute content. Therefore, the man must have increased total body Na$^+$ content with a *proportionately* increased water content. The combination of increased Na$^+$ and water content in the body is responsible for his increased ECF volume.

The man has markedly decreased plasma [K$^+$] concentration with increased urine K$^+$ excretion. Although it would *seem* that renal K$^+$ excretion should decrease in the face of such a low plasma [K$^+$], these observations can be reconciled by concluding that the low plasma [K$^+$] is *caused* by the increased urine K$^+$ excretion.

All of the findings in this patient can be explained by the diagnosis of an aldosterone-secreting tumor of the zona glomerulosa of the adrenal gland, resulting in primary hyperaldosteronism (Conn syndrome). The high circulating levels of aldosterone have two effects on the principal cells of the late distal tubule and collecting ducts: increased Na$^+$ reabsorption and increased K$^+$ secretion. The consequences of the increased K$^+$ secretion are straightforward: Increased K$^+$ secretion by the principal cells causes the urinary K$^+$ excretion to increase and the plasma [K$^+$] to decrease. The observation of a normal urine Na$^+$ excretion is puzzling, however. The direct effect of aldosterone on the principal cells is to increase Na$^+$ reabsorption, and urine Na$^+$ should be decreased. The increased Na$^+$ reabsorption then leads to increased ECF Na$^+$ content and increased ECF volume. There is, however, a secondary effect of this ECF volume expansion on the proximal tubule: ECF volume expansion inhibits proximal tubule reabsorption, which is called "escape from aldosterone," or mineralocorticoid escape. Thus, because of "escape from aldosterone," the urine Na$^+$ in this man is higher than if aldosterone had only a direct effect on the principal cells.

TREATMENT. The man's hypertension is treatable by removal of the adrenal tumor. While awaiting surgery, he is placed on spironolactone, an aldosterone antagonist, and on a sodium-restricted diet. Spironolactone blocks all of the effects of aldosterone on the principal cells. Na$^+$ reabsorption is reduced to normal (reducing his ECF volume) and K$^+$ secretion also is reduced to normal (increasing his plasma [K$^+$]). After surgery, his blood pressure returns to normal levels, and his blood and urine chemistries return to normal.

---

luminal K$^+$ concentration is diluted, which increases the driving force for K$^+$ secretion. (The driving force across the luminal membrane can be increased *either* by increasing the intracellular K$^+$ concentration *or* by decreasing the luminal K$^+$ concentration.)

Loop diuretics (but not thiazide diuretics) also cause increased K$^+$ excretion by inhibiting Na$^+$-K$^+$-2Cl$^-$ cotransport and, as a result, K$^+$ reabsorption in the thick ascending limb. This direct effect in the thick ascending limb, coupled with increased K$^+$ secretion by the principal cells, predicts that loop diuretics will produce a profound kaliuresis and hypokalemia.

♦ The **K$^+$-sparing diuretics** (e.g., spironolactone, amiloride, triamterene) are the only diuretics that do not cause kaliuresis. As explained, these diuretics inhibit all of the actions of aldosterone on the principal cells and, therefore, **inhibit K$^+$ secretion.** The major application of K$^+$-sparing diuretics is in combination with the loop or thiazide diuretics to offset the kaliuresis and hypokalemia produced by those drugs.

♦ **Luminal anions.** The presence of large anions (e.g., sulfate, HCO$_3^-$) in the lumen of the distal tubule and collecting duct increases K$^+$ secretion. Such nonreabsorbable anions increase the electronegativity of the lumen, thereby increasing the electrochemical driving force for K$^+$ secretion.

PHOSPHATE, CALCIUM, AND MAGNESIUM BALANCE

Phosphate

Phosphate plays a critical role in the body as a constituent of bone and as a urinary buffer for H$^+$. Because the kidneys regulate the blood phosphate concentration, the renal mechanisms deserve special attention. (Overall phosphate homeostasis and its hormonal regulation are discussed in Chapter 9.)

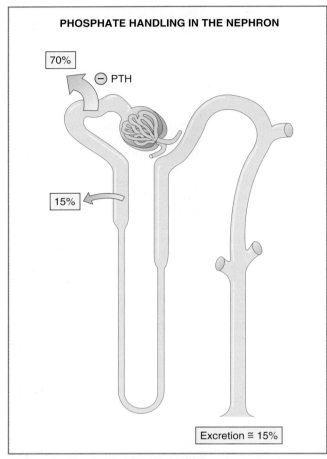

PHOSPHATE HANDLING IN THE NEPHRON

70%

⊖ PTH

15%

Excretion ≅ 15%

Figure 6–33 Phosphate handling in the nephron. *Arrows* show location of phosphate reabsorption; *numbers* are percentages of the filtered load reabsorbed or excreted. PTH, Parathyroid hormone.

Phosphate is localized primarily in bone matrix (85%), and the remainder of the body phosphate is divided between ICF (15%) and ECF (<0.5%). In ICF, phosphate is a component of nucleotides (DNA and RNA), high-energy molecules (e.g., ATP), and metabolic intermediates. In ECF, phosphate is present in its inorganic form and serves as a buffer for H^+. About 10% of the phosphate in plasma is protein bound.

The **renal handling of phosphate** is illustrated in Figure 6-33. Phosphate that is not bound to plasma proteins (90%) is filtered across glomerular capillaries. Subsequently, about 70% of the filtered load is reabsorbed in the **proximal convoluted tubule,** and 15% of the filtered load is reabsorbed in the **proximal straight tubule.** At the cellular level, phosphate reabsorption is accomplished by an Na^+-phosphate cotransporter in the luminal membrane of the proximal tubule cells (see Fig. 6-20). Similar to the reabsorption of glucose, phosphate reabsorption is saturable and exhibits a T_m. When the T_m is reached, any phosphate that is not reabsorbed will be excreted. Whether phosphate is reabsorbed in later segments of the nephron (e.g., distal tubule) is debatable, but it seems to depend on the level of dietary phosphate and parathyroid hormone. When compared with other substances (e.g., Na^+, Cl^-, HCO_3^-, glucose), phosphate excretion of 15% of the filtered load is a high percentage. The comparatively high level of phosphate excretion is physiologically important because unreabsorbed phosphate serves as a **urinary buffer for H^+** (called titratable acid; see Chapter 7).

Parathyroid hormone (**PTH**) regulates the reabsorption of phosphate in the proximal tubule by inhibiting Na^+-phosphate cotransport, thereby decreasing the T_m for phosphate reabsorption. When PTH inhibits phosphate reabsorption, it causes **phosphaturia,** or increased phosphate excretion. In the context of this action, it is significant that little or no phosphate reabsorption occurs beyond the proximal tubule. PTH inhibits phosphate reabsorption in the proximal tubule, and the unreabsorbed phosphate then is excreted because segments beyond the proximal tubule have little or no reabsorptive capacity for phosphate.

At the cellular level, the mechanism of action of PTH involves binding of hormone to a basolateral receptor in the proximal tubule cells, which is coupled to **adenylyl cyclase** via a G_s protein. When activated, adenylyl cyclase catalyzes the conversion of ATP to cyclic adenosine monophosphate (cAMP), the second messenger. cAMP then activates a series of protein kinases, which phosphorylate components of the luminal membrane. The final step in this sequence is inhibition of Na^+-phosphate cotransport. As an aside, the luminal membrane of proximal tubule cells has a transporter for cAMP, so cAMP moves into the lumen and is excreted. Increased **urinary cAMP** and phosphaturia are the hallmarks of PTH action.

A defect in the receptor, G_s protein, or adenylyl cyclase complex causes an inherited disorder called **pseudohypoparathyroidism.** In this disorder, renal cells are resistant to the action of PTH. Although circulating PTH levels are elevated, PTH cannot produce its usual phosphaturic effect, and both urinary phosphate and cyclic AMP are decreased.

Calcium

Like phosphate, most of the body's calcium (Ca^{2+}) is contained in bone (99%). The remaining 1% is present in ICF (mostly in bound form) and in ECF. The total Ca^{2+} concentration in plasma is 5 mEq/L or 10 mg/dL. Of the total plasma Ca^{2+}, 40% is bound to plasma proteins, 10% is bound to other anions such as phosphate and citrate, and 50% is in the free, ionized form. The plasma Ca^{2+} concentration is regulated by PTH, involving a complex interaction of bone, the gastrointestinal tract, and the kidneys. Like phosphate, the renal is reabsorbed (exactly the same percentage as Na$^+$ reabsorption). In fact, Ca^{2+} reabsorption is tightly coupled to Na$^+$ reabsorption in the proximal tubule. For example, when Na$^+$ reabsorption is inhibited by volume expansion, Ca^{2+} reabsorption is simultaneously inhibited; when Na$^+$ reabsorption is stimulated by volume contraction, so is Ca^{2+} reabsorption.

♦ **Thick ascending limb of the loop of Henle.** As with Na$^+$, 25% of the filtered load of Ca^{2+} is reabsorbed in the thick ascending limb of the loop of Henle. In this segment, Ca^{2+} reabsorption occurs along a paracellular route (between cells) and is tightly coupled to Na$^+$ reabsorption. The mechanism of coupling in the thick ascending limb depends on the **lumen-positive potential difference,** which is generated by the Na$^+$-K$^+$-2Cl$^-$ cotransporter. This lumen-positive potential normally drives the reabsorption of divalent cations such as Ca^{2+}, as positive charge repels positive charge. Coupling of Ca^{2+} and Na$^+$ reabsorption in the thick ascending limb has an important implication for diuretic action: **Loop diuretics** such as furosemide inhibit Ca^{2+} reabsorption to the same extent that they inhibit Na$^+$ reabsorption. The mechanism is inhibition of Na$^+$-K$^+$-2Cl$^-$ cotransport and elimination of the lumen-positive potential, thereby eliminating the driving force for paracellular Ca^{2+} reabsorption. This action of loop diuretics underlies their usefulness in the **treatment of hypercalcemia.**

♦ **Distal tubule.** The distal tubule reabsorbs about 8% of the filtered load of Ca^{2+}. Although this is a quantitatively smaller amount than is reabsorbed in the earlier segments of the nephron, the distal tubule is the site of *regulation* of Ca^{2+} reabsorption. The following three points concerning regulation in the distal tubule are relevant: (1) The distal tubule is the only nephron segment in which Ca^{2+} reabsorption is *not* coupled directly to Na$^+$ reabsorption. In other words, Ca^{2+} reabsorption and Na$^+$ reabsorption in the distal tubule are not necessarily parallel (as they are in the proximal tubule and the thick ascending limb). The uncoupling of Ca^{2+} and Na$^+$ reabsorption in the distal tubule is illustrated by the action of thiazide diuretics (see point 3). (2) Not only is distal Ca^{2+} reabsorption uncoupled from Na$^+$ reabsorption, but it has its own regulatory hormone, PTH. In the distal tubule, **PTH** increases Ca^{2+} reabsorption via a basolateral receptor, activation of adenylyl cyclase, and generation of cAMP as the second messenger. This action of PTH on the distal tubule is called its **hypocalciuric** action. Thus, PTH has two effects on the nephron, both of which are mediated by cAMP: a phosphaturic action in the proximal tubule and a hypocalciuric action in the distal tubule. (3) Because of the uncoupling of distal Ca^{2+} and Na$^+$ reabsorption, the effect of thiazide

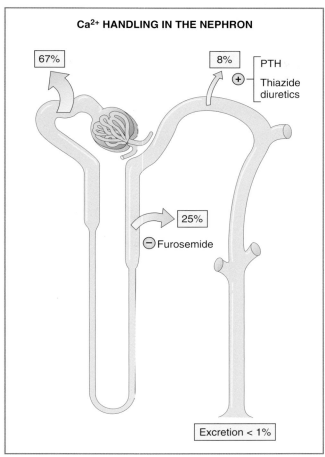

Figure 6-34 **Ca^{2+} handling in the nephron.** *Arrows* show location of Ca^{2+} reabsorption; *numbers* are percentages of the filtered load reabsorbed or excreted. PTH, Parathyroid hormone.

mechanisms are an integral part of overall Ca^{2+} homeostasis, as discussed in Chapter 9.

The **renal handling of Ca^{2+}** is illustrated in Figure 6-34. The pattern of Ca^{2+} reabsorption along the nephron is quite similar to the pattern for Na$^+$ reabsorption (see Fig. 6-19). Like Na$^+$, over 99% of the filtered Ca^{2+} is reabsorbed, leaving less than 1% to be excreted. Ca^{2+} reabsorption is tightly coupled to Na$^+$ reabsorption in the proximal tubule and loop of Henle, and only in the distal tubule is the reabsorption of the two ions dissociated.

♦ **Filtration.** Ca^{2+} differs from Na$^+$ at the filtration step. Any Ca^{2+} bound to plasma proteins (i.e., 40% of the total Ca^{2+}) cannot be filtered across glomerular capillaries; therefore, only 60% is **ultrafilterable.** To calculate the filtered load of Ca^{2+}, a correction is made for protein binding: If GFR is 180 L/day and total plasma Ca^{2+} is 5 mEq/L, then the filtered load of Ca^{2+} is 540 mEq/day (180 L/day × 5 mEq/L × 0.60).

♦ **Proximal tubule.** Ca^{2+} parallels Na$^+$ reabsorption in the proximal tubule in that 67% of the filtered load diuretics on Ca^{2+} reabsorption differs entirely from the effects of diuretics that act in the proximal tubule or thick ascending limb. Thiazide diuretics increase Ca^{2+} reabsorption, whereas the other classes of diuretics decrease it.

Recall that **thiazide diuretics** inhibit Na^+ reabsorption in the early distal tubule by inhibiting Na^+-Cl^- cotransport, thereby increasing Na^+ excretion. However, the effect on Ca^{2+} reabsorption is the exact opposite: Thiazide diuretics increase Ca^{2+} reabsorption, thereby decreasing Ca^{2+} excretion. This action of thiazides forms the basis for their usefulness in the **treatment of idiopathic hypercalciuria** (meaning increased urinary Ca^{2+} excretion of unknown etiology). Administration of thiazide diuretics increases Ca^{2+} reabsorption, decreases urinary Ca^{2+} excretion, and decreases the likelihood of Ca^{2+} stone formation.

Magnesium

In several respects, the pattern of magnesium (Mg^{2+}) reabsorption differs from that of either Na^+ or Ca^{2+}. Overall reabsorption of Mg^{2+} by the nephron is 95%, leaving 5% for excretion, which is a higher percentage than for many other substances (Fig. 6-35). Twenty percent of plasma Mg^{2+} is bound to proteins, and 80% is filterable across glomerular capillaries. In the **proximal tubule,** 30% of the filtered load is reabsorbed, a small percentage when compared with Na^+ and Ca^{2+} (67% for Na^+ and Ca^{2+}). In contrast to the other segments, the major site of Mg^{2+} reabsorption is the **thick ascending limb,** where 60% of the filtered load is reabsorbed. As with Ca^{2+}, Mg^{2+} reabsorption in the thick ascending limb is driven by the lumen-positive potential difference. Here again, **loop diuretics** strongly inhibit Mg^{2+} reabsorption and increase Mg^{2+} excretion, which may lead to **hypomagnesemia.** In the distal tubule, a small percentage (5%) of Mg^{2+} is reabsorbed.

WATER BALANCE—CONCENTRATION AND DILUTION OF URINE

Body fluid osmolarity is maintained at a value of about **290 mOsm/L** (for simplicity, 300 mOsm/L) by processes called **osmoregulation.** Even small deviations in body fluid osmolarity produce a set of hormonal responses that alter water reabsorption by the kidneys, attempting to return osmolarity back toward the normal value. *These renal mechanisms for water reabsorption are responsible for maintaining constant body fluid osmolarity.* As with other renal regulatory mechanisms, control of water balance is exerted at the level of the late distal tubule and collecting duct.

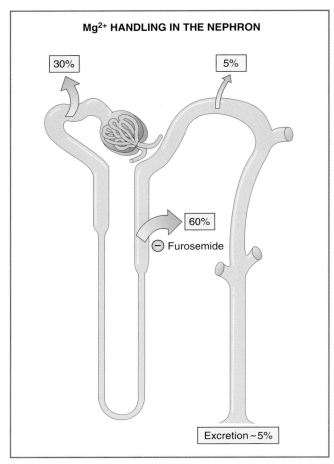

Figure 6–35 Mg^{2+} handling in the nephron. *Arrows* show location of Mg^{2+} reabsorption; *numbers* are percentages of the filtered load reabsorbed or excreted.

Variations in water reabsorption produce variations in urine osmolarity. Urine osmolarity can vary from as low as 50 mOsm/L to as high as 1200 mOsm/L. The following descriptors are used to describe urine osmolarity: When urine osmolarity is equal to blood osmolarity, it is called **isosmotic** urine. When urine osmolarity is higher than blood osmolarity, it is called **hyperosmotic** urine. When urine osmolarity is lower than blood osmolarity, it is called **hyposmotic** urine.

Regulation of Body Fluid Osmolarity

The regulation of body fluid osmolarity is best illustrated by two commonplace examples. The first example is the body's response to water deprivation; the second is the body's response to drinking water.

Response to Water Deprivation

Figure 6-36 shows the events that occur when a person is **deprived of drinking water** (e.g., person is lost in the desert for 12 hours with no source of drinking water). The circled numbers in the figure correlate with the following steps:

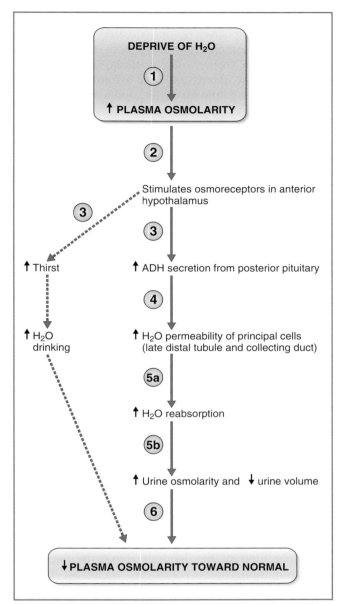

Figure 6-36 **Responses to water deprivation.** See the text for an explanation of the *circled numbers.* ADH, Antidiuretic hormone.

1. Water is continuously lost from the body in sweat and in water vapor from the mouth and nose (called insensible water loss). If this water is not replaced by drinking water, then plasma osmolarity increases.

2. The increase in osmolarity stimulates **osmoreceptors** in the anterior hypothalamus, which are exquisitely sensitive and are stimulated by increases in osmolarity of less than 1 mOsm/L.

3. Stimulation of the hypothalamic osmoreceptors has two effects. It stimulates **thirst,** which drives drinking behavior. It also stimulates secretion of **ADH** from the posterior pituitary gland.

4. The posterior pituitary gland secretes ADH. ADH circulates in the blood to the kidneys, where it produces an increase in water permeability of the principal cells of the late distal tubule and collecting duct.

5. The increase in water permeability results in increased water reabsorption (5a) in the late distal tubule and collecting ducts. As more water is reabsorbed by these segments, **urine osmolarity increases** and **urine volume decreases** (5b).

6. Increased water reabsorption means that more water is returned to the body fluids. Coupled with increased thirst and drinking behavior, plasma osmolarity is decreased, back toward the normal value. This system is an elegant example of negative feedback, in which the original disturbance (increased plasma osmolarity) causes a set of feedback responses (secretion of ADH and increased water reabsorption) that restore plasma osmolarity to its normal value.

Response to Water Drinking

Figure 6-37 shows the series of events that occur when a person drinks water. These responses will be easy to understand because they are the exact opposite of those described for water deprivation. Again, the circled numbers in the figure correspond to the following steps:

1. When a person drinks water, the ingested water is distributed throughout the body fluids. Because the amount of solute in the body is unchanged, the added water will dilute the body fluids and cause a decrease in plasma osmolarity.

2. The decrease in plasma osmolarity inhibits osmoreceptors in the anterior hypothalamus.

3. Inhibition of the osmoreceptors has two effects. It decreases thirst and suppresses water drinking behavior. It also inhibits secretion of ADH from the posterior pituitary gland.

4. When ADH secretion is inhibited, circulating levels of ADH are reduced and less ADH is delivered to the kidneys. As a result of the lower ADH levels, there is a decrease in water permeability of the principal cells of the late distal tubule and collecting ducts.

5. The decrease in water permeability results in decreased water reabsorption by the late distal tubule and collecting ducts (5a). The water that is not reabsorbed by these segments is excreted, **decreasing urine osmolarity** and **increasing urine volume** (5b).

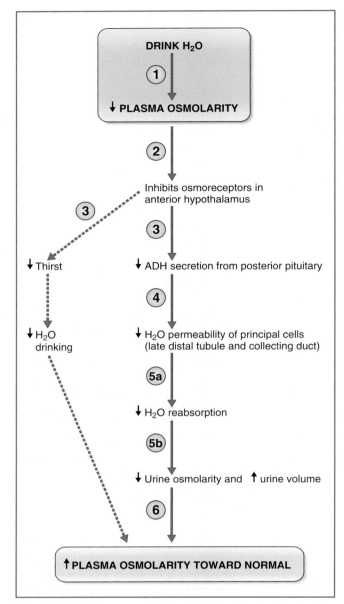

Figure 6–37 **Responses to water drinking.** See the text for an explanation of the *circled numbers.* ADH, Antidiuretic hormone.

6. Because less water is reabsorbed, less water is returned to the circulation. Coupled with the inhibition of thirst and the suppression of water drinking, plasma osmolarity increases back toward the normal value.

Corticopapillary Osmotic Gradient

To understand how the kidneys participate in osmoregulation, it is first necessary to appreciate the creation and role of the **corticopapillary osmotic gradient.** Descriptively, it is a gradient of osmolarity in the interstitial fluid of the kidney from the cortex to the papilla

(see Fig. 6-1 for anatomic divisions of the kidney). The osmolarity of the cortex is approximately 300 mOsm/L, similar to the osmolarity of other body fluids. Moving from the cortex to the outer medulla, inner medulla, and papilla, the interstitial fluid osmolarity progressively increases. At the tip of the papilla, the osmolarity can be as high as 1200 mOsm/L.

The question arises as to the origin of the corticopapillary osmotic gradient. *What solutes contribute to the osmotic gradient, and what mechanisms deposit these solutes in the interstitial fluid?* The answers can be found in two processes: **countercurrent multiplication,** a function of the loop of Henle, which deposits NaCl in the deeper regions of the kidney; and **urea recycling,** a function of the inner medullary collecting ducts, which deposits urea.

Countercurrent Multiplication

Countercurrent multiplication is a function of the **loop of Henle.** Its role in the formation of the corticopapillary osmotic gradient is to deposit **NaCl** in the interstitial fluid of the deeper regions of the kidney. Figure 6-38 shows a single loop of Henle and the process of countercurrent multiplication, explained subsequently in a stepwise fashion. For didactic purposes, the loop of Henle is initially shown with no corticopapillary gradient; osmolarity is 300 mOsm/L throughout the loop and in the surrounding interstitial fluid. Countercurrent multiplication will build up a gradient of osmolarity in the interstitial fluid through a repeating **two-step process.** The first step is called the single effect, and the second step is the flow of tubular fluid.

SINGLE EFFECT

The single effect refers to the function of the thick ascending limb of the loop of Henle. In the **thick ascending limb,** NaCl is reabsorbed via the **Na^+-K^+-$2Cl^-$ cotransporter**. Because the thick ascending limb is impermeable to water, water is not reabsorbed along with NaCl, thereby diluting the tubular fluid in the ascending limb. The NaCl, which is transported out of the thick ascending limb, enters the interstitial fluid, increasing its osmolarity. Because the descending limb is permeable to water, water flows out of the descending limb until its osmolarity increases to the level of the adjacent interstitial fluid. Thus, as a result of the single effect, the osmolarity of the ascending limb decreases and the osmolarities of the interstitial fluid and the descending limb increase. **ADH** increases the activity of Na^+-K^+-$2Cl^-$ cotransporter and, therefore, enhances the single effect. For example, in conditions where circulating levels of ADH are high (e.g., dehydration), the corticopapillary osmotic gradient is augmented; in conditions where circulating levels of ADH are low (e.g., central diabetes insipidus), the corticopapillary osmotic gradient is diminished.

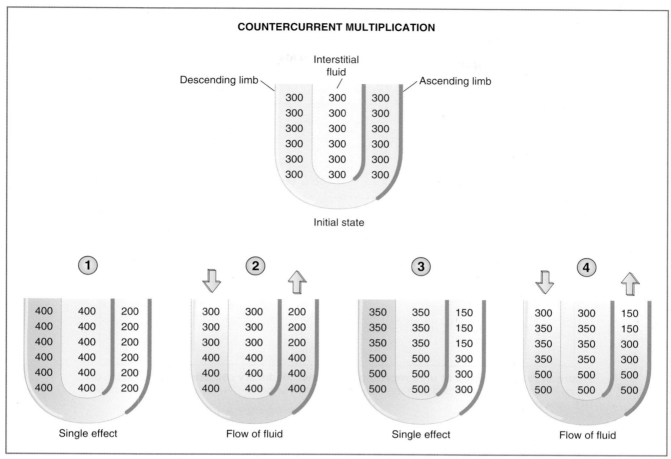

Figure 6–38 **Mechanism of countercurrent multiplication in a loop of Henle.** See the text for an explanation of the *circled numbers*; numbers are osmolarities of tubular fluid or interstitial fluid; *arrows* show the direction of fluid flow; *heavy outline* shows water impermeability of the ascending limb.

FLOW OF TUBULAR FLUID

Since glomerular filtration is an ongoing process, fluid flows continuously through the nephron. As new fluid enters the descending limb from the proximal tubule, an equal volume of fluid must leave the ascending limb and enter the distal tubule. The new fluid that enters the descending limb will have an osmolarity of 300 mOsm/L because it has come from the proximal tubule. At the same time, the high osmolarity fluid in the descending limb (created by the single effect) is pushed down toward the bend of the loop of Henle.

The two-step process for establishing the corticopapillary osmotic gradient is illustrated in Figure 6-37. Again, in the initial state, the loop of Henle and the surrounding interstitial fluid have no corticopapillary osmotic gradient. The circled numbers on the figure correlate with the following steps involved in creating the gradient:

1. **Step 1** is the **single effect.** As NaCl is reabsorbed out of the ascending limb and deposited in the surrounding interstitial fluid, water is left behind in the ascending limb. As a result, interstitial fluid osmolarity increases to 400 mOsm/L and the fluid in the ascending limb is diluted to 200 mOsm/L. Fluid in the descending limb equilibrates with the interstitial fluid, and its osmolarity also becomes 400 mOsm/L.

2. **Step 2** is the **flow of fluid.** New fluid with an osmolarity of 300 mOsm/L enters the descending limb from the proximal tubule, and an equal volume of fluid is displaced from the ascending limb. As a result of this fluid shift, the high osmolarity fluid in the descending limb (400 mOsm/L) is "pushed down" toward the bend of the loop of Henle. Even at this early stage, you can see that the corticopapillary osmotic gradient is beginning to develop.

3. **Step 3** is the **single effect** again. NaCl is reabsorbed out of the ascending limb and deposited in interstitial fluid, and water remains behind in the ascending limb. The osmolarity of the interstitial fluid

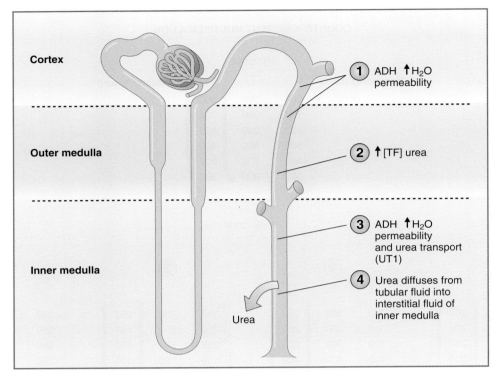

Figure 6–39 **Mechanism of urea recycling from inner medullary collecting ducts.** See the text for an explanation of the *circled numbers.* ADH, Antidiuretic hormone; [TF], tubular fluid concentration; UT1, urea transporter 1.

and descending limb fluid increases, adding to the gradient that was established in the previous steps. The osmolarity of the fluid of the ascending limb decreases further (is diluted).

4. **Step 4** is the **flow of fluid** again. New fluid with an osmolarity of 300 mOsm/L enters the descending limb from the proximal tubule, which displaces fluid from the ascending limb. As a result of the fluid shift, the high osmolarity fluid in the descending limb is pushed down toward the bend of the loop of Henle. The gradient of osmolarity is now larger than it was in step 2.

These two basic steps are repeated until the full corticopapillary gradient is established. As shown in Figure 6-38, each repeat of the two steps increases, or multiplies, the gradient. The size of the corticopapillary osmotic gradient depends on the **length of the loop of Henle.** In humans, the osmolarity of interstitial fluid at the bend of the loop of Henle is 1200 mOsm/L, but in species with longer loops of Henle (e.g., desert rodents), the osmolarity at the bend can be as high as 3000 mOsm/L.

Urea Recycling

Urea recycling from the inner medullary collecting ducts is the second process that contributes to the establishment of the corticopapillary osmotic gradient.

The mechanism of urea recycling is explained in Figure 6-39. The circled numbers on the figure correlate with the following steps:

1. In the **cortical and outer medullary collecting ducts,** ADH increases water permeability, but it does not increase urea permeability. As a result, water is reabsorbed from the cortical and outer medullary collecting ducts, but urea remains behind in the tubular fluid.

2. This differential effect of ADH on water and urea permeability in cortical and outer medullary collecting ducts causes the urea concentration of tubular fluid to increase.

3. In the **inner medullary collecting ducts,** ADH increases water permeability *and* it increases the transporter for facilitated diffusion of urea, **UT1** (in contrast to its effect on only water permeability in cortical and outer medullary collecting ducts).

4. Because the urea concentration of tubular fluid has been elevated by reabsorption of water in the cortical and outer medullary collecting ducts, a large concentration gradient has been created for urea. In the presence of ADH, the inner medullary collecting ducts can transport urea, and urea diffuses down its concentration gradient into the interstitial fluid. Urea that would have otherwise been excreted is

recycled into the inner medulla, where it is added to the corticopapillary osmotic gradient.

As implied in the mechanism, urea recycling also depends on **ADH.** When ADH levels are high, as in water deprivation, the differential permeability effects occur and urea is recycled into the inner medulla, adding to the corticopapillary osmotic gradient. When ADH levels are low, as in water drinking or in central diabetes insipidus, the differential permeability effects do not occur and urea is not recycled. The positive effect of ADH on urea recycling is the second mechanism by which ADH augments the corticopapillary osmotic gradient (the first is stimulation of Na^+-K^+-$2Cl^-$ cotransport and the single effect of countercurrent multiplication). Thus, the corticopapillary osmotic gradient is larger when ADH levels are high (e.g., water deprivation, SIADH) than when ADH levels are low (e.g., water drinking, central diabetes insipidus).

Vasa Recta

The vasa recta are capillaries that serve the medulla and papilla of the kidney. The vasa recta follow the same course as the loop of Henle and have the same hairpin (U) shape. Only 5% of the renal blood flow serves the medulla, and blood flow through the vasa recta is especially low.

The vasa recta participate in **countercurrent exchange,** which differs from countercurrent multiplication as follows: Countercurrent multiplication, as described, is an active process that *establishes* the corticopapillary osmotic gradient. Countercurrent exchange is a purely passive process that helps *maintain* the gradient. The passive properties of the vasa recta are the same as for other capillaries: They are freely permeable to small solutes and water. Blood flow through the vasa recta is slow, and solutes and water can move in and out, allowing for efficient countercurrent exchange.

Countercurrent exchange is illustrated schematically in Figure 6-40. The figure shows a single vasa recta, with its descending limb and ascending limb. Blood entering the descending limb has an osmolarity of 300 mOsm/L. As this blood flows down the **descending limb,** it is exposed to interstitial fluid with increasingly higher osmolarity (the corticopapillary osmotic gradient). Because the vasa recta are capillaries, small solutes such as NaCl and urea diffuse into the descending limb and water diffuses out, allowing blood in the descending limb of the vasa recta to equilibrate osmotically with the surrounding interstitial fluid. At the bend of the vasa recta, the blood has an osmolarity equal to that of interstitial fluid at the tip of the papilla, 1200 mOsm/L. In the **ascending limb,** the opposite events occur. As blood flows up the ascending limb, it is exposed to interstitial fluid with decreasing osmolarity. Small solutes diffuse out of the ascending limb and

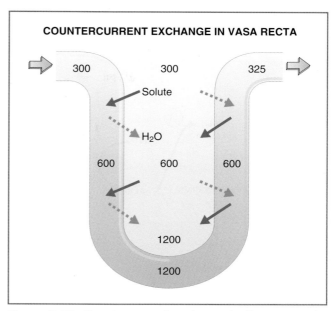

Figure 6–40 Countercurrent exchange in the vasa recta. *Solid dark blue arrows* show the direction of solute movement; *dashed green arrows* show the direction of water movement; *thick light blue arrows* show blood flow through the vasa recta; numbers are osmolarity in mOsm/L.

water diffuses in, and the blood in the ascending limb of the vasa recta equilibrates with the surrounding interstitial fluid.

In Figure 6-40, notice that the blood leaving the vasa recta has an osmolarity of 325 mOsm/L, which is slightly higher than the osmolarity of the original blood that entered it. Some of the solute from the corticopapillary osmotic gradient was picked up and will be carried back to the systemic circulation. With time, this process could dissipate the corticopapillary osmotic gradient. The gradient normally does not dissipate, however, because the mechanisms of countercurrent multiplication and urea recycling continuously replace any solute that is carried away by blood flow.

Antidiuretic Hormone

As described in the preceding section, ADH has three actions on the renal tubule. (1) It increases the water permeability of the principal cells of the late distal tubule and collecting ducts. (2) It increases the activity of the Na^+-K^+-$2Cl^-$ cotransporter of the thick ascending limb, thereby enhancing countercurrent multiplication and the size of the corticopapillary osmotic gradient. (3) It increases urea permeability in the inner medullary collecting ducts (but not in the cortical or outer medullary collecting ducts), enhancing urea recycling and the size of the corticopapillary osmotic gradient.

Of these actions, the effect on **water permeability** of the principal cells is the best known and

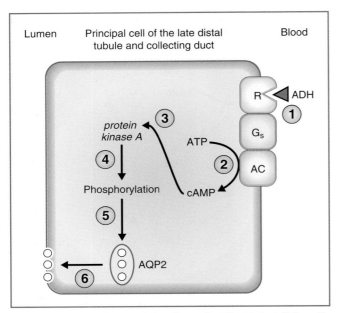

Lumen   Principal cell of the late distal tubule and collecting duct   Blood

Figure 6–41 Cellular mechanism of action of antidiuretic hormone in the principal cell of the late distal tubule and collecting duct. See the text for an explanation of the circled numbers. AC, Adenylyl cyclase; ADH, antidiuretic hormone; AQP2, aquaporin 2; ATP, adenosine triphosphate; cAMP, cyclic adenosine monophosphate, or cyclic AMP; G_s, stimulatory G protein; R, V_2 receptor.

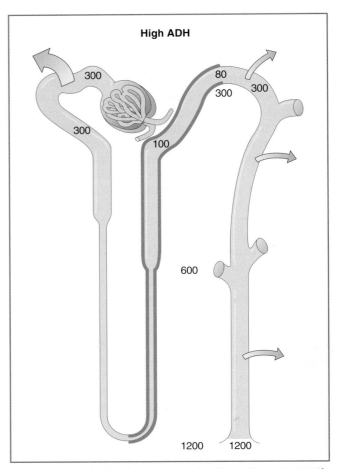

High ADH

Figure 6–42 Mechanisms for production of hyperosmotic (concentrated) urine in the presence of antidiuretic hormone (ADH). *Arrows* show location of water reabsorption; *heavy outline* shows water-impermeable portions of the nephron; numbers are osmolarity of tubular fluid or interstitial fluid.

physiologically is the most important. In the absence of ADH, the principal cells are impermeable to water. In the presence of ADH, **water channels,** or **aquaporins,** are inserted in the luminal membrane of the principal cells, making them permeable to water. The following steps are involved in the action of ADH on the principal cells (Fig. 6-41). These steps correspond to the circled numbers in the figure:

1. When circulating levels of ADH are high, ADH is delivered to the principal cells via the peritubular capillary blood. **V_2 receptors** for ADH, present in the basolateral membrane, are coupled to **adenylyl cyclase** via a stimulatory G protein (G_s).

2. When ADH binds to the receptors, adenylyl cyclase is activated and catalyzes the conversion of ATP to **cAMP.**

3. and 4. cAMP activates **protein kinase A.** Activated protein kinase A then causes **phosphorylation** of intracellular structures. The identity of these structures is uncertain, although possibilities include microtubules and microfilaments, which are involved in intracellular shuttling mechanisms.

5. and 6. After the phosphorylation step, vesicles containing water channels are shuttled to and inserted into the luminal membrane of the principal cell, thus increasing its water permeability. The

specific water channel that is controlled by ADH is **aquaporin 2 (AQP2).** Using freeze-fracture electron microscopy, the water channels in the luminal membrane can be visualized in clusters called **intramembranous particles.** The presence and number of intramembranous particle clusters correlate with the presence and magnitude of water permeability of principal cells, suggesting that the particle clusters are an anatomic representation of the water channels.

Production of Hyperosmotic Urine

By definition, hyperosmotic, or concentrated, urine has an osmolarity that is higher than blood osmolarity. Hyperosmotic urine is produced when the **circulating levels of ADH are high,** as occurs in water deprivation or in SIADH. The mechanisms are shown in Figure 6-42.

Steps in Production of Hyperosmotic Urine

Before the mechanism is described in detail, a few general comments should be made about the format of Figure 6-42. The numbers on the figure give the osmolarity at various points along the nephron and in the interstitial fluid. The *heavily outlined* portion of the thick ascending limb and early distal tubule indicates that these segments are impermeable to water. The *arrows* represent water reabsorption in different segments of the nephron.

Note that the initial glomerular filtrate has the same osmolarity as the blood, 300 mOsm/L, but the urine osmolarity is much higher (1200 mOsm/L) than blood osmolarity. Notice also that the corticopapillary osmotic gradient is in place, having been established by the ongoing processes of countercurrent multiplication and urea recycling. The two basic questions concerning formation of hyperosmotic urine are, *How does the kidney produce urine that is more concentrated than blood, and what determines how high the urine osmolarity will be?* The following steps are involved in producing hyperosmotic urine:

1. The osmolarity of glomerular filtrate is identical to that of blood, 300 mOsm/L, because water and small solutes are freely filtered. The osmolarity remains at 300 mOsm/L along the entire proximal convoluted tubule, even though a significant volume of water is reabsorbed. This occurs because water is always reabsorbed in exact proportion to solute; that is, the process is **isosmotic.** The isosmotic process also can be expressed in terms of $[TF/P]_{osm}$: In glomerular filtrate, $[TF/P]_{osm} = 1.0$ and remains constant along the proximal tubule.

2. In the **thick ascending limb of the loop of Henle,** NaCl is reabsorbed via the **Na$^+$-K$^+$-2Cl$^-$ cotransporter.** However, because the cells of the thick ascending limb are **impermeable to water,** water reabsorption cannot accompany solute reabsorption. As solute is reabsorbed, water is left behind and the tubular fluid is diluted. The osmolarity of tubular fluid leaving this segment is 100 mOsm/L. Thus, the thick ascending limb also is called the **diluting segment.**

3. In the **early distal tubule,** NaCl is reabsorbed by an **Na$^+$-Cl$^-$ cotransporter.** Like the thick ascending limb, cells of the early distal tubule are **impermeable to water** and water reabsorption cannot follow solute reabsorption. Here, the osmolarity of tubular fluid becomes even more dilute, as low as 80 mOsm/L. Thus, the early distal tubule also is called the **cortical diluting segment** (*cortical* because the distal tubule is located in the cortex, rather than in the medulla where the thick ascending limb is found).

4. In the **late distal tubule,** the principal cells are permeable to water in the presence of **ADH.** Recall that the fluid entering the late distal tubule is quite dilute, 80 mOsm/L. Because the cells are now permeable to water, water flows out of the tubular fluid by osmosis, driven by the osmotic gradient across the cells (i.e., is reabsorbed). Water reabsorption will continue until the tubular fluid equilibrates osmotically with the surrounding interstitial fluid. The tubular fluid leaving the distal tubule is equilibrated with the interstitial fluid of the cortex, and it has an osmolarity of 300 mOsm/L.

5. In the **collecting ducts,** the mechanism is the same as that described for the late distal tubule. The principal cells of the collecting ducts are permeable to water in the presence of **ADH.** As tubular fluid flows down the collecting ducts, it is exposed to interstitial fluid with increasingly higher osmolarity (i.e., the corticopapillary osmotic gradient). Water will be reabsorbed until the tubular fluid equilibrates osmotically with surrounding interstitial fluid. The final urine will reach the osmolarity present at the tip of the papilla, which, in this example, is 1200 mOsm/L.

The two questions about production of hyperosmotic urine have been answered. *How is urine rendered hyperosmotic?* Urine becomes hyperosmotic, in the presence of ADH, by equilibration of tubular fluid in the collecting ducts with the high osmolarity of the corticopapillary gradient. The corticopapillary osmotic gradient is established by countercurrent multiplication, a function of the loop of Henle, and by urea recycling, a function of the inner medullary collecting ducts. *How high will the urine osmolarity be?* Final urine osmolarity, in the presence of ADH, will be equal to the osmolarity at the bend of the loop of Henle (the tip of the papilla).

SIADH

As previously described, the *appropriate* response to water deprivation is production of hyperosmotic urine. However, in the syndrome of inappropriate ADH (SIADH), hyperosmotic urine is produced *inappropriately* (Table 6-10). In SIADH, circulating levels of the hormone ADH are abnormally high owing to either excessive secretion from the posterior pituitary following head injury or secretion of ADH from abnormal sites such as **lung tumors.** In these conditions, ADH is secreted autonomously, without an osmotic stimulus; in other words, ADH is secreted when it is not needed. In SIADH, the high levels of ADH increase water reabsorption by the late distal tubule and collecting ducts, making the urine hyperosmotic and diluting the plasma osmolarity. (Normally, a low plasma osmolarity would inhibit secretion of ADH; however, in SIADH,

Table 6–10 Antidiuretic Hormone Examples of Physiology and Pathophysiology

Example	Serum ADH	Plasma Osmolarity	Urine Osmolarity	Urine Flow Rate	Free-Water Clearance (C_{H_2O})
Water deprivation	↑	High-normal	Hyperosmotic	Low	Negative
SIADH	↑↑	Low (reabsorption of excess water)	Hyperosmotic	Low	Negative
Water drinking	↓	Low-normal	Hyposmotic	High	Positive
Central diabetes insipidus	↓↓	High (excretion of excess water)	Hyposmotic	High	Positive
Nephrogenic diabetes insipidus	↑ (stimulated by high plasma osmolarity)	High (excretion of excess water)	Hyposmotic	High	Positive

ADH, Antidiuretic hormone; SIADH, syndrome of inappropriate antidiuretic hormone.

this feedback inhibition does not occur because ADH is secreted autonomously.) Treatment of SIADH consists of administration of a drug such as **demeclocycline,** which inhibits the ADH action on the renal principal cells.

Production of Hyposmotic Urine

By definition, hyposmotic (dilute) urine has an osmolarity lower than blood osmolarity. Hyposmotic urine is produced when there are **low circulating levels of ADH** (e.g., water drinking, central diabetes insipidus) or when **ADH is ineffective** (e.g., nephrogenic diabetes insipidus). The mechanisms for the production of hyposmotic urine are shown in Figure 6-42.

Steps in Production of Hyposmotic Urine

The format of Figure 6-43 is similar to that of Figure 6-42. The numbers give the osmolarity, and the *arrow* shows water reabsorption. The *heavily outlined* portion indicates the nephron segments that are impermeable to water, which now include the thick ascending limb *and* the entire distal tubule and collecting duct. Notice that there is still a corticopapillary osmotic gradient, but it is smaller than in the presence of ADH (see Fig. 6-42). The smaller gradient can be understood from the positive effects that ADH has on countercurrent multiplication and on urea recycling. In the absence of ADH, these processes are diminished and the size of the corticopapillary osmotic gradient also is diminished. The basic questions about formation of hyposmotic urine are, *How does the kidney produce urine that is less concentrated than blood,* and *what determines how low the urine osmolarity will be?* The following steps are involved in producing hyposmotic urine:

1. Reabsorption in the **proximal tubule** is not affected by ADH. Thus, in the absence of ADH, fluid is again reabsorbed isosmotically, tubular fluid osmolarity is 300 mOsm/L, and $[TF/P]_{osm} = 1.0$.

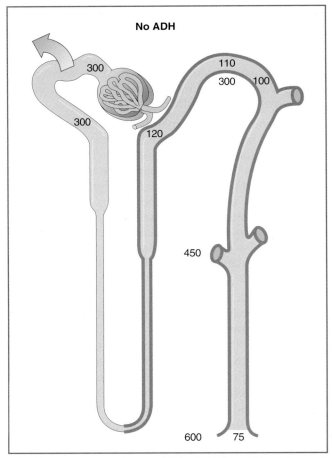

Figure 6–43 **Mechanisms for production of hyposmotic (dilute) urine in the absence of antidiuretic hormone (ADH).** *Arrow* shows location of water reabsorption; *heavy outline* shows water-impermeable portions of the nephron; numbers are osmolarity of tubular fluid or interstitial fluid.

2. In the **thick ascending limb of the loop of Henle,** NaCl is reabsorbed via the Na⁺-K⁺-2Cl⁻ cotransporter. Water is not reabsorbed, however, because of the impermeability of this segment. Thus, the tubular fluid is diluted, and the fluid leaving

the thick ascending limb has an osmolarity of 120 mOsm/L. Notice that this osmolarity is *not quite as low* as in the presence of ADH (see Fig. 6-41) because the dilution step is diminished in the absence of ADH (Na^+-K^+-$2Cl^-$ cotransport is inhibited).

3. In the **early distal tubule,** dilution continues. NaCl is reabsorbed by the Na^+-Cl^- cotransporter, but the cells are impermeable to water. Thus, tubular fluid that leaves the early distal tubule has an osmolarity of 110 mOsm/L.

4. The **late distal tubule and collecting ducts** exhibit the most dramatic and important differences when ADH is low or absent. These segments are now **impermeable to water:** As tubular fluid flows through them, no osmotic equilibration is possible. Although tubular fluid is exposed to the increasingly higher osmolarity of the corticopapillary osmotic gradient, water is not reabsorbed in response to the osmotic driving force. The final urine, which is *not equilibrated* with the osmolarity at the tip of the papilla, has an osmolarity of 75 mOsm/L. (Final urine osmolarity is even less than the tubular fluid osmolarity in the early distal tubule because the late distal tubule and collecting duct reabsorb some NaCl. In effect, the late distal tubule and collecting duct also become diluting segments.)

The two questions about production of hyposmotic urine have been answered. *How is urine rendered hyposmotic?* Tubular fluid is diluted in the "diluting segments," which reabsorb NaCl without water. Osmotic equilibration does not occur in the collecting ducts in the absence of ADH, and the dilute urine is excreted. *How low will urine osmolarity be?* Final urine osmolarity will reflect the combined functions of *all* the diluting segments including the thick ascending limb and the early distal tubule, as well as the remainder of the distal tubule and collecting ducts.

Hyposmotic urine is produced as the normal response to water drinking. There are, however, two abnormal conditions in which dilute urine is produced inappropriately: **central diabetes insipidus** and **nephrogenic diabetes insipidus.** Features of these conditions are summarized in Table 6-10.

Central Diabetes Insipidus

Central diabetes insipidus can follow **head injury,** in which trauma depletes the posterior pituitary gland of ADH stores. The posterior pituitary is, therefore, unable to secrete ADH in response to an osmotic stimulus. Because circulating levels of ADH are low or zero, the entire distal tubule and collecting ducts are impermeable to water. Hence, large volumes (up to 15 L/day) of dilute urine are excreted. Plasma osmolarity increases

to abnormally high values as excessive amounts of water are excreted in the urine (water that would have been reabsorbed if ADH were present). The high plasma osmolarity would normally stimulate ADH secretion, but in central diabetes insipidus, there is no ADH to be secreted from the posterior pituitary gland. Treatment of central diabetes insipidus consists of administration of an ADH analogue, such as 1-deamino-8-D-arginine vasopressin (**dDAVP**).

Nephrogenic Diabetes Insipidus

Nephrogenic diabetes insipidus involves a defect in the response of the kidneys to ADH. Although ADH secretion from the posterior pituitary gland is normal, a defect in the receptor, the G_s protein, or adenylyl cyclase makes the principal cells unresponsive to ADH.

As a result, ADH fails to increase water permeability in the late distal tubule and collecting ducts. As in central diabetes insipidus, water cannot be reabsorbed by these segments and large volumes of dilute urine are excreted. The plasma osmolarity increases, which stimulates the posterior pituitary to secrete even more ADH. Circulating ADH levels are higher than normal in nephrogenic diabetes insipidus, but these high levels of ADH still are ineffective on principal cells.

Nephrogenic diabetes insipidus is treated with **thiazide diuretics.** (Administration of an ADH analogue such as dDAVP would be futile because the defect lies in the response to ADH.) To understand the rationale for using thiazide diuretics, first consider the fundamental problem in nephrogenic diabetes insipidus: Because the principal cells are unresponsive to ADH, there is excretion of large volumes of dilute urine. Thiazide diuretics are helpful as follows: (1) They inhibit Na^+-Cl^- cotransport in the early distal tubule, thereby preventing dilution of the urine in this segment. As more NaCl is excreted, the urine is less dilute than it would be without treatment. (2) Thiazide diuretics produce a decrease in GFR and, secondary to decreased Na^+ reabsorption, a decrease in ECF volume. The decrease in ECF volume causes an increase in proximal tubule reabsorption via effects on Starling forces. The combination of less water filtered and more water reabsorbed in the proximal tubule means that the total volume of water excreted is decreased.

Free-Water Clearance

Free water is defined as distilled water that is free of solutes (or solute-free water). In the nephron, free water is generated in the **diluting segments,** where solute is reabsorbed without water. The diluting segments of the nephron are the water-impermeable segments: the thick ascending limb and the early distal tubule.

Measurement of free-water clearance (C_{H_2O}) provides a method for assessing the ability of the kidneys to dilute or concentrate the urine. The principles underlying this measurement are as follows: When **ADH levels are low,** all of the free water generated in the thick ascending limb and early distal tubule is excreted (because it cannot be reabsorbed by the collecting ducts). The urine is hyposmotic, and free-water clearance is positive. When **ADH levels are high,** all of the free water generated in the thick ascending limb and the early distal tubule is reabsorbed by the late distal tubule and collecting duct. The urine is hyperosmotic, and free-water clearance is negative.

Measurement of C_{H_2O}

Free-water clearance (C_{H_2O}) is calculated by the following equation:

$$C_{H_2O} = \dot{V} - C_{osm}$$
$$= \dot{V} - \frac{[U]_{osm} \times \dot{V}}{[P]_{osm}}$$

where

$$
\begin{aligned}
C_{H_2O} &= \text{Free-water clearance (mL/min)} \\
\dot{V} &= \text{Urine flow rate (mL/min)} \\
C_{osm} &= \text{Clearance of osmoles (mL/min)} \\
[U]_{osm} &= \text{Urine osmolarity (mOsm/L)} \\
[P]_{osm} &= \text{Plasma osmolarity (mOsm/L)}
\end{aligned}
$$

SAMPLE PROBLEM. A man has a urine flow rate of 10 mL/min, a urine osmolarity of 100 mOsm/L, and a plasma osmolarity of 290 mOsm/L. *What is his free-water clearance, and what is its significance?*

SOLUTION. The man's free-water clearance is calculated as follows:

$$C_{H_2O} = \dot{V} - C_{osm}$$

$$= \dot{V} - \frac{[U]_{osm} \times \dot{V}}{[P]_{osm}}$$

$$= 10 \text{ mL/min} - \frac{100 \text{ mOsm/L} \times 10 \text{ mL/min}}{290 \text{ mOsm/}L}$$

$$= 10 \text{ mL/min} - 3.45 \text{ mL/min}$$

$$= +6.55 \text{ mL/min}$$

C_{H_2O} is a positive value, which means that free water is being excreted. The solute-free water generated in the thick ascending limb and early distal tubule is not reabsorbed by the collecting ducts, but it is excreted. This situation occurs when circulating ADH levels are low, as in water drinking or central diabetes insipidus (or if ADH is ineffective, as in nephrogenic diabetes insipidus).

Significance of C_{H_2O}

C_{H_2O} can be zero, positive, or negative. The explanations for these values are as follows:

♦ **C_{H_2O} is zero.** C_{H_2O} is zero when no solute-free water is excreted. Under these conditions, urine is **isosmotic** with plasma (called isosthenuric). It is unusual for C_{H_2O} to be zero, but it can occur during treatment with a **loop diuretic,** where NaCl reabsorption is inhibited in the thick ascending limb. When solute reabsorption is inhibited in the thick ascending limb, no free water is generated at this site: If free water is not generated, it cannot be excreted. Therefore, the ability to dilute the urine during water drinking is impaired in a person who is treated with a loop diuretic. Likewise, the ability to concentrate the urine during water deprivation is impaired because loop diuretics also interfere with generation of the corticopapillary osmotic gradient (by inhibiting Na^+-K^+-$2Cl^-$ cotransport and countercurrent multiplication).

♦ **C_{H_2O} is positive.** C_{H_2O} is positive when **ADH levels are low** or when ADH is ineffective and the urine is **hyposmotic.** The solute-free water, which is generated in the thick ascending limb and early distal tubule, is excreted in the urine because the late distal tubules and collecting ducts are impermeable to water under these conditions (Box 6-3).

♦ **C_{H_2O} is negative.** C_{H_2O} is negative when **ADH levels are high** and the urine is **hyperosmotic.** All of the solute-free water generated in the thick ascending limb and early distal tubule (and more) is reabsorbed by the late distal tubules and collecting ducts. Because negative C_{H_2O} is a cumbersome term, the sign is reversed, and it is called **free-water reabsorption,** or T^c_{H2O} (c stands for collecting ducts).

SUMMARY

■ Total body water is distributed between ICF and ECF. As percentages of body weight, 60% is total body water, 40% is ICF, and 20% is ECF. ECF consists of plasma and interstitial fluid. Volumes of the body fluid compartments are measured by dilution of marker substances.

■ ECF and ICF osmolarity are always equal in the steady state. When there is a disturbance of body fluid osmolarity, water shifts across cell membranes to reestablish the equality of ECF and ICF osmolarity. These shifts produce changes in ECF and ICF volume.

■ Renal clearance is the volume of plasma cleared of a substance per unit time and is determined by its renal

BOX 6–3 Clinical Physiology: Central Diabetes Insipidus

DESCRIPTION OF CASE. A 45-year-old woman is admitted to the hospital following a head injury. She has severe polyuria (producing 1 L of urine every 2 hours) and polydipsia (drinking 3 to 4 glasses of water every hour). During a 24-hour period in the hospital, the woman produces 10 L of urine, containing no glucose. She is placed on overnight water restriction for further evaluation. The following morning, she is weak and confused. Her serum osmolarity is 330 mOsm/L, her serum [Na^+] is 164 mEq/L, and her urine osmolarity is 70 mOsm/L. She is treated with dDAVP by nasal spray. Within 24 hours of initiating the treatment, her serum osmolarity is 295 mOsm/L and her urine osmolarity is 620 mOsm/L.

EXPLANATION OF CASE. Following overnight water restriction, the striking observation is that the woman is still producing dilute (hyposmotic) urine despite a severely elevated serum osmolarity. Diabetes mellitus is ruled out as a cause of her polyuria because no glucose is found in her urine. The diagnosis is that the woman has central diabetes insipidus secondary to a head injury.

The woman's posterior pituitary gland does not secrete ADH, even with a strong osmotic stimulus such as a serum osmolarity of 330 mOsm/L. This absence of ADH results in a profound disturbance of water reabsorption, and she is unable to produce concentrated urine. Her distal tubule and collecting ducts are impermeable to water in the absence of ADH, no water can be reabsorbed by these segments, and her urine is hyposmotic (70 mOsm/L). Because she is excreting excessive amounts of free water, serum osmolarity and serum [Na^+] increase. The high serum osmolarity is an intense stimulus for thirst, causing the woman to drink water almost continuously.

TREATMENT. The woman is treated with dDAVP, an ADH analogue that activates V_2 receptors on the principal cells. When ADH binds to the V_2 receptors, adenylyl cyclase is activated, cAMP is generated, and water channels are inserted in the luminal membrane, which restores water permeability of the principal cells. After initiating dDAVP therapy, the woman produces hyperosmotic urine, restoring her serum osmolarity to normal.

---

handling. Substances with the highest clearances are both filtered and secreted. Substances with the lowest clearances either are not filtered or are filtered and subsequently reabsorbed. Inulin is a glomerular marker whose clearance equals the GFR.

■ RBF is autoregulated over a wide range of arterial pressures by changes in the resistance of the afferent arterioles. Effective RPF is measured by the clearance of PAH, and RBF is calculated from the RPF.

■ GFR is determined by the permeability of the glomerular capillary barrier (K_f) and the net ultrafiltration pressure. Net ultrafiltration pressure is the sum of three Starling pressures across the glomerular capillary: P_{GC}, π_{GC}, and P_{BS}. If any of the Starling pressures change, net ultrafiltration pressure and GFR are altered.

■ Reabsorption and secretion modify the ultrafiltrate that is produced by glomerular filtration. The net reabsorption or secretion rate of a substance is the difference between its filtered load and its excretion rate. Glucose is reabsorbed by a T_m-limited process: When the filtered load of glucose exceeds the T_m, then glucose is excreted in the urine (glucosuria). PAH is secreted by a T_m-limited process.

■ Na^+ reabsorption is greater than 99% of the filtered load and occurs throughout the nephron. In the proximal tubule, 67% of the filtered Na^+ is reabsorbed isosmotically with water. In the early proximal tubule, Na^+ is reabsorbed by Na^+-glucose cotransport, Na^+-amino acid cotransport, and Na^+-H^+ exchange. In the late proximal tubule, NaCl is reabsorbed. ECF volume expansion inhibits proximal tubule reabsorption, and ECF volume contraction stimulates it. In the thick ascending limb of the loop of Henle, a water-impermeable segment, 25% of the filtered Na^+ is reabsorbed by Na^+-K^+-$2Cl^-$ cotransport. Loop diuretics inhibit the Na^+-K^+-$2Cl^-$ cotransporter. In the distal tubule and collecting ducts, 8% of the filtered Na^+ is reabsorbed. In the early distal tubule, the mechanism is Na^+-Cl^- cotransport, which is inhibited by thiazide diuretics. In the late distal tubule and collecting ducts, the principal cells have aldosterone-dependent Na^+ channels, which are inhibited by K^+-sparing diuretics.

■ K^+ balance is maintained by shifts of K^+ across cell membranes and by renal regulation. The renal mechanisms for K^+ balance include filtration, reabsorption in the proximal tubule and thick ascending limb, and secretion by the principal cells of the late distal tubule and collecting ducts. Secretion by the principal cells is influenced by dietary K^+, aldosterone, acid-base balance, and flow rate. Under the conditions of low K^+ intake, K^+ is reabsorbed by α-intercalated cells of the distal tubule.

■ Body fluid osmolarity is maintained at a constant value by changes in water reabsorption in the principal cells of the late distal tubule and collecting duct. During water deprivation, ADH is secreted and acts on the principal cells to increase water reabsorption. During water drinking, ADH secretion is suppressed and the principal cells are impermeable to water.

Challenge Yourself

Answer each question with a word, phrase, sentence, or numerical solution. When a list of possible answers is supplied with the question, one, more than one, or none of the choices may be correct. Correct answers are provided at the end of the book.

1 Constriction of which arteriole leads to decreased renal plasma flow (RPF) and increased glomerular filtration rate (GFR)?

2 In what portion of, or at what point on, the glucose titration curve, is the renal vein glucose concentration equal to the renal artery glucose concentration?

3 What happens to the oncotic pressure of peritubular capillary blood following an increase in filtration fraction?

4 When the clearance of PAH is used to measure effective RPF, is the measurement done at plasma concentrations of PAH that are above or below the T_m for secretion?

5 A person with an ECF volume of 14 L, an ICF volume of 28 L, and a plasma osmolarity of 300 mOsm/L drinks 3 L of water and eats 600 mmoles of NaCl. In the new steady state, what is the plasma osmolarity?

6 If GFR is constant and there is an increase in urine flow rate, how does the plasma inulin concentration change: increased, decreased, or unchanged?

7 An increase in urine pH causes what change in the excretion of a weak acid: increased, decreased, or unchanged?

8 During water diuresis, where in the nephron is $[TF/P]_{inulin}$ lowest?

9 Where in the nephron is fractional excretion of Na^+ highest?

10 What is the effect of a loop diuretic (inhibitor of $Na^+-K^+-2Cl^-$ cotransporter) on maximum urine osmolarity during production of hyperosmotic urine: increased, decreased, unchanged?

11 Which ADH disorder is represented by the following changes: increased plasma osmolarity, dilute urine, decreased ADH?

12 In a person who ingests a bag of potato chips (i.e., NaCl), what happens to intracellular volume: increased, decreased, or unchanged?

13 What are the units of glucose T_m?

14 What is the effect of dilation of the efferent arteriole on filtration fraction: increased, decreased, or unchanged?

15 Which of the following cause(s) hyperkalemia: lack of insulin, hyperaldosteronism, loop diuretics, spironolactone, hyperosmolarity, metabolic alkalosis?

16 Regarding the actions of parathyroid hormone (PTH) on the kidney, which of the following is/are seen: inhibition of Na^+-phosphate cotransport, decreased urinary phosphate excretion, decreased urinary Ca^{2+} excretion, decreased urinary cyclic AMP?

17 GFR is 120 mL/min, the plasma concentration of X is 10 mg/mL, the urine concentration of X is 100 mg/mL, and urine flow rate is 1.0 mL/min. Assuming that X is freely filtered, is there net reabsorption or net secretion of X, and what is the rate?

18 During production of hyperosmotic urine, where in the nephron is $[TF/P]_{osmolarity}$ lowest?

19 Which is highest: clearance of PAH below T_m, clearance of glucose below threshold, or clearance of inulin?

20 Rank the following substances in order of fractional excretion from highest to lowest: inulin, Na^+, glucose (below threshold), K^+ on a high potassium diet, and HCO_3^-.

SELECTED READINGS

Koeppen BM, Stanton BA: Renal Physiology, 3rd ed. St Louis, Mosby, 2001.

Seldin DW, Giebish G: The Kidney: Physiology and Pathophysiology, 2nd ed. New York, Raven Press, 1992.

Valtin H, Schafer JA: Renal Function, 3rd ed. Boston, Little, Brown, 1995.

Windhager EE: Handbook of Physiology: Renal Physiology, New York, American Physiological Society, Oxford University Press, 1992.

Acid-Base Physiology

Acid-base balance is concerned with maintaining a normal hydrogen ion concentration in the body fluids. This balance is achieved by utilization of buffers in extracellular fluid and intracellular fluid, by respiratory mechanisms that excrete carbon dioxide, and by renal mechanisms that reabsorb bicarbonate and secrete hydrogen ions.

pH OF BODY FLUIDS

The hydrogen ion (H^+) concentration of the body fluids is extremely low. In arterial blood, the H^+ concentration is 40×10^{-9} equivalents per liter (or 40 nEq/L), which is more than six orders of magnitude lower than the sodium (Na^+) concentration. Because it is cumbersome to work with such small numbers, H^+ concentration is routinely expressed as a logarithmic function called **pH:**

$$pH = -\log_{10}[H^+]$$

The normal H^+ concentration of 40×10^{-9} Eq/L is converted to pH as follows:

$$pH = -\log_{10}[40 \times 10^{-9} \text{ Eq/L}]$$
$$= 7.4$$

When using pH instead of H^+ concentration, there are two points of caution. First, because of the *minus* sign in the logarithmic expression, a mental reversal is necessary: As H^+ concentration increases, pH decreases, and conversely. Second, the relationship between H^+ concentration and pH is logarithmic, not linear. Thus, equal changes in pH do not reflect equal changes in H^+ concentration. This lack of linearity is illustrated in Figure 7-1, in which the relationship between H^+ concentration and pH is shown over the physiologic range in body fluids. An *increase* in pH from 7.4 to 7.6 (0.2 pH units) reflects a decrease in H^+ concentration of 15 nEq/L; a *decrease* in pH from 7.4 to 7.2 (also 0.2 pH units) reflects a larger increase in H^+ concentration of 23 nEq/L. In other words, a given change in pH in the acidic range (pH < 7.4) reflects a larger change in H^+ concentration than the same change in pH in the alkaline range (pH > 7.4).

The **normal range of arterial pH is 7.37 to 7.42.** When arterial pH is less than 7.37, it is called **acidemia.** When arterial pH is greater than 7.42, it is called **alkalemia.** The pH range compatible with life is 6.8 to 8.0.

The mechanisms that contribute to maintaining pH in the normal range include buffering of H^+ in both extracellular fluid (ECF) and intracellular fluid (ICF), respiratory compensation, and renal compensation. The mechanisms for buffering and respiratory

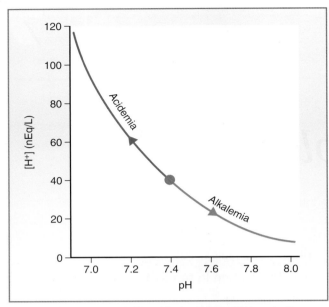

Figure 7–1 **Relationship between [H⁺] and pH.**

compensation occur rapidly, within minutes to hours. The mechanisms for renal compensation are slower, requiring hours to days.

ACID PRODUCTION IN THE BODY

Arterial pH is slightly alkaline (7.4) despite the production of large amounts of acid on a daily basis. This acid production has two forms: volatile acid (carbon dioxide, CO_2) and nonvolatile, or fixed, acid. Both volatile and fixed acids are produced in large quantities and present a challenge to the normally alkaline pH.

CO_2

CO_2, or volatile acid, is the end product of aerobic metabolism in the cells and is generated at a rate of 13,000 to 20,000 millimoles daily (mmol/day). CO_2 itself is not an acid. However, when it reacts with water (H_2O), it is converted to the weak acid carbonic acid, H_2CO_3:

$$CO_2 + H_2O \leftrightarrow H_2CO_3 \leftrightarrow H^+ + HCO_3^-$$
$$\text{carbonic anhydrase}$$

The reactions show that CO_2 combines reversibly with H_2O to form H_2CO_3, catalyzed by the enzyme **carbonic anhydrase.** H_2CO_3 dissociates into H^+ and HCO_3^-, and the H^+ generated by this reaction must be buffered. Recall that CO_2 produced by the cells is added to venous blood, converted to H^+ and HCO_3^- within the red blood cells, and carried to the lungs. In the lungs, the

reactions occur in reverse and CO_2 is regenerated and expired. (CO_2 is therefore called a *volatile* acid.) Thus, buffering of the H^+ that comes from CO_2 is only a temporary problem for venous blood.

Fixed Acid

Catabolism of proteins and phospholipids results in the production of approximately 50 mmol/day of fixed acid. Proteins with the sulfur-containing amino acids (e.g., methionine, cysteine, cystine) generate **sulfuric acid** when they are metabolized, and phospholipids generate **phosphoric acid.** In contrast with CO_2, which is volatile and will be expired by the lungs, sulfuric acid and phosphoric acid are *not* volatile. Therefore, fixed acids first must be buffered in the body fluids until they can be excreted by the kidneys.

In addition to sulfuric and phosphoric acids, which are produced from *normal* catabolic processes, in certain pathophysiologic states, fixed acids can be produced in excessive quantities. These fixed acids include **β-hydroxybutyric acid** and **acetoacetic acid,** both ketoacids that are generated in untreated diabetes mellitus, and **lactic acid,** which may be generated during strenuous exercise or when the tissues are hypoxic. In addition, other fixed acids may be ingested, such as **salicylic acid** (from aspirin overdose), **formic acid** (from methanol ingestion), and **glycolic** and **oxalic acids** (from ethylene glycol ingestion). Overproduction or ingestion of fixed acids causes metabolic acidosis, as discussed later in the chapter.

BUFFERING

Principles of Buffering

A **buffer** is a mixture of a weak acid and its conjugate base *or* a weak base and its conjugate acid. The two forms of the buffer are called the buffer pair. In Brønsted-Lowry nomenclature, for a **weak acid,** the acid form is called HA and is defined as the H^+ donor. The base form is called A^- and is defined as the H^+ acceptor. Likewise, for a **weak base,** the H^+ donor is called BH^+ and the H^+ acceptor is called B.

A buffered solution **resists a change in pH.** Thus, H^+ can be added to or removed from a buffered solution, but the pH of that solution will change only minimally. For example, when H^+ is added to a buffered solution containing a weak acid, it combines with the A^- form of the buffer and converts it to the HA form. Conversely, when H^+ is removed from a buffered solution (or OH^- is added), H^+ is released from the HA form of the buffer, converting it to the A^- form.

The body fluids contain a large variety of buffers, which constitute an important first defense against changes in pH. Robert Pitts demonstrated this buffering capacity experimentally by injecting 150 mEq of H^+ (as hydrochloric acid, HCl) into a dog whose total body water was 11.4 L. In a parallel experiment, Pitts added 150 mEq of H^+ to 11.4 L of distilled water. In the dog, the addition of H^+ caused the blood pH to decrease from 7.44 to 7.14—the dog was acidemic but alive. In the distilled water, addition of the same amount of H^+ caused the pH to drop precipitously to 1.84, a value that would have been instantly fatal to the dog. Pitts concluded that the dog's body fluids contained buffers that protected his pH from the addition of large amounts of H^+. The added H^+ combined with the A^- form of these buffers, and a strong acid was converted to a weak acid. The change in the dog's body fluid pH was minimized, although not totally prevented. The distilled water contained no buffers and had no such protective mechanisms.

Henderson-Hasselbalch Equation

The Henderson-Hasselbalch equation is used to calculate the pH of a buffered solution. This equation is derived from the behavior of weak acids (and bases) in solution, which is described by the kinetics of reversible reactions:

$$HA \underset{K_2}{\overset{K_1}{\rightleftharpoons}} H^+ + A^-$$

The forward reaction, the dissociation of HA into H^+ and A^-, is characterized by a rate constant, K_1, and the reverse reaction is characterized by a rate constant, K_2. When the rates of the forward and reverse reactions are exactly equal, there is a state of **chemical equilibrium**, in which there is no further net change in the concentration of HA or A^-. As shown here, the **law of mass action** states that at chemical equilibrium,

$$K_1[HA] = K_2[H^+][A^-]$$

Rearranging,

$$\frac{K_1}{K_2} = \frac{[H^+][A^-]}{[HA]}$$

The ratio of rate constants can be combined into a single constant, **K**, called the **equilibrium constant**, as follows:

$$K = \frac{[H^+][A^-]}{[HA]}$$

Rearranging again to solve for $[H^+]$:

$$[H^+] = K\frac{[HA]}{[A^-]}$$

To express $[H^+]$ as pH, *take the negative log_{10} of both sides of the previous equation*. Then,

$$-\log[H^+] = -\log K - \log\frac{[HA]}{[A^-]}$$

Recall that $-\log [H^+]$ equals pH, that $-\log K$ equals pK, and that *minus* log HA/A^- equals *plus* log A^-/HA. Thus, the final form of the **Henderson-Hasselbalch equation** is as follows:

$$pH = pK + \log\frac{[A^-]}{[HA]}$$

where

> pH = $-\log_{10}$ $[H^+]$ (pH units)
> pK = $-\log_{10}$ K (pH units)
> $[A^-]$ = Concentration of base form of buffer (mEq/L)
> [HA] = Concentration of acid form of buffer (mEq/L)

Therefore, the pH of a buffered solution can be calculated with the following information: the pK of the buffer, the concentration of the base form of the buffer ($[A^-]$), and the concentration of the acid form of the buffer ([HA]). Conversely, if the pH of the solution and the pK of the buffer are known, it is possible to calculate the relative concentrations of the A^- and HA forms.

pK is a characteristic value for a buffer pair. *What factor, or factors, determine its value?* In the previous derivation, note that the equilibrium constant (K) is the ratio of the rate constant of the forward reaction divided by the rate constant of the reverse reaction. Therefore, **strong acids** such as HCl are *more* dissociated into H^+ and A^-, and they have high equilibrium constants (K) and **low pKs** (because pK is *minus* $\log_{10}$ of the equilibrium constant). On the other hand, **weak acids** such as H_2CO_3 are *less* dissociated and have low equilibrium constants and **high pKs.**

SAMPLE PROBLEM. The pK of the $HPO_4^{-2}/H_2PO_4^-$ buffer pair is 6.8. Answer two questions about this buffer: *(1) At a blood pH of 7.4, what are the relative concentrations of the acid form and the base form of this buffer pair? (2) At what pH would the concentrations of the acid and base forms be equal?*

SOLUTION. The acid form of this buffer is $H_2PO_4^-$, and the base form is HPO_4^{-2}. The relative concentrations of the acid and base forms are set by the pH of the solution and the characteristic pK.

(1) Answering the first question: The relative concentrations of acid and base forms at pH 7.4 are calculated with the Henderson-Hasselbalch equation. (Hint: In the last step of the solution, take the antilog of both sides of the equation!)

$$pH = pK + \log\frac{HPO_4^{-2}}{H_2PO_4^{-}}$$

$$7.4 = 6.8 + \log\frac{HPO_4^{-2}}{H_2PO_4^{-}}$$

$$0.6 = \log\frac{HPO_4^{-2}}{H_2PO_4^{-}}$$

$$3.98 = HPO_4^{-2}/H_2PO_4^{-}$$

Therefore, at pH 7.4, the concentration of the base form (HPO_4^{-2}) is approximately fourfold that of the acid form ($H_2PO_4^{-}$).

(2) Answering the second question: The pH at which there would be equal concentrations of the acid and base forms can also be calculated from the Henderson-Hasselbalch equation. When the acid and base forms are in equal concentrations, $HPO_4^{-2}/H_2PO_4^{-} = 1.0$.

$$pH = pK + \log\frac{HPO_4^{-2}}{H_2PO_4^{-}}$$
$$= 6.8 + \log 1$$
$$= 6.8 + 0$$
$$= 6.8$$

The calculated pH equals the pK of the buffer. This important calculation demonstrates that *when the pH of a solution equals the pK, the concentrations of the acid and base forms of the buffer are equal.* As discussed later in the chapter, a buffer functions best when the pH of the solution is equal (or nearly equal) to the pK, precisely because the concentrations of the acid and base forms are equal, or nearly equal.

Titration Curves

Titration curves are graphic representations of the Henderson-Hasselbalch equation. Figure 7-2 shows the titration curve of a hypothetical weak acid (HA) and its conjugate base (A^-) in solution. As H^+ is added or removed, the pH of the solution is measured.

As previously shown by the Henderson-Hasselbalch equation, the relative concentrations of HA and A^- depend on the pH of the solution and the pK of the buffer. The **pK** of this hypothetical buffer is 6.5. At low (acidic) pH, the buffer exists primarily in the HA form. At high (alkaline) pH, the buffer exists primarily in the A^- form. When the pH equals the pK, there are equal concentrations of HA and A^-: Half of the buffer is in the HA form and half in the A^- form.

A striking feature of the titration curve is its sigmoidal shape. In the **linear portion of the curve,** only small changes in pH occur when H^+ is added or removed; the most effective buffering occurs in this

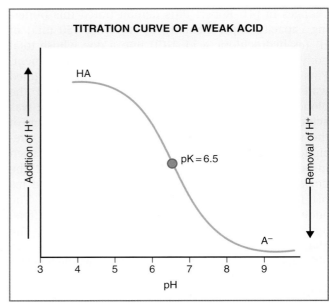

Figure 7-2 **Titration curve of a weak acid (HA) and its conjugate base (A^-).** When pH equals pK, there are equal concentrations of HA and A^-.

range. The linear range of the curve extends 1.0 pH unit above and below the pK (pK ± 1.0). Therefore, the most effective physiologic buffers will have a pK within 1.0 pH unit of 7.4 (7.4 ± 1.0). Outside the effective buffering range, pH changes drastically when small amounts of H^+ are added or removed. For this buffer, when the pH is lower than 5.5, the addition of H^+ causes a large decrease in pH; when the pH is higher than 7.5, the removal of H^+ causes a large increase in pH.

Extracellular Fluid Buffers

The major buffers of the ECF are bicarbonate and phosphate. For **bicarbonate,** the A^- form is HCO_3^- and the HA form is CO_2 (in equilibrium with H_2CO_3). For **phosphate,** the A^- form is HPO_4^{-2} and the HA form is $H_2PO_4^-$. The titration curves of these buffers are shown in Figure 7-3.

HCO_3^-/CO_2 Buffer

The most important extracellular buffer is HCO_3^-/CO_2. It is utilized as the first line of defense when H^+ is gained or lost from the body. The following characteristics account for the preeminence of HCO_3^-/CO_2 as an ECF buffer: (1) The concentration of the A^- form, HCO_3^-, is high at 24 mEq/L. (2) The pK of the HCO_3^-/CO_2 buffer is 6.1, which is fairly close to the pH of ECF. (3) CO_2, the acid form of the buffer, is volatile and can be expired by the lungs (see Fig. 7-3).

The function of the HCO_3^-/CO_2 buffer is illustrated in the previous example of HCl injection into a dog. To

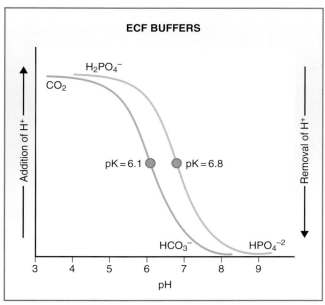

ECF BUFFERS

Figure 7–3 Comparison of titration curves for $H_2PO_4^-$/HPO_4^{-2} and CO_2/HCO_3^-. ECF, Extracellular fluid.

understand this example, assume that ECF is a simple solution of $NaHCO_3$, ignoring its other constituents. When HCl is added to ECF, H^+ combines with some of the HCO_3^- to form H_2CO_3. Thus, a strong acid (HCl) is converted to a weak acid (H_2CO_3). H_2CO_3 then dissociates into CO_2 and H_2O, both of which are expired by the lungs. The pH of the dog's blood decreases, but not as dramatically as if no buffer were available. The reactions are as follows:

$$H^+ + Cl^- + Na^+ + HCO_3^- \leftrightarrow Na^+ + Cl^- + H_2CO_3$$
$$\updownarrow$$
$$CO_2 + H_2O$$

The Henderson-Hasselbalch equation can be applied to the HCO_3^-/CO_2 buffer. The base form (A^-) is HCO_3^- and the acid form (HA) is H_2CO_3, which is in equilibrium with CO_2. In the presence of carbonic anhydrase, most of the H_2CO_3 is present in the CO_2 form (i.e., 400 CO_2:1 H_2CO_3); thus, the H_2CO_3 concentration usually is so low that it is ignored.

The pH of arterial blood can be calculated with the **Henderson-Hasselbalch equation** by substituting the normal concentrations of HCO_3^- and CO_2 and by knowing the pK. Note that because values of CO_2 usually are reported as partial pressures, P_{CO_2} must be converted to CO_2 concentration by multiplying by the solubility of CO_2 in blood (0.03 mmol/L/mm Hg). The final form of the equation is as follows:

$$pH = pK + \log \frac{HCO_3^-}{0.03 \times P_{CO_2}}$$

Substituting the following normal values, the pH of arterial blood can be calculated as follows:

$$pK = 6.1$$
$$[HCO_3^-] = 24 \text{ mmol/L}$$
$$P_{CO_2} = 40 \text{ mm Hg}$$

Thus,

$$pH = 6.1 + \log \frac{24 \text{ mmol/L}}{0.03 \times 40 \text{ mm Hg}}$$
$$= 6.1 + \log 20$$
$$= 7.4$$

The Henderson-Hasselbalch equation also can be represented on an **acid-base map,** which shows the relationships between P_{CO_2}, HCO_3^- concentration, and pH (Fig. 7-4). The lines radiating from the origin on the map are called the **isohydric lines** (meaning same H^+ concentration or same pH); each isohydric line gives all of the combinations of P_{CO_2} and HCO_3^- that yield the same value of pH. The **ellipse** in the center shows the normal values for arterial blood. Any point on the graph can be calculated by substituting the appropriate values into the Henderson-Hasselbalch equation. For example, the previous calculations show that a P_{CO_2} of 40 mm Hg and an HCO_3^- concentration of 24 mEq/L yields a pH of 7.4. The acid-base map confirms that when the P_{CO_2} is 40 mm Hg and the HCO_3^- concentration is 24 mEq/L, the pH is 7.4.

It is important to note that *abnormal combinations of P_{CO_2} and HCO_3^- concentration can yield normal (or nearly normal) values of pH.* For example, the combination of a P_{CO_2} of 60 mm Hg and an HCO_3^- concentration of 36 mEq/L also corresponds to a pH of 7.4, although both the HCO_3^- concentration and the P_{CO_2} clearly are higher than normal. For another example, the combination of a P_{CO_2} of 20 mm Hg and an HCO_3^- concentration of 12 mEq/L also corresponds to a pH of 7.4, although both the HCO_3^- concentration and the P_{CO_2} are lower than normal. (This important principle underlies the processes of respiratory and renal compensation that attempt to normalize the pH when there is an acid-base disorder.)

The importance of the HCO_3^-/CO_2 buffer system in protecting the pH can be illustrated by imagining that **12 mmol/L of HCl is added to ECF.** The initial HCO_3^- concentration of ECF is 24 mmol/L. Then, 12 mmol/L of added H^+ combines with 12 mmol/L of HCO_3^- to form 12 mmol/L of H_2CO_3, which is converted to 12 mmol/L of CO_2 in the presence of carbonic anhydrase. After this **buffering** reaction occurs, the *new* HCO_3^- concentration will be 12 mmol/L instead of the original 24 mmol/L. The *new* CO_2 concentration will be the original concentration of 1.2 mmol/L (i.e., 40 mm Hg × 0.03) *plus* the 12 mmol/L that is

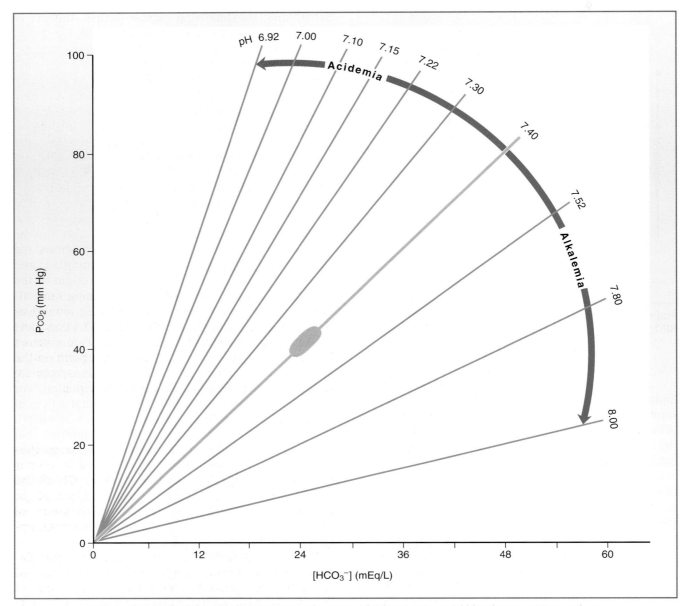

Figure 7–4 Acid-base map. The relationships shown are between arterial blood P_{CO_2}, $[HCO_3^-]$, and pH. The *ellipse* in the center gives the range of normal values. (Modified from Cohen JJ, Kassirer JP: Acid/ Base. Boston, Little, Brown, 1982.)

generated in the buffering reaction. Assuming for a moment that the additional CO_2 generated cannot be expired by the lungs, the *new* pH will be

$$pH = 6.1 + \log \frac{12 \text{ mmol/L}}{1.2 \text{ mmol/L} + 12 \text{ mmol/L}}$$

$$= 6.1 + \log \frac{12 \text{ mmol/L}}{13.2 \text{ mmol/L}}$$

$$= 6.06$$

Clearly, a pH this low (6.06) would be fatal! There is, however, a second protective mechanism, **respiratory compensation,** which prevents the pH from falling to this fatally low value. Acidemia stimulates

chemoreceptors in the carotid bodies that produce an immediate increase in the ventilation rate **(hyperventilation):** All of the excess CO_2, *plus more,* is expired by the lungs. This response, called respiratory compensation, drives the P_{CO_2} down to lower than normal values (e.g., to 24 mm Hg). Substituting these values in the Henderson-Hasselbalch equation, another pH can be calculated:

$$pH = 6.1 + \log \frac{12 \text{ mmol/L}}{0.03 \times 24 \text{ mm Hg}}$$

$$= 6.1 + \log \frac{12 \text{ mmol/L}}{0.72}$$

$$= 7.32$$

The combination of buffering by HCO_3^- and respiratory compensation (i.e., hyperventilation) results in an almost normal pH (normal = 7.4). Although both the HCO_3^- concentration and the P_{CO_2} are severely reduced, the pH is nearly normal. Full restoration of acid-base balance depends on the kidneys. Eventually, by processes described later in this chapter, the kidneys secrete H^+ and synthesize "new" HCO_3^- to replace the HCO_3^- that was consumed in buffering the added fixed H^+.

$HPO_4^{-2}/H_2PO_4^-$ Buffer

Inorganic phosphate also serves as a buffer. Its titration curve can be compared with that for HCO_3^- (see Fig. 7-3). Recall that the pK for HCO_3^-/CO_2 is 6.1, with the linear portion of the titration curve extending from pH 5.1 to 7.1; technically, the linear portion is outside the buffering range for a pH of 7.4. On the other hand, the pK of the $HPO_4^{-2}/H_2PO_4^-$ buffer is 6.8, with the linear portion of its curve extending from pH 5.8 to 7.8. It *seems* that inorganic phosphate would be a more important physiologic buffer than HCO_3^-, because its effective buffering range is closer to 7.4, the pH of blood. However, two features of the HCO_3^-/CO_2 buffer make it the more effective buffer: (1) HCO_3^- is in much higher concentration (24 mmol/L) than phosphate (1 to 2 mmol/L). (2) The acid form of the HCO_3^-/CO_2 buffer is CO_2, which is volatile and can be expired by the lungs.

Intracellular Fluid Buffers

There are vast quantities of intracellular buffers, which include **organic phosphates and proteins.** To utilize these ICF buffers in acid-base disturbances, H^+ first must cross the cell membrane by one of the following three mechanisms: (1) In conditions where there is an excess or a deficit of CO_2, as in respiratory acid-base disturbances, CO_2 *itself* can cross the cell membranes. For example, in respiratory acidosis, there is excess CO_2, which generates H^+ that must be buffered. CO_2 rapidly enters the cells, and the H^+ it generates is buffered by intracellular buffers. (2) In conditions where there is an excess or a deficit of fixed acid, H^+ can enter or leave the cell with an organic anion such as lactate. For example, in metabolic acidosis caused by increased levels of lactic acid, excess H^+ is produced along with lactate and H^+ and lactate enter the cells together, preserving electroneutrality. (3) In other cases of excess or deficit of fixed H^+ in which there is no accompanying organic anion, H^+ exchanges with K^+ to preserve electroneutrality.

Although they are not present in ICF, **plasma proteins** also buffer H^+. A relationship exists between plasma proteins, H^+, and calcium (Ca^{2+}), which results in changes in ionized Ca^{2+} concentration when there is an acid-base disturbance. (See Chapter 9, Fig. 9-34.) The mechanism is as follows: Negatively charged groups on plasma proteins (e.g., albumin) can bind either H^+ or Ca^{2+}. (Protein-binding of Ca^{2+} is extensive and accounts for 40% of total Ca^{2+}.) In **acidemia,** there is an excess of H^+ in blood. Because more H^+ is bound to plasma proteins, less Ca^{2+} is bound, producing an increase in free Ca^{2+} concentration. In **alkalemia,** there is a deficit of H^+ in blood. Because less H^+ is bound to plasma proteins, more Ca^{2+} is bound, producing a decrease in free Ca^{2+} concentration (hypocalcemia). Symptoms of hypocalcemia commonly occur in respiratory alkalosis and include tingling, numbness, and tetany.

Organic Phosphates

Organic phosphates in ICF include adenosine triphosphate (ATP), adenosine diphosphate (ADP), adenosine monophosphate (AMP), glucose-1-phosphate, and 2,3-diphosphoglycerate (2,3-DPG). H^+ is buffered by the phosphate moiety of these organic molecules. The pKs for these organic phosphates range from 6.0 to 7.5, ideal for effective physiologic buffering.

Proteins

Intracellular proteins serve as buffers because they contain a large number of acidic or basic groups such as $-COOH/-COO^-$ or $-NH_3^+/-NH_2$. Of all the dissociable groups on proteins, those with a pK in the physiologic range are the imidazole group of histidine (pK 6.4 to 7.0) and the α amino groups (pK 7.4 to 7.9).

The most significant intracellular buffer is **hemoglobin,** which is present in high concentration inside red blood cells. Each hemoglobin molecule has a total of 36 histidine residues (9 on each of the 4 polypeptide chains). The pK of oxyhemoglobin is 6.7, which is in the range for effective physiologic buffering. **Deoxyhemoglobin,** however, is an even more effective buffer with a pK of 7.9. The change in the pK of hemoglobin when it releases oxygen (O_2) has physiologic significance. As blood flows through the systemic capillaries, oxyhemoglobin releases O_2 to the tissues and is converted to deoxyhemoglobin. At the same time, CO_2 is added to systemic capillary blood from the tissues. This CO_2 diffuses into the red blood cells and combines with H_2O to form H_2CO_3. The H_2CO_3 then dissociates into H^+ and HCO_3^-. The H^+ generated is buffered by hemoglobin, which now is conveniently in its deoxygenated form. Deoxyhemoglobin certainly must be an excellent buffer for H^+: The pH of venous blood is 7.37, which is only 0.03 pH units more acidic than the pH of arterial blood despite the addition of large amounts of acid as CO_2.

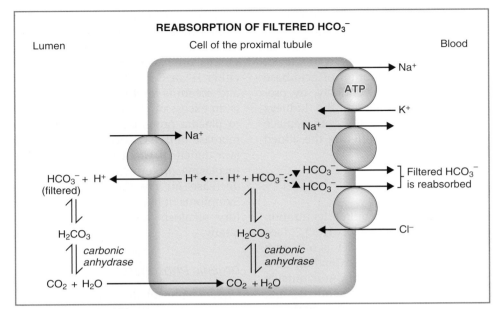

Figure 7-5 **Mechanism for reabsorption of filtered HCO$_3^-$ in a cell of the proximal tubule.** ATP, Adenosine triphosphate.

RENAL MECHANISMS IN ACID-BASE BALANCE

The kidneys play two major roles in the maintenance of normal acid-base balance: reabsorption of HCO$_3^-$ and excretion of H$^+$. The first role of the kidneys is to **reabsorb the filtered HCO$_3^-$** so that this important extracellular buffer is not excreted in urine. The second role of the kidneys is to **excrete fixed H$^+$** that is produced from protein and phospholipid catabolism. There are two mechanisms for excretion of this fixed H$^+$: (1) excretion of H$^+$ as titratable acid (i.e., buffered by urinary phosphate) and (2) excretion of H$^+$ as NH$_4^+$. Excretion of H$^+$ by either mechanism is accompanied by synthesis and reabsorption of *new* HCO$_3^-$. The purpose of synthesis and reabsorption of new HCO$_3^-$ is to replenish the HCO$_3^-$ stores that were used in buffering fixed H$^+$.

Reabsorption of Filtered HCO$_3^-$

Almost 99.9% of the filtered HCO$_3^-$ is reabsorbed, ensuring that the major extracellular buffer is conserved, rather than excreted. The reabsorption rate can be calculated (as explained in Chapter 6) by comparing the filtered load of HCO$_3^-$ with the excretion rate of HCO$_3^-$. If the glomerular filtration rate (GFR) is 180 L/day and the plasma HCO$_3^-$ concentration is 24 mEq/L, then the filtered load is 4320 mEq/day (180 L/day × 24 mEq/L). The measured excretion rate of HCO$_3^-$ is merely 2 mEq/day. Therefore, the reabsorption rate of HCO$_3^-$ is 4318 mEq/day, which is 99.9% of the filtered load. Most filtered HCO$_3^-$ reabsorption occurs in the **proximal tubule,** and only small quantities are reabsorbed in the loop of Henle, distal tubule, and collecting duct.

Mechanism of HCO$_3^-$ Reabsorption in the Proximal Tubule

Figure 7-5 is a diagram of a cell of the early proximal tubule, where filtered HCO$_3^-$ is reabsorbed. Reabsorption of filtered HCO$_3^-$ involves the following steps and includes conversion of HCO$_3^-$ to CO$_2$ in the lumen, diffusion of CO$_2$ into the cell, conversion back to HCO$_3^-$ in the cell, and reabsorption of HCO$_3^-$ into the blood:

1. The luminal membrane contains an **Na$^+$-H$^+$ exchanger,** which is one of several Na$^+$-dependent secondary active transport mechanisms in the early proximal tubule. As Na$^+$ moves from the lumen into the cell down its electrochemical gradient, H$^+$ moves from the cell into the lumen against its electrochemical gradient.

2. The H$^+$ secreted into the lumen combines with filtered HCO$_3^-$ to form H$_2$CO$_3$. The H$_2$CO$_3$ then decomposes into CO$_2$ and H$_2$O, catalyzed by a **brush border carbonic anhydrase.** (Carbonic anhydrase inhibitors such as acetazolamide inhibit the reabsorption of filtered HCO$_3^-$ by interfering with this step.) The CO$_2$ and H$_2$O that are formed in this reaction readily cross the luminal membrane and enter the cell.

3. Inside the cell, the reactions occur in reverse. CO$_2$ and H$_2$O recombine to form H$_2$CO$_3$, catalyzed by *intracellular* carbonic anhydrase. H$_2$CO$_3$ is

converted back to H^+ and HCO_3^-. The fates of the H^+ and HCO_3^- are different. H^+ is secreted by the Na^+-H^+ exchanger to aid in the reabsorption of another filtered HCO_3^-. The HCO_3^- is transported across the basolateral membrane into the blood (i.e., the HCO_3^- is reabsorbed) by two mechanisms: Na^+-HCO_3^- cotransport and Cl^--HCO_3^- exchange. Special features of the mechanism for reabsorption of filtered HCO_3^- include the following:

♦ The process results in **net reabsorption of Na^+ and HCO_3^-.** Thus, a portion of the Na^+ reabsorption in the proximal tubule is linked directly to the reabsorption of filtered HCO_3^-. (The rest of the Na^+ reabsorption is linked to reabsorption of glucose, amino acids, Cl^-, and phosphate.)

♦ There is *no* **net secretion of H^+** via this mechanism. Each H^+ secreted by the Na^+-H^+ exchanger in the luminal membrane combines with a filtered HCO_3^- to form CO_2 and H_2O, which enter the cell and are converted back to H^+ and HCO_3^-. The H^+ is recycled across the luminal membrane on the Na^+-H^+ exchanger to reabsorb more filtered HCO_3^-.

♦ Because there is no net secretion of H^+ by this mechanism, it produces **little change in tubular fluid pH.**

Effect of Filtered Load of HCO_3^-

The filtered load of HCO_3^- is the product of GFR and the plasma HCO_3^- concentration. Over a wide range of filtered loads, virtually all of the HCO_3^- is reabsorbed. However, when the plasma HCO_3^- concentration is greater than 40 mEq/L, the filtered load becomes so high that the reabsorption mechanism is saturated; any filtered HCO_3^- that cannot be reabsorbed is excreted. For example, in metabolic alkalosis where the blood HCO_3^- concentration is elevated, restoration of normal acid-base balance requires excretion of the excess HCO_3^- in the urine. This is accomplished because, as the concentration of HCO_3^- in the blood increases, the filtered load increases and exceeds the reabsorptive capacity. The nonreabsorbed HCO_3^- is excreted, lowering the blood HCO_3^- concentration to normal.

Effect of Extracellular Fluid Volume

Most of the filtered HCO_3^- is reabsorbed in the proximal tubule, where changes in ECF volume alter isosmotic reabsorption via changes in the Starling forces in the peritubular capillaries (see Chapter 6). Because HCO_3^- is part of this isosmotic reabsorption, changes in ECF volume alter HCO_3^- reabsorption in a predictable way. For example, **ECF volume expansion** inhibits isosmotic reabsorption in the proximal tubule and, therefore,

inhibits HCO_3^- reabsorption. Conversely, **ECF volume contraction** stimulates isosmotic reabsorption in the proximal tubule and stimulates HCO_3^- reabsorption.

A second mechanism, involving angiotensin II, participates in the response of HCO_3^- reabsorption to ECF volume contraction. Recall that decreases in ECF volume activate the renin–angiotensin II–aldosterone system. **Angiotensin II** stimulates Na^+-H^+ exchange in the proximal tubule, thus stimulating HCO_3^- reabsorption and increasing the blood HCO_3^- concentration. This mechanism explains the phenomenon of **contraction alkalosis,** which literally means metabolic alkalosis that occurs secondary to ECF volume contraction. Contraction alkalosis occurs during treatment with **loop diuretics** or **thiazide diuretics,** and it is a complicating factor in the metabolic alkalosis caused by **vomiting.** Contraction alkalosis is treated by infusing isotonic NaCl to restore ECF volume.

Effect of P_{CO_2}

Chronic changes in P_{CO_2} alter the reabsorption of filtered HCO_3^- and explain the phenomenon of renal compensation for chronic respiratory acid-base disorders. Increases in P_{CO_2} increase the reabsorption of HCO_3^-, and decreases in P_{CO_2} decrease the reabsorption of HCO_3^-.

The mechanism underlying the effect of CO_2 is not completely understood. One explanation, however, involves the *supply* of CO_2 to the renal cells. In **respiratory acidosis,** the P_{CO_2} is increased. Because more CO_2 is available in the renal cells to generate H^+ for secretion by the Na^+-H^+ exchanger, more HCO_3^- can be reabsorbed. Thus, the plasma HCO_3^- concentration increases, which increases the arterial pH (a compensation). In **respiratory alkalosis,** the P_{CO_2} is decreased. As less CO_2 is available in the renal cells to generate H^+ for secretion, less HCO_3^- is reabsorbed. In this case, the plasma HCO_3^- concentration decreases, which decreases the arterial pH (a compensation).

Excretion of H^+ as Titratable Acid

By definition, titratable acid is H^+ excreted with urinary buffers. Inorganic phosphate is the most important of these buffers because of its relatively high concentration in urine and its ideal pK. Recall that there is a significant amount of phosphate in urine because only 85% of the filtered phosphate is reabsorbed; 15% of the filtered phosphate is left to be excreted as titratable acid.

Mechanism of Excretion of Titratable Acid

Titratable acid is excreted throughout the nephron, but primarily in the α-intercalated cells of the late distal tubule and collecting ducts. The cellular mechanism for

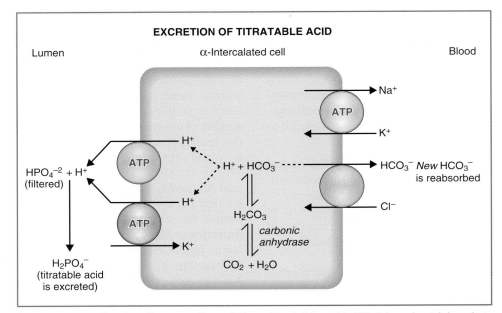

EXCRETION OF TITRATABLE ACID

Figure 7–6 **Mechanism for excretion of H⁺ as titratable acid.** ATP, Adenosine triphosphate.

this process is illustrated in Figure 7-6 and is described as follows:

1. The luminal membrane of α-intercalated cells of the late distal tubule and collecting ducts has two primary active transport mechanisms for secreting H⁺ into tubular fluid. The first mechanism for H⁺ secretion is **H⁺ ATPase,** which is stimulated by **aldosterone.** Aldosterone not only acts on the principal cells in stimulation of Na⁺ reabsorption and K⁺ secretion but also stimulates H⁺ secretion in the α-intercalated cells. The other mechanism for H⁺ secretion is **H⁺-K⁺ ATPase,** the transporter responsible for K⁺ reabsorption in α-intercalated cells (see Chapter 6). In the lumen, the secreted H⁺ combines with the A⁻ form of the phosphate buffer, HPO_4^{-2}, to produce the HA form of the buffer, $H_2PO_4^-$. **$H_2PO_4^-$ is titratable acid,** which is excreted.

   For this mechanism to be useful, it is essential that most of the filtered phosphate be in the form that can accept an H⁺ (i.e., in the HPO_4^{-2} form). *Is this so?* By calculating the relative concentrations of HPO_4^{-2} and $H_2PO_4^-$ at pH 7.4, it can be confirmed that the concentration of HPO_4^{-2} is almost fourfold the concentration of $H_2PO_4^-$ in the glomerular filtrate (pH = pK + log $HPO_4^{-2}/H_2PO_4^-$, where pK = 6.8; at pH 7.4, $HPO_4^{-2}/H_2PO_4^-$ = 3.98).

2. The H⁺ secreted by the H⁺ ATPase is produced in the renal cells from CO_2 and H_2O, which combine to form H_2CO_3 in the presence of intracellular carbonic anhydrase. H_2CO_3 dissociates into H⁺, which is secreted, and HCO_3^-, which is reabsorbed into the blood via Cl^--HCO_3^- exchange.

3. For each H⁺ excreted as titratable acid, one ***new*** **HCO_3^- is synthesized and reabsorbed.** This new HCO_3^- replenishes extracellular HCO_3^- stores, which previously had been depleted from buffering fixed H⁺. Because the generation, or synthesis, of new HCO_3^- is an ongoing process, HCO_3^- is continuously replaced as it is used for buffering the fixed acids produced from protein and phospholipid catabolism.

Amount of Urinary Buffer

The amount of H⁺ excreted as titratable acid depends on the *amount* of urinary buffer available. Although it may not be immediately obvious why this is so, the underlying principle is that the **minimum urine pH is 4.4.** Because blood pH is 7.4, a urine pH of 4.4 represents a 1000-fold difference in H⁺ concentration across the renal tubular cells. This 1000-fold difference is the largest concentration gradient against which H⁺ can be secreted by the H⁺ ATPase. When the urine pH is reduced to 4.4, net secretion of H⁺ ceases.

To understand this principle, it is important to distinguish between *the amount of H⁺ excreted* and the *value for urine pH.* To illustrate this distinction, consider the following two examples: First, imagine that there are *no* urinary buffers. In that case, the first few H⁺ secreted, finding no urinary buffers, would be free in solution and cause the pH to decrease to the minimum value of 4.4, and thereafter, no additional H⁺ could be secreted. Next, imagine that urinary buffers are plentiful. In that case, large quantities of H⁺ could be secreted and buffered in urine before the pH would be reduced to 4.4.

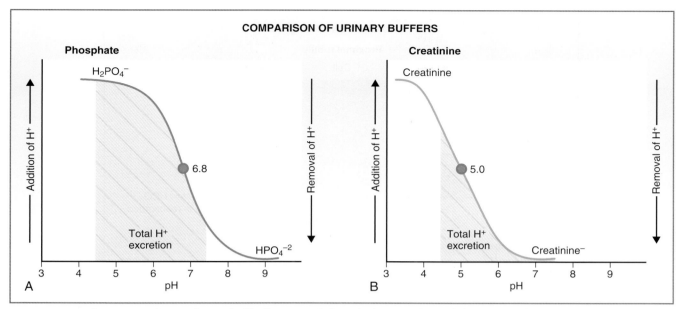

Figure 7–7 **Comparison of effectiveness of phosphate (A) and creatinine (B) as urinary buffers.** The pK of the phosphate buffer is 6.8; the pK of the creatinine buffer is 5.0. The *shaded areas* show the total amount of H⁺ that is secreted into tubular fluid between the glomerular filtrate (pH 7.4) and the final urine (pH 4.4).

This point is further illustrated in Figure 7-7. Figure 7-7A shows the range of tubular fluid pH (shaded area) superimposed on the phosphate titration curve. Begin with the glomerular filtrate, which has a pH of 7.4: Both HPO_4^{-2} and $H_2PO_4^-$ are present, with the concentration of HPO_4^{-2} considerably higher than that of $H_2PO_4^-$. As H⁺ is secreted into tubular fluid, it combines with the HPO_4^{-2} form of the phosphate buffer and converts it to $H_2PO_4^-$. In the linear portion of the titration curve (pH 7.8 to 5.8), the addition of H⁺ to tubular fluid causes the pH to decrease only modestly. However, once most of the HPO_4^{-2} has been converted to $H_2PO_4^-$, further secretion of H⁺ causes the tubular fluid pH to decrease precipitously to 4.4. At that point, no additional H⁺ can be secreted. The only way to secrete more H⁺ would be to provide more HPO_4^{-2}. Thus, the *amount* of H⁺ excreted as titratable acid depends on the *amount* of available urinary buffer.

pK of Urinary Buffers

The pK of the urinary buffers also affects the amount of H⁺ that is excreted. Robert Pitts demonstrated the importance of pK by comparing the effectiveness of creatinine (with a pK of 5.0) as a urinary buffer with the effectiveness of phosphate (with a pK of 6.8). He found that for a given quantity of urinary buffer, more H⁺ was excreted when the buffer was phosphate than when the buffer was creatinine (see Fig. 7-7).

The difference in the amount of H⁺ excreted is attributed to the different pKs of the two buffers. Remember that **phosphate** is an *almost ideal* urinary buffer. The linear range of its titration curve overlaps almost

perfectly with the range of tubular fluid pH. In Figure 7-7A, the shaded area under the phosphate titration curve represents the total amount of H⁺ secreted as the tubular fluid pH decreases from pH 7.4 in glomerular filtrate to pH 4.4 in the final urine.

Figure 7-7B shows the titration curve for **creatinine.** Again, the pH of tubular fluid ranges from 7.4 (in glomerular filtrate) to 4.4 in the final urine. The pK of creatinine, at 5.0, is close to the minimum urine pH; therefore, the total amount of H⁺ that can be secreted (*shaded area*) before the pH falls to 4.4 is *much less* than the amount secreted when phosphate is the buffer.

Excretion of H⁺ as NH₄⁺

If titratable acid were the only mechanism for excreting H⁺, then excretion of fixed H⁺ would be limited by the amount of phosphate in urine. Recall that fixed H⁺ production from protein and phospholipid catabolism is approximately 50 mEq/day. On average, however, only 20 mEq/day of this fixed H⁺ is excreted as titratable H⁺. The remaining 30 mEq/day is excreted by a second mechanism, as NH_4^+.

Mechanism of Excretion of H⁺ as NH₄⁺

Three segments of the nephron participate in the excretion of H⁺ as NH_4^+: the proximal tubule, the thick ascending limb of Henle's loop, and α-intercalated cells of the collecting ducts. In the **proximal tubule,** NH_4^+ is secreted by the Na⁺-H⁺ exchanger. In the **thick ascending limb,** NH_4^+ that was previously secreted by

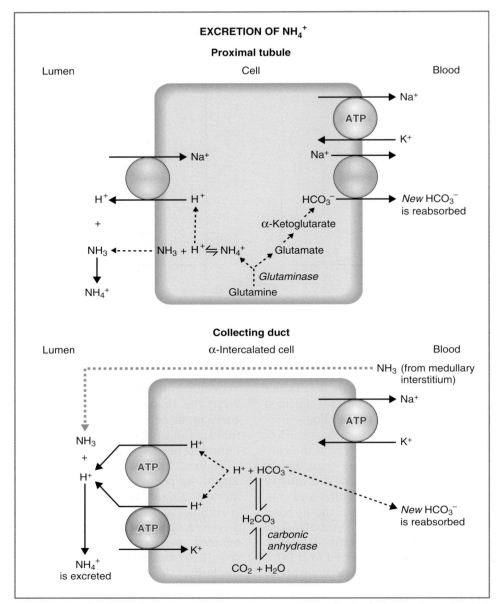

Figure 7–8 **Mechanism of excretion of H⁺ as NH₄⁺.** In the proximal tubule, NH_3 is produced from glutamine in the renal cells. H^+ is secreted by Na^+-H^+ exchanger and NH_3 diffuses into the lumen. NH_4^+ is reabsorbed by Na^+-K^+-$2Cl^-$ cotransporter in the TALH and deposited in the medullary interstitial fluid (not shown). In the collecting ducts, NH_3 diffuses from the medullary interstitium into the lumen, combines with secreted H^+ in the lumen, and is excreted as NH_4^+. ATP, Adenosine triphosphate. TALH, thick ascending limb of loop of Henle.

the proximal tubules is reabsorbed and added to the corticopapillary osmotic gradient. In the α-intercalated cells of the **collecting duct,** NH_3 and H^+ are secreted into the lumen, combine to form NH_4^+, and are excreted.

♦ **Proximal tubule.** In the cells of the proximal tubule, the enzyme **glutaminase** metabolizes **glutamine** to glutamate and NH_4^+ (Fig. 7-8). The glutamate is metabolized to α-ketoglutarate, which is ultimately metabolized to CO_2 and H_2O and then to HCO_3^-. The HCO_3^- is reabsorbed across the basolateral membrane into the blood via Na^+-HCO_3^- cotransport.

Similar to the titratable acid mechanism, this HCO_3^- is newly synthesized and helps to replenish HCO_3^- stores in the ECF. For each NH_4^+ generated (and ultimately excreted), one new HCO_3^- is reabsorbed.

The fate of the NH_4^+ requires several additional steps. In the proximal tubule cell, NH_4^+ is in equilibrium with NH_3 and H^+. The NH_3 form, being lipid soluble, diffuses down its concentration gradient from cell to lumen, and the H^+ is secreted into the lumen on the Na^+-H^+ exchanger. Once in the lumen, NH_3 and H^+ recombine into NH_4^+. The fate of the NH_4^+, once in the lumen of the proximal tubule, is as follows. A portion of the NH_4^+ is excreted *directly* in the urine. The remainder follows a circuitous route and is excreted *indirectly:* It is first reabsorbed by the thick ascending limb, then deposited in the medullary interstitial fluid, and then secreted from the medullary interstitial fluid into the collecting ducts for final excretion.

♦ **Thick ascending limb.** As previously noted but not shown in Figure 7-8, a portion of the NH_4^+ that is secreted in the proximal tubule and delivered to the loop of Henle is reabsorbed by the thick ascending limb. At the cellular level, NH_4^+ is reabsorbed by substituting for K^+ on the Na^+-K^+-$2Cl^-$ cotransporter. As a result of this substitution, NH_4^+ participates in **countercurrent multiplication** (much like NaCl) and is concentrated in the interstitial fluid of the inner medulla and papilla of the kidney.

♦ **Collecting duct.** As described for the titratable acid mechanism, the luminal membrane of α-intercalated cells of the collecting duct contains two transporters that secrete H^+ into tubular fluid (see Fig. 7-8): H^+ ATPase and H^+-K^+ ATPase. The **H^+ ATPase** is stimulated by **aldosterone.**

As H^+ is secreted into tubular fluid, **NH_3 diffuses** from its high concentration in the medullary interstitial fluid into the lumen of the collecting duct, where it combines with the secreted H^+ to form NH_4^+. The question that arises is *Why does only the NH_3 form of the NH_3/NH_4^+ buffer diffuse from the medullary interstitium?* The answer is that although both NH_4^+ and NH_3 are present in the medullary interstitial fluid, only the NH_3 form is lipid soluble and can diffuse across the collecting duct cells into tubular fluid. Once in the tubular fluid, NH_3 combines with the secreted H^+ to form NH_4^+. NH_4^+ is not lipid soluble and, thus, is trapped in the tubular fluid and excreted. The overall process is termed **diffusion trapping** because the lipid-soluble form of the buffer (NH_3) *diffuses* and the water-soluble form of the buffer (NH_4^+) is *trapped* and excreted.

Note that the source of the H^+ secreted by the α-intercalated cells is CO_2 and H_2O. For each H^+ produced in the cells and secreted, one *new* **HCO_3^- is synthesized and reabsorbed.** As with the titratable acid mechanism, this new HCO_3^- helps to replenish depleted HCO_3^- stores.

Effect of Urinary pH on Excretion of NH_4^+

As urinary pH decreases, the excretion of H^+ as NH_4^+ increases. The effect of urine pH on the excretion of NH_4^+ is advantageous: In acidosis, where urine pH tends to be low, there are large quantities of H^+ to be excreted. The mechanism underlying the effect of urine pH is based on diffusion trapping of NH_3/NH_4^+. As the pH of urine decreases, more of the urinary buffer is present in the NH_4^+ form and less is present in the NH_3 form. The lower the luminal concentration of NH_3, the larger the gradient for diffusion of NH_3 from medullary interstitial fluid into tubular fluid. Thus, the lower the pH of tubular fluid, the greater the amount of NH_3 diffusion and the greater the amount of H^+ excreted as NH_4^+.

Effect of Acidosis on NH_3 Synthesis

The rate of NH_3 synthesis changes, depending on the quantity of H^+ that must be excreted. In **chronic acidosis,** there is an **adaptive increase in NH_3 synthesis** in the cells of the proximal tubule. The mechanism involves a decrease in intracellular pH, which induces the synthesis of enzymes involved in glutamine metabolism. When NH_3 synthesis is augmented in this way, more H^+ is excreted as NH_4^+ and more new HCO_3^- is reabsorbed. For example, in diabetic ketoacidosis, fixed acid production is increased. The ability of the kidneys to excrete this additional fixed acid load is attributable, in large part, to an adaptive increase in NH_3 synthesis.

Effect of Plasma K^+ Concentration on NH_3 Synthesis

Plasma K^+ concentration also alters NH_3 synthesis. **Hyperkalemia** inhibits NH_3 synthesis and reduces the ability to excrete H^+ as NH_4^+, causing **type 4 renal tubular acidosis** (RTA). **Hypokalemia** stimulates NH_3 synthesis and increases the ability to excrete H^+ as NH_4^+. These effects are most likely mediated by the exchange of H^+ and K^+ across renal cell membranes, which in turn alters intracellular pH. In hyperkalemia, K^+ enters the renal cells and H^+ leaves. The resulting increase in intracellular pH inhibits NH_3 synthesis from glutamine. In hypokalemia, K^+ leaves renal cells and H^+ enters. The resulting decrease in intracellular pH stimulates NH_3 synthesis from glutamine.

Comparison of Titratable Acid and NH_4^+ Excretion

On a daily basis, H^+ is excreted as both titratable acid and NH_4^+ so that normally all of the fixed H^+ produced from protein and phospholipid catabolism is eliminated from the body (and all of the HCO_3^- used to buffer that fixed H^+ is replaced). Table 7-1 summarizes and compares the rates of excretion of H^+ as titratable acid and NH_4^+ in normal persons and in those with different types of metabolic acidosis (i.e., diabetic ketoacidosis and chronic renal failure).

♦ In **normal** persons eating a relatively high protein diet, approximately 50 mEq of fixed H^+ is produced daily. The kidneys excrete *all* (100%) of the fixed acid that is produced: 40% is excreted as titratable acid (20 mEq/day) and 60% as NH_4^+ (30 mEq/day).

Table 7-1 Comparison of H⁺ Excretion as Titratable Acid and NH₄⁺

Condition	Total Production of Fixed H^+ (mEq/day)	Excretion of H^+ as Titratable Acid (mEq/day)	Excretion of H^+ as NH_4^+ (mEq/day)
Normal	50	20	30
Diabetic ketoacidosis	500	100	400
Chronic renal failure	50	10	5

♦ In persons with **diabetic ketoacidosis,** fixed acid production may be increased as much as 10-fold, to 500 mEq/day. To excrete this additional acid load, excretion of both titratable acid and NH₄⁺ is increased. NH₄⁺ excretion is increased because acidosis induces the enzymes involved in glutamine metabolism, thereby increasing NH₃ synthesis. As more NH₃ is produced by the renal cells, more H⁺ is excreted as NH₄⁺.

It is less apparent why titratable acid excretion is increased. In diabetic ketoacidosis, β-OH butyric acid and acetoacetic acid are overproduced, which causes metabolic acidosis. The salts of these keto-acids (i.e., butyrate and acetoacetate) are themselves filtered and serve as urinary buffers, similar to phosphate, increasing the total amount of H⁺ excreted as titratable acid.

♦ **Chronic renal failure** is another cause of metabolic acidosis. A person in chronic renal failure who continues to eat a relatively high protein diet will produce 50 mEq of fixed acid daily. In this disease, there is a progressive loss of nephrons, and the renal mechanisms for excreting fixed acid are severely impaired for two reasons: (1) Titratable acid excretion is reduced because glomerular filtration is reduced, which reduces the filtered load of phosphate and, thus, the amount of phosphate that can serve as a urinary buffer; (2) NH₄⁺ excretion is reduced because synthesis of NH₃ is impaired in the diseased nephrons.

Notice that the total fixed acid excretion in chronic renal failure is only 15 mEq/day (10 mEq as titratable acid plus 5 mEq as NH₄⁺), which is much less than the amount of fixed acid produced from protein catabolism (50 mEq/day). In chronic renal failure, the *cause* of the metabolic acidosis is, in fact, the inability of the kidneys to excrete all of the fixed acid produced daily. Logically, persons with chronic renal failure are placed on a low-protein diet to reduce daily fixed acid production and thereby reduce the demand on the kidneys for fixed acid excretion and new HCO₃⁻ reabsorption.

ACID-BASE DISORDERS

Disturbances of acid-base balance are among the most common conditions in all of clinical medicine. Acid-base disorders are characterized by an abnormal concentration of H⁺ in blood, reflected as abnormal pH. **Acidemia** is an increase in H⁺ concentration in blood (decrease in pH) and is caused by a pathophysiologic process called acidosis. **Alkalemia,** on the other hand, is a decrease in H⁺ concentration in blood (increase in pH) and is caused by a pathophysiologic process called *alkalosis.*

Disturbances of blood pH can be caused by a *primary* disturbance of HCO₃⁻ concentration or a *primary* disturbance of Pco₂. Such disturbances are best understood by considering the Henderson-Hasselbalch equation for the HCO₃⁻/CO₂ buffer. Recall that the equation states that blood pH is determined by the ratio of the HCO₃⁻ concentration to the CO₂ concentration. Thus, changes in either HCO₃⁻ concentration or Pco₂ will produce a change in pH.

Disturbances of acid-base balance are described as either *metabolic* or *respiratory,* depending on whether the primary disturbance is in HCO₃⁻ or CO₂. There are four **simple acid-base disorders,** where *simple* means that only one acid-base disorder is present. When there is more than one acid-base disorder present, the condition is called a *mixed* acid-base disorder.

Metabolic acid-base disturbances are primary disorders involving HCO₃⁻. **Metabolic acidosis** is caused by a decrease in HCO₃⁻ concentration that, according to the Henderson-Hasselbalch equation, leads to a decrease in pH. This disorder is caused by gain of fixed H⁺ in the body (through overproduction of fixed H⁺, ingestion of fixed H⁺, or decreased excretion of fixed H⁺) or loss of HCO₃⁻. **Metabolic alkalosis** is caused by an increase in HCO₃⁻ concentration that, according to the Henderson-Hasselbalch equation, leads to an increase in pH. This disorder is caused by loss of fixed H⁺ from the body or gain of HCO₃⁻.

Respiratory acid-base disturbances are primary disorders of CO₂ (i.e., disorders of respiration). **Respiratory acidosis** is caused by hypoventilation, which results in CO₂ retention, increased Pco₂, and decreased pH. **Respiratory alkalosis** is caused by hyperventilation, which results in CO₂ loss, decreased Pco₂, and increased pH.

When there is an acid-base disturbance, several mechanisms are utilized in an attempt to keep the blood pH in the normal range. The first line of defense is buffering in ECF and ICF. In addition to buffering,

Table 7-2   Summary of Acid-Base Disorders

Disorder	$CO_2 + H_2O$	$\leftrightarrow$	H^+	$+$	HCO_3^-	Respiratory Compensation	Renal Compensation or Correction
Metabolic Acidosis	↓		↑		**↓**	Hyperventilation	↑ HCO_3^- reabsorption (correction)
Metabolic Alkalosis	↑		↓		**↑**	Hypoventilation	↑ HCO_3^- excretion (correction)
Respiratory Acidosis	**↑**		↑		↑	None	↑ HCO_3^- reabsorption (compensation)
Respiratory Alkalosis	**↓**		↓		↓	None	↓ HCO_3^- reabsorption (compensation)

Bold arrows indicate initial disturbance.

two types of compensatory responses attempt to normalize the pH: **respiratory compensation** and **renal compensation.** A helpful rule of thumb to learn is this: If the acid-base disturbance is metabolic (i.e., disturbance of HCO_3^-), then the compensatory response is respiratory to adjust the P_{CO_2}; if the acid-base disturbance is respiratory (i.e., disturbance of CO_2), then the compensatory response is renal (or metabolic) to adjust the HCO_3^- concentration. Another helpful rule is this: The compensatory response is always in the same direction as the original disturbance. For example, in metabolic acidosis, the primary disturbance is a *decrease* in the blood HCO_3^- concentration. The respiratory compensation is hyperventilation, which *decreases* the P_{CO_2}. In respiratory acidosis, the primary disturbance is *increased* P_{CO_2}. The renal compensation *increases* the HCO_3^- concentration.

As each acid-base disorder is presented, the buffering and compensatory responses are discussed in detail. Table 7-2 presents a summary of the four simple acid-base disorders and the expected compensatory responses that occur in each.

Anion Gap of Plasma

A measurement that is useful in the diagnosis of acid-base disorders is the **anion gap of plasma** (or simply **anion gap**). The anion gap is based on the principle of electroneutrality: For any body fluid compartment such as plasma, the concentration of cations and anions must be equal. In routine analysis of plasma, some cations and anions are measured and others are not. The cation that usually is measured is Na^+; the anions that usually are measured are HCO_3^- and Cl^-. When the Na^+ concentration (in mEq/L) is compared with the sum of the HCO_3^- and Cl^- concentrations (in mEq/L), there is an anion gap; that is, the Na^+ concentration is greater than the sum of the HCO_3^- concentration and the Cl^- concentration (Fig. 7-9). Because electroneutrality is never violated, plasma must contain **unmeasured anions** that make up this difference, or "gap." The unmeasured anions of plasma include plasma proteins, phosphate, citrate, and sulfate.

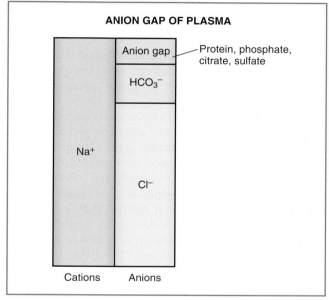

ANION GAP OF PLASMA

Figure 7-9   **Anion gap of plasma.**

The anion gap of plasma is calculated as follows:

$$\text{Plasma anion gap} = [Na^+] - ([HCO_3^-] + [Cl^-])$$

where

$$\text{Plasma anion gap} = \text{Unmeasured anions (mEq/L)}$$
$$[Na^+] = \text{Measured cation (mEq/L)}$$
$$[HCO_3^-] \text{ and } [Cl^-] = \text{Measured anions (mEq/L)}$$

The range of normal values for the plasma anion gap is **8 to 16 mEq/L.** The normal value for anion gap can be obtained by substituting normal values for plasma Na^+ concentration, HCO_3^- concentration, and Cl^- concentration into the equation. Thus, if the Na^+ concentration is 140 mEq/L, the HCO_3^- concentration is 24 mEq/L, and the Cl^- concentration is 105 mEq/L, then the plasma anion gap is 11 mEq/L.

The plasma anion gap is useful primarily in the differential diagnosis of **metabolic acidosis.** Metabolic acidosis is, by definition, associated with a decrease in plasma HCO_3^- concentration. Assuming that the Na^+

concentration is unchanged, to preserve electroneutrality of the plasma compartment, the concentration of an anion must increase to replace the "lost" HCO_3^-. That anion can be one of the unmeasured anions, or it can be Cl^-. If HCO_3^- is replaced by unmeasured anions, the calculated anion gap is increased. If HCO_3^- is replaced by Cl^-, the calculated anion gap is normal.

Increased Anion Gap

In several forms of metabolic acidosis, an organic anion (e.g., ketoacid, lactate, formate, salicylate) is accumulated. In these cases, the decrease in HCO_3^- concentration is offset by an increase in the concentration of an unmeasured organic anion. Thus, there is an increased anion gap, and this type of metabolic acidosis is called *metabolic acidosis with an increased anion gap*. Examples of increased anion gap metabolic acidosis are diabetic ketoacidosis, lactic acidosis, salicylate poisoning, methanol poisoning, ethylene glycol poisoning, and chronic renal failure.

In certain causes of metabolic acidosis with increased anion gap (i.e., methanol and ethylene glycol poisoning), there is also an **osmolar gap.** Osmolar gap is the difference between the *measured* plasma osmolarity and the *estimated* plasma osmolarity. (Recall from Chapter 6 that plasma osmolarity is estimated by summing the major solutes in plasma; that is, Na^+ [and its accompanying anions Cl^- and HCO_3^-], glucose, and urea. As explained in Chapter 6, estimated plasma osmolarity = $2 \times Na^+$ + glucose/18 + BUN/2.8.) Normally, there is little difference between measured and estimated plasma osmolarity because the estimation method accounts for almost all solutes normally present. However, in the case of methanol poisoning or ethylene glycol poisoning, because these substances have low molecular weight, there is significant addition of moles of solute to plasma, thus increasing the measured plasma osmolarity. Because the estimated plasma osmolarity does not count these unusual solutes, an osmolar gap is present. Theoretically, other substances that cause metabolic acidosis with increased anion gap (e.g., ketoacids, lactic acid, salicylic acid) could produce an osmolar gap. However, because of their relatively high molecular weights, toxic concentrations contribute little to the total osmolarity of plasma.

Normal Anion Gap

In a few causes of metabolic acidosis (e.g., diarrhea, renal tubular acidosis), no organic anion is accumulated. In these cases, the decrease in HCO_3^- concentration is offset by an increase in the concentration of Cl^-, which is a measured anion. Because one measured anion (HCO_3^-) is replaced by another measured anion (Cl^-), there is no change in the anion gap. This type of metabolic acidosis is called *hyperchloremic metabolic acidosis with a normal anion gap*. (Some may use the term "nonanion gap," but this is a misnomer. In such cases, an anion gap is still present, but it is normal, rather than increased.)

Acid-Base Map

Each of the four simple acid-base disorders is associated with a range of values for pH, Pco_2, and HCO_3^- concentration. These values can be superimposed as shaded areas on the acid-base map, as shown in Figure 7-10. This map provides a convenient method for assessing a patient's acid-base status.

♦ **Metabolic disorders.** Each of the simple metabolic disorders has *one* range of expected values, since respiratory compensation for metabolic acidosis or metabolic alkalosis occurs immediately.

♦ **Respiratory disorders.** Each of the simple respiratory disorders has *two* ranges of expected values, one for the acute disorder and one for the chronic disorder. The **acute** disorder is present before renal compensation has occurred, and, therefore, values for blood pH tend to be more abnormal. The **chronic** disorder is present once renal compensation has occurred, which takes several days. Because of the compensatory process, values for blood pH tend to be more normal in the chronic phase.

The acid-base map is used as follows: If a patient's values fall *within a shaded area,* it can be concluded that only one acid-base disorder is present. If a patient's values fall *outside the shaded areas* (e.g., between two areas), then it can be concluded that more than one disorder is present (i.e., mixed disorder). As each simple acid-base disorder is described subsequently, refer to Table 7-2 and the acid-base map shown in Figure 7-10.

Rules for Compensatory Responses

The acid-base map is useful pictorially, but it may be inconvenient to use at the patient's bedside. Therefore, "rules of thumb," or "renal rules," have been developed to determine if the patient's pH, Pco_2, and HCO_3^- concentrations are consistent with a simple acid-base disorder. These rules are summarized in Table 7-3. For each **metabolic disorder,** the rules predict the expected compensatory change in Pco_2 (i.e., respiratory compensation) for a given change in HCO_3^- concentration. For each **respiratory disorder,** the rules predict the expected compensatory change in HCO_3^- concentration (i.e., renal compensation) for a given change in Pco_2. As with the acid-base map, for each respiratory disorder there are two sets of predictions: one for the *acute* phase and one for the *chronic* phase.

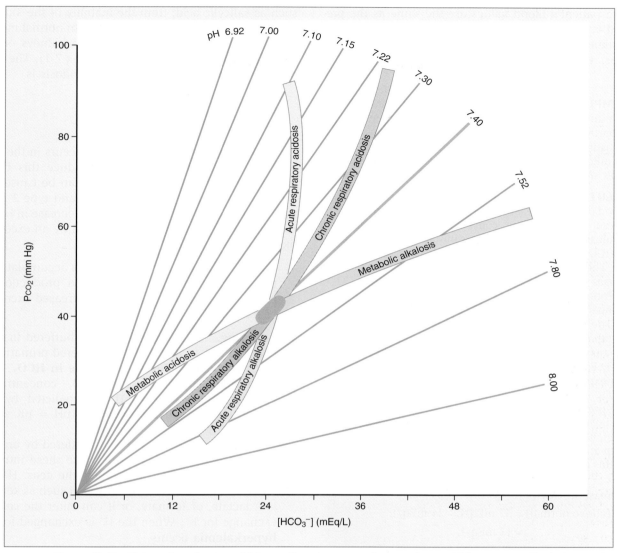

Figure 7–10 **Values for simple acid-base disorders superimposed on acid-base map.** *Shaded areas* show the range of values usually seen for each of the simple acid-base disorders. There are two *shaded areas* for each respiratory disorder: one for the acute phase and one for the chronic phase.

Table 7–3 Renal Rules for Predicting Compensatory Responses in Simple Acid-Base Disorders

Acid-Base Disturbance	Primary Disturbance	Compensation	Predicted Compensatory Response
Metabolic Acidosis	↓ $[HCO_3^-]$	↓ P_{CO_2}	1 mEq/L decrease in HCO_3^- → 1.3 mm Hg decrease in P_{CO_2}
Metabolic Alkalosis	↑ $[HCO_3^-]$	↑ P_{CO_2}	1 mEq/L increase in HCO_3^- → 0.7 mm Hg increase in P_{CO_2}
Respiratory Acidosis			
Acute	↑ P_{CO_2}	↑ $[HCO_3^-]$	1 mm Hg increase in P_{CO_2} → 0.1 mEq/L increase in HCO_3^-
Chronic	↑ P_{CO_2}	↑ $[HCO_3^-]$	1 mm Hg increase in P_{CO_2} → 0.4 mEq/L increase in HCO_3^-
Respiratory Alkalosis			
Acute	↓ P_{CO_2}	↓ $[HCO_3^-]$	1 mm Hg decrease in P_{CO_2} → 0.2 mEq/L decrease in HCO_3^-
Chronic	↓ P_{CO_2}	↓ $[HCO_3^-]$	1 mm Hg decrease in P_{CO_2} → 0.4 mEq/L decrease in HCO_3^-

If a patient's blood values are the same as the predicted values, a single acid-base disorder is present. If a patient's values are different from the predicted values, a mixed acid-base disorder is present.

SAMPLE PROBLEM. A woman who had been vomiting for 3 days was taken to the emergency department, where the following blood values were measured: pH, 7.5; P_{CO_2}, 48 mm Hg; and HCO_3^-, 37 mEq/L. *What acid-base disorder does she have? Does she have a simple or mixed acid-base disorder?*

SOLUTION. The woman has an increased (alkaline) blood pH and increased P_{CO_2} and HCO_3^- concentration. These values all are consistent with a metabolic alkalosis. Metabolic alkalosis is initiated by an increase in HCO_3^- concentration, which leads to an increase in pH. The increase in pH, acting through chemoreceptors, causes hypoventilation. Hypoventilation leads to CO_2 retention and increased P_{CO_2}, which is the respiratory compensation for metabolic alkalosis.

The question of whether the woman has simple metabolic alkalosis or a mixed acid-base disorder can be answered by applying the renal rules (see Table 7-3). For metabolic alkalosis, the renal rules predict the expected increase in P_{CO_2} for a given increase in HCO_3^- concentration. If the actual P_{CO_2} is the same as the predicted P_{CO_2}, the person has simple metabolic alkalosis. If the actual P_{CO_2} differs from the predicted P_{CO_2}, the person has metabolic alkalosis combined with another acid-base disorder (i.e., mixed disorder). In this example, the renal rules are applied as follows:

Increase in HCO_3^-

   (above normal) = 37 mEq/L − 24 mEq/L

               = 13 mEq/L

Predicted increase in P_{CO_2}

   (above normal) = 0.7 mm Hg/mEq/L × 13 mEq/L

               = 9.1 mm Hg

   Predicted P_{CO_2} = 40 mm Hg + 9.1 mm Hg

               = 49.1 mm Hg

To interpret this calculation, in simple metabolic alkalosis with an HCO_3^- concentration of 37 mEq/L, compensatory hypoventilation is expected to raise the P_{CO_2} to 49.1 mm Hg. The woman's actual P_{CO_2} of 48 mm Hg is virtually identical. Thus, she has the expected degree of respiratory compensation for simple metabolic alkalosis, and no other acid-base disorder is present.

Metabolic Acidosis

Metabolic acidosis is caused by a **decreased HCO_3^- concentration** in the blood. Metabolic acidosis can result from increased production of fixed acids such as ketoacids or lactic acid; from ingestion of fixed acids

such as salicylic acid; from the inability of the kidneys to excrete the fixed acids produced from normal metabolism; or from loss of HCO_3^- via the kidneys or the gastrointestinal tract (Table 7-4 and Box 7-1). The arterial blood profile seen in metabolic acidosis is

$$pH\downarrow$$
$$[HCO_3^-]\downarrow$$
$$P_{CO_2}\downarrow$$

The following sequence of events occurs in the generation of metabolic acidosis to produce this blood profile. Although metabolic acidosis can be caused by a frank loss of HCO_3^-, as in diarrhea and type 2 renal tubular acidosis (leading directly to a decrease in HCO_3^- concentration), most often it is caused by an excess of fixed acid in the body.

1. **Gain of fixed H^+.** Excess fixed H^+ is accumulated in the body either through increased production or ingestion of fixed acid or from decreased excretion of fixed acid.

2. **Buffering.** The excess fixed H^+ is buffered in both ECF and ICF. In ECF, the H^+ is buffered primarily by HCO_3^-, which produces a **decrease in HCO_3^- concentration.** The decrease in HCO_3^- concentration causes a **decrease in pH,** as predicted by the Henderson-Hasselbalch equation (pH = pK + log HCO_3^-/CO_2).

   In ICF, the excess fixed H^+ is buffered by organic phosphates and proteins. To utilize these intracellular buffers, H^+ first must enter the cells. H^+ can enter the cells with an organic anion such as ketoanion, lactate, or formate, or it can enter the cells in exchange for K^+. When the H^+ is exchanged for K^+, **hyperkalemia** occurs.

3. **Respiratory compensation.** Decreased arterial pH stimulates peripheral chemoreceptors in the carotid bodies, which respond by causing **hyperventilation.** In turn, hyperventilation produces a **decreased P_{CO_2},** which is the respiratory compensation for metabolic acidosis. To appreciate *why* this is a compensatory response, examine the Henderson-Hasselbalch equation:

$$pH = pK + \log \frac{[HCO_3^-]}{P_{CO_2}} \quad \begin{matrix} (\downarrow = \textit{Primary disturbance}) \\ (\downarrow = \textit{Respiratory compensation}) \end{matrix}$$

   The primary disturbance is decreased HCO_3^- concentration, which, by itself, would lead to a profound decrease in pH. The respiratory compensation, hyperventilation, decreases the P_{CO_2}, which tends to normalize the ratio of HCO_3^-/CO_2 and to normalize the pH.

4. **Renal correction.** Buffering and respiratory compensation occur quickly. However, the ultimate *correction* of metabolic acidosis (that will return the

Table 7–4 Causes of Metabolic Acidosis

Cause	Examples	Comments
Excessive production or ingestion of fixed H^+	Diabetic ketoacidosis	Accumulation of β-OH butyric acid and acetoacetic acid ↑ Anion gap
	Lactic acidosis	Accumulation of lactic acid during hypoxia ↑ Anion gap
	Salicylate poisoning	Also causes respiratory alkalosis ↑ Anion gap
	Methanol/formaldehyde poisoning	Converted to formic acid ↑ Anion gap ↑ Osmolar gap
	Ethylene glycol poisoning	Converted to glycolic and oxalic acids ↑ Anion gap ↑ Osmolar gap
Loss of HCO_3^-	Diarrhea	Gastrointestinal loss of HCO_3^- Normal anion gap Hyperchloremia
	Type 2 renal tubular acidosis (type 2 RTA)	Renal loss of HCO_3^- (failure to reabsorb filtered HCO_3^-) Normal anion gap Hyperchloremia
Inability to excrete fixed H^+	Chronic renal failure	↓ Excretion of H^+ as NH_4^+ ↑ Anion gap
	Type 1 renal tubular acidosis (type 1 RTA)	↓ Excretion of H^+ as titratable acid and NH_4^+ ↓ Ability to acidify urine Normal anion gap
	Type 4 renal tubular acidosis (type 4 RTA)	Hypoaldosteronism ↓ Excretion of NH_4^+ Hyperkalemia inhibits NH_3 synthesis Normal anion gap

---

BOX 7–1 Clinical Physiology: Diabetic Ketoacidosis

DESCRIPTION OF CASE. A 56-year-old woman has a 15-year history of type I diabetes mellitus, which has been controlled by careful dietary monitoring and treatment with subcutaneous injections of insulin twice a day. A recent viral illness results in loss of appetite, fever, and vomiting. She becomes short of breath and is admitted to the intensive care unit of the hospital.

Physical examination reveals that the woman is acutely ill. Her mucous membranes are dry, and she has decreased skin turgor. She is breathing deeply and rapidly. A urine sample contains glucose and ketones. Laboratory tests on her blood yield the following information:

Arterial blood	Venous plasma
pH, 7.07	$[Na^+]$, 132 mEq/L
Pco_2, 18 mm Hg	$[Cl^-]$, 94 mEq/L
$[HCO_3^-]$, 5 mEq/L	$[K^+]$, 5.9 mEq/L
	[Glucose], 650 mg/dL

The woman is given an insulin injection and an intravenous infusion of isotonic saline solution. Her blood values and her breathing return to normal within 12 hours after beginning treatment.

EXPLANATION OF CASE. The woman's diabetes mellitus was well controlled until an acute viral illness precipitated an episode of diabetic ketoacidosis. Her elevated blood glucose level of 650 mg/dL (normal, 80 mg/dL) and the presence of glucose in her urine are evidence that her diabetes mellitus is not being controlled. She is excreting glucose in her urine because the blood glucose concentration is so high that the filtered load has exceeded the reabsorptive capacity of the renal tubule.

On admission, the woman has arterial blood values consistent with metabolic acidosis: decreased pH, decreased $[HCO_3^-]$, and decreased Pco_2. Metabolic acidosis in uncontrolled type I diabetes mellitus is caused by excessive production of the fixed acids β-OH butyric acid and acetoacetic acid. The absence of insulin causes increased lipolysis (increased fat breakdown); fatty acids, the products of lipolysis, then are converted to the ketoacids β-OH butyric acid and acetoacetic acid. (The presence of ketones in her urine supports the

Continued

BOX 7–1   Clinical Physiology: Diabetic Ketoacidosis—cont'd

diagnosis of ketoacidosis.) These excess fixed acids are buffered by extracellular HCO_3^-, which decreases the blood $[HCO_3^-]$ and decreases blood pH. The decreased P_{CO_2} is a result of hyperventilation (rapid, deep breathing), a respiratory compensation for metabolic acidosis known as Kussmaul's respiration.

Does the woman have **simple** *metabolic acidosis (one acid-base disorder), or does she have a* **mixed** *acid-base disorder?* To answer this question, the rules of thumb are used to calculate the predicted change in P_{CO_2} (respiratory compensation) for the measured change in $[HCO_3^-]$ (refer to Table 7-3 for this calculation). For simple metabolic acidosis, the rules state that a decrease in $[HCO_3^-]$ of 1 mEq/L will produce a decrease in P_{CO_2} of 1.3 mm Hg. The woman's $[HCO_3^-]$ is 5 mEq/L, which is a decrease of 19 mEq/L from the normal value of 24 mEq/L; thus, the predicted change in P_{CO_2} for this change in $[HCO_3^-]$ is 25 mm Hg (19 × 1.3). The predicted change in P_{CO_2} now is compared with the actual change in P_{CO_2}. The woman's P_{CO_2} is 18 mm Hg, which is 22 mm Hg lower than the normal value of 40 mm Hg. The predicted change in P_{CO_2} (25 mm Hg) and the actual change in P_{CO_2} (22 mm Hg) are close and suggest that only one acid-base disorder is present, metabolic acidosis.

The plasma anion gap provides useful information in the differential diagnosis of metabolic acidosis. The woman's anion gap is calculated as follows:

$$Anion\ gap = [Na^+] - ([Cl^-] + [HCO_3^-])$$
$$= 132 - (94 + 5)$$
$$= 33\ mEq/L$$

The normal range for plasma anion gap is 8 to 16 mEq/L. At 33 mEq/L, the woman's anion gap is severely elevated due to the presence of unmeasured anions. In other words, HCO_3^-, a measured anion, is decreased and is replaced by unmeasured anions to maintain electroneutrality of the plasma compartment. Considering the woman's history of diabetes mellitus and the presence of ketones in her urine, these unmeasured anions most likely are β-OH butyrate and acetoacetate.

The decreased skin turgor and dry mucous membranes suggest ECF volume contraction. The cause of her ECF volume contraction is loss of solute and water in urine due to an osmotic diuresis of glucose. Because the woman's blood glucose is so high, a portion of the filtered glucose cannot be reabsorbed. The unreabsorbed glucose then acts as an osmotic diuretic, and NaCl and water are excreted along with it to cause ECF volume contraction.

Hyponatremia, or decreased blood $[Na^+]$, is often seen in diabetic ketoacidosis and can be explained as follows: Because the woman's ECF [glucose] is markedly elevated, her ECF osmolarity also is elevated (glucose is an osmotically active solute). As a result of this hyperosmolarity of ECF, water shifts out of the cells to achieve osmotic equilibration between ECF and ICF, diluting the solutes in the ECF and decreasing the blood $[Na^+]$.

The woman has hyperkalemia (increased blood $[K^+]$). The relationship between acid-base balance and K^+ balance is often complicated, but particularly so in cases of diabetic ketoacidosis. The most likely cause of her hyperkalemia is the lack of insulin. Recall from Chapter 6 that insulin is a major factor causing a shift of K^+ into cells. In the absence of insulin, K^+ shifts out of cells and produces hyperkalemia. The other factor contributing to her hyperkalemia is hyperosmolarity, which is presumed to be a result of the elevated blood glucose. As water shifts out of the cells to achieve osmotic equilibration, it carries K^+ along with it, causing further hyperkalemia. The metabolic acidosis is most likely not a factor in causing her hyperkalemia, because when H^+ enters the cells to be buffered, it enters with the ketoanions; it need not exchange for K^+.

TREATMENT. Treatment consists of an injection of insulin, which decreases the woman's blood glucose level, corrects her ketoacidosis, and corrects her hyperkalemia. She also is given an intravenous saline solution to replace the losses of Na^+ and water resulting from the osmotic diuresis.

person's acid-base status to normal) occurs in the kidneys and takes several days. The excess fixed H^+ will be excreted as titratable acid and NH_4^+. Simultaneously, new HCO_3^- will be synthesized and reabsorbed by the kidneys to replace the HCO_3^- that was consumed earlier in buffering. In this way, the blood HCO_3^- concentration will be returned to normal.

Metabolic Alkalosis

Metabolic alkalosis is caused by an **increased HCO_3^-** concentration in the blood. Metabolic alkalosis is the result of loss of fixed H^+ from the gastrointestinal tract; loss of fixed H^+ from the kidney (e.g., hyperaldosteronism); administration of solutions containing HCO_3^-; or ECF volume contraction (e.g., administration of diuretics) (Table 7-5 and Box 7-2). The arterial blood profile seen in metabolic alkalosis is

$$pH \uparrow$$
$$[HCO_3^-] \uparrow$$
$$P_{CO_2} \uparrow$$

The following sequence of events occurs in the generation of metabolic alkalosis to produce this blood

BOX 7–2   Clinical Physiology: Metabolic Alkalosis due to Vomiting

DESCRIPTION OF CASE. A 35-year-old man is admitted to the hospital for evaluation of severe epigastric pain. For several days prior to admission, he has had persistent nausea and vomiting. On physical examination, he has midepigastric tenderness. His blood pressure is 120/80 mm Hg when supine and 100/60 mm Hg when standing. Upper gastrointestinal endoscopy reveals a pyloric ulcer with partial gastric outlet obstruction. The following blood values are obtained on admission:

Arterial blood	Venous blood
pH, 7.53	[Na$^+$], 137 mEq/L
Pco$_2$, 45 mm Hg	[Cl$^-$], 82 mEq/L
[HCO$_3^-$], 37 mEq/L	[K$^+$], 2.8 mEq/L

The man is treated with intravenous isotonic saline solution and K$^+$, and surgery is recommended.

EXPLANATION OF CASE. In this patient, the pyloric ulcer has created a gastric outlet obstruction. Because the gastric contents could not pass easily to the small intestine, the man started vomiting. Arterial blood values are consistent with metabolic alkalosis: increased pH, increased [HCO$_3^-$], and increased Pco$_2$. The man has vomited and lost H$^+$ from his stomach, leaving HCO$_3^-$ behind in the blood. Note that his blood [Cl$^-$] is decreased (normal, 100 mEq/L), because H$^+$ is lost from the stomach as HCl. His Pco$_2$ is elevated as a result of hypoventilation, which is the expected respiratory compensation for metabolic alkalosis.

The anion gap is calculated with any acid-base disorder. The man's plasma anion gap is elevated, at 18 mEq/L:

$$\text{Anion gap} = [Na^+] - ([Cl^-] + [HCO_3^-])$$
$$= 137 - (82 + 37)$$
$$= 18 \text{ mEq/L}$$

This case shows that an increased anion gap *does not* necessarily mean that there is metabolic acidosis. In this man, the acid-base disorder is metabolic *alkalosis*. His anion gap is elevated because he has not eaten for several days. Fat is being catabolized, and the resulting fatty acids are generating ketoacids, which are unmeasured anions.

The man has orthostatic hypotension (his blood pressure falls when he stands), which is consistent with ECF volume contraction. His ECF volume contraction activates the renin–angiotensin II–aldosterone system, which worsens his metabolic alkalosis. The increased angiotensin II increases HCO$_3^-$ reabsorption by stimulating Na$^+$-H$^+$ exchange, and the increased aldosterone increases H$^+$ secretion. Together, these two effects on the renal tubule exacerbate the metabolic alkalosis. To summarize this point, the loss of gastric H$^+$ generated the metabolic alkalosis and volume contraction maintained it by not allowing the excess HCO$_3^-$ to be excreted in the urine.

The hypokalemia has several explanations. First, some K$^+$ is lost in gastric fluids. Second, in metabolic alkalosis, H$^+$ shifts out of cells and K$^+$ shifts into cells, causing hypokalemia. Finally, the most important factor is that ECF volume contraction has caused increased secretion of aldosterone. This secondary hyperaldosteronism causes increased K$^+$ secretion by the renal principal cells (see Chapter 6), which leads to further hypokalemia.

TREATMENT. Immediate treatment consists of intravenous saline and K$^+$. To correct the metabolic alkalosis, ECF volume must be restored even if the vomiting stops.

Table 7–5   Causes of Metabolic Alkalosis

Cause	Examples	Comments
Loss of H$^+$	Vomiting	Loss of gastric H$^+$ HCO$_3^-$ remains in the blood Maintained by volume contraction Hypokalemia
	Hyperaldosteronism	Increased H$^+$ secretion by intercalated cells Hypokalemia
Gain of HCO$_3^-$	Ingestion of NaHCO$_3$ Milk-alkali syndrome	Ingestion of large amounts of HCO$_3^-$ in conjunction with renal failure
Volume contraction alkalosis	Loop or thiazide diuretics	↑ HCO$_3^-$ reabsorption due to ↑ angiotensin II and aldosterone

profile. Although metabolic alkalosis can be caused by administration of HCO_3^-, most often it is caused by loss of fixed acid from the body.

1. **Loss of fixed acid.** The classic example of metabolic alkalosis is **vomiting,** in which HCl is lost from the stomach. The gastric parietal cells produce H^+ and HCO_3^- from CO_2 and H_2O. The H^+ is secreted with Cl^- into the lumen of the stomach to aid in digestion, and the HCO_3^- enters the blood. In normal persons, the secreted H^+ moves from the stomach to the small intestine, where a low pH triggers the secretion of HCO_3^- by the pancreas. Thus, normally, the HCO_3^- added to blood by the parietal cells is later removed from blood in the pancreatic secretions. However, when vomiting occurs, H^+ is lost from the stomach and never reaches the small intestine. HCO_3^- secretion from the pancreas, therefore, is not stimulated, and the HCO_3^- remains in the blood, resulting in an **increase in HCO_3^- concentration.** The increase in HCO_3^- concentration causes an **increase in pH,** as predicted by the Henderson-Hasselbalch equation (pH = pK + log HCO_3^-/CO_2).

2. **Buffering.** As with metabolic acidosis, buffering occurs in both ECF and ICF. To utilize ICF buffers, H^+ leaves the cells in exchange for K^+, and **hypokalemia** occurs.

3. **Respiratory compensation.** Increased arterial pH inhibits the peripheral chemoreceptors, which respond by causing **hypoventilation.** In turn, hypoventilation produces an **increased P_{CO_2},** which is the respiratory compensation for metabolic alkalosis. As before, examine the Henderson-Hasselbalch equation to understand the compensation:

$$pH = pK + log\frac{[HCO_3^-]\,(\uparrow = \textit{Primary disturbance})}{P_{CO_2}}\;(\uparrow = \textit{Respiratory compensation})$$

The primary disturbance in metabolic alkalosis is an increased HCO_3^- concentration that, by itself, would lead to a profound increase in pH. The respiratory compensation, hypoventilation, increases P_{CO_2}, which tends to normalize the ratio of HCO_3^-/CO_2 and to normalize the pH.

4. **Renal correction.** The correction of metabolic alkalosis *should be* the most straightforward of all the acid-base disorders. Because the primary disturbance is increased HCO_3^- concentration, restoration of acid-base balance will take place when the excess HCO_3^- is excreted by the kidneys. This can be accomplished because the renal tubule has a finite reabsorptive capacity for filtered HCO_3^-. When the filtered load of HCO_3^- exceeds the reabsorptive capacity, HCO_3^- is excreted in the urine, eventually reducing the HCO_3^- concentration to normal. However, the correction of metabolic alkalosis is

often *not so straightforward.* It is complicated when there is associated **ECF volume contraction** (e.g., due to vomiting). ECF volume contraction produces three secondary effects on the kidney, all of which conspire to *maintain* the metabolic alkalosis **(contraction alkalosis)** by not allowing the excess HCO_3^- to be excreted in urine (Fig. 7-11): (1) ECF volume contraction, via the Starling forces, causes increased HCO_3^- reabsorption in the proximal tubule; (2) ECF volume contraction, via the renin–angiotensin II–aldosterone system, produces increased levels of angiotensin II; **angiotensin II** stimulates Na^+-H^+ exchange and promotes reabsorption of filtered HCO_3^-; (3) Increased levels of **aldosterone** stimulate secretion of H^+ and reabsorption of "new" HCO_3^-. When combined, these effects, all of which are secondary to ECF volume contraction, increase the HCO_3^- concentration and maintain the metabolic alkalosis, even when vomiting has stopped.

Respiratory Acidosis

Respiratory acidosis is caused by **hypoventilation,** which results in **retention of CO_2.** The retention of CO_2 can be caused by inhibition of the medullary respiratory center, paralysis of respiratory muscles, airway obstruction, or failure to exchange CO_2 between pulmonary capillary blood and alveolar gas (Table 7-6 and Box 7-3). The arterial blood profile seen in respiratory acidosis is

$$pH\downarrow$$
$$[HCO_3^-]\uparrow$$
$$P_{CO_2}\uparrow$$

The following sequence of events occurs in the generation of respiratory acidosis to produce this blood profile:

1. **Retention of CO_2.** Hypoventilation causes retention of CO_2 and an **increase in P_{CO_2}.** The increased P_{CO_2} is the primary disturbance in respiratory acidosis and, as predicted by the Henderson-Hasselbalch equation, causes a **decrease in pH** (pH = 6.1 + log HCO_3^-/CO_2). The increased P_{CO_2}, by mass action, also causes an increased concentration of HCO_3^-.

2. **Buffering.** Buffering of the excess CO_2 occurs exclusively in ICF, especially in red blood cells. To utilize these intracellular buffers, CO_2 diffuses across the cell membranes. Within the cells, CO_2 is converted to H^+ and HCO_3^- and the H^+ is buffered by intracellular proteins (e.g., hemoglobin) and by organic phosphates.

3. **Respiratory compensation.** There is *no* respiratory compensation for respiratory acidosis, since respiration is the *cause* of this disorder.

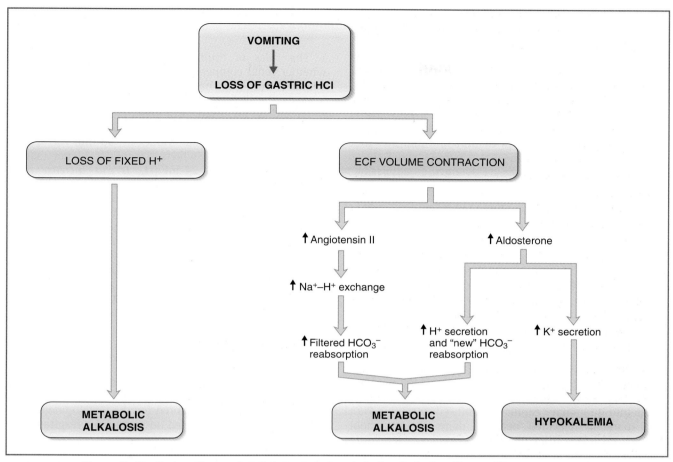

Figure 7–11 **Generation and maintenance of metabolic alkalosis with vomiting.** ECF, Extracellular fluid.

Table 7–6 Causes of Respiratory Acidosis

Cause	Examples	Comments
Inhibition of the medullary respiratory center	Opiates, barbiturates, anesthetics Lesions of the central nervous system Central sleep apnea Oxygen therapy	Inhibition of peripheral chemoreceptors
Disorders of respiratory muscles	Guillain-Barré syndrome, polio, amyotrophic lateral sclerosis (ALS), multiple sclerosis	
Airway obstruction	Aspiration Obstructive sleep apnea Laryngospasm	
Disorders of gas exchange	Acute respiratory distress syndrome (ARDS) Chronic obstructive pulmonary disease (COPD) Pneumonia Pulmonary edema	$\downarrow$ Exchange of CO_2 between pulmonary capillary blood and alveolar gas

---

BOX 7–3   Clinical Physiology: Chronic Obstructive Pulmonary Disease

DESCRIPTION OF CASE. A 68-year-old man has smoked three packs of cigarettes per day for 40 years. He has a history of producing morning sputum, cough, and dyspnea (shortness of breath), and he has had frequent episodes of asthmatic bronchitis. He is admitted to the hospital with a low-grade fever, dyspnea, and wheezing. His physical examination indicates that he is cyanotic and that he has a barrel-shaped chest. The following blood values are obtained on admission:

Arterial blood	Venous blood
pH, 7.29	[Na$^+$], 139 mEq/L
P$_{CO_2}$, 70 mm Hg	[Cl$^-$], 95 mEq/L
P$_{O_2}$, 54 mm Hg	
[HCO$_3^-$], 33 mEq/L	

EXPLANATION OF CASE. The man's history of smoking combined with asthma and bronchitis suggests chronic obstructive pulmonary disease (COPD). The arterial blood values are consistent with respiratory acidosis: decreased pH, increased P$_{CO_2}$, and increased [HCO$_3^-$]. When obstructive lung disease is present, alveolar ventilation is inadequate. Thus, his P$_{O_2}$ is markedly depressed, at 54 mm Hg (normal P$_{O_2}$, 100 mm Hg) because there is insufficient O$_2$ transfer from alveolar gas into pulmonary capillary blood. Likewise, his P$_{CO_2}$ is markedly elevated because there is insufficient transfer of CO$_2$ from pulmonary capillary blood into alveolar gas (i.e., respiratory acidosis). The [HCO$_3^-$] is elevated because of mass action and possibly, in addition, because of renal compensation.

The rules of thumb can be used to determine whether renal compensation has taken place; that is, whether this man has *acute* or *chronic* respiratory acidosis. Recall that in respiratory acidosis, the change in [HCO$_3^-$] is predicted for a given change in P$_{CO_2}$. In this man, the P$_{CO_2}$ is 70 mm Hg, which is 30 mm Hg higher than the normal value of 40 mm Hg. His [HCO$_3^-$] is 33 mEq/L, which is 9 mEq/L higher than the normal value of 24 mEq/L. *Is this increase in HCO$_3^-$ consistent with acute or chronic respiratory acidosis?* For a 30 mm Hg increase in P$_{CO_2}$, the rules for acute respiratory acidosis predict an increase in [HCO$_3^-$] of 3 mEq/L; for chronic respiratory acidosis, the rules predict an increase of 12 mEq/L. Thus, the change in the man's [HCO$_3^-$] is closer to that predicted for compensated chronic respiratory acidosis (he has a history of *chronic* lung disease). Because the change in [HCO$_3^-$] is not exactly the value predicted by the rules, a second acid-base disorder may be present, which may be lactic acidosis due to poor tissue oxygenation.

The anion gap is 11 mEq/L anion gap = Na$^+$ − (Cl$^-$ + HCO$_3^-$) = 139 − 95 − 33 = 11 mEq/L, which is within the normal range, suggesting that if any lactic acidosis is present, it is not yet significant. The anion gap should be carefully monitored for the development of lactic acidosis superimposed on his chronic respiratory acidosis.

TREATMENT. The man is treated with antibiotics and his lungs are mechanically ventilated.

---

4. **Renal compensation.** Renal compensation for respiratory acidosis consists of increased H$^+$ excretion as titratable acid and NH$_4^+$ and increased synthesis and reabsorption of new HCO$_3^-$. Reabsorption of new HCO$_3^-$ increases the HCO$_3^-$ concentration even further than the effect of mass action alone. The Henderson-Hasselbalch equation can be used to understand why the increased HCO$_3^-$ concentration is a compensatory response. Thus,

$$pH = pK + \log \frac{[HCO_3^-]}{P_{CO_2}} \frac{(\uparrow = Renal\ compensation)}{(\uparrow = Primary\ disturbance)}$$

In **acute respiratory acidosis**, renal compensation has not yet occurred, and the pH tends to be quite low (there is an increase in the denominator in the Henderson-Hasselbalch equation but little increase in the numerator). On the other hand, in **chronic respiratory acidosis,** renal compensation is occurring, which increases the HCO$_3^-$ concentration and tends to normalize both the ratio of HCO$_3^-$/CO$_2$ and the pH. The *difference* between acute and chronic respiratory acidosis lies in the renal compensation. Accordingly, based on the absence or presence of renal compensation, the renal rules give different calculations for the expected change in HCO$_3^-$ concentration that occurs in acute and chronic respiratory acidosis (see Table 7-3).

Respiratory Alkalosis

Respiratory alkalosis is caused by **hyperventilation,** which results in **excessive loss of CO$_2$.** Hyperventilation can be caused by direct stimulation of the medullary respiratory center, by hypoxemia (which stimulates peripheral chemoreceptors), or by mechanical ventilation (Table 7-7). The arterial blood profile seen in respiratory alkalosis is

$$pH \uparrow$$
$$[HCO_3^-] \downarrow$$
$$P_{CO_2} \downarrow$$

The following sequence of events occurs in the generation of respiratory alkalosis to produce this blood profile:

Table 7-7 Causes of Respiratory Alkalosis

Cause	Examples	Comments
Stimulation of the medullary respiratory center	Hysterical hyperventilation Gram-negative septicemia Salicylate poisoning Neurologic disorders (tumor; stroke)	Also causes metabolic acidosis
Hypoxemia	High altitude Pneumonia; pulmonary embolism	Hypoxemia stimulates peripheral chemoreceptors
Mechanical ventilation		

1. **Loss of CO_2.** Hyperventilation causes an excessive loss of CO_2 and a **decrease in P_{CO_2}**. The decreased P_{CO_2} is the primary disturbance in respiratory alkalosis and, as predicted by the Henderson-Hasselbalch equation, causes an **increase in pH** (pH = 6.1 + log HCO_3^-/CO_2). The decreased P_{CO_2}, by mass action, also causes a decreased concentration of HCO_3^-.

2. **Buffering.** Buffering occurs exclusively in ICF, particularly in red blood cells. In this case, CO_2 leaves the cells and intracellular pH increases.

3. **Respiratory compensation.** As with respiratory acidosis, there is *no* respiratory compensation for respiratory alkalosis because respiration is the *cause* of the disorder.

4. **Renal compensation.** Renal compensation for respiratory alkalosis consists of decreased excretion of H^+ as titratable acid and NH_4^+ and decreased synthesis and reabsorption of new HCO_3^-. Decreased reabsorption of HCO_3^- decreases the HCO_3^- concentration even further than did the effect of mass action alone. The Henderson-Hasselbalch equation can be used to understand why the decreased HCO_3^- concentration is a compensatory response:

$$pH = pK + \log \frac{[HCO_3^-]\,(\downarrow = Renal\ compensation)}{P_{CO_2}\ \ (\downarrow = Primary\ disturbance)}$$

In **acute respiratory alkalosis,** renal compensation has not yet occurred and pH is quite high (there is a decrease in the denominator of the Henderson-Hasselbalch equation but little decrease in the numerator). In **chronic respiratory alkalosis,** renal compensation is occurring, which further decreases the blood HCO_3^- concentration and tends to normalize both the ratio of HCO_3^-/CO_2 and the pH. The difference between acute and chronic respiratory alkalosis lies in renal compensation. Again, on the basis of the absence or presence of renal compensation, the renal rules give different calculations for the expected change in HCO_3^- concentration in acute and chronic respiratory alkalosis (see Table 7-3).

SAMPLE PROBLEM. A patient has the following arterial blood values: pH, 7.33; $[HCO_3^-]$, 36 mEq/L; P_{CO_2}, 70 mm Hg. *What is the patient's acid-base disorder? Is it acute or chronic? Are the blood values consistent with a simple or mixed acid-base disorder?*

SOLUTION. With a pH of 7.33, the patient is acidemic. The $[HCO_3^-]$ and P_{CO_2} are consistent with respiratory acidosis rather than metabolic acidosis. The P_{CO_2} is elevated due to primary hypoventilation. (If it was metabolic acidosis, the P_{CO_2} would be decreased due to compensatory hyperventilation.)

Whether the respiratory acidosis is acute or chronic can be determined by comparing the patient's values with the ranges on the acid-base map. Using the acid-base map, it can be concluded that the patient has *chronic* respiratory acidosis.

The rules of thumb also can be used to distinguish between acute and chronic respiratory acidosis by calculating the predicted change in $[HCO_3^-]$ for the change in P_{CO_2}. The patient's P_{CO_2} is 70 mm Hg, which is 30 mm Hg above normal (normal P_{CO_2}, 40 mm Hg). The compensatory response is an increased $[HCO_3^-]$. The patient's $[HCO_3^-]$ is 36 mEq/L, which is 12 mEq/L above normal (normal $[HCO_3^-]$, 24 mEq/L). The change in $[HCO_3^-]$ relative to the change in P_{CO_2} is therefore 12/30, or 0.4 mEq/L/mm Hg. The compensation is exactly as predicted by the rules of thumb for chronic respiratory acidosis. It can be concluded that the patient has *simple* **chronic respiratory acidosis** with the expected level of renal compensation.

SUMMARY

■ The pH of body fluids is normally maintained at 7.4 in spite of the daily production of large amounts of CO_2 (volatile acid) and fixed acids (nonvolatile acids). The mechanisms that maintain a constant pH include buffering, respiratory compensation, and renal compensation.

■ Buffering represents the first line of defense in protecting the pH. A buffered solution is a mixture of a weak acid and its conjugate base. The most effective physiologic buffers have a pK near 7.4. Extracellular buffers include HCO_3^-/CO_2 (the most important) and $HPO_4^{-2}/H_2PO_4^-$. Intracellular buffers include organic phosphates and proteins (e.g., deoxyhemoglobin).

■ Renal mechanisms in acid-base balance include reabsorption of virtually all of the filtered HCO_3^- and excretion of H^+ as titratable acid and NH_4^+. For each H^+ excreted as titratable acid or NH_4^+, one new HCO_3^- is synthesized and reabsorbed.

■ Simple acid-base disorders can be metabolic or respiratory in origin. Metabolic disorders involve a primary disturbance of the $[HCO_3^-]$, caused by gain or loss of fixed H^+. When there is a gain of fixed H^+, metabolic acidosis occurs; when there is a loss of fixed H^+, metabolic alkalosis occurs. Respiratory disorders involve a primary disturbance of P_{CO_2}, caused by hypoventilation (respiratory acidosis) or hyperventilation (respiratory alkalosis).

■ Compensation for acid-base disorders is either respiratory or renal. When the primary disorder is metabolic, compensation is respiratory. When the primary disorder is respiratory, compensation is renal (metabolic).

Challenge Yourself

Answer each question with a word, phrase, sentence, or numerical solution. When a list of possible answers is supplied with the question, one, more than one, or none of the choices may be correct. Correct answers are provided at the end of the book.

1 Weak acid "A" has a pK of 5.5 and weak acid "B" has a pK of 7.5. At pH 7, which weak acid is predominantly in its A^- form?

2 If a person's arterial blood has a pH of 7.22 and P_{CO_2} of 20 mm Hg, what is the HCO_3^- concentration?

3 For the person described in question 2, is ventilation increased, decreased, or unchanged (compared with normal)?

4 A person's arterial blood pH is 7.25, P_{CO_2} is 24 mm Hg, and HCO_3^- is 10.2 mEq/L. Which of the following might cause this pattern: diarrhea, vomiting, obstructive pulmonary disease, hysterical hyperventilation, salicylate overdose, chronic renal failure?

5 Which class(es) of diuretics cause(s) metabolic alkalosis: carbonic anhydrase inhibitors, loop diuretics, thiazide diuretics, K^+-sparing diuretics?

6 A patient is seen in the emergency department with the following blood values: pH, 7.1; HCO_3^-, 10 mEq/L; Na^+, 142 mEq/L; and Cl^-, 103 mEq/L. What is the acid-base disorder, and what is the value of the anion gap?

7 What are the units of osmolar gap?

8 Among patients with the following disorders, which is/are hypoventilating: diarrhea, vomiting, ascent to high altitude, morphine overdose, obstructive lung disease, hyperaldosteronism, ethylene glycol poisoning, salicylate poisoning?

9 What is the correct sequence of these events: Na^+-H^+ exchange, filtration of HCO_3^- across glomerular capillaries, facilitated diffusion of HCO_3^-, conversion of H_2CO_3 to CO_2 and H_2O, conversion of H_2CO_3 to H^+ and HCO_3^-, conversion of HCO_3^- to H_2CO_3?

10 If, in one day, 25 mEq of H^+ is excreted as $H_2PO_4^-$ and 45 mEq of H^+ is excreted as NH_4^+, how much new HCO_3^- is synthesized?

11 Two patients have an elevated arterial P_{CO_2} of 70 mm Hg. One has acute respiratory acidosis and the other has chronic respiratory acidosis. Which patient has the higher blood HCO_3^- concentration? Which patient has the higher pH?

12 A patient has the following blood values: pH, 7.22; HCO_3^-, 18 mEq/L; and P_{CO_2}, 45 mm Hg. Are these values consistent with a simple acid-base disorder? If yes, which one? If no, what acid-base disorders are present?

13 In the conversion from acute to chronic respiratory alkalosis, what happens to blood pH?

14 Which is the best indicator of total H^+ excreted in the urine: urine pH, filtered load of HPO_4^{-2}, filtered load of NH_3?

15 Which condition has the highest excretion of NH_4^+: diabetic ketoacidosis, chronic renal failure, vomiting, hysterical hyperventilation?

SELECTED READINGS

Cohen JJ, Kassirer JP: Acid/Base. Boston, Little, Brown, 1982.

Davenport HW: The ABC of Acid-Base Chemistry, 6th ed. Chicago, University of Chicago Press, 1974.

Rose BD: Clinical Physiology of Acid-Base and Electrolyte Disorders, 5th ed. New York, McGraw-Hill, 2000.

Valtin H, Gennari FJ: Acid-Base Disorders. Boston, Little, Brown, 1987.

Gastrointestinal Physiology

The functions of the gastrointestinal tract are digestion and absorption of nutrients. To serve these functions, there are four major activities of the gastrointestinal tract. (1) Motility propels ingested food from the mouth toward the rectum and mixes and reduces the size of the food. The rate at which food is propelled through the gastrointestinal tract is regulated to optimize the time for digestion and absorption. (2) Secretions from the salivary glands, pancreas, and liver add fluid, electrolytes, enzymes, and mucus to the lumen of the gastrointestinal tract. These secretions further aid in digestion and absorption. (3) Ingested foods are digested into absorbable molecules. (4) Nutrients, electrolytes, and water are absorbed from the intestinal lumen into the bloodstream.

STRUCTURE OF THE GASTROINTESTINAL TRACT

The gastrointestinal tract is arranged linearly in the following sequence: mouth, esophagus, stomach, small intestine (including the duodenum, jejunum, and ileum), large intestine, and anus. Other structures of the gastrointestinal tract are the salivary glands, pancreas, liver, and gallbladder, all of which serve secretory functions.

The wall of the gastrointestinal tract has two surfaces, mucosal and serosal. The **mucosal** surface faces the lumen, and the **serosal** surface faces the blood (Fig. 8-1). The layers of the gastrointestinal wall are as follows, starting from the lumen and moving toward the blood: A **mucosal layer** consists of a layer of epithelial cells, a lamina propria, and a muscularis mucosae. The epithelial cells are specialized to carry out absorptive and secretory functions. The lamina propria consists primarily of connective tissue, but it also includes blood and lymph vessels. The muscularis mucosae consists of smooth muscle cells; contraction of the muscularis mucosae changes the shape and surface area of the epithelial cell layer. Beneath the mucosal layer is a **submucosal layer,** which consists of collagen, elastin, glands, and the blood vessels of the gastrointestinal tract. Motility of the gastrointestinal tract is provided by two layers of smooth muscle, **circular muscle** and **longitudinal muscle,** which are interposed between the submucosa and the serosa. The longitudinal muscle layer is thin and contains few nerve fibers, whereas the circular muscle layer is thick and more densely innervated. Neurons do not make true synapses on the gastrointestinal smooth muscle fibers; rather they release transmitters from varicosities along the length of their axons. Two plexuses, the submucosal plexus and the myenteric plexus, contain the nervous system of the gastrointestinal tract.

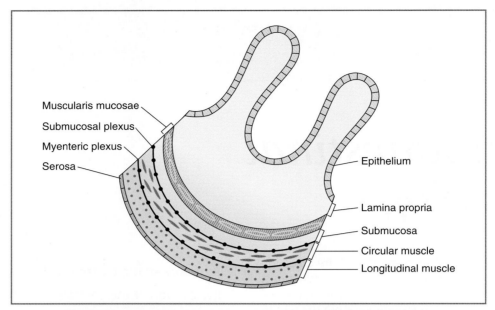

Figure 8-1 The structure of the wall of the gastrointestinal tract.

The **submucosal plexus** (Meissner's plexus) lies between the submucosa and the circular muscle. The **myenteric plexus** lies between the circular muscle and the longitudinal muscle.

INNERVATION OF THE GASTROINTESTINAL TRACT

The gastrointestinal tract is regulated, in part, by the **autonomic nervous system,** which has an extrinsic component and an intrinsic component. The **extrinsic component** is the sympathetic and parasympathetic innervation of the gastrointestinal tract. The **intrinsic component** is called the **enteric nervous system.** The enteric nervous system is wholly contained within the submucosal and myenteric plexuses in the wall of the gastrointestinal tract; it communicates extensively with the parasympathetic and sympathetic nervous systems.

Parasympathetic Innervation

Parasympathetic innervation is supplied by the vagus nerve (cranial nerve [CN] X) and the pelvic nerve (see Chapter 2, Fig. 2-3). The pattern of parasympathetic innervation of the gastrointestinal tract is consistent with its function. The **vagus nerve** innervates the *upper* gastrointestinal tract including the striated muscle of the upper third of the esophagus, the wall of the stomach, the small intestine, and the ascending colon. The **pelvic nerve** innervates the *lower* gastrointestinal tract including the striated muscle of the external anal canal and the walls of the transverse, descending, and sigmoid colons.

Recall from Chapter 2 that the parasympathetic nervous system has long preganglionic fibers that synapse in ganglia *in or near* the target organs. In the gastrointestinal tract, these ganglia actually are located in the walls of the organs within the myenteric and submucosal plexuses. Information relayed from the parasympathetic nervous system is coordinated in these plexuses and then relayed to smooth muscle, endocrine, and secretory cells (Figs. 8-2 and 8-3).

Postganglionic neurons of the parasympathetic nervous system are classified as either cholinergic or peptidergic. **Cholinergic neurons** release acetylcholine (ACh) as the neurotransmitter. **Peptidergic neurons** release one of several peptides including substance P and vasoactive inhibitory peptide (VIP); in some instances, the neuropeptide has not yet been identified.

The vagus nerve is a mixed nerve in which 75% of the fibers are afferent and 25% are efferent. Afferent fibers deliver sensory information from the periphery (e.g., from mechanoreceptors and chemoreceptors in the wall of the gastrointestinal tract) to the central nervous system (CNS). Efferent fibers deliver motor information from the CNS to target tissues in the periphery (e.g., smooth muscle, secretory, and endocrine cells) (see Fig. 8-2). Thus, mechanoreceptors and chemoreceptors in the gastrointestinal mucosa relay afferent information to the CNS via the vagus nerve, which triggers reflexes whose efferent limb is also in the vagus nerve. Such reflexes, in which both afferent and efferent limbs are contained in the vagus nerve, are called **vagovagal reflexes.**

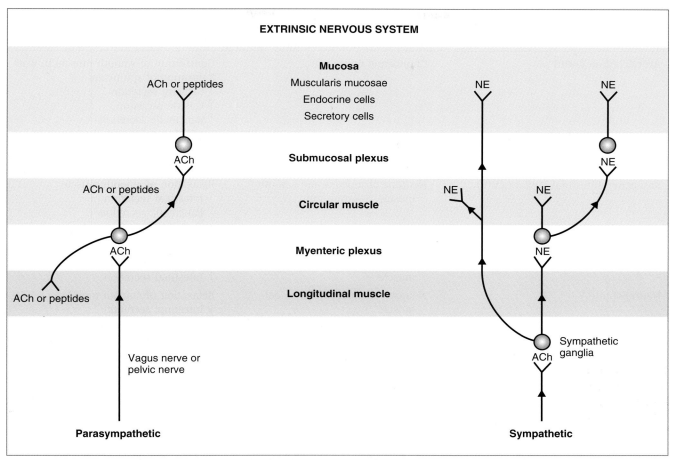

Figure 8–2 **The extrinsic nervous system of the gastrointestinal tract.** Efferent neurons of the parasympathetic and sympathetic nervous systems synapse in the myenteric and submucosal plexuses, in the smooth muscle, and in the mucosa. ACh, Acetylcholine; NE, norepinephrine.

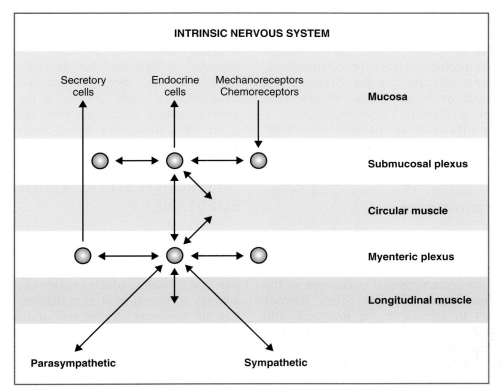

Figure 8–3 Intrinsic nervous system of the gastrointestinal tract.

Table 8–1 Neurotransmitters and Neuromodulators in the Enteric Nervous System

Substance	Source	Actions
Acetylcholine (ACh)	Cholinergic neurons	Contraction of smooth muscle in wall Relaxation of sphincters ↑ Salivary secretion ↑ Gastric secretion ↑ Pancreatic secretion
Norepinephrine (NE)	Adrenergic neurons	Relaxation of smooth muscle in wall Contraction of sphincters ↑ Salivary secretion
Vasoactive Intestinal Peptide (VIP)	Neurons of mucosa and smooth muscle	Relaxation of smooth muscle ↑ Intestinal secretion ↑ Pancreatic secretion
Gastrin-Releasing Peptide (GRP), or Bombesin	Neurons of gastric mucosa	↑ Gastrin secretion
Enkephalins (opiates)	Neurons of mucosa and smooth muscle	Contraction of smooth muscle ↓ Intestinal secretion
Neuropeptide Y	Neurons of mucosa and smooth muscle	Relaxation of smooth muscle ↓ Intestinal secretion
Substance P	Cosecreted with ACh	Contraction of smooth muscle ↑ Salivary secretion

Sympathetic Innervation

Preganglionic fibers of the sympathetic nervous system are relatively short and synapse in ganglia *outside* the gastrointestinal tract. (Contrast the preganglionic fibers of the parasympathetic nervous system, which are long and synapse in ganglia *inside* the wall of the gastrointestinal tract.) Four sympathetic ganglia serve the gastrointestinal tract: celiac, superior mesenteric, inferior mesenteric, and hypogastric (see Chapter 2, Fig. 2-2). Postganglionic nerve fibers, which are adrenergic (i.e., release norepinephrine), leave these sympathetic ganglia and synapse on ganglia in the myenteric and submucosal plexuses, or they directly innervate smooth muscle, endocrine, or secretory cells (see Fig. 8-2).

Approximately 50% of the sympathetic nerve fibers are afferent and 50% are efferent. Thus, as with the parasympathetic innervation, sensory and motor information is relayed back and forth between the gastrointestinal tract and the CNS, coordinated by the submucosal and myenteric plexuses.

Intrinsic Innervation

The intrinsic or **enteric nervous system** can direct all functions of the gastrointestinal tract, even in the absence of extrinsic innervation. The enteric nervous system is located in ganglia in the myenteric and submucosal plexuses and controls the contractile, secretory, and endocrine functions of the gastrointestinal tract (see Fig. 8-3). As shown in Figure 8-2, these ganglia receive input from the parasympathetic and sympathetic nervous systems, which modulate their activity. These ganglia also receive sensory information directly *from* mechanoreceptors and chemoreceptors in the mucosa and send motor information directly *to* smooth muscle, secretory, and endocrine cells. Information is also relayed *between* ganglia by interneurons.

A large number of neurochemicals, or **neurocrines,** have been identified in neurons of the enteric nervous system (Table 8-1). Some of the substances listed are classified as neurotransmitters and some are neuromodulators (i.e., they *modulate* the activity of neurotransmitters). Most neurons of the enteric nervous system contain more than one neurochemical, and upon stimulation, they may cosecrete two or more neurocrines.

GASTROINTESTINAL REGULATORY SUBSTANCES

Gastrointestinal peptides, including hormones, neurocrines, and paracrines, regulate the functions of the gastrointestinal tract. These functions include contraction and relaxation of the smooth muscle wall and the sphincters; secretion of enzymes for digestion; secretion of fluid and electrolytes; and trophic (growth) effects on the tissues of the gastrointestinal tract. In addition, some gastrointestinal peptides regulate the secretion of *other* gastrointestinal peptides; for example,

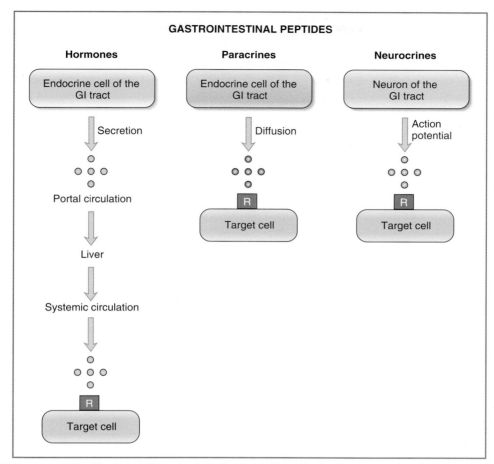

Figure 8–4 **Classification of gastrointestinal peptides as hormones, paracrines, or neurocrines.** GI, Gastrointestinal; R, receptor.

somatostatin inhibits secretion of all the gastrointestinal hormones.

Characteristics of Gastrointestinal Peptides

The gastrointestinal peptides are classified as hormones, paracrines, or neurocrines. The designation is based on whether the peptide is released from an endocrine cell or from a neuron of the gastrointestinal tract and the route the peptide takes to reach its target cell (Fig. 8-4).

♦ **Hormones** are peptides released from endocrine cells of the gastrointestinal tract. They are secreted into the portal circulation, pass through the liver, and enter the systemic circulation. The systemic circulation then delivers the hormone to target cells with receptors for that hormone. The target cells may be located in the gastrointestinal tract itself (e.g., gastrin acts on the parietal cells of the stomach to cause acid secretion), or the target cells may be located elsewhere in the body (e.g., gastric inhibitory peptide acts on the beta [β] cells of the pancreas to cause insulin secretion). Endocrine cells of the gastrointestinal mucosa are not concentrated in glands but are single cells or groups of cells dispersed over large areas. Four gastrointestinal peptides are classified as hormones: gastrin, cholecystokinin (CCK), secretin, and glucose-dependent insulinotropic peptide (or gastric inhibitory peptide, GIP).

♦ **Paracrines,** like hormones, are peptides secreted by endocrine cells of the gastrointestinal tract. In contrast to hormones, however, paracrines act *locally* within the same tissue that secretes them. Paracrine substances reach their target cells by diffusing short distances through interstitial fluid, or they are carried short distances in capillaries. Thus, for a substance to have a paracrine action, the site of secretion must be only a *short distance* from the site of action. The major gastrointestinal peptide with a known paracrine function is somatostatin, which has inhibitory actions throughout the gastrointestinal tract. (Histamine, another gastrointestinal paracrine, is not a peptide.)

Table 8-2 Summary of Gastrointestinal Hormones

Hormone	Hormone Family	Site of Secretion	Stimuli for Secretion	Actions
Gastrin	Gastrin-CCK	G cells of stomach	Small peptides and amino acids Distention of the stomach Vagal stimulation (GRP)	↑ Gastric H^+ secretion Stimulates growth of gastric mucosa
Cholecystokinin (CCK)	Gastrin-CCK	I cells of duodenum and jejunum	Small peptides and amino acids Fatty acids	↑ Pancreatic enzyme secretion ↑ Pancreatic HCO_3^- secretion Stimulates contraction of the gallbladder and relaxation of the sphincter of Oddi Stimulates growth of the exocrine pancreas and gallbladder Inhibits gastric emptying
Secretin	Secretin-glucagon	S cells of duodenum	H^+ in the duodenum Fatty acids in the duodenum	↑ Pancreatic HCO_3^- secretion ↑ Biliary HCO_3^- secretion ↓ Gastric H^+ secretion Inhibits trophic effect of gastrin on gastric mucosa
Glucose-Dependent Insulinotropic Peptide (GIP)	Secretin-glucagon	Duodenum and jejunum	Fatty acids Amino acids Oral glucose	↑ Insulin secretion from pancreatic β cells ↓ Gastric H^+ secretion

GRP, Gastrin-releasing peptide.

♦ **Neurocrines** are substances that are synthesized in neurons of the gastrointestinal tract and released following an action potential. After release, the neurocrine diffuses across the synapse and acts on its target cell. Neurocrine substances of the gastrointestinal tract include ACh, norepinephrine, vasoactive intestinal peptide (VIP), gastrin-releasing peptide (GRP) or bombesin, enkephalins, neuropeptide Y, and substance P. The sources and actions of these substances are summarized in Table 8-1.

Gastrointestinal Hormones

Several criteria must be met for a substance to qualify as a gastrointestinal hormone: (1) The substance must be secreted in response to a physiologic stimulus and be carried in the bloodstream to a distant site, where it produces a physiologic action; (2) its function must be independent of any neural activity; and (3) it must have been isolated, purified, chemically identified, and synthesized. After applying these stringent criteria, only the following four substances qualify as gastrointestinal hormones: gastrin, CCK, secretin, and GIP. In addition, several candidate hormones, including motilin, pancreatic polypeptide, and enteroglucagon, meet some, but not all, of the criteria.

Table 8-2 describes the four "official" gastrointestinal hormones with respect to hormone family, site of secretion, stimuli producing secretion, and physiologic actions. Use Table 8-2 as a reference for discussions later in the chapter about motility, secretion, and absorption.

Gastrin

The functions of gastrin are coordinated to promote **hydrogen ion (H^+) secretion** by the gastric parietal cells. Gastrin, a 17-amino acid straight chain peptide, is secreted by G (gastrin) cells in the antrum of the stomach. The 17-amino acid form of gastrin, which is called G_{17} or *"little" gastrin,* is the form of gastrin secreted in response to a meal. A 34-amino acid form of gastrin, which is called G_{34} or *"big" gastrin,* is secreted during the interdigestive period (between meals). Thus, during the interdigestive period, most of the serum gastrin is in the G_{34} form, which is secreted at low basal levels. When a meal is ingested, G_{17} is secreted. G_{34} is *not* a dimer of G_{17}, nor is G_{17} formed from G_{34}. Rather, each form of gastrin has its own biosynthetic pathway, beginning with its own precursor, a progastrin molecule.

The minimum fragment necessary for biologic activity of gastrin is the **C-terminal tetrapeptide** (Fig. 8-5). (The C-terminal phenylalanine contains an NH_2 group,

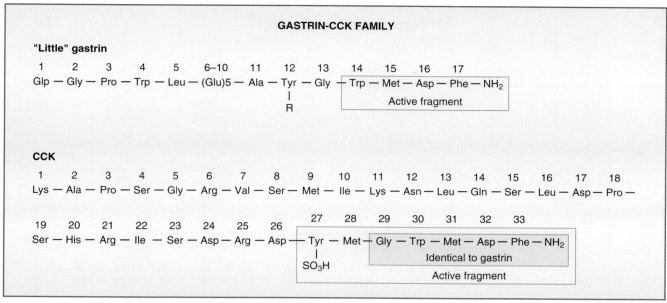

Figure 8–5 Structures of human gastrin and porcine cholecystokinin (CCK). The *blue-shaded boxes* show the fragments necessary for minimal biologic activity. The *green-shaded box* shows the portion of the CCK molecule that is identical to gastrin. Glp, Pyroglutamyl residue.

which simply means that it is phenylalamide.) Although the C-terminal tetrapeptide is the minimum fragment necessary for activity, it still is only one sixth as active as the entire gastrin molecule.

♦ **Secretion of gastrin.** In response to eating a meal, gastrin is secreted from **G cells** located in the antrum of the stomach. The physiologic stimuli that initiate gastrin secretion all are related to ingestion of food. These stimuli include the products of protein digestion (e.g., small peptides and amino acids), distention of the stomach by food, and vagal stimulation. Among the products of protein digestion, the amino acids phenylalanine and tryptophan are the most potent stimuli for gastrin secretion. Local vagal reflexes also stimulate gastrin secretion. In these local reflexes, the neurocrine released from vagal nerve endings onto the G cells is **gastrin-releasing peptide (GRP),** or bombesin. In addition to these positive stimuli, gastrin secretion is *inhibited* by a low pH of the gastric contents and by somatostatin.

♦ **Actions of gastrin.** Gastrin has two major actions: (1) It stimulates **H⁺ secretion** by gastric parietal cells, and (2) it stimulates **growth of the gastric mucosa,** a trophic effect. The physiologic actions of gastrin are nicely illustrated in conditions of gastrin excess or deficiency. For example, in persons with gastrin-secreting tumors (Zollinger-Ellison syndrome), H⁺ secretion is increased and the trophic effect of gastrin causes the gastric mucosa to hypertrophy. Conversely, in persons whose gastric antrum is resected (which removes the source of gastrin, the

G cells), H⁺ secretion is decreased and the gastric mucosa atrophies.

♦ **Zollinger-Ellison syndrome** is caused by a gastrin-secreting tumor or **gastrinoma,** usually in the non–β-cell pancreas. The signs and symptoms of Zollinger-Ellison syndrome all are attributable to high circulating levels of gastrin: increased H⁺ secretion by parietal cells, hypertrophy of the gastric mucosa (the trophic effect of gastrin), and **duodenal ulcers** caused by the unrelenting secretion of H⁺. The increased H⁺ secretion also results in acidification of the intestinal lumen, which inactivates pancreatic lipase, an enzyme necessary for fat digestion. As a result, dietary fats are not adequately digested or absorbed, and fat is excreted in the stool **(steatorrhea).** Treatment of Zollinger-Ellison syndrome includes administration of H₂ receptor–blocking drugs (e.g., **cimetidine);** administration of inhibitors of the H⁺ pump (e.g., **omeprazole);** removal of the tumor; or, as the last resort, gastric resection, which removes gastrin's target tissue.

Cholecystokinin

The functions of cholecystokinin (CCK) are coordinated to promote **fat digestion and absorption.** CCK is a 33-amino acid peptide, which is structurally related to gastrin and a member of the "gastrin-CCK family" (see Fig. 8-5). The C-terminal five amino acids (CCK-5) are identical to those of gastrin and include the tetrapeptide that is minimally necessary for gastrin activity. Thus, CCK has *some* gastrin activity. CCK$_A$ receptors

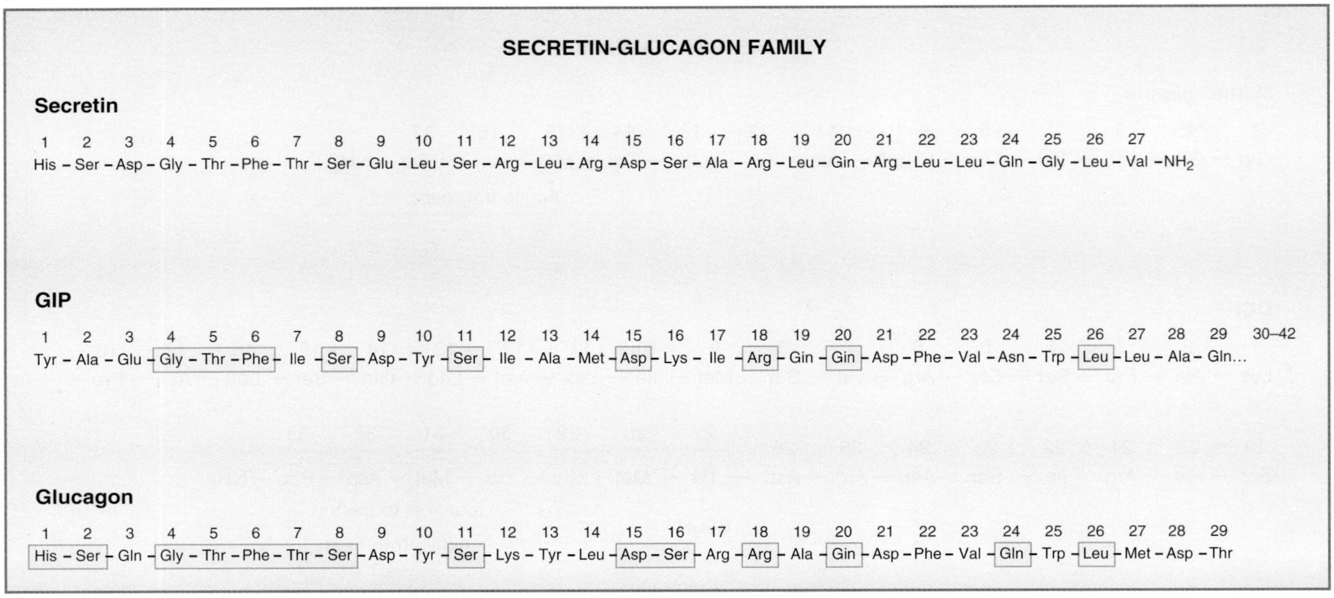

SECRETIN-GLUCAGON FAMILY

Secretin

1	2	3	4	5	6	7	8	9	10	11	12	13	14	15	16	17	18	19	20	21	22	23	24	25	26	27
His	Ser	Asp	Gly	Thr	Phe	Thr	Ser	Glu	Leu	Ser	Arg	Leu	Arg	Asp	Ser	Ala	Arg	Leu	Gin	Arg	Leu	Leu	Gin	Gly	Leu	Val –NH₂

GIP

1	2	3	4	5	6	7	8	9	10	11	12	13	14	15	16	17	18	19	20	21	22	23	24	25	26	27	28	29	30–42
Tyr	Ala	Glu	Gly	Thr	Phe	Ile	Ser	Asp	Tyr	Ser	Ile	Ala	Met	Asp	Lys	Ile	Arg	Gin	Gin	Asp	Phe	Val	Asn	Trp	Leu	Leu	Ala	Gin...

Glucagon

1	2	3	4	5	6	7	8	9	10	11	12	13	14	15	16	17	18	19	20	21	22	23	24	25	26	27	28	29
His	Ser	Gin	Gly	Thr	Phe	Thr	Ser	Asp	Tyr	Ser	Lys	Tyr	Leu	Asp	Ser	Arg	Arg	Ala	Gin	Asp	Phe	Val	Gin	Trp	Leu	Met	Asp	Thr

Figure 8–6 **Structures of secretin, glucose-dependent insulinotropic peptide (GIP), and glucagon.** The *blue-shaded fragments* (amino acids) show the portions of GIP and glucagon that are homologous with secretin.

are selective for CCK, while CCK_B receptors are equally sensitive to CCK and gastrin. The minimum fragment of CCK necessary for its biologic activity is the **C-terminal heptapeptide** (seven amino acids [CCK-7]).

CCK is secreted by the **I cells** of the duodenal and jejunal mucosa in response to two types of physiologic stimuli: (1) monoglycerides and fatty acids (but not triglycerides) and (2) small peptides and amino acids. These stimuli alert the I cells to the presence of a meal containing fat and protein, which must be digested and absorbed. CCK will then ensure that appropriate pancreatic enzymes and bile salts are secreted to aid in this digestion and absorption.

There are five major **actions of CCK,** and each contributes to the overall process of fat, protein, and carbohydrate digestion and absorption.

♦ **Contraction of the gallbladder** with simultaneous relaxation of the sphincter of Oddi ejects bile from the gallbladder into the lumen of the small intestine. Bile is needed for emulsification and solubilization of dietary lipids.

♦ **Secretion of pancreatic enzymes.** Pancreatic lipases digest ingested lipids to fatty acids, monoglycerides, and cholesterol, all of which can be absorbed. Pancreatic amylase digests carbohydrates, and pancreatic proteases digest protein.

♦ **Secretion of bicarbonate (HCO₃⁻) from the pancreas.** This is not a major effect of CCK, but it potentiates the effects of secretin on HCO₃⁻ secretion.

♦ **Growth of the exocrine pancreas and gallbladder.** Because the major target organs for CCK are the

exocrine pancreas and the gallbladder, it is logical that CCK also has trophic effects on these organs.

♦ **Inhibition of gastric emptying.** CCK inhibits or slows gastric emptying and *increases gastric emptying time.* This action is critical for the processes of fat digestion and absorption, which require a considerable amount of time. CCK slows the delivery of chyme (partially digested food) from the stomach to the small intestine, ensuring adequate time for the subsequent digestive and absorptive steps.

Secretin

Secretin, a 27-amino acid peptide, is structurally homologous to glucagon and is a member of the secretin-glucagon family (Fig. 8-6). Fourteen of the 27 amino acids of secretin are identical and in the same position as those of glucagon. In contrast to gastrin and CCK, which have active fragments, all 27 amino acids of secretin are required for its biologic activity. For activity, the entire secretin molecule must fold into its tertiary structure, an α helix.

Secretin is secreted by the **S cells** (secretin cells) of the duodenum in response to H⁺ and fatty acids in the lumen of the small intestine. Thus, secretion of secretin is initiated when the acidic gastric contents (pH < 4.5) arrive in the small intestine.

The function of secretin is to promote the **secretion of pancreatic and biliary HCO₃⁻,** which then neutralizes H⁺ in the lumen of the small intestine. Neutralization of H⁺ is essential for fat digestion; pancreatic lipases have pH optimums between 6 and 8, and they are inactivated or denatured when the pH is less than 3.

Secretin also inhibits the effects of gastrin on the parietal cells (H^+ secretion and growth).

Glucose-Dependent Insulinotropic Peptide

Glucose-dependent insulinotropic peptide (GIP), a 42-amino acid peptide, is also a member of the secretin-glucagon family (see Fig. 8-6). GIP has 9 amino acids in common with secretin and 16 amino acids in common with glucagon. Because of this homology, pharmacologic levels of GIP produce most of the actions of secretin.

GIP is secreted by K cells of the duodenal and jejunal mucosa. It is the only gastrointestinal hormone that is secreted in response to all three types of nutrients: glucose, amino acids, and fatty acids.

The major physiologic action of GIP is **stimulation of insulin secretion** by the pancreatic β cells; because of this action, it is classified as an **incretin** (i.e., a gastrointestinal hormone that promotes the secretion of insulin). This action explains the observation that an oral glucose load is utilized by cells more rapidly than an equivalent intravenous glucose load. Oral glucose stimulates GIP secretion, which stimulates insulin secretion (in addition to the direct stimulatory action of absorbed glucose on the β cells). Glucose given intravenously stimulates insulin secretion only by the direct action on the β cells. The other actions of GIP are **inhibition of gastric H^+ secretion** and inhibition of gastric emptying.

Candidate Hormones

Candidate, or putative, hormones also are secreted by the gastrointestinal tract. They are considered to be *candidate* hormones because they fail to meet one or more of the criteria necessary to be classified as "official" gastrointestinal hormones.

Motilin, a 22-amino acid peptide, is not a member of the gastrin-CCK family or the secretin-glucagon family. It is secreted from the upper duodenum during fasting states. Motilin is believed to increase gastrointestinal motility and, specifically, to initiate the **interdigestive myoelectric complexes** that occur at 90-minute intervals.

Pancreatic polypeptide is a 36-amino acid peptide secreted by the pancreas in response to ingestion of carbohydrates, proteins, or lipids. Pancreatic polypeptide inhibits pancreatic secretion of HCO_3^- and enzymes, although its physiologic role is uncertain.

Enteroglucagon is released from intestinal cells in response to a decrease in blood glucose concentration. It then directs the liver to increase glycogenolysis and gluconeogenesis.

Glucagon-like peptide-1 (GLP-1) is produced from the selective cleavage of proglucagon. It is synthesized and secreted by the L cells of the small intestine. Like GIP, GLP-1 is classified as an **incretin,** because it binds to receptors on the pancreatic beta cells and **stimulates insulin secretion.** In complementary actions, it also inhibits glucagon secretion, increases the sensitivity of pancreatic beta cells to secretagogues such as glucose, decreases gastric emptying, and inhibits appetite (i.e., increases satiety). For these reasons, analogues of GLP-1 have been considered as possible treatments for type 2 diabetes mellitus.

Paracrines

As with the gastrointestinal hormones, paracrines are synthesized in endocrine cells of the gastrointestinal tract. The paracrines do not enter the systemic circulation but *act locally,* reaching their target cells by diffusing over short distances.

Somatostatin is secreted by D cells (both endocrine and paracrine) of the gastrointestinal mucosa in response to decreased luminal pH. In turn, somatostatin *inhibits* secretion of the other gastrointestinal hormones and *inhibits* gastric H^+ secretion. In addition to these paracrine functions in the gastrointestinal tract, somatostatin is secreted by the hypothalamus and by the delta (δ) cells of the endocrine pancreas.

Histamine is secreted by endocrine-type cells of the gastrointestinal mucosa, particularly in the H^+-secreting region of the stomach. Histamine, along with gastrin and ACh, stimulates H^+ secretion by the gastric parietal cells.

Neurocrines

Neurocrines are synthesized in cell bodies of gastrointestinal neurons. An action potential in the neuron causes release of the neurocrine, which diffuses across the synapse and interacts with receptors on the postsynaptic cell.

Table 8-1 presents a summary of neurocrines including nonpeptides such as ACh and norepinephrine and peptides such as VIP, GRP, the enkephalins, neuropeptide Y, and substance P. The best-known neurocrines are ACh (released from cholinergic neurons) and norepinephrine (released from adrenergic neurons). The other neurocrines are released from postganglionic *noncholinergic* parasympathetic neurons (also called peptidergic neurons).

Satiety

The centers that control appetite and feeding behavior are located in the hypothalamus. A **satiety center,** which inhibits appetite even in the presence of food, is located in the ventromedial nucleus (VPN) of the hypothalamus and a **feeding center** is located in the lateral hypothalamic area (LHA). Information feeds into these centers from the **arcuate nucleus** of the hypothalamus.

The arcuate nucleus has various neurons that project onto the satiety feeding centers. **Anorexigenic neurons** release pro-opiomelanocortin (POMC) and cause decreased appetite; **orexigenic neuron**s release neuropeptide Y and cause increased appetite. The following substances influence the anorexigenic and orexigenic neurons of the arcuate nucleus and, accordingly, decrease or increase appetite and feeding behavior.

♦ **Leptin.** Leptin is secreted by **fat cells** in proportion to the amount of fat stored in adipose tissue. Thus, leptin senses body fat levels, is secreted into the circulation, crosses the blood-brain barrier, and acts on neurons of the arcuate nucleus of the hypothalamus. It stimulates anorexigenic neurons and inhibits orexigenic neurons, thereby **decreasing appetite** and increasing energy expenditure. Because leptin detects stored body fat, it has chronic (long-term) effects to decrease appetite.

♦ **Insulin.** Insulin has similar actions to leptin, in that it stimulates anorexigenic neurons and inhibits orexigenic neurons, thus decreasing appetite. In contrast to leptin, insulin levels fluctuate during the day, thus it has acute (short-term) effects to decrease appetite.

♦ **GLP-1.** As discussed earlier, GLP-1 is synthesized and secreted by intestinal L cells. Among its actions (like leptin and insulin), it decreases appetite.

♦ **Ghrelin.** Ghrelin is secreted by **gastric cells** just before ingestion of a meal. It acts oppositely to leptin and insulin to stimulate orexigenic neurons and inhibit anorexigenic neurons, thus **increasing appetite** and food intake. Periods of starvation and weight loss strongly stimulate ghrelin secretion.

♦ **Peptide YY (PYY).** PYY is secreted by intestinal L cells following a meal. It acts to decrease appetite, both through a direct effect on the hypothalamus and by inhibiting ghrelin secretion.

MOTILITY

Motility is a general term that refers to contraction and relaxation of the walls and sphincters of the gastrointestinal tract. Motility grinds, mixes, and fragments ingested food to prepare it for digestion and absorption, and then it propels the food along the gastrointestinal tract.

All of the contractile tissue of the gastrointestinal tract is smooth muscle, *except* for that in the pharynx, the upper one third of the esophagus, and the external anal sphincter, which is striated muscle. The smooth muscle of the gastrointestinal tract is **unitary smooth muscle,** in which the cells are electrically coupled via low-resistance pathways called **gap junctions.** Gap junctions permit rapid cell-to-cell spread of action potentials that provide for coordinated and smooth contraction.

The circular and longitudinal muscles of the gastrointestinal tract have different functions. When **circular muscle** contracts, it results in shortening of a ring of smooth muscle, which decreases the diameter of that segment. When **longitudinal muscle** contracts, it results in shortening in the longitudinal direction, which decreases the length of that segment.

Contractions of gastrointestinal smooth muscle can be either phasic or tonic. **Phasic contractions** are periodic contractions followed by relaxation. Phasic contractions are found in the esophagus, gastric antrum, and small intestine, all tissues involved in mixing and propulsion. **Tonic contractions** maintain a constant level of contraction or tone without regular periods of relaxation. They are found in the orad (upper) region of the stomach and in the lower esophageal, ileocecal, and internal anal sphincters.

Slow Waves

Like all muscle, contraction in gastrointestinal smooth muscle is preceded by electrical activity, the action potentials. Slow waves are a unique feature of the electrical activity of gastrointestinal smooth muscle. Slow waves are *not action potentials* but rather **oscillating depolarization and repolarization** of the membrane potential of the smooth muscle cells (Fig. 8-7). During the depolarization phase of the slow wave, the membrane potential becomes less negative and moves toward threshold; during the repolarization phase, the membrane potential becomes more negative and moves away from threshold. If, at the plateau or the peak of the slow wave, the membrane potential is depolarized all the way to threshold, then action potentials occur "on top of" the slow wave. For example, the slow waves shown in Figure 8-7 reach threshold and result in bursts of six action potentials at the plateau. As in other types of muscle, the mechanical response (contraction or tension) follows the electrical response. In Figure 8-7, notice that the contraction, or tension, occurs slightly after the burst of action potentials.

♦ **Frequency of slow waves.** The intrinsic rate, or frequency, of slow waves varies along the gastrointestinal tract, from 3 to 12 slow waves per minute. Each portion of the gastrointestinal tract has a characteristic frequency, with the stomach having the lowest rate (3 slow waves per minute) and the duodenum having the highest rate (12 slow waves per minute). The frequency of slow waves sets the frequency of action potentials and, therefore, sets the frequency of contractions. (Action potentials cannot occur unless the slow wave brings the membrane

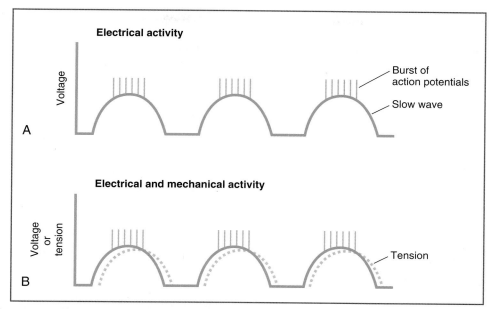

Figure 8–7 **Slow waves of the gastrointestinal tract superimposed by action potentials and contraction.** A burst of action potentials is followed by contraction. **A,** Electrical activity; **B,** electrical and mechanical activity.

potential to threshold.) The characteristic frequency of slow waves is not influenced by neural or hormonal input, although neural activity and hormonal activity do modulate both the production of action potentials and the strength of contractions.

◆ **Origin of slow waves.** It is believed that slow waves originate in the **interstitial cells of Cajal,** which are abundant in the myenteric plexus. Cyclic depolarizations and repolarizations occur spontaneously in the interstitial cells of Cajal and spread rapidly to adjacent smooth muscle via low-resistance gap junctions. Just as the sinoatrial node is the pacemaker of the heart, the interstitial cells of Cajal can be considered the **pacemaker** for gastrointestinal smooth muscle. In each region of the gastrointestinal tract, the pacemaker drives the frequency of slow waves, which determines the rate at which action potentials and contractions can occur.

◆ **Mechanism of slow waves.** The depolarizing phase of the slow wave is caused by the cyclic opening of calcium (Ca^{2+}) channels, which produces an inward Ca^{2+} current that depolarizes the cell membrane. During the plateau of the slow wave, Ca^{2+} channels open, producing an inward Ca^{2+} current that maintains the membrane potential at the depolarized level. The repolarizing phase of the slow wave is caused by opening of potassium (K^+) channels, which produces an outward K^+ current that repolarizes the cell membrane.

◆ **Relationship between slow waves, action potentials, and contraction.** In gastrointestinal smooth muscle, even subthreshold slow waves produce a weak contraction. Thus, even without the occurrence of action potentials, the smooth muscle is not completely relaxed but exhibits basal contractions, or **tonic contractions.** However, if slow waves depolarize the membrane potential to threshold, then action potentials occur on top of the slow waves, followed by much stronger contractions, or **phasic contractions.** The greater the number of action potentials on top of the slow waves, the larger the phasic contraction. In contrast to skeletal muscle (where each action potential is followed by a separate contraction or twitch), in smooth muscle individual action potentials are not followed by separate twitches; instead, the twitches summate into one long contraction (see Fig. 8-7*B*).

Chewing and Swallowing

Chewing and swallowing are the first steps in the processing of ingested food as it is prepared for digestion and absorption.

Chewing

Chewing has three functions: (1) It mixes food with saliva, lubricating it to facilitate swallowing; (2) it reduces the size of food particles, which facilitates swallowing (although the size of the swallowed particles has no effect on the digestive process); and (3) it mixes ingested carbohydrates with salivary amylase to begin carbohydrate digestion.

Chewing has both voluntary and involuntary components. The involuntary component involves reflexes

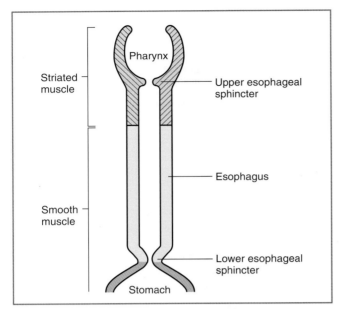

Figure 8-8 **Structures of the upper gastrointestinal tract.** The pharynx, upper esophageal sphincter, and upper third of the esophagus are composed of striated muscle. The lower two thirds of the esophagus and lower esophageal sphincter are composed of smooth muscle.

initiated by food in the mouth. Sensory information is relayed from mechanoreceptors in the mouth to the **brain stem,** which orchestrates a reflex oscillatory pattern of activity to the muscles involved in chewing. Voluntary chewing can override involuntary or reflex chewing at any time.

Swallowing

Swallowing is initiated voluntarily in the mouth, but thereafter it is under involuntary or reflex control. The reflex portion is controlled by the **swallowing center,** which is located in the **medulla.** Sensory information (e.g., food in the mouth) is detected by somatosensory receptors located near the pharynx. This sensory, or afferent, information is carried to the medullary swallowing center via the vagus and glossopharyngeal nerves. The medulla coordinates the sensory information and directs the motor, or efferent, output to the striated muscle of the pharynx and upper esophagus (Fig. 8-8).

Three phases are involved in swallowing: oral, pharyngeal, and esophageal. The oral phase is voluntary, and the pharyngeal and esophageal phases are controlled by reflexes.

- **Oral phase.** The oral phase is initiated when the tongue forces a bolus of food back toward the pharynx, which contains a high density of somatosensory receptors. As previously noted, activation of these receptors then initiates the involuntary swallowing reflex in the medulla.

- **Pharyngeal phase.** The purpose of the pharyngeal phase is to propel the food bolus from the mouth through the pharynx to the esophagus in the following steps: (1) The soft palate is pulled upward, creating a narrow passage for food to move into the pharynx so that food cannot reflux into the nasopharynx. (2) The epiglottis moves to cover the opening to the larynx, and the larynx moves upward against the epiglottis to prevent food from entering the trachea. (3) The upper esophageal sphincter relaxes, allowing food to pass from the pharynx to the esophagus. (4) A peristaltic wave of contraction is initiated in the pharynx and propels food through the open sphincter. Breathing is inhibited during the pharyngeal phase of swallowing.

- **Esophageal phase.** The esophageal phase of swallowing is controlled in part by the swallowing reflex and in part by the enteric nervous system. In the esophageal phase, food is propelled through the esophagus to the stomach. Once the bolus has passed through the upper esophageal sphincter in the pharyngeal phase, the swallowing reflex closes the sphincter so that food cannot reflux into the pharynx. A **primary peristaltic wave,** also coordinated by the swallowing reflex, travels down the esophagus (see discussion of peristalsis), propelling the food along. If the primary peristaltic wave does not clear the esophagus of food, a **secondary peristaltic wave** is initiated by the continued distention of the esophagus. The secondary wave, which is mediated by the enteric nervous system, begins at the site of distention and travels downward.

Esophageal Motility

The function of motility in the esophagus is to propel the food bolus from the pharynx to the stomach (see Fig. 8-8). There is overlap between the esophageal phase of swallowing and esophageal motility. The path of the food bolus through the esophagus is as follows:

1. The **upper esophageal sphincter** opens, mediated by the swallowing reflex, allowing the bolus to move from the pharynx to the esophagus. Once the bolus enters the esophagus, the upper esophageal sphincter closes, which prevents reflux into the pharynx.

2. A **primary peristaltic contraction,** also mediated by the swallowing reflex, involves a series of coordinated sequential contractions (Fig. 8-9). As each segment of esophagus contracts, it creates an area of high pressure just behind the bolus, pushing it down the esophagus. Each sequential contraction pushes the bolus further along. If the person is sitting or standing, this action is accelerated by **gravity.**

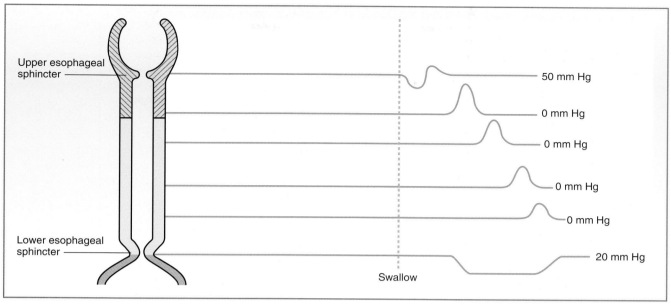

Figure 8–9 **Pressures in esophagus during swallowing.**

3. As the peristaltic wave and the food bolus approach the lower esophageal sphincter, the sphincter opens. Opening of the **lower esophageal sphincter** is mediated by peptidergic fibers in the vagus nerve that release **VIP** as their neurotransmitter. VIP produces relaxation in the smooth muscle of the lower esophageal sphincter.

At the same time that the lower esophageal sphincter relaxes, the orad region of the stomach also relaxes, a phenomenon called **receptive relaxation.** Receptive relaxation decreases pressure in the orad stomach and facilitates movement of the bolus into the stomach. As soon as the bolus enters the orad stomach, the lower esophageal sphincter contracts, returning to its high resting tone. At this resting tone, the pressure at the sphincter is higher than the pressure in the esophagus or in the orad stomach.

4. If the primary peristaltic contraction does not clear the esophagus of food, a **secondary peristaltic contraction,** mediated by the enteric nervous system, clears the esophagus of any remaining food. The secondary peristaltic contraction begins at the point of distention and travels downward.

An interesting problem is posed by the **intrathoracic location of the esophagus** (only the lower esophagus is located in the abdomen). The thoracic location means that intraesophageal pressure is equal to intrathoracic pressure, which is lower than atmospheric pressure. It also means that intraesophageal pressure is lower than abdominal pressure. The lower intraesophageal pressure creates two problems: (1) keeping air out of the esophagus at the upper end and (2) keeping the acidic gastric contents out at the lower end. It is the function of the upper esophageal sphincter to prevent air from entering the upper esophagus, and the lower esophageal sphincter functions to prevent the acidic gastric contents from entering the lower esophagus. Both the upper and lower esophageal sphincters are closed, except when food is passing from the pharynx into the esophagus or from the esophagus into the stomach. Conditions in which intra-abdominal pressure is increased (e.g., pregnancy or morbid obesity) may cause **gastroesophageal reflux,** in which the contents of the stomach reflux into the esophagus.

Gastric Motility

There are three components of gastric motility: (1) relaxation of the orad region of the stomach to receive the food bolus from the esophagus, (2) contractions that reduce the size of the bolus and mix it with gastric secretions to initiate digestion, and (3) gastric emptying that propels chyme into the small intestine. The rate of delivery of chyme to the small intestine is hormonally regulated to ensure adequate time for digestion and absorption of nutrients in the small intestine.

Structure and Innervation of the Stomach

The stomach has three layers of muscle: an outer longitudinal layer, a middle circular layer, and an inner oblique layer that is unique to the stomach. The thickness of the muscle wall increases from the proximal stomach to the distal stomach.

The innervation of the stomach includes extrinsic innervation by the autonomic nervous system and

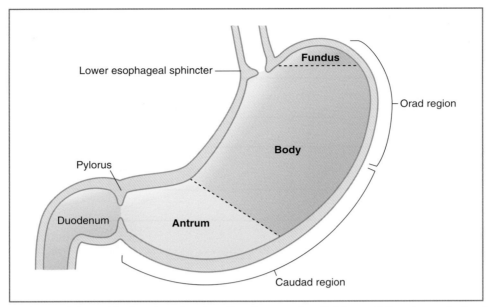

Figure 8–10 **Schematic drawing showing the three major divisions of the stomach: fundus, body, and antrum.** The orad region includes the fundus and the upper body. The caudad region includes the lower body and the antrum.

intrinsic innervation from the myenteric and submucosal plexuses. The myenteric plexus serving the stomach receives parasympathetic innervation via the vagus nerve and sympathetic innervation via fibers originating in the celiac ganglion.

Figure 8-10 shows the three anatomic divisions of the stomach: **fundus, body,** and **antrum.** On the basis of differences in motility, the stomach also can be divided into two regions, orad and caudad. The **orad region** is proximal, contains the fundus and the proximal portion of the body, and is thin walled. The **caudad region** is distal, contains the distal portion of the body and the antrum, and is thick walled to generate much stronger contractions than the orad region. Contractions of the caudad region mix the food and propel it into the small intestine.

Receptive Relaxation

The orad region of the stomach has a thin muscular wall. Its function is to receive the food bolus. As noted in the discussion about esophageal motility, distention of the lower esophagus by food produces relaxation of the lower esophageal sphincter and, simultaneously, relaxation of the orad stomach, called **receptive relaxation.** Receptive relaxation reduces the pressure and increases the volume of the orad stomach, which, in its relaxed state, can accommodate as much as 1.5 L of food.

Receptive relaxation is a **vagovagal reflex,** meaning that both afferent and efferent limbs of the reflex are carried in the vagus nerve. Mechanoreceptors detect distention of the stomach and relay this information to the CNS via sensory neurons. The CNS then sends efferent information to the smooth muscle wall of the orad stomach, causing it to relax. The neurotransmitter released from these postganglionic peptidergic vagal nerve fibers is **VIP.** Vagotomy eliminates receptive relaxation.

Mixing and Digestion

The caudad region of the stomach has a thick muscular wall and produces the contractions necessary for mixing and digesting food. These contractions break the food into smaller pieces and mix it with gastric secretions to begin the digestive process.

Waves of contraction begin in the middle of the body of the stomach and move distally along the caudad stomach. These are vigorous contractions that increase in strength as they approach the pylorus. The contractions mix the gastric contents and periodically propel a portion of the gastric contents through the pylorus into the duodenum. Much of the chyme is not immediately injected into the duodenum, however, because the wave of contraction also closes the pylorus. Therefore, most of the gastric contents are propelled back into the stomach for further mixing and further reduction of particle size, a process known as **retropulsion.**

The frequency of **slow waves** in the caudad stomach is from 3 to 5 waves per minute. Recall that slow waves bring the membrane potential to threshold so that action potentials can occur. Because the frequency of slow waves sets the maximal frequency of action potentials and contractions, the caudad stomach contracts 3 to 5 times per minute.

Although neural input and hormonal input *do not* influence the frequency of slow waves, they *do* influence the frequency of action potentials and the force of contraction. **Parasympathetic stimulation** and the hormones gastrin and motilin *increase* the frequency of action potentials and the force of gastric contractions. **Sympathetic stimulation** and the hormones secretin and GIP *decrease* the frequency of action potentials and the force of contractions.

During fasting, there are periodic gastric contractions, called the **migrating myoelectric complexes,** which are mediated by **motilin.** These contractions occur at 90-minute intervals and function to clear the stomach of any residue remaining from the previous meal.

Gastric Emptying

After a meal, the stomach contains about 1.5 L, which is composed of solids, liquids, and gastric secretions. Emptying of the gastric contents to the duodenum takes approximately 3 hours. The rate of gastric emptying must be closely regulated to provide adequate time for neutralization of gastric H^+ in the duodenum and adequate time for digestion and absorption of nutrients.

Liquids empty more rapidly than solids, and isotonic contents empty more rapidly than either hypotonic or hypertonic contents. To enter the duodenum, solids must be reduced to particles of 1 mm^3 or less; retropulsion in the stomach continues until solid food particles are reduced to the required size.

Two major factors slow or inhibit gastric emptying (i.e., *increase gastric emptying time*): the presence of fat and the presence of H^+ ions (low pH) in the duodenum. The effect of **fat** is mediated by **CCK,** which is secreted when fatty acids arrive in the duodenum. In turn, CCK slows gastric emptying, ensuring that gastric contents are delivered slowly to the duodenum and providing adequate time for fat to be digested and absorbed. The effect of H^+ is mediated by reflexes in the **enteric nervous system.** H^+ receptors in the duodenal mucosa detect low pH of the intestinal contents and relay this information to gastric smooth muscle via interneurons in the myenteric plexus. This reflex also ensures that the gastric contents are delivered slowly to the duodenum, permitting time for neutralization of H^+ by pancreatic HCO_3^-, as is necessary for optimal function of pancreatic enzymes.

Small Intestinal Motility

The functions of the small intestine are digestion and absorption of nutrients. In this context, motility of the small intestine serves to mix the chyme with digestive enzymes and pancreatic secretions, expose the nutrients to the intestinal mucosa for absorption, and propel the unabsorbed chyme along the small intestine into the large intestine.

In the small intestine, as with other gastrointestinal smooth muscle, the frequency of **slow waves** determines the rate at which action potentials and contractions occur. Slow waves are more frequent in the duodenum (12 waves per minute) than in the stomach. In the ileum, the frequency of slow waves decreases slightly, to 9 waves per minute. As in the stomach, contractions (called **migrating myoelectric complexes**) occur every 90 minutes to clear the small intestine of residual chyme.

There is both parasympathetic and sympathetic innervation of the small intestine. Parasympathetic innervation occurs via the vagus nerve, and sympathetic innervation occurs via fibers that originate in the celiac and superior mesenteric ganglia. **Parasympathetic** stimulation *increases* contraction of intestinal smooth muscle, and **sympathetic** activity *decreases* contraction. Although many of the parasympathetic nerves are cholinergic (i.e., they release ACh), some of the parasympathetic nerves release other neurocrines (i.e., they are peptidergic). Neurocrines released from parasympathetic peptidergic neurons of the small intestine include VIP, enkephalins, and motilin.

There are two patterns of contractions in the small intestine: segmentation contractions and peristaltic contractions. Each pattern is coordinated by the **enteric nervous system** (Fig. 8-11).

Segmentation Contractions

Segmentation contractions serve to **mix the chyme** and expose it to pancreatic enzymes and secretions, as shown in Figure 8-11*A*. Step 1 shows a bolus of chyme in the intestinal lumen. A section of small intestine contracts, splitting the chyme and sending it in both orad and caudad directions (Step 2). That section of intestine then relaxes, allowing the bolus of chyme that was split to merge back together (Step 3). This back-and-forth movement serves to mix the chyme but produces no forward, propulsive movement along the small intestine.

Peristaltic Contractions

In contrast to segmentation contractions, which are designed to mix the chyme, peristaltic contractions are designed to **propel the chyme** along the small intestine toward the large intestine (see Fig. 8-11*B*). Step 1 shows a bolus of chyme. A contraction occurs at a point orad to (behind) the bolus; simultaneously, the portion of intestine caudad to (in front of) the bolus relaxes (Step 2). The chyme is thereby propelled in the caudad direction. A wave of peristaltic contractions occurs down the small intestine, repeating the sequence of contractions

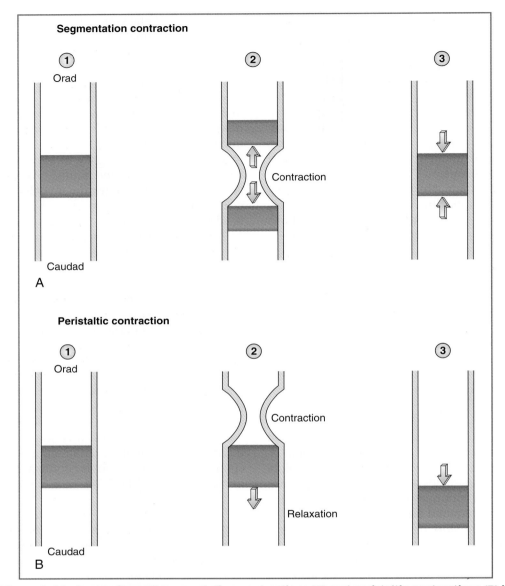

Figure 8–11 **Comparison of segmentation contractions (A) and peristaltic contractions (B) in the small intestine.** Segmentation contractions mix the chyme. Peristalsis moves the chyme in the caudad direction. For the peristaltic contraction, behind the bolus (orad) circular muscle contracts and longitudinal muscle relaxes; in front of the bolus (caudad), circular muscle relaxes and longitudinal muscle contracts.

behind the bolus and relaxation in front of the bolus, which moves the chyme along (Step 3).

To accomplish such propulsive movements along the small intestine, circular and longitudinal muscles must function oppositely to complement each other's actions. (Recall that contraction of circular muscle decreases the *diameter* of that small intestinal segment, whereas contraction of longitudinal muscle decreases the *length* of that small intestinal segment.) To prevent the conflict that would occur if circular and longitudinal muscle contracted at the same time, they are reciprocally innervated. Consequently, when the circular muscle of a segment contracts, the longitudinal muscle simultaneously relaxes; when the longitudinal muscle contracts, the circular muscle simultaneously relaxes.

Peristalsis therefore occurs as follows. The food bolus in the intestinal lumen is sensed by enterochromaffin cells of the intestinal mucosa, which release serotonin (5-hydroxytyptamine, 5-HT). The 5-HT binds to receptors on intrinsic primary afferent neurons (IPANs) that, when activated, initiate the **peristaltic reflex** in that segment of small intestine. **Behind the bolus,** excitatory transmitters (e.g., ACh, substance P, neuropeptide Y) are released in circular muscle, while these pathways are simultaneously inhibited in the longitudinal muscle; thus, this segment of small intestine narrows and lengthens. **In front of the bolus,** inhibitory pathways (e.g., vasoactive intestinal peptide, nitric oxide) are activated in circular muscle, while excitatory pathways are activated in longitudinal muscle; thus, this segment of small intestine widens and shortens.

Vomiting

A **vomiting center** in the medulla coordinates the vomiting reflex. Afferent information comes to the vomiting center from the vestibular system, the back of the throat, the gastrointestinal tract, and the chemoreceptor trigger zone in the fourth ventricle.

The **vomiting reflex** includes the following events in this temporal sequence: **reverse peristalsis** that begins in the small intestine; relaxation of the stomach and pylorus; forced inspiration to increase abdominal pressure; movement of the larynx upward and forward and relaxation of the lower esophageal sphincter; closure of the glottis; and forceful expulsion of gastric, and sometimes duodenal, contents. In **retching,** the upper esophageal sphincter remains closed, and because the lower esophageal sphincter is open, the gastric contents return to the stomach when the retch is over.

Large Intestinal Motility

Material that is not absorbed in the small intestine enters the large intestine. The contents of the large intestine, called **feces,** are destined for excretion. After the contents of the small intestine enter the cecum and proximal colon, the ileocecal sphincter contracts, preventing reflux into the ileum. Fecal material then moves from the cecum through the colon (i.e., ascending, transverse, descending, and sigmoid colons), to the rectum, and on to the anal canal.

Segmentation Contractions

Segmentation contractions occur in the cecum and proximal colon. As in the small intestine, these contractions function to mix the contents of the large intestine. In the large intestine, the contractions are associated with characteristic saclike segments called **haustra.**

Mass Movements

Mass movements occur in the colon and function to move the contents of the large intestine over long distances, such as from the transverse colon to the sigmoid colon. Mass movements occur anywhere from **1 to 3 times per day.** Water absorption occurs in the distal colon, making the fecal contents of the large intestine semisolid and increasingly difficult to move. A final mass movement propels the fecal contents into the rectum, where they are stored until defecation occurs.

Defecation

As the rectum fills with feces, the smooth muscle wall of the rectum contracts and the internal anal sphincter relaxes in the **rectosphincteric reflex.** Defecation will not occur at this time, however, because the external anal sphincter (composed of striated muscle and under voluntary control) is still tonically contracted. However, once the rectum fills to 25% of its capacity, there is an urge to defecate. When it is appropriate, the external anal sphincter is relaxed voluntarily, the smooth muscle of the rectum contracts to create pressure, and feces are forced out through the anal canal. The intra-abdominal pressure created for defecation can be increased by a **Valsalva maneuver** (expiring against a closed glottis).

Gastrocolic Reflex

Distention of the stomach by food increases the motility of the colon and increases the frequency of mass movements in the large intestine. This long arc reflex, called the **gastrocolic reflex,** has its afferent limb in the stomach, which is mediated by the parasympathetic nervous system. The efferent limb of the reflex, which produces increased motility of the colon, is mediated by the hormones CCK and gastrin.

SECRETION

Secretion is the *addition* of fluids, enzymes, and mucus to the lumen of the gastrointestinal tract. These secretions are produced by salivary glands (saliva), the cells of the gastric mucosa (gastric secretion), the exocrine cells of the pancreas (pancreatic secretion), and the liver (bile) (Table 8-3).

Salivary Secretion

Saliva, which is produced by the salivary glands at the rate of 1 L per day, is secreted into the mouth. The **functions of saliva** include initial digestion of starches and lipids by salivary enzymes; dilution and buffering of ingested foods, which may otherwise be harmful; and lubrication of ingested food with mucus to aid its movement through the esophagus.

Structure of the Salivary Glands

The three major salivary glands are the parotid glands, the submandibular glands, and the sublingual glands. Each gland is a paired structure that produces saliva and delivers it to the mouth through a duct. The **parotid glands** are composed of serous cells and secrete an aqueous fluid composed of water, ions, and enzymes. The **submaxillary and sublingual glands** are mixed glands and have both serous and mucous cells. The

Table 8-3 Summary of Gastrointestinal Secretions

Secretion	Characteristics of Secretion	Factors That Increase Secretion	Factors That Decrease Secretion
Saliva	High [HCO_3^-] High [K^+] Hypotonic α-Amylase and lingual lipase	Parasympathetic (prominent) Sympathetic	Sleep Dehydration Atropine
Gastric	HCl	Gastrin Acetylcholine Histamine	H^+ in the stomach Chyme in the duodenum Somatostatin Atropine Cimetidine Omeprazole
	Pepsinogen Intrinsic factor	Parasympathetic	
Pancreatic	High [HCO_3^-] Isotonic	Secretin Cholecystokinin (CCK) (potentiates secretin) Parasympathetic	
	Pancreatic lipase, amylase, proteases	CCK Parasympathetic	
Bile	Bile salts Bilirubin Phospholipids Cholesterol	CCK (contraction of the gallbladder and relaxation of the sphincter of Oddi) Parasympathetic	Ileal resection

serous cells secrete an aqueous fluid, and the mucous cells secrete mucin glycoproteins for lubrication.

Each salivary gland has the appearance of a "bunch of grapes," where a single grape corresponds to a single acinus (Fig. 8-12). The **acinus** is the blind end of a branching duct system and is lined with acinar cells. The **acinar cells** produce an initial saliva composed of water, ions, enzymes, and mucus. This initial saliva passes through a short segment, called an intercalated duct, and then through a striated duct, which is lined with ductal cells. The **ductal cells** modify the initial saliva to produce the final saliva by altering the concentrations of various electrolytes. **Myoepithelial cells** are present in the acini and intercalated ducts. When stimulated by neural input, the myoepithelial cells contract to eject saliva into the mouth.

Salivary acinar cells and ductal cells have **both parasympathetic and sympathetic innervation.** Although many organs have such dual innervation, the unusual feature of the salivary glands is that saliva production is *stimulated by both* parasympathetic and sympathetic nervous systems (although parasympathetic control is dominant).

The salivary glands have an unusually **high blood flow** that increases when saliva production is stimulated. When corrected for organ size, maximal blood flow to the salivary glands is more than 10 times the blood flow to exercising skeletal muscle!

Formation of Saliva

Saliva is an aqueous solution whose volume is very high considering the small size of the glands. Saliva is composed of water, electrolytes, α-amylase, lingual lipase, kallikrein, and mucus. When compared with plasma, saliva is **hypotonic** (i.e., has a lower osmolarity), has higher K^+ and bicarbonate (HCO_3^-) concentrations, and has lower Na^+ and chloride (Cl^-) concentrations. Saliva, therefore, is not a simple ultrafiltrate of plasma, but it is formed in a two-step process that involves several transport mechanisms. The first step is the formation of an isotonic plasma-like solution by the acinar cells. The second step is modification of this plasma-like solution by the ductal cells.

The acinar and ductal steps in saliva production are shown in Figure 8-12. The circled numbers in the figure correspond to the following steps:

1. The **acinar cells** secrete the initial saliva, which is **isotonic** and has approximately the same electrolyte composition as plasma. Thus, in initial saliva, osmolarity, Na^+, K^+, Cl^-, and HCO_3^- concentrations are similar to those in plasma.

2. The **ductal cells** modify the initial saliva. The transport mechanisms involved in this modification are complex, but they can be simplified by considering events in the luminal and basolateral membranes separately and then by determining the net result

SALIVARY SECRETION

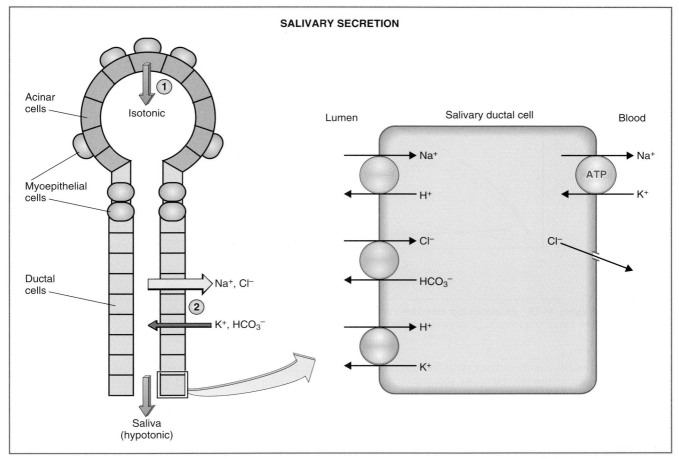

Figure 8–12 **Mechanism of salivary secretion.** Initial saliva is produced by acinar cells (1) and subsequently modified by ductal epithelial cells (2). ATP, Adenosine triphosphate.

of all the transport mechanisms. The luminal membrane of the ductal cells contains three transporters: Na^+-H^+ exchange, Cl^--HCO_3^- exchange, and H^+-K^+ exchange. The basolateral membrane contains the Na^+-K^+ ATPase and Cl^- channels. The combined action of these transporters working together is *absorption* of Na^+ and Cl^- and *secretion* of K^+ and HCO_3^-. Net absorption of Na^+ and Cl^- causes the Na^+ and Cl^- concentrations of saliva to become lower than their concentrations in plasma, and net secretion of K^+ and HCO_3^- causes the K^+ and HCO_3^- concentrations of saliva to become higher than those in plasma. Because more NaCl is absorbed than $KHCO_3$ is secreted, there is **net absorption of solute.**

A final question is *How does saliva, which was initially isotonic, become hypotonic as it flows through the ducts?* The answer lies in the relative **water impermeability** of the ductal cells. As noted, there is net absorption of solute because more NaCl is absorbed than $KHCO_3$ is secreted. Because ductal cells are water impermeable, water is not absorbed along with the solute, making the final saliva **hypotonic.**

The acinar cells also secrete organic constituents such as α-amylase, lingual lipase, mucin glycoproteins, IgA (immunoglobulin A), and kallikrein. **α-Amylase** begins the initial digestion of carbohydrates, and **lingual lipase** begins the initial digestion of lipids. The mucus component serves as a lubricant. **Kallikrein** is an enzyme that cleaves high-molecular-weight kininogen into bradykinin, a potent vasodilator. During periods of high salivary gland activity, kallikrein is secreted and produces bradykinin. Bradykinin then causes local vasodilation, which accounts for the high salivary blood flow during periods of increased salivary activity.

Effect of Flow Rate on Composition of Saliva

The ionic composition of saliva changes as the salivary flow rate changes (Fig. 8-13). At the **highest flow rates** (4 mL/min), the final saliva most closely resembles plasma and the initial saliva produced by the acinar cells. At the **lowest flow rates** (<1 mL/min), the final saliva is most dissimilar to plasma (it has lower concentrations of Na^+ and Cl^- and a higher concentration of K^+). The mechanism of the flow-rate–dependent changes in concentration is based primarily on the

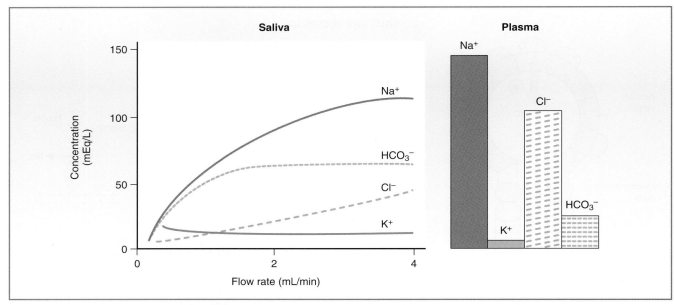

Figure 8-13 **Relationship between the composition of saliva and the salivary flow rate.** The ionic composition of saliva is compared with that of plasma.

amount of time saliva is in contact with the ductal cells. At high flow rates, the ductal cells have *less time* to modify the saliva; at low flow rates, they have *more time* to modify the saliva. Under conditions of low flow rate, where there is the greatest contact time, more Na^+ and Cl^- are reabsorbed, which decreases their concentrations relative to the initial saliva, and more K^+ is secreted, which increases its concentration.

The only electrolyte that is not described by this "contact-time" explanation is HCO_3^-. According to the contact time explanation, because HCO_3^- is secreted by ductal cells, its concentration should be highest at low flow rates. However, as shown in Figure 8-13, the HCO_3^- concentration of saliva is lowest at low flow rates and highest at high flow rates. This occurs because HCO_3^- secretion is *selectively* stimulated when saliva production is stimulated (e.g., by parasympathetic stimulation). Thus, as the flow rate of saliva increases, the HCO_3^- concentration also increases.

Regulation of Salivary Secretion

There are two unusual features in the regulation of salivary secretion. (1) Salivary secretion is exclusively under neural control by the autonomic nervous system, whereas the other gastrointestinal secretions are under both neural and hormonal control. (2) Salivary secretion is increased by *both* **parasympathetic and sympathetic** stimulation, although parasympathetic stimulation is dominant. (Usually, the parasympathetic and sympathetic nervous systems have opposite actions.)

Regulation of saliva secretion by the autonomic nervous system is summarized in Figure 8-14. As illustrated, there is parasympathetic and sympathetic innervation of acinar and ductal cells. Stimulation of salivary cells results in increased saliva production, increased HCO_3^- and enzyme secretions, and contraction of myoepithelial cells.

♦ **Parasympathetic innervation.** The parasympathetic input to the salivary glands is carried on the facial (CN VII) and glossopharyngeal (CN IX) nerves. Postganglionic parasympathetic neurons release ACh, which interacts with **muscarinic receptors** on the acinar and ductal cells. At the cellular level, activation of muscarinic receptors leads to production of inositol 1,4,5-triphosphate (**IP₃**) and increased intracellular calcium (Ca^{2+}) concentration, which produce the physiologic action of increased saliva secretion, primarily increasing the volume of saliva and the enzymatic component. Several factors modulate the parasympathetic input to the salivary glands. Parasympathetic activity to the salivary glands is increased by food, smell, and nausea and by conditioned reflexes (e.g., as demonstrated by Pavlov's salivating dogs). Parasympathetic activity is decreased by fear, sleep, and dehydration.

♦ **Sympathetic innervation.** The sympathetic input to the salivary glands originates in thoracic segments T1 to T3 with preganglionic nerves that synapse in the superior cervical ganglion. The postganglionic sympathetic neurons release norepinephrine, which interacts with **β-adrenergic receptors** on the acinar and ductal cells. Activation of β-adrenergic receptors leads to stimulation of adenylyl cyclase and production of **cyclic adenosine monophosphate (cAMP).**

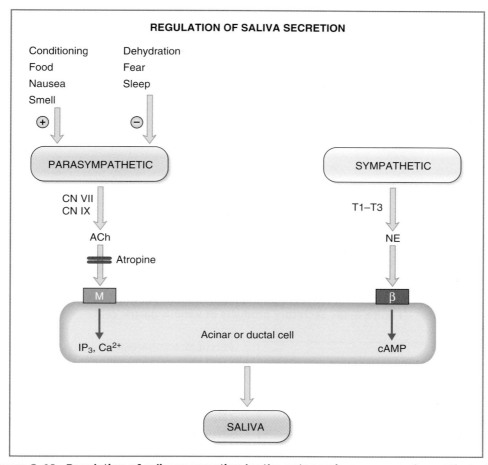

Figure 8–14 **Regulation of salivary secretion by the autonomic nervous system.** ACh, Acetylcholine; β, β receptor; cAMP, cyclic adenosine monophosphate; CN, cranial nerve; M, muscarinic receptor; NE, norepinephrine; T1–T3, thoracic segments.

The physiologic action of cAMP, like that of the parasympathetic IP_3/Ca^{2+} mechanism, is to increase saliva secretion. Sympathetic stimulation also activates α-adrenergic receptors on acinar cells, although the activation of β-adrenergic receptors is considered more important.

Gastric Secretion

The cells of the gastric mucosa secrete a fluid called **gastric juice.** The four major components of gastric juice are hydrochloric acid (HCl), pepsinogen, intrinsic factor, and mucus. Together, **HCl** and **pepsinogen** initiate the process of protein digestion. **Intrinsic factor** is required for the absorption of vitamin B_{12} in the ileum, and it is the only *essential* component of gastric juice. **Mucus** protects the gastric mucosa from the corrosive action of HCl and also lubricates the gastric contents.

Structure and Cell Types of the Gastric Mucosa

The anatomic divisions of the stomach (fundus, body, and antrum) have been discussed in the section on motility. In addition to these gross anatomic divisions, the gastric mucosa contains several cell types that secrete the various components of gastric juice. The cell types and their secretory products are illustrated in Figure 8-15.

The body of the stomach contains **oxyntic glands** that empty their secretory products, via ducts, into the lumen of the stomach (Fig. 8-16). The openings of the ducts on the gastric mucosa are called pits, which are lined with epithelial cells. Deeper in the gland are mucous neck cells, parietal (oxyntic) cells, and chief (peptic) cells. The **parietal cells** have two secretory products, HCl and intrinsic factor. The **chief cells** have one secretory product, pepsinogen.

The antrum of the stomach contains the **pyloric glands,** which are configured similar to the oxyntic glands but with deeper pits. The pyloric glands contain two cell types: the G cells and the mucous cells. The **G cells** secrete gastrin, not into the pyloric ducts but *into the circulation.* The **mucous neck cells** secrete mucus, HCO_3^-, and pepsinogen. Mucus and HCO_3^- have a protective, neutralizing effect on the gastric mucosa.

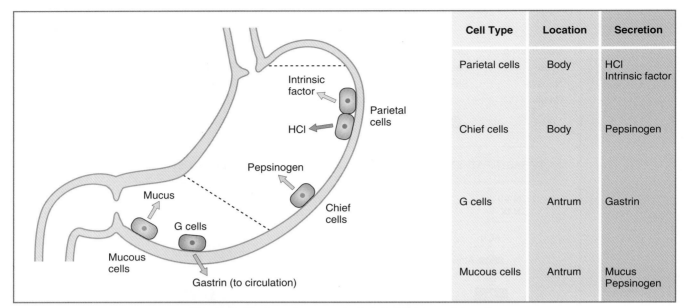

Cell Type	Location	Secretion
Parietal cells	Body	HCl Intrinsic factor
Chief cells	Body	Pepsinogen
G cells	Antrum	Gastrin
Mucous cells	Antrum	Mucus Pepsinogen

Figure 8–15 Secretory products of various gastric cells.

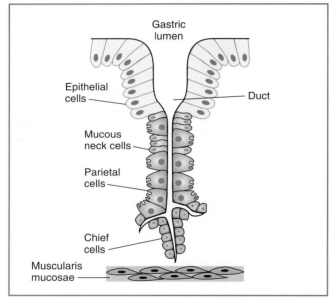

Figure 8–16 Structure of a gastric oxyntic gland showing the various cell types lining the gland. The ducts open into pits on the surface of the gastric mucosa.

HCl Secretion

A major function of the **parietal cells** is secretion of **HCl,** which acidifies the gastric contents to between pH 1 and 2. Physiologically, the function of this low gastric pH is to convert *inactive* pepsinogen, which is secreted by the nearby chief cells, to its *active* form, pepsin, a protease that begins the process of protein digestion. The cellular mechanism of HCl secretion by parietal cells will be described first, followed by discussion of the mechanisms that regulate HCl secretion and the pathophysiology of H+ secretion.

CELLULAR MECHANISM

The cellular mechanism of HCl secretion by gastric parietal cells is illustrated in Figure 8-17. As in renal cells, the cell membranes facing the lumen of the stomach are called the apical or luminal membranes and the cell membranes facing the bloodstream are called the basolateral membranes. The **apical membranes** contain H+-K+ ATPase and Cl− channels, and the **basolateral membranes** contain Na+-K+ ATPase and Cl−-HCO3− exchangers. The cells contain carbonic anhydrase.

HCl secretion is illustrated in Figure 8-17 and is described as follows:

1. In intracellular fluid, carbon dioxide (CO_2) produced from aerobic metabolism combines with H_2O to form H_2CO_3, catalyzed by **carbonic anhydrase.** H_2CO_3 dissociates into H+ and HCO3−. The H+ is secreted with Cl− into the lumen of the stomach, and the HCO3− is absorbed into the blood, as described in steps 2 and 3, respectively.

2. At the **apical membrane,** H+ is secreted into the lumen of the stomach via the **H+-K+ ATPase.** The H+-K+ ATPase is a primary active process that transports H+ and K+ against their electrochemical gradients (uphill). H+-K+ ATPase is inhibited by the drug **omeprazole,** which is used in the treatment of ulcers to reduce H+ secretion. Cl− follows H+ into the lumen by diffusing through **Cl− channels** in the apical membrane.

3. At the **basolateral membrane,** HCO3− is absorbed from the cell into the blood via a Cl−-HCO3− exchanger. The absorbed HCO3− is responsible for the "alkaline tide" (high pH) that can be observed

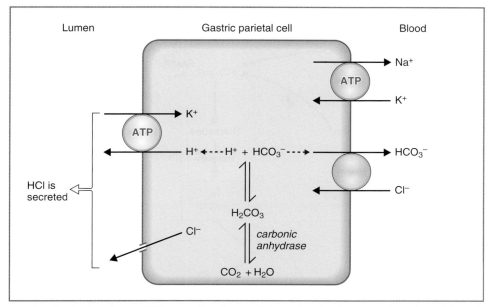

Figure 8–17 **Mechanism of HCl secretion by gastric parietal cells.** ATP, Adenosine triphosphate.

in gastric venous blood after a meal. Eventually, this HCO_3^- will be secreted back into the gastrointestinal tract in pancreatic secretions.

4. In combination, the events occurring at the apical and basolateral membranes of gastric parietal cells result in **net secretion of HCl** and **net absorption of HCO_3^-.**

SUBSTANCES THAT ALTER HCL SECRETION

Three substances stimulate H^+ secretion by gastric parietal cells: histamine (a paracrine), ACh (a neurocrine), and gastrin (a hormone). Each substance binds to a different receptor on the parietal cell and has a different cellular mechanism of action (Fig. 8-18). In addition, there are indirect effects of ACh and gastrin via stimulation of histamine release.

♦ **Histamine** is released from enterochromaffin-like (ECL) cells in the gastric mucosa and diffuses via a paracrine mechanism to the nearby parietal cells, where it binds to **H_2 receptors.** The second messenger for histamine is **cAMP.** Histamine binds to H_2 receptors, which are coupled to adenylyl cyclase by a G_s protein. When adenylyl cyclase is activated, there is increased production of cAMP. cAMP activates protein kinase A, leading to secretion of H^+ by the parietal cells. **Cimetidine** blocks H_2 receptors and blocks the action of histamine on parietal cells.

♦ **ACh** is released from vagus nerves innervating the gastric mucosa and binds directly to **muscarinic (M_3) receptors** on the parietal cells. The second messengers for ACh are **IP_3/Ca^{2+}.** When ACh binds to muscarinic receptors, phospholipase C is activated.

Phospholipase C liberates diacylglycerol and IP_3 from membrane phospholipids, and IP_3 then releases Ca^{2+} from intracellular stores. Ca^{2+} and diacylglycerol activate protein kinases that produce the final physiologic action: H^+ secretion by the parietal cells. **Atropine** blocks muscarinic receptors on parietal cells and, accordingly, blocks the action of ACh.

ACh also increases H^+ secretion indirectly by stimulating ECL cells to release histamine, which then acts on the parietal cells as described earlier.

♦ **Gastrin** is secreted into the circulation by G cells in the stomach antrum. Gastrin reaches the parietal cells by an endocrine mechanism, *not* by local diffusion within the stomach. Thus, gastrin is secreted from the stomach antrum into the systemic circulation and then delivered *back* to the stomach via the circulation. Gastrin binds to cholecystokinin B (CCK_B) receptors on the parietal cells. (The CCK_B receptor has equal affinity for gastrin and CCK, whereas the CCK_A receptor is specific for CCK.) Like ACh, gastrin stimulates H^+ secretion through the **IP_3/Ca^{2+}** second messenger system. The stimuli that trigger gastrin secretion from the G cells are discussed in detail subsequently. Briefly, these stimuli are distention of the stomach, presence of small peptides and amino acids, and stimulation of the vagus nerves.

Like ACh, gastrin also stimulates H^+ secretion indirectly by causing release of histamine from ECL cells.

The rate of H^+ secretion is regulated by the independent actions of histamine, ACh, and gastrin, as well as by *interactions* among the three agents. The interaction

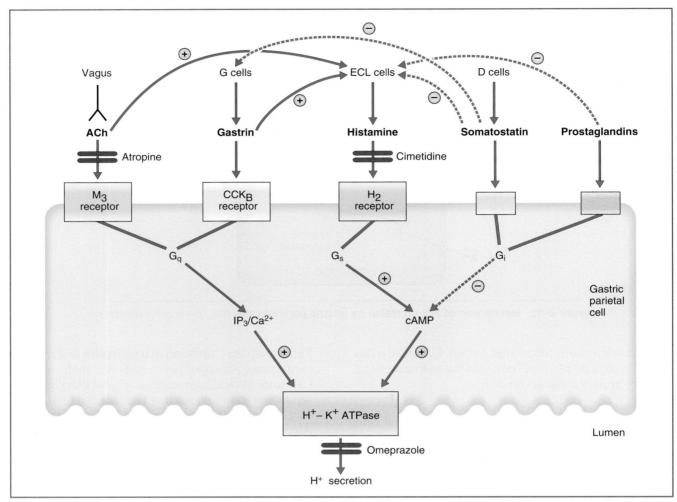

Figure 8–18 **Agents that stimulate and inhibit H⁺ secretion by gastric parietal cells.** ACh, Acetyl-choline; cAMP, cyclic adenosine monophosphate; CCK, cholecystokinin; ECL, enterochromaffin-like; IP₃, inositol 1,4,5-triphosphate; M, muscarinic.

is called **potentiation,** which refers to the ability of two stimuli to produce a combined response that is greater than the sum of the individual responses. One explanation for potentiation in the parietal cells is that each agent stimulates H⁺ secretion via a different receptor and, in the case of histamine, a different second messenger. Another explanation derives from the fact that both ACh and gastrin stimulate histamine release from ECL cells and thereby induce H⁺ secretion by a second, indirect, route. This phenomenon of potentiation has consequences for the actions of the various drugs that inhibit H⁺ secretion. For example, because histamine potentiates the actions of ACh and gastrin, H₂ receptor–blocking agents such as **cimetidine** have a greater effect than expected: They block the direct action of histamine *and* they also block the histamine-potentiated effects of ACh and gastrin. In another example, ACh potentiates the actions of histamine and gastrin. A consequence of this potentiation is that

muscarinic-blocking agents such as **atropine** block the direct effects of ACh *and* the ACh-potentiated effects of histamine and gastrin.

STIMULATION OF H⁺ SECRETION

Having established that histamine, ACh, and gastrin all stimulate HCl secretion by parietal cells, the control of HCl secretion in response to a meal now can be discussed in an integrated fashion. Figure 8-19 depicts the gastric parietal cells, which secrete HCl, and the G cells, which secrete gastrin. Vagus nerves innervate parietal cells directly, where they release ACh as the neurotransmitter. Vagus nerves also innervate G cells, where they release GRP as the neurotransmitter.

As shown in Figure 8-19, the second path, the G cell path, provides an *indirect* route for vagal stimulation of the parietal cells: Vagal stimulation releases gastrin from the G cells, and gastrin enters the systemic circulation and is delivered back to the stomach to stimulate

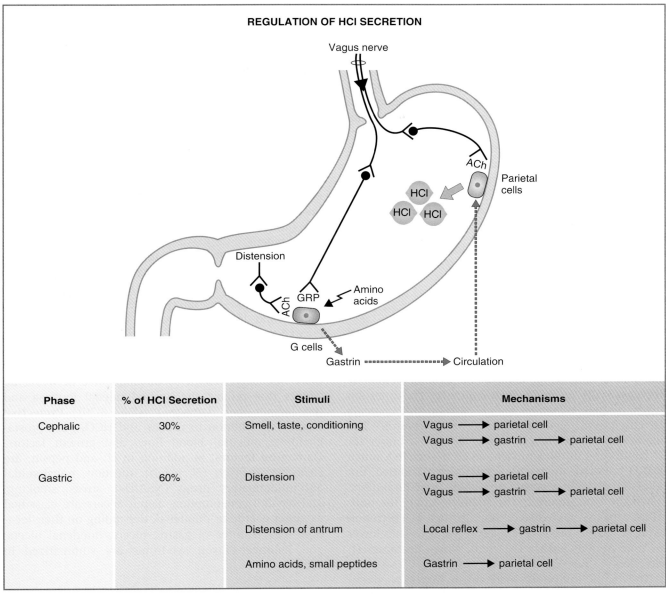

REGULATION OF HCl SECRETION

Phase	% of HCl Secretion	Stimuli	Mechanisms
Cephalic	30%	Smell, taste, conditioning	Vagus ⟶ parietal cell Vagus ⟶ gastrin ⟶ parietal cell
Gastric	60%	Distension	Vagus ⟶ parietal cell Vagus ⟶ gastrin ⟶ parietal cell
		Distension of antrum	Local reflex ⟶ gastrin ⟶ parietal cell
		Amino acids, small peptides	Gastrin ⟶ parietal cell

Figure 8–19 **Regulation of HCl secretion during cephalic and gastric phases.** ACh, Acetylcholine; GRP, gastrin-releasing peptide (bombesin).

H⁺ secretion by the parietal cells. One consequence of this dual action of vagal stimulation is that muscarinic-blocking agents such as **atropine** do not block HCl secretion completely. Atropine *will* block the direct vagal effects on the parietal cells, which are mediated by ACh, but it *will not* block the vagal effects on gastrin secretion because the neurotransmitter at the synapses on G cells is GRP, not ACh.

Gastric HCl secretion is divided into three phases: cephalic, gastric, and intestinal. The cephalic and gastric phases are illustrated in Figure 8-19.

♦ The **cephalic phase** accounts for approximately **30%** of the total HCl secreted in response to a meal. The stimuli for HCl secretion in the cephalic phase are **smelling** and **tasting,** chewing, swallowing, and **conditioned reflexes** in anticipation of food. Two mechanisms promote HCl secretion in the cephalic phase. The first mechanism is direct stimulation of the parietal cell by vagus nerves, which release ACh. The second mechanism is indirect stimulation of the parietal cells by gastrin. In the indirect path, vagus nerves release GRP at the G cells, stimulating gastrin secretion; gastrin enters the circulation and stimulates the parietal cells to secrete HCl.

♦ The **gastric phase** accounts for approximately **60%** of the total HCl secreted in response to a meal. The stimuli for HCl secretion in the gastric phase are **distention** of the stomach and the presence of breakdown products of protein, **amino acids and small peptides.** Four physiologic mechanisms are involved in the gastric phase. The first two mechanisms, which are initiated by distention of the stomach, are similar to those utilized in the cephalic phase: Distention causes direct vagal stimulation of the parietal cells and indirect stimulation of the parietal cells via gastrin release. The third mechanism is initiated by distention of the stomach antrum and involves local reflexes that stimulate gastrin release. The fourth mechanism is a direct effect of amino acids and small peptides on the G cells to stimulate gastrin release. In addition to these physiologic mechanisms, **alcohol** and **caffeine** also stimulate gastric HCl secretion.

♦ The **intestinal phase** accounts for only **10%** of HCl secretion (not shown in Figure 8-19) and is mediated by products of protein digestion.

INHIBITION OF HCL SECRETION

HCl secretion is inhibited when HCl is no longer needed for the activation of pepsinogen to pepsin (i.e., when chyme has moved to the small intestine). Logically, the major inhibitory control of HCl secretion is **decreased pH** of the gastric contents. The question arises, though: *Why does the pH of the gastric contents decrease when chyme moves to the small intestine?* The answer lies in the fact that food is itself a buffer for H^+. With food in the stomach, as H^+ is secreted, much of it is buffered; the gastric contents are acidified, but not as much as they would be if there were no buffers. When the food moves to the small intestine, the buffering capacity is reduced, and further H^+ secretion reduces gastric pH to even lower values. This lower pH then inhibits gastrin secretion, which decreases H^+ secretion.

The major inhibitory mechanism for H^+ secretion by parietal cells involves **somatostatin.** Somatostatin inhibits gastric H^+ secretion through both a direct pathway and indirect pathways (see Fig. 8-18). In the **direct pathway,**, somatostatin binds to receptors on parietal cells that are coupled to adenylyl cyclase via a G_i protein. When somatostatin binds to its receptor, G_i is activated, adenylyl cyclase is inhibited, and cAMP levels are reduced; in this way, somatostatin antagonizes the stimulatory effect of histamine on H^+ secretion. In the **indirect pathways,** somatostatin inhibits both histamine release from ECL cells and gastrin release from G cells; the net result of these indirect actions is to reduce the stimulatory actions of histamine and gastrin. In similar fashion to somatostatin, **prostaglandins** also antagonize histamine's stimulatory action on H^+ secretion by activating a G_i protein and inhibiting adenylyl cyclase (see Fig. 8-18).

PEPTIC ULCER DISEASE

It seems that the gastric mucosal epithelium would be in direct contact with potentially damaging gastric luminal contents—the gastric contents are very acidic and contain the digestive enzyme pepsin. What prevents the gastric contents from eroding and digesting the mucosal epithelial cells? First, mucous neck glands secrete **mucus,** which forms a gel-like protective barrier between the cells and the gastric lumen. Second, gastric epithelial cells secrete HCO_3^-, which is trapped in the mucus. Should any H^+ penetrate the mucus, it is neutralized by HCO_3^- before reaching the epithelial cells. Furthermore, should any pepsin penetrate the mucus, it is inactivated in the relatively alkaline (high HCO_3^-) environment.

Peptic ulcer disease is an ulcerative lesion of the gastric or duodenal mucosa. The ulceration is caused by the erosive and digestive action of H^+ and pepsin on the mucosa (normally protected by the layer of mucus and HCO_3^-). Thus, for a peptic ulcer to be created there must be (1) loss of the protective mucous barrier, (2) excessive H^+ and pepsin secretion, or (3) a combination of the two. Stated differently, peptic ulcer disease is caused by an imbalance between the factors that protect the gastroduodenal mucosa and the factors that damage it (Fig. 8-20). **Protective factors,** in addition to mucus and HCO_3^-, are prostaglandins, mucosal blood flow, and growth factors. **Damaging factors,** in addition to H^+ and pepsin, are *Helicobacter pylori* (*H. pylori*) infection, nonsteroidal anti-inflammatory drugs (NSAIDs), stress, smoking, and alcohol consumption. Peptic ulcers are classified as either gastric or duodenal, depending on their location. The features of gastric ulcers, duodenal ulcers, and Zollinger-Ellison syndrome are summarized in Table 8-4.

♦ **Gastric ulcers.** Gastric ulcers form primarily because the mucosal barrier is defective, which allows H^+ and pepsin to digest a portion of the mucosa. A major causative factor in gastric ulcers is the **gram-negative bacterium *H. pylori*.** In producing gastric ulcer, the causation is fairly direct: *H. pylori* colonizes the gastric mucus (often in the antrum), attaches to gastric epithelial cells, and releases cytotoxins (e.g., cagA toxin) that break down the protective mucous barrier and the underlying cells. *H. pylori* is allowed to colonize the gastric mucus because it contains the enzyme **urease,** which converts urea to NH_3. The NH_3 generated alkalinizes the local environment, permitting the bacteria to survive in the otherwise acidic gastric lumen. Because the local environment is hospitable, the bacteria bind to the gastric epithelium instead of being shed. An additional damaging factor is NH_4^+, which is in

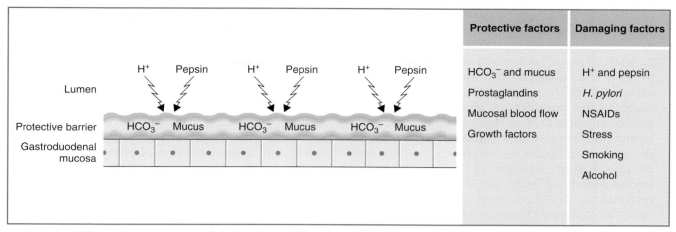

Figure 8-20 **Balance of protective and damaging factors on gastroduodenal mucosa.** *H. pylori,* Helicobacter pylori; NSAIDs, nonsteroidal anti-inflammatory drugs.

Table 8-4 Disorders of Gastric H⁺ Secretion

Disorder	H⁺ Secretion	Gastrin Levels	Comments
Gastric ulcer	↓	↑ (because of decreased H⁺ secretion)	Causes damage to protective barrier of gastric mucosa
Duodenal ulcer	↑	↑ (gastrin response to ingestion of food)	Increased parietal cell mass due to increased gastrin levels
Zollinger-Ellison syndrome	↑↑	↑↑	Gastrin is secreted by pancreatic tumor Increased parietal cell mass due to trophic effect of increased gastrin levels

equilibrium with NH_3. A **diagnostic test** for *H. pylori* is based on its urease activity. In the test, the patient drinks a solution containing ^{13}C-urea, which is converted to $^{13}CO_2$ and NH_3 in the stomach; the $^{13}CO_2$ is absorbed into blood, expired by the lungs, and measured in a breath test. Surprisingly, in persons with gastric ulcers, net H⁺ secretory rates are lower than normal because some of the secreted H⁺ leaks into the damaged mucosa. In gastric ulcer disease, the secretion rate of gastrin is increased as a result of the reduced net H⁺ secretion. (Recall that gastrin secretion is inhibited by H⁺.)

♦ **Duodenal ulcers.** Duodenal ulcers are more common than gastric ulcers and form because H⁺ secretory rates are higher than normal. If excess H⁺ is delivered to the duodenum, it may overwhelm the buffering capacity of HCO_3^- in pancreatic juice. Acting with pepsin, this excess H⁺ digests and damages the duodenal mucosa. *H. pylori* infection also causes duodenal ulcer, but its role is indirect. (If the bacteria colonize *gastric* mucosa, how do they cause *duodenal* ulcer?) (1) As described previously, *H. pylori* colonizes gastric mucus. One consequence of this colonization is to **inhibit somatostatin secretion**

from D cells in the gastric antrum. Because somatostatin normally inhibits gastrin secretion from G cells, "inhibition of inhibition" results in increased gastrin secretion, which leads to increased H⁺ secretion by gastric parietal cells. In this way, there is an increased H⁺ load delivered to the duodenum. (2) The gastric *H. pylori* infection spreads to the duodenum and **inhibits duodenal HCO_3^- secretion.** Normally, duodenal HCO_3^- is sufficient to neutralize the H⁺ load delivered from the stomach. However, in this case, not only is excess H⁺ delivered to the duodenum, but less HCO_3^- is secreted to neutralize it. In summary, neutralization of H⁺ in the duodenum is insufficient, the duodenal contents become abnormally acidic, and there is an erosive action of H⁺ and pepsin on the duodenal mucosa. In persons with duodenal ulcers, baseline gastrin levels may be normal, but gastrin secretion in response to a meal is increased. The increased gastrin levels also exert a trophic effect on the stomach, which increases parietal cell mass.

♦ **Zollinger-Ellison syndrome (gastrinoma).** The highest rates of H⁺ secretion are those seen in Zollinger-Ellison syndrome, in which a tumor (usually in the pancreas) secretes large quantities of gastrin. The high levels of gastrin have two direct effects: increased H⁺ secretion by parietal cells and increased parietal cell mass. The delivery of excessive amounts of H⁺ to the duodenum overwhelms the buffering capacity of HCO_3^- in pancreatic juices, erodes the mucosa, and produces an **ulcer.** Delivery of increased amounts of H⁺ to the duodenum also causes **steatorrhea** because low duodenal pH inactivates the pancreatic lipases necessary for fat digestion. Because gastrin secretion by the tumor is *not* feedback-inhibited by H⁺ (as is physiologic gastrin secretion by G cells), it continues unabated. Treatment of Zollinger-Ellison syndrome includes inhibitors of H⁺ secretion such as **cimetidine** and **omeprazole** and surgical removal of the tumor.

Pepsinogen Secretion

Pepsinogen, the inactive precursor to pepsin, is secreted by chief cells and by mucous cells in the oxyntic glands. When the pH of gastric contents is lowered by H⁺ secretion from parietal cells, pepsinogen is converted to pepsin, beginning the process of protein digestion. In the cephalic and gastric phases of H⁺ secretion, **vagal stimulation** is the most important stimulus for pepsinogen secretion. H⁺ also triggers local reflexes, which stimulate the chief cells to secrete pepsinogen. These complementary reflexes ensure that pepsinogen is secreted only when the gastric pH is low enough to convert it to pepsin.

Intrinsic Factor Secretion

Intrinsic factor, a mucoprotein, is the "other" secretory product of the parietal cells. Intrinsic factor is required for absorption of vitamin B_{12} in the ileum, and its absence causes **pernicious anemia.** Intrinsic factor is the only *essential* secretion of the stomach. Thus, following gastrectomy (removal of the stomach), patients must receive injections of vitamin B_{12} to bypass the absorption defect caused by the loss of gastric intrinsic factor.

Pancreatic Secretion

The exocrine pancreas secretes approximately 1 L of fluid per day into the lumen of the duodenum. The secretion consists of an aqueous component that is high in HCO_3^- and an enzymatic component. The HCO_3^--containing aqueous portion functions to neutralize the H⁺ delivered to the duodenum from the stomach. The **enzymatic portion** functions to digest carbohydrates, proteins, and lipids into absorbable molecules.

Structure of the Pancreatic Exocrine Glands

The exocrine pancreas constitutes approximately 90% of the pancreas. The rest of the pancreatic tissue is the endocrine pancreas (2%), blood vessels, and interstitial fluid. (The endocrine pancreas is discussed in Chapter 9.)

The exocrine pancreas is organized much like the salivary glands: It resembles a bunch of grapes, with each grape corresponding to a single acinus (Fig. 8-21). The **acinus,** which is the blind end of a branching duct system, is lined with acinar cells that secrete the enzymatic portion of the pancreatic secretion. The ducts are lined with **ductal cells.** Ductal epithelial cells extend into a special region of **centroacinar cells** in the acinus. The centroacinar and ductal cells secrete the aqueous HCO_3^--containing component of the pancreatic secretion.

The exocrine pancreas is innervated by both parasympathetic and sympathetic nervous systems. Sympathetic innervation is provided by postganglionic nerves from the celiac and superior mesenteric plexuses. Parasympathetic innervation is provided by the vagus nerve; parasympathetic preganglionic fibers synapse in the enteric nervous system, and postganglionic fibers synapse on the exocrine pancreas. **Parasympathetic** activity stimulates pancreatic secretion, and **sympathetic** activity inhibits pancreatic secretion. (Contrast the exocrine pancreas with the salivary glands, in which both parasympathetic and sympathetic activity are stimulatory.)

Formation of Pancreatic Secretion

The enzymatic and aqueous components of pancreatic secretion are produced by separate mechanisms. Enzymes are secreted by the acinar cells, and the aqueous component is secreted by the centroacinar cells and then modified by the ductal cells.

Pancreatic secretion occurs in the following steps and is illustrated in Figure 8-21:

1. **Enzymatic component of pancreatic secretion (acinar cells).** Most of the enzymes required for digestion of carbohydrates, proteins, and lipids are secreted by the pancreas (Table 8-5). Pancreatic **amylase** and **lipases** are secreted as active enzymes. Pancreatic **proteases** are secreted in inactive forms and converted to their active forms in the lumen of the duodenum; for example, the pancreas secretes trypsinogen, which is converted in the intestinal lumen to its active form, trypsin. The functions of the pancreatic enzymes are discussed later in the chapter in the section on digestion of nutrients.

   The pancreatic enzymes are synthesized on the **rough endoplasmic reticulum** of the acinar cells. They are transferred to the Golgi complex and then to condensing vacuoles, where they are concentrated in zymogen granules. The enzymes are stored in the zymogen granules until a stimulus (e.g., parasympathetic activity or CCK) triggers their secretion.

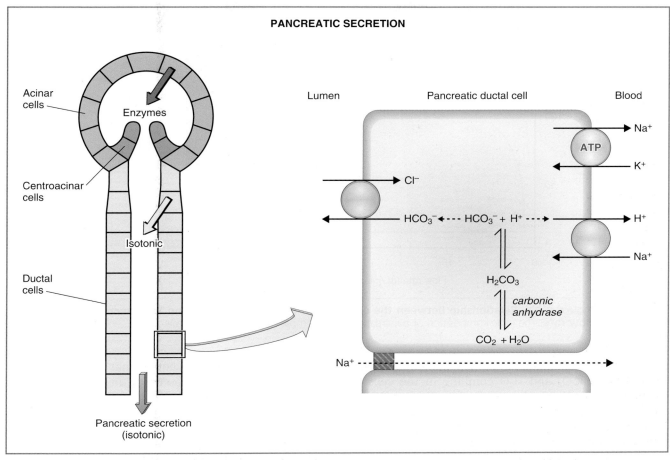

Figure 8-21 Mechanism of pancreatic secretion. The enzymatic component is produced by acinar cells, and the aqueous component is produced by centroacinar and ductal cells. ATP, Adenosine triphosphate.

Table 8-5 Sources of Digestive Enzymes

Nutrient Group	Saliva	Stomach	Pancreas	Intestinal Mucosa
Carbohydrates	Amylase	—	Amylase	Sucrase Maltase Lactase Trehalase α-Dextrinase
Proteins	—	Pepsin	Trypsin Chymotrypsin Carboxypeptidase Elastase	Amino-oligopeptidase Dipeptidase Enterokinase
Lipids	Lingual lipase	—	Lipase-colipase Phospholipase A_2 Cholesterol ester hydrolase	—

2. **Aqueous component of pancreatic secretion (centroacinar and ductal cells).** Pancreatic juice is an isotonic solution containing Na^+, Cl^-, K^+, and HCO_3^- (in addition to the enzymes). The Na^+ and K^+ concentrations are the same as their concentrations in plasma, but the Cl^- and HCO_3^- concentrations vary with pancreatic flow rate.

Centroacinar and ductal cells produce the initial aqueous secretion, which is **isotonic** and contains Na^+, K^+, Cl^-, and HCO_3^-. This initial secretion is then modified by transport processes in the ductal epithelial cells as follows: The apical membrane of ductal cells contains a Cl^--HCO_3^- exchanger, and the basolateral membrane contains Na^+-K^+ ATPase and

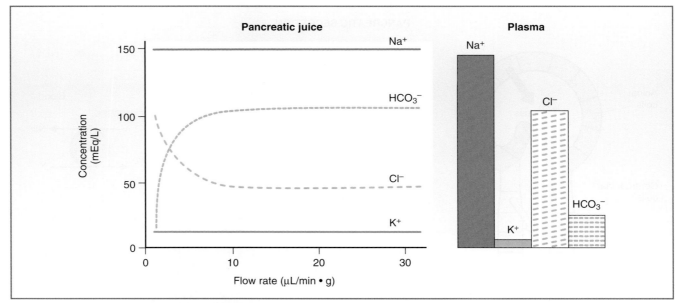

Figure 8–22 **Relationship between the composition of pancreatic juice and the pancreatic flow rate.** The ionic composition of pancreatic juice is compared with that of plasma.

an Na^+-H^+ exchanger. In the presence of carbonic anhydrase, CO_2 and H_2O combine in the cells to form H_2CO_3. H_2CO_3 dissociates into H^+ and HCO_3^-. The HCO_3^- is secreted into pancreatic juice by the Cl^--HCO_3^- exchanger in the apical membrane. The H^+ is transported into the blood by the Na^+-H^+ exchanger in the basolateral membrane. The net result, or sum, of these transport processes is net secretion of HCO_3^- into pancreatic ductal juice and net absorption of H^+; absorption of H^+ causes acidification of pancreatic venous blood.

Effect of Flow Rate on Composition of Pancreatic Juice

When the pancreatic flow rate changes, the Na^+ and K^+ concentrations in pancreatic juice remain constant, whereas the concentrations of HCO_3^- and Cl^- change (Fig. 8-22). (Recall that a similar, but not identical, relationship is observed between saliva composition and salivary flow rate.) In pancreatic juice, there is a reciprocal relationship between the Cl^- and HCO_3^- concentrations, which is maintained by the Cl^--HCO_3^- exchanger in the apical membrane of ductal cells (see Fig. 8-21). At the highest pancreatic flow rates (more than 30 $\mu L/min \cdot g$), the HCO_3^- concentration of pancreatic juice is highest (and much higher than plasma HCO_3^-) and the Cl^- concentration is lowest. At the lowest flow rates, HCO_3^- is lowest and Cl^- is highest.

The relationship between flow rate and the relative concentrations of Cl^- and HCO_3^- is explained as follows: At low (basal) rates of pancreatic secretion, the pancreatic cells secrete an isotonic solution composed mainly of Na^+, Cl^-, and H_2O. However, when stimulated (e.g., by secretin), the centroacinar and ductal cells secrete even greater amounts of an isotonic solution with a different composition, mainly Na^+, HCO_3^-, and H_2O.

Regulation of Pancreatic Secretion

Pancreatic secretion has two functions: (1) to secrete the enzymes necessary for digestion of carbohydrates, proteins, and lipids; the enzymatic portion of pancreatic secretion performs these digestive functions; and (2) to neutralize H^+ in the chyme delivered to the duodenum from the stomach. The aqueous portion of pancreatic secretion contains HCO_3^-, which performs the neutralizing function. Therefore, it is logical that the enzymatic and aqueous portions are regulated separately: The aqueous secretion is stimulated by the arrival of H^+ in the duodenum, and the enzymatic secretion is stimulated by products of digestion (small peptides, amino acids, and fatty acids).

Like gastric secretion, pancreatic secretion is divided into cephalic, gastric, and intestinal phases. In the pancreas, the cephalic and gastric phases are less important than the intestinal phase. Briefly, the **cephalic phase** is initiated by smell, taste, and conditioning and is mediated by the vagus nerve. The cephalic phase produces mainly an enzymatic secretion. The **gastric phase** is initiated by distention of the stomach and is also mediated by the vagus nerve. The gastric phase produces mainly an enzymatic secretion.

The **intestinal phase** is the most important phase and accounts for approximately **80%** of the pancreatic secretion. During this phase, *both* enzymatic and aqueous secretions are stimulated. The hormonal and

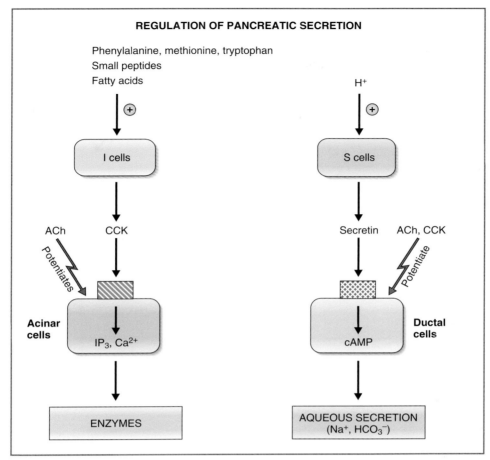

REGULATION OF PANCREATIC SECRETION

Phenylalanine, methionine, tryptophan
Small peptides
Fatty acids

H⁺

I cells

S cells

ACh   CCK   Potentiates

Secretin   ACh, CCK   Potentiate

Acinar cells

IP_3, Ca^{2+}

Ductal cells

cAMP

ENZYMES

AQUEOUS SECRETION
(Na^+, HCO_3^-)

Figure 8–23 **Regulation of pancreatic secretion.** ACh, Acetylcholine; cAMP, cyclic adenosine mono-phosphate; CCK, cholecystokinin; IP_3, inositol 1,4,5-triphosphate.

neural regulation of the acinar and ductal cells in the intestinal phase is shown in Figure 8-23.

♦ **Acinar cells (enzymatic secretion).** The pancreatic acinar cells have receptors for CCK (CCK_A receptors) and muscarinic receptors for ACh. During the intestinal phase, **CCK** is the most important stimulant for the enzymatic secretion. The I cells are stimulated to secrete CCK by the presence of amino acids, small peptides, and fatty acids in the intestinal lumen. Of the amino acids stimulating CCK secretion, phenyl-alanine, methionine, and tryptophan are most potent. In addition, **ACh** stimulates enzyme secre-tion and potentiates the action of CCK by vagovagal reflexes.

♦ **Ductal cells (aqueous secretion of Na^+, HCO_3^-, and H_2O).** The pancreatic ductal cells have receptors for CCK, ACh, and secretin. **Secretin,** which is secreted by the S cells of the duodenum, is the major stimu-lant of the aqueous HCO_3^--rich secretion. Secretin is secreted in response to H⁺ in the lumen of the intes-tine, which signals the arrival of acidic chyme from the stomach. To ensure that pancreatic lipases will

be active (because they are inactivated at low pH), the acidic chyme requires rapid neutralization by the HCO_3^--containing pancreatic juice. The effects of secretin are potentiated by both CCK and ACh.

Bile Secretion

Bile is necessary for the **digestion and absorption of lipids** in the small intestine. Compared with carbohy-drates and proteins, lipids pose special problems for digestion and absorption because they are insoluble in water. Bile, a mixture of bile salts, bile pigments, and cholesterol, solves this problem of insolubility. Bile is produced and secreted by the liver, stored in the gall-bladder, and ejected into the lumen of the small intes-tine when the gallbladder is stimulated to contract. In the lumen of the intestine, bile salts emulsify lipids to prepare them for digestion and then solubilize the prod-ucts of lipid digestion in packets called micelles.

Overview of the Biliary System

The components of the biliary system are the liver, gallbladder and bile duct, duodenum, ileum, and portal

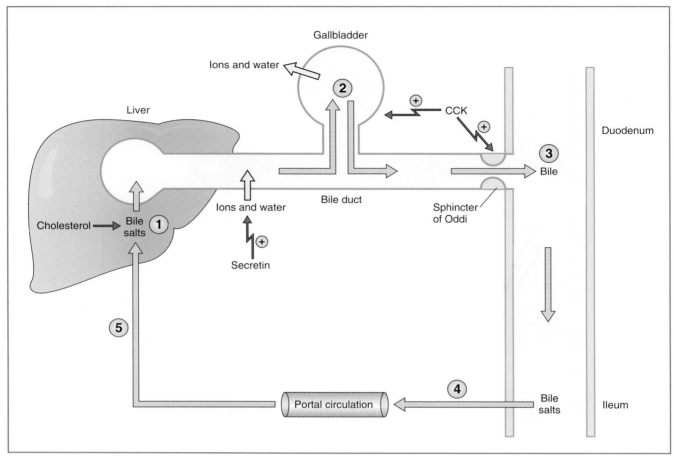

Figure 8-24 **Secretion and enterohepatic circulation of bile salts.** *Light blue arrows* show the path of bile flow; *yellow arrows* show the movement of ions and water. CCK, Cholecystokinin.

circulation, as illustrated in Figure 8-24. An overview of the system is presented in this section, with detailed descriptions of the steps in later sections.

The hepatocytes of the liver continuously synthesize and secrete the constituents of bile (Step 1). The components of bile are the **bile salts,** cholesterol, phospholipids, bile pigments, ions, and water. Bile flows out of the liver through the bile ducts and fills the gallbladder, where it is stored (Step 2). The gallbladder then concentrates the bile salts by absorption of water and ions.

When chyme reaches the small intestine, **CCK** is secreted. CCK has two separate but coordinated actions on the biliary system: It stimulates contraction of the gallbladder and relaxation of the sphincter of Oddi, causing stored bile to flow from the gallbladder into the lumen of the duodenum (Step 3). In the small intestine, the bile salts emulsify and solubilize dietary lipids.

When lipid absorption is complete, the bile salts are recirculated to the liver via the **enterohepatic circulation** (Step 4). The steps involved in the enterohepatic circulation include absorption of bile salts from the ileum into the portal circulation, delivery back to

the liver, and extraction of bile salts from the portal blood by the hepatocytes (Step 5). The recirculation of bile salts to the liver reduces the demand to synthesize *new* bile salt. The liver must replace only the small percentage of the bile salt pool that is excreted in feces.

Composition of Bile

As noted previously, bile is secreted continuously by the hepatocytes. The organic constituents of bile are bile salts (50%), bile pigments such as bilirubin (2%), cholesterol (4%), and phospholipids (40%). Bile also contains electrolytes and water, which are secreted by hepatocytes lining the bile ducts.

♦ **Bile salts** (including bile acids) constitute 50% of the organic component of bile. The total bile salt pool is approximately 2.5 g, which includes bile salts in the liver, bile ducts, gallbladder, and intestine. As shown in Figure 8-25, the hepatocytes synthesize two **primary bile acids** from cholesterol: cholic acid and chenodeoxycholic acid. When these primary bile acids are secreted into the lumen of the intestine, a portion of each is dehydroxylated at

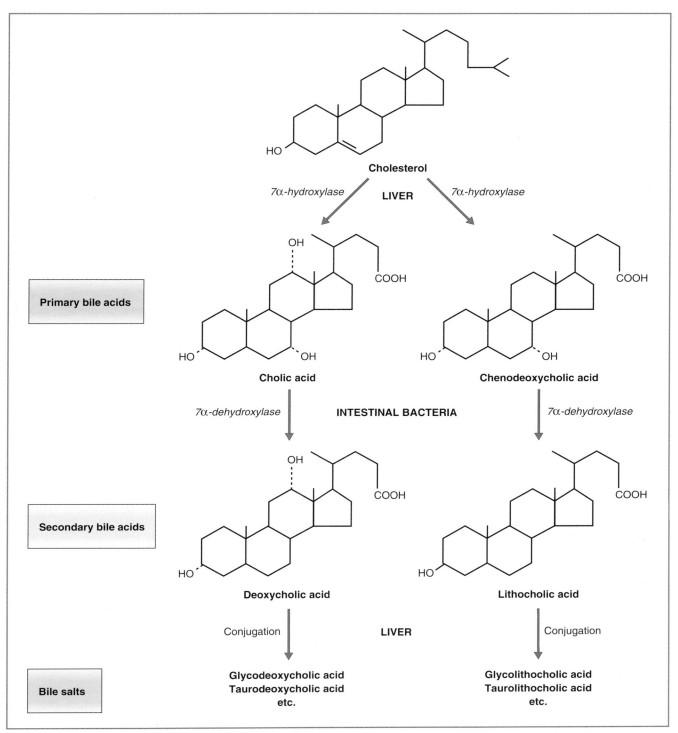

Figure 8-25 **Biosynthetic pathways for bile acids.** The liver conjugates primary and secondary bile acids with glycine or taurine to their respective bile salts. The resulting bile salt is named for the bile acid and the conjugating amino acid (e.g., glycodeoxycholic acid is deoxycholic acid conjugated with glycine).

C-7 by intestinal bacteria to produce two **secondary bile acids,** deoxycholic acid and lithocholic acid. Thus, a total of four bile acids are present in the following relative amounts: Cholic acid > chenodeoxycholic acid > deoxycholic acid > lithocholic acid.

The liver conjugates the bile acids with the amino acids glycine or taurine to form **bile salts.** Consequently, there are a total of eight bile salts, each named for the parent bile acid and the conjugating amino acid (e.g., glycocholic acid, taurocholic acid). This conjugation step changes the pKs of bile acids and causes them to become *much more water soluble,* which is explained as follows: The pH of duodenal contents ranges between pH 3 and 5. Bile acids have pKs of approximately 7. Thus, at duodenal pH, most bile acids will be in their nonionized form, HA, which is insoluble in water. On the other hand, bile salts have pKs ranging between 1 and 4. At duodenal pH, most bile salts will be in their ionized form, A⁻, which is soluble in water. It follows from this discussion that bile salts are more soluble than bile acids in the aqueous duodenal contents. (See Chapter 7 for a discussion of pH and pK.)

The critical property of bile salts is that they are **amphipathic,** meaning the molecules have both hydrophilic (water-soluble) and hydrophobic (lipid-soluble) portions. Hydrophilic, negatively charged groups point outward from a hydrophobic steroid nucleus such that, at an oil-water interface, the hydrophilic portion of a bile salt molecule dissolves in the aqueous phase and the hydrophobic portion dissolves in the oil phase.

The function of bile salts, which depends on their amphipathic properties, is to solubilize dietary lipids. Without the bile salts, lipids would be insoluble in the aqueous solution in the intestinal lumen and less amenable to digestion and absorption. In this regard, the first role of bile salts is to **emulsify** dietary lipids. The negatively charged bile salts surround the lipids, creating small lipid droplets in the intestinal lumen. The negative charges on the bile salts repel each other, so the droplets disperse, rather than coalesce, thereby increasing the surface area for digestive enzymes. (Without emulsification, dietary lipids would coalesce into large "blobs," with relatively little surface area for digestion.) The second role of bile salts is to form **micelles** with the products of lipid digestion including monoglycerides, lysolecithin, and fatty acids. The core of the micelle contains these lipid products, and the surface of the micelle is lined with bile salts. The hydrophobic portions of the bile salt molecules are dissolved in the lipid core of the micelle, and the hydrophilic portions are dissolved in the aqueous solution in the intestinal lumen. In this way,

hydrophobic lipid digestion products are dissolved in an otherwise "unfriendly" aqueous environment. The primary bile salts, having more hydroxyl groups than the secondary bile salts, are more effective at solubilizing lipids.

♦ **Phospholipids** and **cholesterol** also are secreted into bile by the hepatocytes and are included in the micelles with the products of lipid digestion. Like the bile salts, phospholipids are amphipathic and aid the bile salts in forming micelles. The hydrophobic portions of the phospholipids point to the interior of the micelle, and the hydrophilic portions dissolve in the aqueous intestinal solution.

♦ **Bilirubin,** a yellow-colored byproduct of hemoglobin metabolism, is the major bile **pigment.** The cells of the reticuloendothelial system degrade hemoglobin, yielding bilirubin, which is carried in blood bound to albumin. The liver extracts bilirubin from blood and conjugates it with glucuronic acid to form **bilirubin glucuronide,** which is secreted into bile and accounts for bile's yellow color. Bilirubin glucuronide, or conjugated bilirubin, is secreted into the intestine as a component of bile. In the intestinal lumen, bilirubin glucuronide is converted back to bilirubin, which is then converted to **urobilinogen** by the action of intestinal bacteria. A portion of the urobilinogen is recirculated to the liver, a portion is excreted in the urine, and a portion is oxidized to **urobilin** and **stercobilin,** the compounds that give stool its dark color.

♦ **Ions and water** are secreted into bile by epithelial cells lining the bile ducts. The secretory mechanisms are the same as those in the pancreatic ductal cells. Secretin stimulates ion and water secretion by the bile ducts just as it does in the pancreatic ducts.

Function of the Gallbladder

The gallbladder serves the following three functions: It stores bile, it concentrates bile, and when stimulated to contract, it ejects bile into the lumen of the small intestine.

♦ **Filling of the gallbladder.** As previously described, the hepatocytes and ductal cells produce bile continuously. As bile is produced by the liver, it flows through the bile ducts into the gallbladder, where it is stored for later release. During the interdigestive periods, the gallbladder can fill because it is relaxed and the sphincter of Oddi is closed.

♦ **Concentration of bile.** The epithelial cells of the gallbladder absorb ions and water in an isosmotic fashion, similar to the isosmotic reabsorptive process in the proximal tubule of the kidney. Because the organic components of bile are not absorbed, they become concentrated as the isosmotic fluid is removed.

♦ **Ejection of bile.** Ejection of bile from the gallbladder begins within 30 minutes after a meal is ingested. The major stimulus for ejection of bile is CCK, which is secreted by the I cells in response to amino acids, small peptides, and fatty acids. As noted, **CCK** has two simultaneous effects that result in ejection of bile from the gallbladder: (1) **contraction of the gallbladder** and (2) **relaxation of the sphincter of Oddi** (a thickening of the smooth muscle of the bile duct at its entrance to the duodenum). Bile is ejected in pulsatile "spurts," not in a steady stream. The pulsatile pattern is caused by the rhythmic contractions of the duodenum. When the duodenum is relaxed and duodenal pressure is low, bile is ejected; when the duodenum is contracting and duodenal pressure is higher, bile is not ejected against the higher pressure.

Enterohepatic Circulation of Bile Salts

Normally, most of the secreted bile salts are recirculated to the liver via an enterohepatic circulation (meaning circulation between the intestine and the liver), rather than being excreted in feces. The steps involved in the enterohepatic circulation are as follows (see Fig. 8-24):

1. In the **ileum,** the bile salts are transported from the intestinal lumen into the portal blood by **Na⁺-bile salt cotransporters** (Step 4, Fig. 8-24). Significantly, this recirculation step is located in the *terminal* small intestine (ileum), so bile salts are present in high concentration for the *entire* length of small intestine to maximize lipid digestion and absorption.

2. The portal blood carries bile salts to the liver (Step 5, Fig. 8-24).

3. The liver extracts the bile salts from portal blood and adds them to the hepatic bile salt/bile acid pool. Therefore, the liver must replace, by synthesis, only the small percentage of the bile salts that is not recirculated (i.e., excreted in feces); the fecal loss is about **600 mg/day** (out of the total bile salt pool of 2.5 g). The liver "knows" how much new bile acid to synthesize daily because bile acid synthesis is under negative feedback control by the bile salts. The rate-limiting enzyme in the biosynthetic pathway, **cholesterol 7α-hydroxylase,** is inhibited by bile salts. When greater quantities of bile salts are recirculated to the liver, there is decreased demand for synthesis and the enzyme is inhibited. When smaller quantities of bile salts are recirculated, there is increased demand for synthesis and

the enzyme is stimulated. Recirculation of bile salts to the liver also stimulates biliary secretion, which is called a **choleretic effect.**

In persons who have had an **ileal resection** (removal of the ileum), the recirculation of bile salts to the liver is interrupted and large quantities of bile salts are excreted in feces. Excessive fecal loss diminishes the total bile salt/bile acid pool because synthesis of new bile acids, even though it is strongly stimulated, cannot keep pace with the loss. One consequence of decreased bile salt content of bile is impaired absorption of dietary lipids and steatorrhea (Box 8-1).

DIGESTION AND ABSORPTION

Digestion and absorption are the ultimate functions of the gastrointestinal tract.

Digestion is the chemical breakdown of ingested foods into absorbable molecules. The digestive enzymes are secreted in salivary, gastric, and pancreatic juices and also are present on the apical membrane of intestinal epithelial cells. The sources of the various digestive enzymes are summarized in Table 8-5, and the digestive and absorptive functions are summarized in Table 8-6.

Absorption is the movement of nutrients, water, and electrolytes from the lumen of the intestine into the blood. There are two paths for absorption: a cellular path and a paracellular path. In the **cellular** path, the substance must cross the apical (luminal) membrane, enter the intestinal epithelial cell, and then be extruded from the cell across the basolateral membrane into blood. Transporters in the apical and basolateral membranes are responsible for the absorptive processes. In the **paracellular** path, substances move across the tight junctions between intestinal epithelial cells, through the lateral intercellular spaces, and into the blood.

The structure of the intestinal mucosa is ideally suited for absorption of large quantities of nutrients. Structural features called villi and microvilli increase the surface area of the small intestine, maximizing the exposure of nutrients to digestive enzymes and creating a large absorptive surface. The surface of the small intestine is arranged in longitudinal folds, called folds of Kerckring. Fingerlike **villi** project from these folds. The villi are longest in the duodenum, where most digestion and absorption occurs, and shortest in the terminal ileum. The surfaces of the villi are covered with **epithelial cells** (enterocytes) interspersed with mucus-secreting cells (goblet cells). The apical surface of the epithelial cells is further expanded by tiny enfoldings called **microvilli.** This microvillar surface is called the **brush border** because of its "brushlike" appearance under light microscopy. Together, the folds of

BOX 8–1 Clinical Physiology: Resection of the Ileum

DESCRIPTION OF CASE. A 36-year-old woman had 75% of her ileum resected following a perforation caused by severe Crohn disease (chronic inflammatory disease of the intestine). Her postsurgical management included monthly injections of vitamin B_{12}. After surgery, she experienced diarrhea and noted oil droplets in her stool. Her physician prescribed the drug cholestyramine to control her diarrhea, but she continues to have steatorrhea.

EXPLANATION OF CASE. The woman's severe Crohn disease caused an intestinal perforation, which necessitated a subtotal ileectomy, removal of the terminal portion of the small intestine. Consequences of removing the ileum include decreased recirculation of bile acids to the liver and decreased absorption of the intrinsic factor–vitamin B_{12} complex.

In normal persons with an intact ileum, 95% of the bile acids secreted in bile are returned to the liver, via the enterohepatic circulation, rather than being excreted in feces. This recirculation decreases the demand on the liver for the synthesis of new bile acids. In a patient who has had an ileectomy, most of the secreted bile acids are lost in feces, increasing the demand for synthesis of new bile acids. The liver is unable to keep pace with the demand, causing a decrease in the total bile acid pool. Because the pool is decreased, inadequate quantities of bile acids are secreted into the small intestine and both emulsification of dietary lipids for digestion and micelle formation for absorption of lipids are compromised. As a result, dietary lipids are excreted in feces, seen as oil droplets in the stool (steatorrhea).

This patient has lost another important function of the ileum, the absorption of vitamin B_{12}. Normally, the ileum is the site of absorption of the intrinsic factor–vitamin B_{12} complex. Intrinsic factor is secreted by gastric parietal cells, forms a stable complex with dietary vitamin B_{12}, and the complex is absorbed in the ileum. The patient cannot absorb vitamin B_{12} and must receive monthly injections, bypassing the intestinal absorptive pathway.

The woman's diarrhea is caused, in part, by high concentrations of bile acids in the lumen of the colon (because they are not recirculated). Bile acids stimulate cAMP-dependent Cl^- secretion in colonic epithelial cells. When Cl^- secretion is stimulated, Na^+ and water follow Cl^- into the lumen, producing a secretory diarrhea (sometimes called bile acid diarrhea).

TREATMENT. The drug cholestyramine, used to treat bile acid diarrhea, binds bile acids in the colon. In bound form, the bile acids do not stimulate Cl^- secretion or cause secretory diarrhea. However, the woman will continue to have steatorrhea.

Table 8–6 Summary of Mechanisms of Digestion and Absorption of Nutrients

Nutrient	Products of Digestion	Site of Absorption	Mechanism
Carbohydrates	Glucose Galactose Fructose	Small intestine	Na^+-glucose cotransport Na^+-galactose cotransport Facilitated diffusion
Proteins	Amino acids Dipeptides Tripeptides	Small intestine	Na^+-amino acid cotransport H^+-dipeptide cotransport H^+-tripeptide cotransport
Lipids	Fatty acids Monoglycerides Cholesterol	Small intestine	Bile salts form micelles in the small intestine Diffusion of fatty acids, monoglycerides, and cholesterol into intestinal cells Reesterification in the cell to triglycerides and phospholipids Chylomicrons form in the cell (requiring apoprotein) and are transferred to lymph
Fat-soluble vitamins		Small intestine	Micelles form with bile salts and products of lipid digestion Diffusion into the intestinal cell
Water-soluble vitamins Vitamin B_{12}		Small intestine Ileum	Na^+-dependent cotransport Intrinsic factor
Bile salts		Ileum	Na^+–bile salt cotransport
Ca^{2+}		Small intestine	Vitamin D–dependent Ca^{2+}-binding protein
Fe^{2+}	Fe^{3+} reduced to Fe^{2+}	Small intestine	Binds to apoferritin in the intestinal cell Binds to transferrin in blood

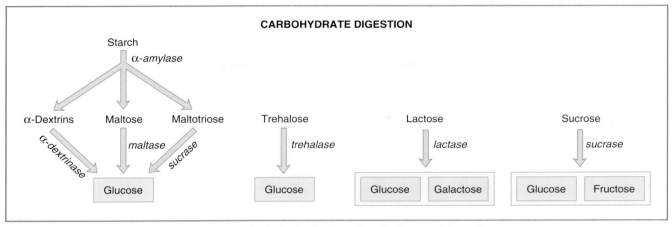

Figure 8-26 **Carbohydrate digestion in the small intestine.**

Kerckring, the villi, and the microvilli increase total surface area by 600-fold!

The epithelial cells of the small intestine have some of the highest turnover rates of any cells in the body—they are replaced every 3 to 6 days. The high turnover rate of the intestinal mucosal cells makes them particularly susceptible to the effects of irradiation and chemotherapy.

Carbohydrates

Carbohydrates constitute about 50% of the typical American diet. Ingested carbohydrates are polysaccharides, disaccharides (sucrose, lactose, maltose, and trehalose), and small amounts of monosaccharides (glucose and fructose).

Digestion of Carbohydrates

Only monosaccharides are absorbed by the intestinal epithelial cells. Therefore, to be absorbed, all ingested carbohydrates must be digested to monosaccharides: glucose, galactose, or fructose. The pathways for carbohydrate digestion are shown in Figure 8-26. Starch is first digested to disaccharides, and then disaccharides are digested to monosaccharides.

Digestion of **starch** begins with **α-amylase.** Salivary amylase starts the process of starch digestion in the mouth; it plays little role overall, however, because it is inactivated by the low pH of the gastric contents. Pancreatic amylase digests interior 1,4-glycosidic bonds in starch, yielding three disaccharides, α-limit dextrins, maltose, and maltotriose. These disaccharides are further digested to monosaccharides by the intestinal brush-border enzymes, **α-dextrinase, maltase,** and **sucrase.** The product of each of these final digestive steps is glucose. Glucose, a monosaccharide, can be absorbed by the epithelial cells.

The three **disaccharides** in food are trehalose, lactose, and sucrose. They do not require the amylase digestive step because they already are in the disaccharide form. Each molecule of disaccharide is digested to two molecules of monosaccharide by the enzymes **trehalase, lactase,** and **sucrase.** Thus, trehalose is digested by trehalase to two molecules of glucose; lactose is digested by lactase to glucose and galactose; and sucrose is digested by sucrase to glucose and fructose.

To summarize, there are three end products of carbohydrate digestion: glucose, galactose, and fructose; each is absorbable by intestinal epithelial cells.

Absorption of Carbohydrates

The mechanism of monosaccharide absorption by intestinal epithelial cells is shown in Figure 8-27. Glucose and galactose are absorbed by mechanisms involving Na^+-dependent cotransport. Fructose is absorbed by facilitated diffusion.

Glucose and galactose are absorbed across the apical membrane by secondary active transport mechanisms similar to those found in the early proximal convoluted tubule. Both glucose and galactose move from the intestinal lumen into the cell on the Na^+-**glucose cotransporter** (**SGLT 1**), against an electrochemical gradient. The energy for this step does not come directly from adenosine triphosphate (ATP) but from the Na^+ gradient across the apical membrane; the Na^+ gradient is, of course, created and maintained by the Na^+-K^+ ATPase on the basolateral membrane. Glucose and galactose are extruded from the cell into the blood, across the basolateral membrane, by facilitated diffusion (**GLUT 2**).

Fructose is handled differently from glucose and galactose. Its absorption does not involve an energy-requiring step or a cotransporter in the apical membrane. Rather, fructose is transported across both the apical and basolateral membranes by facilitated diffusion; in the apical membrane, the fructose-specific transporter is called GLUT 5, and in the basolateral

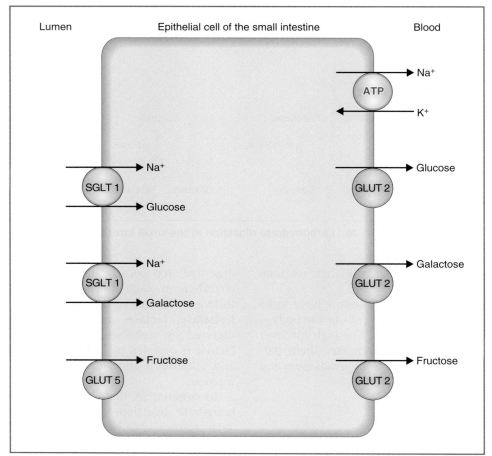

Figure 8–27 **Mechanism of absorption of monosaccharides by epithelial cells of the small intestine.** ATP, Adenosine triphosphate.

membrane, fructose is transported by GLUT 2. Because only facilitated diffusion is involved, fructose cannot be absorbed against an electrochemical gradient (in contrast to glucose and galactose).

Disorders of Carbohydrate Digestion and Absorption

Most disorders of carbohydrate absorption are the result of a failure to break down ingested carbohydrates to an absorbable form (i.e., to monosaccharides). If nonabsorbable carbohydrates (e.g., disaccharides) remain in the gastrointestinal lumen, they "hold" an equivalent amount of water to keep the intestinal contents isosmotic. Retention of this solute and water in the intestine causes osmotic diarrhea.

Lactose intolerance, which is caused by **lactase deficiency,** is a common example of failure to digest a carbohydrate to an absorbable form. In this disorder, the brush-border lactase is deficient or lacking and lactose is not digested to glucose and galactose. If lactose is ingested in milk or milk products, the lactose remains undigested in the lumen of the intestine.

Lactose, a disaccharide, is nonabsorbable, holds water in the lumen, and causes **osmotic diarrhea.** Persons with lactose intolerance either may avoid ingesting milk products or may ingest milk products supplemented with lactase (Box 8-2).

Proteins

Dietary proteins are digested to absorbable forms (i.e., amino acids, dipeptides, and tripeptides) by proteases in the stomach and small intestine and then absorbed into the blood. The proteins contained in gastrointestinal secretions (e.g., pancreatic enzymes) are similarly digested and absorbed.

Digestion of Proteins

The digestion of protein begins in the stomach with the action of pepsin and is completed in the small intestine with pancreatic and brush-border proteases (Figs. 8-28 and 8-29). The two classes of proteases are endopeptidases and exopeptidases. **Endopeptidases** hydrolyze the interior peptide bonds of proteins. The

BOX 8–2 Clinical Physiology: Lactose Intolerance

DESCRIPTION OF CASE. An 18-year-old college student reports to her physician complaining of diarrhea, bloating, and gas when she drinks milk. She thinks that she has always had difficulty digesting milk. The physician suspects that the woman has lactose intolerance. He requests that she consume no milk products for a 2-week period and note the presence of diarrhea or excessive gas. Neither symptom is noted during this period.

EXPLANATION OF CASE. The woman has lactase deficiency, a partial or total absence of the intestinal brush-border enzyme lactase. Lactase is essential for the digestion of dietary lactose (a disaccharide present in milk) to glucose and galactose. When lactase is deficient, lactose cannot be digested to the absorbable monosaccharide forms and intact lactose remains in the intestinal lumen. There, it behaves as an osmotically active solute: It retains water isosmotically, and it produces osmotic diarrhea. Excess gas is caused by fermentation of the undigested, unabsorbed lactose to methane and hydrogen gas.

TREATMENT. Apparently, this defect is specific only for lactase; the other brush-border enzymes (e.g., α-dextrinase, maltase, sucrase, trehalase) are normal in this woman. Therefore, only lactose must be eliminated from her diet by having her avoid milk products. Alternatively, lactase tablets can be ingested along with milk to ensure adequate digestion of lactose to monosaccharides. No further testing or treatment is necessary.

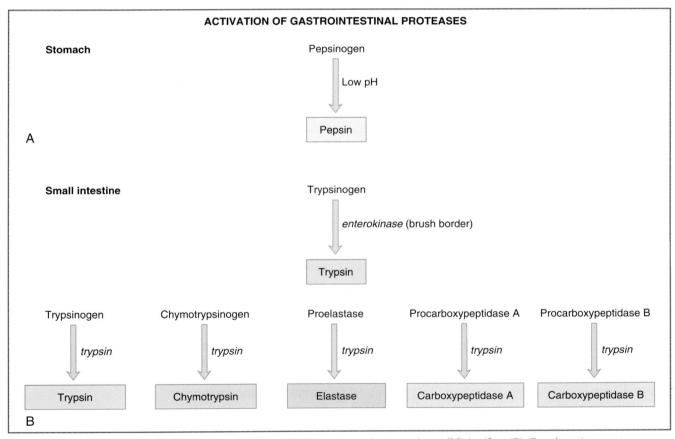

Figure 8–28 Activation of proteases in the stomach (A) and small intestine (B). Trypsin autocatalyzes its own activation and the activation of the other proenzymes.

endopeptidases of the gastrointestinal tract are pepsin, trypsin, chymotrypsin, and elastase. **Exopeptidases** hydrolyze one amino acid at a time from the C-terminal ends of proteins and peptides. The exopeptidases of the gastrointestinal tract are carboxypeptidases A and B.

As noted, protein digestion begins with the action of **pepsin** in the **stomach.** The gastric chief cells secrete the inactive precursor of pepsin, pepsinogen. At low gastric pH, pepsinogen is activated to pepsin. There are three isozymes of pepsin, each of which has

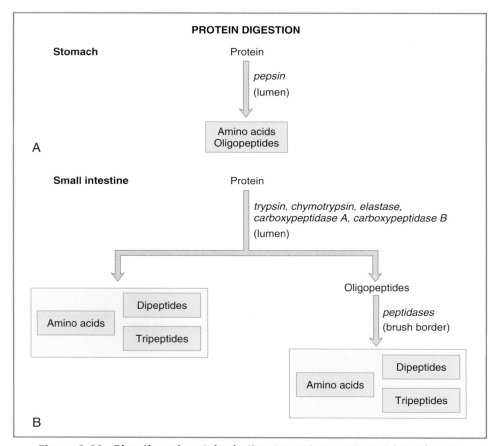

Figure 8–29 **Digestion of proteins in the stomach (A) and small intestine (B).**

a pH optimum ranging between pH 1 and 3; above pH 5, pepsin is denatured and inactivated. Therefore, pepsin is active at the low pH of the stomach, and its actions are terminated in the duodenum, where pancreatic HCO_3^- secretions neutralize gastric H^+ and increase the pH. Interestingly, pepsin is *not essential* for normal protein digestion. In persons whose stomach has been removed or persons who do not secrete gastric H^+ (and cannot activate pepsinogen to pepsin), protein digestion and absorption are normal. These examples demonstrate that pancreatic and brush-border proteases *alone* can adequately digest ingested protein.

Protein digestion continues in the **small intestine** with the combined actions of pancreatic and brush-border proteases. Five major pancreatic proteases are secreted as inactive precursors: trypsinogen, chymotrypsinogen, proelastase, procarboxypeptidase A, and procarboxypeptidase B (see Fig. 8-28).

The first step in intestinal protein digestion is the activation of trypsinogen to its active form, **trypsin,** by the brush-border enzyme **enterokinase.** Initially, a small amount of trypsin is produced, which then catalyzes the conversion of all of the other inactive precursors to their active enzymes. Even the remaining trypsinogen is *autocatalyzed* by trypsin to form more trypsin. The activation steps yield five active enzymes for protein digestion: trypsin, chymotrypsin, elastase, carboxypeptidase A, and carboxypeptidase B. These pancreatic proteases then hydrolyze dietary protein to amino acids, dipeptides, tripeptides, and larger peptides called oligopeptides. Only the amino acids, dipeptides, and tripeptides are absorbable. The oligopeptides are further hydrolyzed by brush-border proteases, yielding the smaller absorbable molecules (see Fig. 8-29). Finally, the pancreatic proteases digest themselves and each other!

Absorption of Proteins

As previously described, the products of protein digestion are amino acids, dipeptides, and tripeptides. Each form can be absorbed by intestinal epithelial cells. Especially note the contrast between proteins and carbohydrates: Carbohydrates are absorbable in the monosaccharide form *only*, whereas proteins are absorbable in larger units.

The **L-amino acids** are absorbed by mechanisms analogous to those for monosaccharide absorption

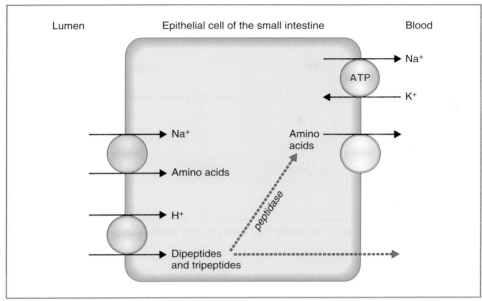

Figure 8–30 **The mechanism of absorption of amino acids, dipeptides, and tripeptides in the small intestine.** ATP, Adenosine triphosphate.

(Fig. 8-30). The amino acids are transported from the lumen into the cell by Na⁺-amino acid cotransporters in the apical membrane, energized by the Na⁺ gradient. There are four separate cotransporters: one each for neutral, acidic, basic, and imino amino acids. The amino acids then are transported across the basolateral membrane into the blood by facilitated diffusion, again by separate mechanisms for neutral, acidic, basic, and imino amino acids.

Most ingested protein is absorbed by intestinal epithelial cells in the **dipeptide** and **tripeptide** forms rather than as free amino acids. Separate H⁺-dependent cotransporters in the apical membrane transport dipeptides and tripeptides from the intestinal lumen into the cell, utilizing an H⁺ ion gradient created by an Na⁺-H⁺ exchanger in the apical membrane (not shown in Fig. 8-30). Once inside the cell, most of the dipeptides and tripeptides are hydrolyzed to amino acids by cytosolic peptidases, producing amino acids that exit the cell by facilitated diffusion; the remaining dipeptides and tripeptides are absorbed unchanged.

Disorders of Protein Digestion and Absorption

Disorders of protein digestion or absorption occur when there is a deficiency of pancreatic enzymes *or* when there is a defect in the transporters of the intestinal epithelial cells.

In disorders of the exocrine pancreas such as **chronic pancreatitis** and **cystic fibrosis,** there is a deficiency of all pancreatic enzymes including the proteases.

Dietary protein cannot be absorbed if it is not digested by proteases to amino acids, dipeptides, and tripeptides. The absence of trypsin *alone* makes it *appear* as if all of the pancreatic enzymes are missing because trypsin is necessary for the activation of all precursor enzymes (including trypsin itself) to their active forms (see Fig. 8-28).

Several diseases are caused by a defect in or absence of an Na⁺-amino acid cotransporter. **Cystinuria** is a genetic disorder in which the transporter for the dibasic amino acids cystine, lysine, arginine, and ornithine is absent in both the small intestine and the kidney. As a result of this deficiency, none of these amino acids is absorbed by the intestine or reabsorbed by the kidney. The intestinal defect results in failure to absorb the amino acids, which are excreted in feces. The renal defect results in increased excretion of these specific amino acids and gives the disease its name, cystinuria or excess cystine excretion.

Lipids

The dietary lipids include triglycerides, cholesterol, and phospholipids. A factor that greatly complicates lipid digestion and absorption is their insolubility in water (their hydrophobicity). Because the gastrointestinal tract is filled with an aqueous fluid, the lipids must somehow be solubilized to be digested and absorbed. Thus, the mechanisms for processing lipids are more complicated than those for carbohydrates and proteins, which are water soluble.

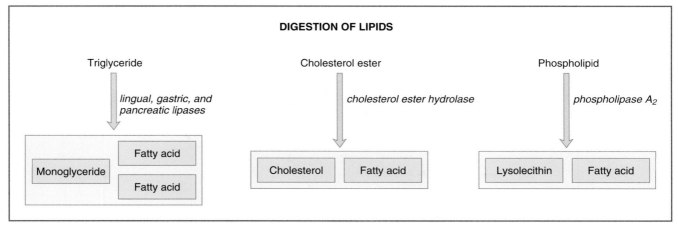

Figure 8-31 **Digestion of lipids in the small intestine.**

Digestion of Lipids

The digestion of dietary lipids begins in the stomach with the action of lingual and gastric lipases and is completed in the small intestine with the actions of the pancreatic enzymes pancreatic lipase, cholesterol ester hydrolase, and phospholipase A_2 (Fig. 8-31).

STOMACH

The function of the stomach in lipid digestion is to churn and mix dietary lipids and to initiate enzymatic digestion. The churning action breaks the lipids into small droplets, increasing the surface area for digestive enzymes. In the stomach, the lipid droplets are emulsified (kept apart) by dietary proteins. (Bile acids, the primary emulsifying agents in the small intestine, are not present in the gastric contents.) **Lingual and gastric lipases** initiate lipid digestion by hydrolyzing approximately 10% of ingested triglycerides to glycerol and free fatty acids. One of the most important contributions of the stomach to overall lipid digestion (and absorption) is that it empties chyme *slowly* into the small intestine, allowing adequate time for pancreatic enzymes to digest lipids. The rate of **gastric emptying,** which is so critical for subsequent intestinal digestive and absorptive steps, is **slowed by CCK.** CCK is secreted when dietary lipids first appear in the small intestine.

SMALL INTESTINE

Most lipid digestion occurs in the small intestine, where conditions are more favorable than in the stomach. **Bile salts** are secreted into the lumen of small intestine. These bile salts, together with lysolecithin and products of lipid digestion, surround and emulsify dietary lipids. **Emulsification** produces small droplets of lipid dispersed in the aqueous solution of the intestinal lumen, creating a large surface area for the action of pancreatic enzymes. The **pancreatic enzymes** (pancreatic lipase, cholesterol ester hydrolase, and phospholipase A_2) and one special protein (colipase) are secreted into the small intestine to accomplish the digestive work (see Fig. 8-31).

♦ **Pancreatic lipase** is secreted as the active enzyme. It hydrolyzes triglyceride molecules to one molecule of monoglyceride and two molecules of fatty acid. A potential problem in the action of pancreatic lipase is that it is inactivated by bile salts. Bile salts displace pancreatic lipase at the lipid-water interface of the emulsified lipid droplets. This "problem" is solved by colipase. **Colipase** is secreted in pancreatic juices in an inactive form, procolipase, which is activated in the intestinal lumen by trypsin. Colipase then displaces bile salts at the lipid-water interface and binds to pancreatic lipase. With the inhibitory bile salts displaced, pancreatic lipase can proceed with its digestive functions.

♦ **Cholesterol ester hydrolase** is secreted as an active enzyme and hydrolyzes cholesterol ester to free cholesterol and fatty acids. It also hydrolyzes ester linkages of triglycerides, yielding glycerol.

♦ **Phospholipase A_2** is secreted as a proenzyme and, like many other pancreatic enzymes, is activated by trypsin. Phospholipase A_2 hydrolyzes phospholipids to lysolecithin and fatty acids.

The final products of lipid digestion are monoglycerides, fatty acids, cholesterol, lysolecithin, and glycerol (from hydrolysis of ester bonds of triglycerides). With the exception of glycerol, each end product is hydrophobic and therefore is not soluble in water. Now the hydrophobic digestive products must be solubilized in micelles and transported to the apical membrane of the intestinal cells for absorption.

Absorption of Lipids

Absorption of lipids occurs in a series of steps illustrated in Figure 8-32 and is described as follows. The

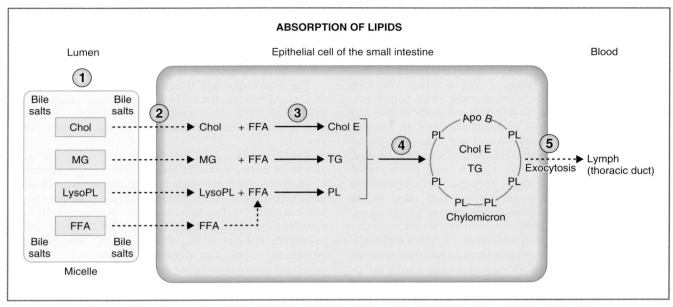

Figure 8–32 **Mechanism of absorption of lipids in the small intestine.** The circled numbers correspond to the steps described in the text. Apo B, β-Lipoprotein; Chol, cholesterol; Chol E, cholesterol ester; FFA, free fatty acids; LysoPL, lysolecithin; MG, monoglycerides; PL, phospholipids; TG, triglycerides.

circled numbers on the figure correlate with the following steps:

1. The products of lipid digestion (cholesterol, monoglycerides, lysolecithin, and free fatty acids) are solubilized in the intestinal lumen in mixed **micelles,** except glycerol, which is water soluble. Mixed micelles are cylindrically shaped disks with an average diameter of 50 Å. As discussed earlier, the core of a micelle contains products of lipid digestion and the exterior is lined with bile salts, which are **amphipathic.** The hydrophilic portion of the bile salt molecules dissolves in the aqueous solution of the intestinal lumen, thus solubilizing the lipids in the micellar core.

2. The micelles diffuse to the apical (brush-border) membrane of the intestinal epithelial cells. At the apical membrane, the lipids are released from the micelle and diffuse down their concentration gradients into the cell. The micelles per se do not enter the cell, however, and the bile salts are left behind in the intestinal lumen to be absorbed downstream in the ileum. Because most ingested lipid is absorbed by the midjejunum, the "work" of the bile salts is completed long before they are returned to the liver via the enterohepatic circulation.

3. Inside the intestinal epithelial cells, the products of lipid digestion are **reesterified** with free fatty acids on the smooth endoplasmic reticulum to form the original ingested lipids, triglycerides, cholesterol ester, and phospholipids.

4. Inside the cells, the reesterified lipids are packaged with apoproteins in lipid-carrying particles called **chylomicrons.** The chylomicrons, with an average diameter of 1000 Å, are composed of triglycerides and cholesterol at the core and phospholipids and apoproteins on the outside. Phospholipids cover 80% of the outside of the chylomicron surface, and the remaining 20% of the surface is covered with **apoproteins.** Apoproteins, which are synthesized by the intestinal epithelial cells, are essential for the absorption of chylomicrons. Failure to synthesize **Apo B** (or β-lipoprotein) results in **abetalipoproteinemia,** a condition in which a person is unable to absorb chylomicrons and, therefore, is also unable to absorb dietary lipids.

5. The chylomicrons are packaged in secretory vesicles on the Golgi apparatus. The secretory vesicles migrate to the basolateral membranes, and there is **exocytosis** of the chylomicrons. The chylomicrons are too large to enter vascular capillaries, but they can enter the **lymphatic capillaries** (lacteals) by moving between the endothelial cells that line the lacteals. The lymphatic circulation carries the chylomicrons to the **thoracic duct,** which empties into the bloodstream.

Abnormalities of Lipid Digestion and Absorption

The mechanisms for lipid digestion and absorption are more complex and involve more steps than those for

BOX 8–3   Clinical Physiology: Zollinger-Ellison Syndrome

DESCRIPTION OF CASE. A 52-year-old man visits his physician complaining of abdominal pain, nausea, loss of appetite, frequent belching, and diarrhea. The man reports that his pain is worse at night and is sometimes relieved by eating food or taking antacids containing HCO_3^-. Gastrointestinal endoscopy reveals an ulcer in the duodenal bulb. Stool samples are positive for blood and fat. Because Zollinger-Ellison syndrome is suspected in this patient, his serum gastrin level is measured and found to be markedly elevated. A computerized tomographic (CT) scan reveals a 1.5-cm mass in the head of the pancreas. The man is referred to a surgeon. While awaiting surgery, the man is treated with the drug omeprazole, which inhibits H^+ secretion by gastric parietal cells. During a laparotomy, a pancreatic tumor is located and excised. After surgery the man's symptoms diminish, and subsequent endoscopy shows that the duodenal ulcer has healed.

EXPLANATION OF CASE. All of the man's symptoms and clinical manifestations are caused, directly or indirectly, by a gastrin-secreting tumor of the pancreas. In Zollinger-Ellison syndrome, the tumor secretes large amounts of gastrin into the circulation. The target cell for gastrin is the gastric parietal cell, where it stimulates H^+ secretion.

The gastric G cells, the physiologic source of gastrin, are under negative feedback control. Thus, normally, gastrin secretion and H^+ secretion are inhibited when the gastric contents are acidified (i.e., when no more H^+ is needed). In Zollinger-Ellison syndrome, however, this negative feedback control mechanism does not operate: Gastrin secretion by the tumor is not inhibited when the gastric contents are acidified. Therefore,

gastrin secretion continues unabated, as does H^+ secretion by the parietal cells.

The man's diarrhea is caused by the large volume of fluid delivered from the stomach (stimulated by gastrin) to the small intestine; the volume is so great that it overwhelms the capacity of the intestine to absorb it.

The presence of fat in the stool (steatorrhea) is abnormal because mechanisms in the small intestine normally ensure that dietary fat is completely absorbed. Steatorrhea is present in Zollinger-Ellison syndrome for two reasons: (1) The first reason is that excess H^+ is delivered from the stomach to the small intestine and overwhelms the buffering ability of HCO_3^--containing pancreatic juices. The duodenal contents remain at acidic pH rather than being neutralized, and the acidic pH inactivates pancreatic lipase. When pancreatic lipase is inactivated, it cannot digest dietary triglycerides to monoglycerides and fatty acids. Undigested triglycerides are not absorbed by intestinal epithelial cells, and thus they are excreted in the stool. (2) The second reason for steatorrhea is that the acidity of the duodenal contents damages the intestinal mucosa (evidenced by the duodenal ulcer) and reduces the microvillar surface area for absorption of lipids.

TREATMENT. While the man is awaiting surgery to remove the gastrin-secreting tumor, he is treated with omeprazole, which directly blocks the H^+-K^+ ATPase in the apical membrane of gastric parietal cells. This ATPase is responsible for gastric H^+ secretion. The drug is expected to reduce H^+ secretion and decrease the H^+ load to the duodenum. Later, the gastrin-secreting tumor is surgically removed.

---

carbohydrate and protein. Thus, there are also more steps at which an abnormality of lipid digestion or absorption can occur. Each step in the normal process is essential: pancreatic enzyme secretion and function, bile acid secretion, emulsification, micelle formation, diffusion of lipids into intestinal epithelial cells, chylomicron formation, and transfer of chylomicrons into lymph. An abnormality at *any one of the steps* will interfere with lipid absorption and result in **steatorrhea** (fat excreted in feces).

♦ **Pancreatic insufficiency.** Diseases of the exocrine pancreas (e.g., **chronic pancreatitis** and **cystic fibrosis**) result in failure to secrete adequate amounts of pancreatic enzymes including those involved in lipid digestion, pancreatic lipase and colipase, cholesterol ester hydrolase, and phospholipase A_2. For example, in the absence of pancreatic lipase, triglycerides cannot be digested to monoglycerides and

free fatty acids. Undigested triglycerides are not absorbable and are excreted in feces.

♦ **Acidity of duodenal contents.** If the acidic chyme delivered to the duodenum is not adequately neutralized by the HCO_3^--containing pancreatic secretions, then pancreatic enzymes are inactivated (i.e., the pH optimum for pancreatic lipase is 6). The gastric chyme, which is delivered to the duodenum, has a pH ranging from 2 at the pylorus to 4 at the duodenal bulb. Sufficient HCO_3^- must be secreted in pancreatic juice to neutralize the H^+ and increase the pH to the range where pancreatic enzymes function optimally.

There are two reasons that all of the H^+ delivered from the stomach might not be neutralized: (1) Gastric parietal cells may be secreting excessive quantities of H^+, causing an overload to the duodenum; or (2) the pancreas may fail to secrete sufficient quantities of HCO_3^- in pancreatic juice. The first reason is illustrated by **Zollinger-Ellison syndrome,** in which a tumor secretes large quantities of gastrin (Box 8-3). The elevated levels of gastrin stimulate excessive secretion of H^+ by the gastric parietal cells, and this H^+ is delivered to the duodenum, overwhelming the ability of pancreatic juices to neutralize it. The second reason is illustrated by disorders of the exocrine pancreas (e.g., pancreatitis) in which there is impaired HCO_3^- secretion (in addition to impaired enzyme secretion).

♦ **Deficiency of bile salts.** Deficiency of bile salts interferes with the ability to form micelles, which are necessary for solubilization of the products of lipid digestion. **Ileal resection** (removal of the ileum) interrupts the enterohepatic circulation of bile salts, which then are excreted in feces rather than being returned to the liver. Because the synthesis of new bile salts cannot keep pace with the fecal loss, the total bile salt pool is reduced.

♦ **Bacterial overgrowth.** Bacterial overgrowth reduces the effectiveness of bile salts by deconjugating them. In other words, bacterial actions remove glycine and taurine from bile salts, converting them to bile acids. Recall that at intestinal pH, bile acids are primarily in the nonionized form (because their pKs are higher than intestinal pH); the nonionized form is lipid soluble and readily absorbed by diffusion across the intestinal epithelial cells. For this reason, the bile acids are absorbed "too early" (before reaching the ileum), before micelle formation and lipid absorption is completed. Similarly, **decreased pH** in the intestinal lumen promotes "early" absorption of bile acids by converting them to their nonionized form.

♦ **Decreased intestinal cells for absorption.** In conditions such as **tropical sprue,** the number of intestinal epithelial cells is reduced, which reduces the microvillar surface area. Because lipid absorption across the apical membrane occurs by diffusion, which depends on surface area, lipid absorption is impaired because the surface area for absorption is decreased.

♦ **Failure to synthesize apoproteins.** Failure to synthesize Apo B (β-lipoprotein) causes **abetalipoproteinemia.** In this disease, chylomicrons either do not form or are unable to be transported out of intestinal cells into lymph. In either case, there is decreased absorption of lipids into blood and a buildup of lipid within the intestinal cells.

Vitamins

Vitamins are required in small amounts to act as coenzymes or cofactors for various metabolic reactions. Because vitamins are not synthesized in the body, they must be acquired from the diet and absorbed by the gastrointestinal tract. The vitamins are categorized as either fat soluble or water soluble.

Fat-Soluble Vitamins

The fat-soluble vitamins are vitamins A, D, E, and K. The mechanism of absorption of fat-soluble vitamins is easily understood: They are processed in the same manner as dietary lipids. In the intestinal lumen, fat-soluble vitamins are incorporated into **micelles** and transported to the apical membrane of the intestinal cells. They diffuse across the apical membrane into the cells, are incorporated in **chylomicrons,** and then are extruded into lymph, which delivers them to the general circulation.

Water-Soluble Vitamins

The water-soluble vitamins include vitamins B_1, B_2, B_6, B_{12}, C, biotin, folic acid, nicotinic acid, and pantothenic acid. In most cases, absorption of the water-soluble vitamins occurs via an **Na^+-dependent cotransport** mechanism in the small intestine.

The *exception* is the absorption of **vitamin B_{12}** (cobalamin), which is more complicated than the absorption of the other water-soluble vitamins. Absorption of vitamin B_{12} requires **intrinsic factor** and occurs in the following steps: (1) Dietary vitamin B_{12} is released from foods by the digestive action of pepsin in the stomach. (2) Free vitamin B_{12} binds to **R proteins,** which are secreted in salivary juices. (3) In the duodenum, pancreatic proteases degrade the R proteins, causing vitamin B_{12} to be transferred to intrinsic factor, a glycoprotein secreted by the gastric parietal cells. (4) The vitamin B_{12}-intrinsic factor complex is resistant to the degradative actions of pancreatic proteases and travels to the ileum, where there is a specific transport mechanism for its absorption.

A consequence of **gastrectomy** is loss of the source of intrinsic factor, the parietal cells. Therefore, after a gastrectomy, patients fail to absorb vitamin B_{12} from the ileum, eventually become vitamin B_{12} deficient, and may develop **pernicious anemia.** To prevent pernicious anemia, vitamin B_{12} must be administered by injection; orally supplemented vitamin B_{12} cannot be absorbed in the absence of intrinsic factor.

Calcium

Ca^{2+} is absorbed in the small intestine and depends on the presence of the active form of vitamin D, **1,25-dihydroxycholecalciferol,** which is produced as follows: Dietary vitamin D_3 (cholecalciferol) is inactive. In the liver, cholecalciferol is converted to 25-hydroxycholecalciferol, which also is inactive but is the principal circulating form of vitamin D_3. In the proximal tubules of the kidney, 25-hydroxycholecalciferol is converted to 1,25-dihydroxycholecalciferol, catalyzed by **1α-hydroxylase.** 1,25-Dihydroxycholecalciferol, the biologically metabolite of vitamin D, has actions on intestine, kidney, and bone. The role of 1,25-dihydroxycholecalciferol in calcium homeostasis is discussed in Chapter 9. Briefly, its most important action is to promote Ca^{2+} absorption from the small intestine by inducing the synthesis of vitamin D–dependent Ca^{2+}-binding protein (**calbindin D-28 K**) in intestinal epithelial cells.

In vitamin D deficiency or when there is failure to convert vitamin D to 1,25-dihydroxycholecalciferol (as occurs in chronic renal failure), there is inadequate Ca^{2+} absorption from the gastrointestinal tract. In children, inadequate Ca^{2+} absorption causes **rickets,** and in adults, it causes **osteomalacia.**

Iron

Iron is absorbed across the apical membrane of intestinal epithelial cells as free iron (Fe^{2+}) or as heme iron (i.e., iron bound to hemoglobin or myoglobin). Inside the intestinal cells, heme iron is digested by lysosomal enzymes, releasing free iron. Free iron then binds to **apoferritin** and is transported across the basolateral membrane into the blood. In the circulation, iron is bound to a β-globulin called **transferrin,** which transports it from the small intestine to storage sites in the liver. From the liver, iron is transported to the bone marrow, where it is released and utilized in the synthesis of hemoglobin.

INTESTINAL FLUID AND ELECTROLYTE TRANSPORT

The gastrointestinal tract absorbs vast quantities of fluid and electrolytes. Together, the small and large intestines absorb approximately 9 L of fluid daily, an amount almost equal to the entire extracellular fluid volume! *What is the source of this large volume of fluid that is absorbed?*

Figure 8-33 shows that there is slightly more than 9 L of fluid in the lumen of the gastrointestinal tract, which is the sum of the volume of liquid in the diet (2 L) *plus* the combined volume of salivary, gastric, pancreatic, biliary, and intestinal secretions (7 L). Of this 9 L, most is absorbed by the epithelial cells of the small intestine and colon. The small remaining volume that is not absorbed (100 to 200 mL) is excreted in feces. Clearly, a disturbance in the absorptive mechanisms can lead to excessive fluid loss from the gastrointestinal tract **(diarrhea).** The *potential* for loss of total body water and electrolytes in diarrhea is enormous.

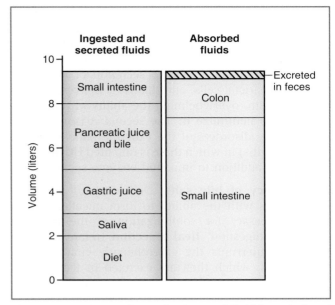

Figure 8–33 **Comparison of volume of fluid ingested and secreted with that absorbed by the intestine.** The hatched area shows the small amount of fluid excreted in feces.

The small intestine and colon not only *absorb* large quantities of electrolytes (Na^+, Cl^-, HCO_3^-, and K^+) and water, but the epithelial cells lining the crypts of the small intestine also *secrete* fluid and electrolytes. This additional secretion contributes to the volume already in the intestinal lumen, which then must be absorbed.

The mechanisms for fluid and electrolyte absorption and secretion in the intestine involve cellular and paracellular routes. The permeability of **tight junctions** between the epithelial cells determines whether fluid and electrolytes will move via the paracellular route or whether they will move via the cellular route. The tight junctions in the small intestine are "leaky" (have low resistance) and permit significant paracellular movement, whereas the tight junctions in the colon are "tight" (have a high resistance) and do not permit paracellular movement.

Intestinal Absorption

Intestinal epithelial cells lining the **villi** absorb large volumes of fluid. The first step in this process is the absorption of solute, followed by the absorption of water. The absorbate (the fluid absorbed) is *always* **isosmotic,** meaning that solute and water absorption occur in proportion to each other. The mechanism of this isosmotic absorption is similar to that in the renal proximal tubule. The solute absorptive mechanisms vary among the jejunum, the ileum, and the colon.

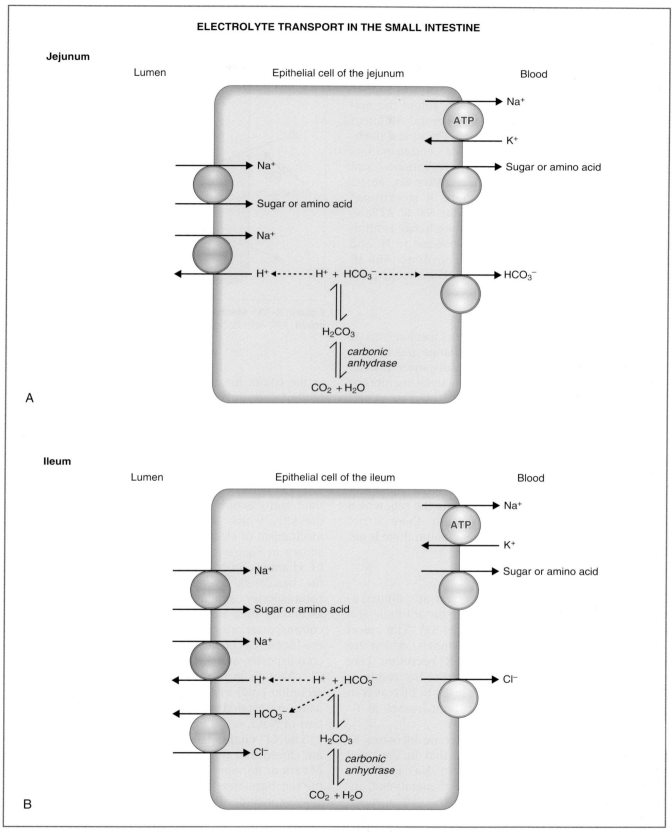

Figure 8–34 **Mechanisms of electrolyte transport in the jejunum (A) and in the ileum (B).**
ATP, Adenosine triphosphate.

Jejunum

The jejunum is the major site for Na⁺ absorption in the small intestine (Fig. 8-34). The mechanisms for electrolyte transport in the jejunum are identical to those in the early proximal tubule of the kidney and are shown in Figure 8-34*A*. Na⁺ enters the epithelial cells of the jejunum via several different Na⁺-dependent coupled transporters. The apical membrane contains Na⁺-monosaccharide cotransporters (Na⁺-glucose and Na⁺-galactose), Na⁺-amino acid cotransporters, and Na⁺-H⁺ exchange. After Na⁺ enters the cell on the coupled transporters, it is extruded across the basolateral membrane via the Na⁺-K⁺ ATPase. Note that the source of H⁺ for Na⁺-H⁺ exchange is intracellular CO_2 and H_2O, which are converted to H⁺ and HCO_3^- in the presence of carbonic anhydrase. The H⁺ is secreted into the lumen on the Na⁺-H⁺ exchanger, and the HCO_3^- is absorbed into blood.

Ileum

The ileum contains the same transport mechanisms as the jejunum *plus* a Cl^--HCO_3^- exchange mechanism in the apical membrane and a Cl^- transporter, instead of an HCO_3^- transporter, in the basolateral membrane (see Fig. 8-34*B*). Thus, when H⁺ and HCO_3^- are generated inside the epithelial cells in the ileum, the H⁺ is secreted into the lumen via the Na⁺-H⁺ exchanger, and the HCO_3^- *also* is secreted into the lumen via the Cl^--HCO_3^- exchanger (rather than being absorbed into blood, as in the jejunum). The result of the combined Na⁺-H⁺ exchange and Cl^--HCO_3^- exchange in the apical membrane is net movement of NaCl into the cell, which then is absorbed. Thus, in the ileum, there is net absorption of NaCl, whereas in the jejunum there is net absorption of $NaHCO_3$.

Colon

The cellular mechanisms in the colon are similar to those in the principal cells of the late distal tubule and collecting ducts of the kidney (Fig. 8-35). The apical membrane contains Na⁺ and K⁺ channels, which are responsible for **Na⁺ absorption** and **K⁺ secretion.** Like the renal principal cells, synthesis of the Na⁺ channels is induced by **aldosterone,** which leads to increases in Na⁺ absorption and, secondarily, to increases in K⁺ secretion.

The mechanism by which aldosterone increases K⁺ secretion in the colon is similar to that in the renal principal cells: increased number of Na⁺ channels, increased Na⁺ entry across the apical membrane, increased Na⁺ pumped out across the basolateral membrane by the Na⁺-K⁺ ATPase, increased K⁺ pumped into the cell, and, finally, increased K⁺ secretion across the apical membrane. Even the flow-rate dependence of K⁺ secretion seen in the renal principal cells is present

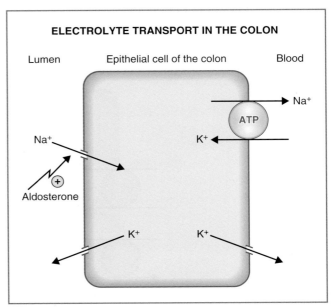

Figure 8-35 **Mechanism of electrolyte transport in the colon.** ATP, Adenosine triphosphate.

in the colon; for example, in **diarrhea,** the high flow rate of intestinal fluid causes increased colonic K⁺ secretion, resulting in increased K⁺ loss in feces and **hypokalemia.**

Intestinal Secretion

The epithelial cells lining the intestinal **crypts** secrete fluid and electrolytes (compared with the cells lining the villi, which absorb fluid and electrolytes). The mechanism of electrolyte secretion in the crypt cells is shown in Figure 8-36. The apical membrane contains Cl^- channels. In addition to having the Na⁺-K⁺ ATPase, the basolateral membrane also has an Na⁺-K⁺-2Cl^- cotransporter similar to that found in the thick ascending limb of the loop of Henle. This three-ion cotransporter brings Na⁺, Cl^-, and K⁺ into the cells from the blood. Cl^- moves into the cells on the Na⁺-K⁺-2Cl^- cotransporter, and then diffuses into the lumen through Cl^- channels in the apical membrane. Na⁺ follows Cl^- secretion passively, moving between the cells. Finally, water is secreted into the lumen, following the secretion of NaCl.

The **Cl^- channels** of the apical membrane usually are closed, but they may open in response to binding of various hormones and neurotransmitters to receptors on the basolateral membrane. These activating substances include, but are not limited to, **ACh** and **VIP.** The neurotransmitter or hormone binds to the basolateral receptor, activating adenylyl cyclase and generating cAMP in the crypt cells. **cAMP** opens the Cl^- channels in the apical membrane, initiating Cl^- secretion; Na⁺

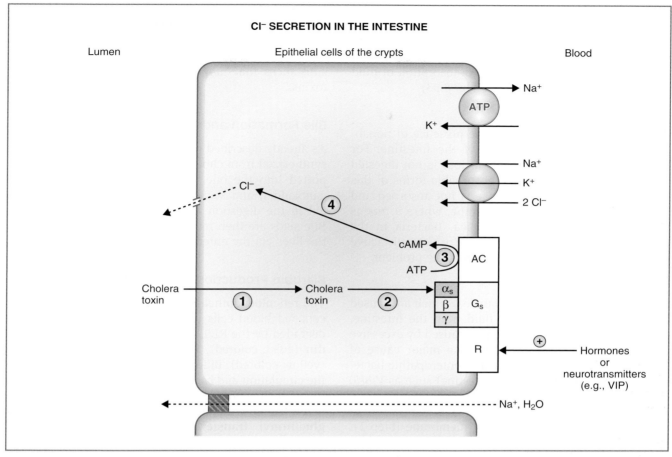

CI⁻ SECRETION IN THE INTESTINE

Figure 8–36 **Mechanism of Cl⁻ and fluid secretion by epithelial cells in intestinal crypts.** The circled numbers correspond to steps described in the text. Cholera toxin activates adenylyl cyclase (AC), increasing cyclic adenosine monophosphate (cAMP) production and opening Cl⁻ channels in the apical membrane. ATP, Adenosine triphosphate; R, receptor; VIP, vasoactive intestinal peptide.

and water follow Cl⁻ into the lumen. Normally, the electrolytes and water secreted by intestinal crypt cells are absorbed by intestinal villar cells. However, in diseases in which adenylyl cyclase is maximally stimulated (e.g., **cholera**), fluid secretion by the crypt cells overwhelms the absorptive capacity of the villar cells and causes severe, life-threatening diarrhea (see later, Secretory Diarrhea).

Diarrhea

Diarrhea, which means "to run through," is a major cause of death worldwide. Serious illness or death may be caused by the rapid loss of large volumes of extracellular-type fluid from the gastrointestinal tract. The previous discussion emphasizes the enormous *potential* for fluid loss from the gastrointestinal tract, as much as 9 L or more per day.

In diarrhea, the loss of extracellular-type fluid results in decreased extracellular fluid volume, decreased intravascular volume, and **decreased arterial pressure.**

The baroreceptor mechanisms and the renin–angiotensin II–aldosterone system will attempt to restore blood pressure, but these attempts will be futile if the volume of fluid lost from the gastrointestinal tract is too great or if the loss is too rapid.

In addition to circulatory collapse, other disturbances caused by diarrhea are related to the specific electrolytes lost from the body in the diarrheal fluid, particularly HCO_3^- and K^+. Diarrheal fluid has a relatively high concentration of HCO_3^- because the fluids secreted into the gastrointestinal tract have a high HCO_3^- content including salivary, pancreatic, and intestinal juices. Loss of HCO_3^- (relative to Cl⁻) causes **hyperchloremic metabolic acidosis with normal anion gap** (see Chapter 7). Diarrheal fluid also has a high concentration of K^+ because of flow-rate–dependent K^+ secretion by the colon. Excessive loss of K^+ from the gastrointestinal tract results in **hypokalemia.**

The causes of diarrhea include decreased absorptive surface area, osmotic diarrhea, and secretory diarrhea.

Decreased Surface Area for Absorption

Disease processes that result in a decreased absorptive surface area including infection and inflammation of the small intestine cause decreased absorption of fluid by the gastrointestinal tract (see Fig. 8-33).

Osmotic Diarrhea

Osmotic diarrhea is caused by the presence of nonabsorbable solutes in the lumen of the intestine. For example, in **lactase deficiency,** lactose is not digested to glucose and galactose, the absorbable forms of this carbohydrate. Undigested lactose is not absorbed and remains in the lumen of the intestine, where it retains water and causes osmotic diarrhea. Bacteria in the intestine may degrade lactose to more osmotically active solute particles, further compounding the problem.

Secretory Diarrhea

In contrast to other forms of diarrhea, which are caused by inadequate absorption of fluid from the intestine, secretory diarrhea (e.g., cholera) is caused by excessive *secretion* of fluid by crypt cells. The major cause of secretory diarrhea is overgrowth of enteropathic bacteria (pathogenic bacteria of the intestine) such as *Vibrio cholerae* or *Escherichia coli.* For example, the bacterial toxin **cholera toxin** (see Fig. 8-36) enters intestinal crypt cells by crossing the apical membrane (Step 1). Inside the cells, the A subunit of the toxin detaches and moves across the cell to the basolateral membrane. There, it catalyzes **adenosine diphosphate (ADP) ribosylation** of the α_s subunit of the G_s protein that is coupled to adenylyl cyclase (Step 2). ADP-ribosylation of the α_s subunit inhibits its GTPase activity, and as a result, GTP cannot be converted back to GDP. With GTP permanently bound to the α_s subunit, adenylyl cyclase is permanently activated (Step 3), cAMP levels remain high, and the Cl^- channels in the apical membrane are kept open (Step 4). The resulting Cl^- secretion is accompanied by secretion of Na^+ and H_2O. The volume of fluid secreted into the intestinal lumen overwhelms the absorptive mechanisms of the small intestine and colon, leading to massive diarrhea.

LIVER PHYSIOLOGY

The liver is located in the abdominal cavity and receives portal blood from the stomach, small and large intestines, pancreas, and spleen. The functions of the liver include processing of absorbed substances; synthesis and secretion of bile acids; bilirubin production and excretion; participation in metabolism of key nutrients including carbohydrates, proteins, and lipids; and detoxification and excretion of waste products.

   The majority of the liver's blood supply is venous blood from the gastrointestinal tract (spleen, stomach, small and large intestines, and pancreas), which is delivered to the liver via the portal vein, as shown in Figure 8-37. Therefore, the liver is ideally located to receive absorbed nutrients and to detoxify absorbed substances that may be harmful such as drugs and toxins.

Bile Formation and Secretion

As already described (see Bile Secretion), bile acids are synthesized from cholesterol by the hepatocytes, transported into the bile, stored and concentrated in the gallbladder, and secreted into the intestinal lumen to aid in the digestion and absorption of dietary lipids. Bile acids are then recirculated from the ileum back to the liver via the enterohepatic circulation.

Bilirubin Production and Excretion

The reticuloendothelial system (RES) processes senescent red blood cells (Fig. 8-38). When hemoglobin is degraded by the RES, one of the byproducts is **biliverdin** (green-colored), which is converted to **bilirubin** (yellow-colored). Bilirubin is then bound to albumin in the circulation and carried to the liver, where it is taken up by the hepatocytes. In hepatic microsomes, bilirubin is conjugated with glucuronic acid via the enzyme **UDP glucuronyl transferase.** (Because UDP glucuronyl transferase is synthesized slowly after birth, some newborn babies develop "newborn jaundice.") Conjugated bilirubin is water soluble, and a portion of it is excreted in the urine. The remainder of the conjugated bilirubin is secreted into bile and then, via bile, into the small intestine. The conjugated bilirubin travels down to the terminal ileum and colon, where it is deconjugated by bacterial enzymes and metabolized to **urobilinogen,** some of which is absorbed via the enterohepatic circulation and delivered back to the liver; the remainder is converted to urobilin and **stercobilin,** which are excreted in the feces.

   Jaundice is a yellow discoloration of the skin and sclera of the eyes due to accumulation of either free or conjugated bilirubin. Jaundice can occur when there is increased destruction of red blood cells that results in increased production of unconjugated bilirubin. Jaundice also occurs with obstruction of bile ducts or with liver disease; in these cases, conjugated bilirubin cannot be excreted in the bile and thus is absorbed into the circulation. In obstructive jaundice, the urine is dark, owing to the high urinary concentration of conjugated bilirubin, and the stool is light ("clay-colored"), owing to the decreased amount of fecal stercobilin.

Metabolic Functions of the Liver

The liver participates in the metabolism of carbohydrates, proteins, and lipids. In **carbohydrate**

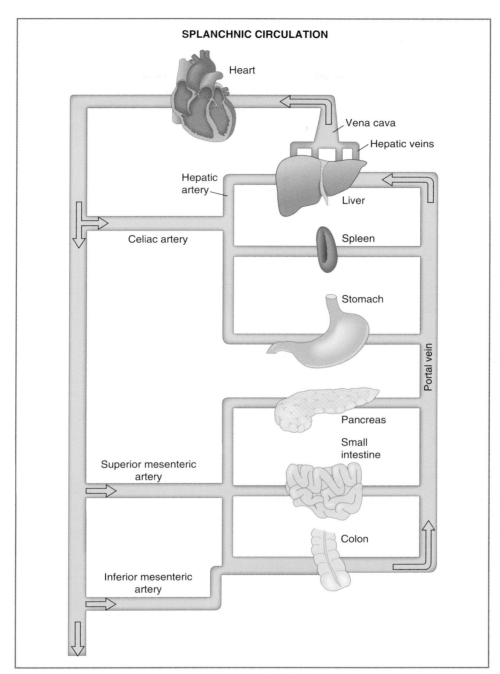

SPLANCHNIC CIRCULATION

Heart

Vena cava

Hepatic veins

Hepatic artery

Liver

Celiac artery

Spleen

Stomach

Portal vein

Pancreas

Small intestine

Superior mesenteric artery

Colon

Inferior mesenteric artery

Figure 8–37 **Blood flow in the splanchnic circulation.**

metabolism, the liver performs gluconeogenesis, stores glucose as glycogen, and releases stored glucose into the bloodstream, when needed.

In **protein metabolism,** the liver synthesizes the nonessential amino acids and modifies amino acids so that they may enter biosynthetic pathways for carbohydrates. The liver also synthesizes almost all plasma proteins including albumin and the clotting factors. Persons with liver failure develop hypoalbuminemia (which may lead to edema due to loss of plasma protein oncotic pressure) and clotting disorders. The liver also converts ammonia, a byproduct of protein catabolism, to urea, which is then excreted in the urine.

In **lipid metabolism,** the liver participates in fatty acid oxidation and synthesizes lipoproteins, cholesterol, and phospholipids. As previously described, the liver converts a portion of the cholesterol to bile acids, which participate in lipid digestion and absorption.

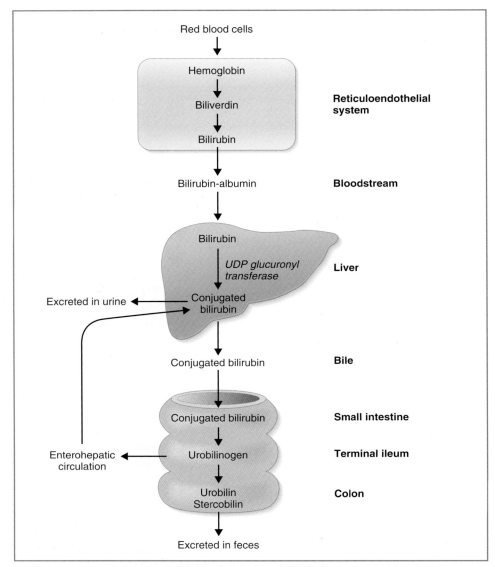

Red blood cells

Hemoglobin

Biliverdin

Bilirubin

Reticuloendothelial system

Bilirubin-albumin

Bloodstream

Bilirubin

UDP glucuronyl transferase

Liver

Conjugated bilirubin

Excreted in urine

Conjugated bilirubin

Bile

Conjugated bilirubin

Small intestine

Urobilinogen

Terminal ileum

Enterohepatic circulation

Urobilin Stercobilin

Colon

Excreted in feces

Figure 8–38   Bilirubin metabolism. UDP, uridine diphosphate.

Detoxification of Substances

The liver protects the body from potentially toxic substances that are absorbed from the GI tract. These substances are presented to the liver via the portal circulation, and the liver modifies them in so-called "first pass metabolism," ensuring that little or none of the substances make it into the systemic circulation. For example, bacteria absorbed from the colon are phagocytized by hepatic Kupffer cells and thus never enter the systemic circulation. In another example, liver enzymes modify both endogenous and exogenous toxins to render them water soluble and thus capable of being excreted in either bile or urine. **Phase I reactions,** which are catalyzed by cytochrome P-450 enzymes, are followed by **phase II reactions** that conjugate the substances with glucuronide, sulfate, amino acids, or glutathione.

SUMMARY

■ The gastrointestinal tract is innervated by both the parasympathetic and sympathetic nervous systems, which converge on the intrinsic nervous system in the myenteric and submucosal plexuses.

■ Gastrointestinal peptides are secreted by cells of the gastrointestinal tract and include the hormones gastrin, CCK, secretin, and GIP, which are released into the circulation; the paracrines somatostatin and histamine, which act locally; and neurocrines, which are released from nerves.

■ Slow waves in gastrointestinal smooth muscle cells are spontaneous depolarizations and repolarizations of the membrane potential. Action potentials are fired *if* the membrane potential reaches threshold as a result of a slow wave. Thus, the frequency of slow waves determines the frequency of action potentials and, consequently, the frequency of contractions.

■ Gastric motility includes mixing and grinding of ingested food. Small intestinal motility includes segmentation contractions, which mix chyme with digestive enzymes, and peristaltic contractions, which move the chyme in the caudad direction. In the large intestine, mass movements push the fecal material over long distances and eventually into the rectum, where it is stored until defecation occurs.

■ Salivary secretion is utilized for buffering and dilution of foods and for initial digestion of starch and lipids. Saliva is hypotonic and is produced by a two-step process involving formation of an initial saliva by acinar cells and its modification by ductal epithelial cells.

■ Pancreatic secretion contains HCO_3^- for the neutralization of H^+ from the stomach and enzymes for digestion of carbohydrates, proteins, and lipids. Pancreatic juice is isotonic and is produced by a two-step process. The acinar cells secrete the enzymatic component, centroacinar and ductal epithelial cells secrete the aqueous HCO_3^--containing component, and ductal cells modify the secretion.

■ Bile salts, the major constituents of bile, are used for emulsification and solubilization of lipids, aiding in their digestion and absorption. Bile is produced by hepatocytes, stored in the gallbladder, and secreted into the intestine when the gallbladder contracts. Bile salts solubilize and form micelles with the products of lipid digestion. Approximately 95% of bile acids are recirculated to the liver via the enterohepatic circulation.

■ Carbohydrates must be digested to monosaccharides for absorption. The digestive steps are carried out by salivary and pancreatic amylases and disaccharidases in the intestinal brush border. Glucose and galactose are absorbed by intestinal epithelial cells by Na^+-dependent cotransporters, and fructose is absorbed by facilitated diffusion.

■ Proteins are digested to amino acids, dipeptides, and tripeptides for absorption. The digestive steps are carried out by pepsin, trypsin, and other pancreatic and brush-border proteases. Amino acids, dipeptides, and tripeptides are absorbed by intestinal epithelial cells by Na^+- or H^+-dependent cotransporters.

■ Lipids are digested to monoglycerides, fatty acids, cholesterol, and lysolecithin by pancreatic enzymes. The products of lipid digestion are solubilized in micelles with bile acids. At the apical membrane of intestinal epithelial cells, the lipids are released from the micelles and diffuse into the cells. Within the cells,

they are packaged in chylomicrons and transferred into lymph vessels by exocytosis.

■ Approximately 9 L of fluid is absorbed daily by the gastrointestinal tract. The volume of fluid absorbed is approximately equal to the sum of the volume ingested and the volume secreted in salivary, gastric, pancreatic, and intestinal juices. Diarrhea results if absorption is decreased or if secretion is increased.

■ The liver conjugates bilirubin, a metabolite of hemoglobin, with glucuronic acid to form conjugated bilirubin, which is excreted into urine and bile. In the intestine, conjugated bilirubin is converted to urobilinogen, which recirculates to the liver, and to urobilin and stercobilin, which are excreted in the stool.

Challenge Yourself

Answer each question with a word, phrase, sentence, or numerical solution. When a list of possible answers is supplied with the question, one, more than one, or none of the choices may be correct. Correct answers are provided at the end of the book.

1 *Which of the following is/are (an) action(s) of cholecystokinin (CCK): contraction of the gallbladder, acceleration of gastric emptying, stimulation of HCO_3^- secretion, stimulation of pancreatic enzyme secretion?*

2 *A patient with a duodenal ulcer is treated with cimetidine, a drug that inhibits H^+ secretion in parietal cells. Which of the following is the mechanism of cimetidine's action: inhibition of H^+-K^+ATPase, inhibition of muscarinic receptors, stimulation of muscarinic receptors, decreased intracellular cyclic AMP (cAMP) levels, inhibition of somatostatin?*

3 *During the rising phase (upstroke) of a slow wave, which change in membrane potential is occurring: more negative, less negative, more positive, less positive?*

4 *Which phenomenon in salivary ducts explains why the final salivary secretion is hypotonic relative to the primary secretion of the acinar cells: secretion of water, absorption of water, absorption of more solute than water, secretion of more solute than water?*

5 *Cholera toxin has which of the following direct or indirect actions: opens Na^+ channels, closes Cl^- channels, increases cAMP levels,* *activates α_s subunit of GTP-binding protein, increases GTPase activity?*

6 *Which of the following substances must be digested before being absorbed by the small intestine: Ca^{2+}, alanine, fructose, sucrose, cholesterol?*

7 *What is the correct sequence of events in lipid absorption: formation of cholesterol ester, action of pancreatic lipase, emulsification of lipids in the intestinal lumen, micelles, chylomicrons?*

8 *As pancreatic flow rate increases, which of the following has/have increased concentration in pancreatic juice: Na^+, K^+, HCO_3^-, Cl^-, osmolarity?*

9 *Which reaction(s) is/are catalyzed by trypsin: pepsinogen to pepsin, trypsinogen to trypsin, procarboxypeptidase to carboxypeptidase?*

10 *Where is the frequency of slow waves the highest: stomach, duodenum, ileum?*

11 *Where am I? For each item in the following list, give its correct location in the gastrointestinal system. The location may be anatomic, a graph or portion of a graph, or a concept.*
Gastrin secretion
Na^+-bile salt cotransport
H^+-K^+ ATPase
Intrinsic factor secretion
Omeprazole action
Na^+-glucose cotransporter
Secondary bile acids (or bile salts)

12 *A patient with H. pylori infection develops a gastric ulcer and is treated with omeprazole. Which of the following is/are mechanism(s) of action of omeprazole? Inhibition of ACh action on parietal cells, stimulation of somatostatin action on parietal cells, inhibition of CCK_B receptors, inhibition of H^+-K^+ ATPase, inhibition of Na^+-K^+ ATPase.*

13 *Which of the following suppresses appetite? Increased body fat, increased insulin levels, increased ghrelin levels.*

14 *In the peristaltic reflex, which of the following occurs orad to (behind) the food bolus? Release of 5-hydroxytryptamine (5-HT) from IPAN neurons, contraction of circular muscle, contraction of longitudinal muscle, action of acetylcholine on circular muscle, action of vasoactive intestinal peptide (VIP) on circular muscle.*

SELECTED READINGS

Johnson LR: Physiology of the Gastrointestinal Tract, 2nd ed. New York, Raven Press, 1987.

Johnson LR: Gastrointestinal Physiology, 6th ed. St Louis, Mosby, 2001.

Schultz SG, Wood JD, Raunder BB: Handbook of Physiology: The Gastrointestinal System. Bethesda, Md, American Physiological Society, 1989.

Endocrine Physiology

The endocrine system, in concert with the nervous system, is responsible for homeostasis. Growth, development, reproduction, blood pressure, concentrations of ions and other substances in blood, and even behavior are all regulated by the endocrine system. Endocrine physiology involves the secretion of hormones and their subsequent actions on target tissues.

A hormone is a chemical substance that is classified as a peptide, steroid, or amine. Hormones are secreted into the circulation in small amounts and delivered to target tissues, where they produce physiologic responses. Hormones are synthesized and secreted by endocrine cells usually found in endocrine glands. Table 9-1 is a list of hormones and their abbreviations, which are used throughout Chapters 9 and 10.

The classical endocrine glands are the hypothalamus, anterior and posterior lobes of the pituitary, thyroid, parathyroid, adrenal cortex, adrenal medulla, gonads, placenta, and pancreas. The kidney also is considered to be an endocrine gland, and endocrine cells are found throughout the gastrointestinal tract. Table 9-2 summarizes the major hormones, their glands of origin, their chemical nature, and their major actions. Its companion, Figure 9-1, is a pictorial summary of the endocrine glands and their hormonal secretions.

HORMONE SYNTHESIS

Hormones are categorized in one of three classes: peptides and proteins, steroids, or amines. Each class differs in its biosynthetic pathway: Peptide and protein hormones are synthesized from amino acids; steroid hormones are derivatives of cholesterol; and amine hormones are derivatives of tyrosine.

Peptide and Protein Hormone Synthesis

Most hormones are peptide or protein in nature. The biosynthetic pathways are familiar from biochemistry. The primary amino acid sequence of the peptide is dictated by a specific messenger ribonucleotide (mRNA), which has been transcribed from the gene

Table 9–1 Commonly Used Abbreviations in Endocrine Physiology

Abbreviation	Hormone	Abbreviation	Hormone
ACTH	Adrenocorticotropic hormone	LH	Luteinizing hormone
ADH	Antidiuretic hormone	MIT	Monoiodotyrosine
CRH	Corticotropin-releasing hormone	MSH	Melanocyte-stimulating hormone
DHEA	Dehydroepiandrosterone	PIF	Prolactin-inhibiting factor (dopamine)
DIT	Diiodotyrosine	POMC	Pro-opiomelanocortin
DOC	11-Deoxycorticosterone	PTH	Parathyroid hormone
FSH	Follicle-stimulating hormone	PTU	Propylthiouracil
GHRH	Growth hormone–releasing hormone	SRIF	Somatotropin release–inhibiting factor
GnRH	Gonadotropin-releasing hormone	T_3	Triiodothyronine
HCG	Human chorionic gonadotropin	T_4	Thyroxine
HGH	Human growth hormone	TBG	Thyroxine-binding globulin
HPL	Human placental lactogen	TRH	Thyrotropin-releasing hormone
IGF	Insulin-like growth factor	TSH	Thyroid-stimulating hormone

Table 9–2 Summary of Endocrine Glands and Actions of Hormones

Gland of Origin	Hormones*	Chemical Classification†	Major Actions
Hypothalamus	Thyrotropin-releasing hormone (TRH)	Peptide	Stimulates secretion of TSH and prolactin
	Corticotropin-releasing hormone (CRH)	Peptide	Stimulates secretion of ACTH
	Gonadotropin-releasing hormone (GnRH)	Peptide	Stimulates secretion of LH and FSH
	Somatostatin or somatotropin release–inhibiting hormone (SRIF)	Peptide	Inhibits secretion of growth hormone
	Dopamine or prolactin-inhibiting factor (PIF)	Amine	Inhibits secretion of prolactin
	Growth hormone–releasing hormone (GHRH)	Peptide	Stimulates secretion of growth hormone
Anterior Pituitary	Thyroid-stimulating hormone (TSH)	Peptide	Stimulates synthesis and secretion of thyroid hormones
	Follicle-stimulating hormone (FSH)	Peptide	Stimulates sperm maturation in Sertoli cells of testes
			Stimulates follicular development and estrogen synthesis in ovaries
	Luteinizing hormone (LH)	Peptide	Stimulates testosterone synthesis in Leydig cells of testes
			Stimulates ovulation, formation of corpus luteum, estrogen and progesterone synthesis in ovaries
	Growth hormone	Peptide	Stimulates protein synthesis and overall growth
	Prolactin	Peptide	Stimulates milk production and secretion in breast
	Adrenocorticotropic hormone (ACTH)	Peptide	Stimulates synthesis and secretion of adrenal cortical hormones (cortisol, androgens, and aldosterone)
	Melanocyte-stimulating hormone (MSH)	Peptide	Stimulates melanin synthesis (? humans)

Table 9–2 Summary of Endocrine Glands and Actions of Hormones—cont'd

Gland of Origin	Hormones*	Chemical Classification[†]	Major Actions
Posterior Pituitary	Oxytocin	Peptide	Stimulates milk ejection from breasts and uterine contractions
	Vasopressin or antidiuretic hormone (ADH)	Peptide	Stimulates water reabsorption in principal cells of collecting ducts and constriction of arterioles
Thyroid	Triiodothyronine (T_3) and L-thyroxine (T_4)	Amine	Stimulates skeletal growth; oxygen consumption; heat production; protein, fat, and carbohydrate utilization; perinatal maturation of the central nervous system
	Calcitonin	Peptide	Decreases serum $[Ca^{2+}]$
Parathyroid	Parathyroid hormone (PTH)	Peptide	Increases serum $[Ca^{2+}]$
Adrenal Cortex	Cortisol (glucocorticoid)	Steroid	Stimulates gluconeogenesis; inhibits inflammatory response; suppresses immune response; enhances vascular responsiveness to catecholamines
	Aldosterone (mineralocorticoid)	Steroid	Increases renal Na^+ reabsorption, K^+ secretion, and H^+ secretion
	Dehydroepiandrosterone (DHEA) and androstenedione (adrenal androgens)	Steroid	See actions of testosterone from testes (see below)
Testes	Testosterone	Steroid	Stimulates spermatogenesis; stimulates male secondary sex characteristics
Ovaries	Estradiol	Steroid	Stimulates growth and development of female reproductive system, follicular phase of menstrual cycle, development of breasts, prolactin secretion; maintains pregnancy
	Progesterone	Steroid	Stimulates luteal phase of menstrual cycle; maintains pregnancy
Corpus Luteum	Estradiol and progesterone	Steroid	See actions of estradiol and progesterone from ovaries (see above)
Placenta	Human chorionic gonadotropin (HCG)	Peptide	Stimulates estrogen and progesterone synthesis in corpus luteum of early pregnancy
	Human placental lactogen (HPL), or human chorionic somatomammotropin	Peptide	Has growth hormone–like and prolactin-like actions during pregnancy
	Estriol	Steroid	See actions of estradiol from ovaries (see above)
	Progesterone	Steroid	See actions of progesterone from ovaries (see above)
Pancreas	Insulin (β cells)	Peptide	Decreases blood [glucose]
	Glucagon (α cells)	Peptide	Increases blood [glucose]
Kidney	Renin	Peptide	Catalyzes conversion of angiotensinogen to angiotensin I
	1,25-Dihydroxycholecalciferol	Steroid	Increases intestinal absorption of Ca^{2+}; bone mineralization
Adrenal Medulla	Norepinephrine, epinephrine	Amine	See actions of sympathetic nervous system (see Chapter 2)

*Standard abbreviations for hormones are given in parentheses.
[†]Peptide refers to both peptides and proteins.

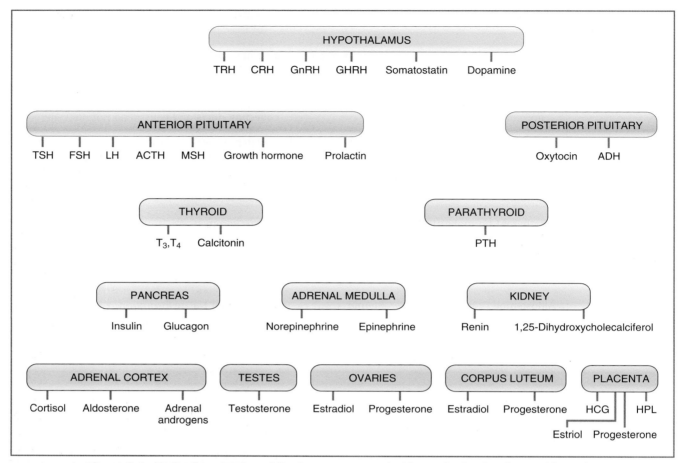

Figure 9–1 Endocrine glands and the hormones secreted by each gland. Refer to Table 9-1 for abbreviations used in this figure.

for that hormone. The biosynthetic pathway for peptide hormones is summarized in Figure 9-2. The circled numbers in the figure correspond to the following steps:

1. In the **nucleus,** the gene for the hormone is transcribed into an **mRNA.** Generally, a single gene is responsible for directing the primary structure of each peptide hormone. (Because the genes for almost all peptide hormones have been cloned, recombinant DNA technology makes it possible to synthesize human peptide hormones.)

2. The mRNA is transferred to the cytoplasm and translated on the **ribosomes** to the first protein product, a **preprohormone.** Translation of the mRNA begins with a signal peptide at the N terminus. Translation ceases, and the signal peptide attaches to receptors on the endoplasmic reticulum via "docking proteins." Translation then continues on the endoplasmic reticulum until the entire peptide sequence is produced (i.e., the preprohormone).

3. The signal peptide is removed in the **endoplasmic reticulum,** converting the preprohormone to a **prohormone.** The prohormone contains the

complete hormone sequence plus other peptide sequences, which will be removed in a final step. Some of the "other" peptide sequences in the prohormone are necessary for proper folding of the hormone (e.g., formation of intramolecular linkages).

4. The prohormone is transferred to the **Golgi apparatus,** where it is packaged in secretory vesicles. In the secretory vesicles, proteolytic enzymes cleave peptide sequences from the prohormone to produce the final **hormone.** Other functions of the Golgi apparatus include glycosylation and phosphorylation of the hormone.

5. The final hormone is stored in **secretory vesicles** until the endocrine cell is stimulated. For example, parathyroid hormone (PTH) is synthesized and stored in vesicles in the chief cells of the parathyroid gland. The stimulus for secretion of PTH is low extracellular calcium (Ca^{2+}) concentration. When sensors on the parathyroid gland detect a low extracellular Ca^{2+} concentration, the secretory vesicles are translocated to the cell membrane, where they extrude PTH into the blood by exocytosis. The other constituents of the secretory vesicles, including

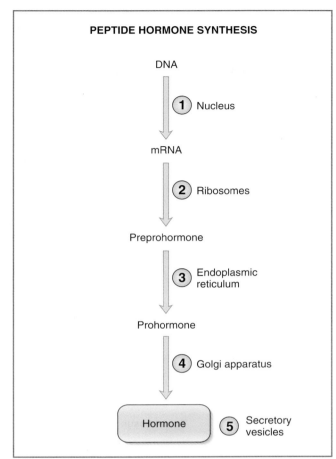

PEPTIDE HORMONE SYNTHESIS

DNA

(1) Nucleus

mRNA

(2) Ribosomes

Preprohormone

(3) Endoplasmic reticulum

Prohormone

(4) Golgi apparatus

Hormone (5) Secretory vesicles

Figure 9–2 **Steps involved in the synthesis of peptide hormones.** See the text for an explanation of the circled numbers. DNA, Deoxyribonucleic acid; mRNA, messenger ribonucleic acid.

copeptides and cleavage enzymes, are extruded with PTH.

Steroid Hormone Synthesis

Steroid hormones are synthesized and secreted by the adrenal cortex, gonads, corpus luteum, and placenta. The steroid hormones are cortisol, aldosterone, estradiol and estriol, progesterone, testosterone, and 1,25-dihydroxycholecalciferol. All steroid hormones are derivatives of **cholesterol,** which is modified by removal or addition of side chains, hydroxylation, or aromatization of the steroid nucleus. The biosynthetic pathways for the adrenocortical hormones and for 1,25-dihydroxycholecalciferol are discussed in this chapter. The pathways for the sex steroid hormones are discussed in Chapter 10.

Amine Hormone Synthesis

The amine hormones are catecholamines (epinephrine, norepinephrine, and dopamine) and thyroid hormones. The amine hormones are derivatives of the amino acid **tyrosine.** The biosynthetic pathway for catecholamines

is discussed in Chapter 1. The pathway for thyroid hormones is discussed in this chapter.

REGULATION OF HORMONE SECRETION

To maintain homeostasis, the secretion of hormones must be turned on and off as needed. Adjustments in secretory rates may be accomplished by neural mechanisms or by feedback mechanisms. **Neural mechanisms** are illustrated by the secretion of catecholamines, where preganglionic sympathetic nerves synapse on the adrenal medulla and, when stimulated, cause secretion of catecholamines into the circulation. **Feedback mechanisms** are more common than neural mechanisms. The term "feedback" means that some element of the physiologic response to a hormone "feeds back," either directly or indirectly, on the endocrine gland that secreted the hormone, changing its secretion rate. Feedback can be negative or positive. Negative feedback is the most important and common mechanism for regulating hormone secretion; positive feedback is rare.

Negative Feedback

The principles of negative feedback underlie the homeostatic regulation of virtually all organ systems. For example, in Chapter 4, negative feedback is discussed in the regulation of arterial blood pressure in which small changes in blood pressure turn on, or activate, mechanisms that will restore blood pressure back to normal. A decrease in arterial blood pressure is detected by baroreceptors, which activate coordinated mechanisms that increase blood pressure. As blood pressure returns to normal, a disturbance is no longer sensed by the baroreceptors and those mechanisms previously activated will be turned off. The more sensitive the feedback mechanism, the smaller the "excursions" of blood pressure above or below normal.

In endocrine systems, negative feedback means that *some feature of hormone action, directly or indirectly, inhibits further secretion of the hormone.* Negative feedback loops are illustrated in Figure 9-3. For illustrative purposes, the hypothalamus is shown in relation to the anterior pituitary, which is shown in relation to a peripheral endocrine gland. In the figure, the hypothalamus secretes a releasing hormone, which stimulates secretion of an anterior pituitary hormone. The anterior pituitary hormone then acts on a peripheral endocrine gland (e.g., the testis) to cause secretion of the hormone (e.g., testosterone), which acts on target tissues (e.g., skeletal muscle) to produce physiologic actions. The hormones "feed back" on the anterior pituitary and the hypothalamus to inhibit their hormonal secretions. **Long-loop feedback** means that the hormone feeds back *all the way* to the hypothalamic-pituitary axis.

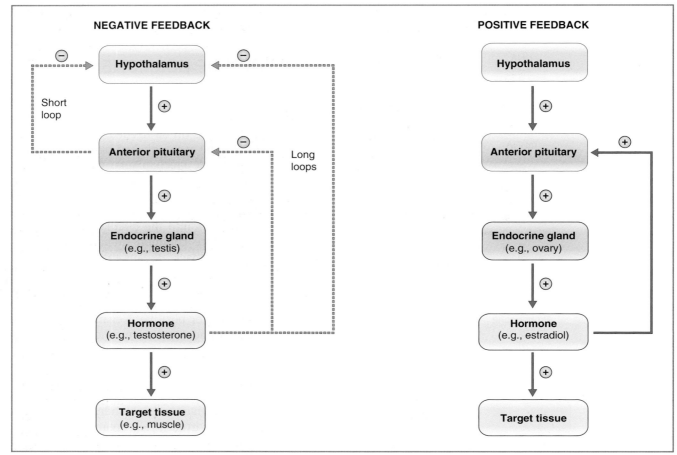

Figure 9–3 **Negative and positive feedback mechanisms.** The hypothalamic-pituitary axis is used as an example in this illustration. *Solid lines* and *plus* (+) *signs* indicate stimulation; *dashed lines* and *minus* (−) *signs* indicate inhibition.

Short-loop feedback means that the anterior pituitary hormone feeds back on the hypothalamus to inhibit secretion of hypothalamic-releasing hormone. Not shown in the figure is a third possibility called **ultrashort-loop feedback,** in which the hypothalamic hormone inhibits its own secretion (e.g., growth hormone–releasing hormone [GHRH] inhibits GHRH secretion).

The net result of any version of negative feedback is that when hormone levels are judged (by their physiologic actions) to be adequate or high, further secretion of the hormone is inhibited. When hormone levels are judged to be inadequate or low, secretion of the hormone is stimulated.

There are other examples of negative feedback that do not utilize the hypothalamic-pituitary axis. For example, **insulin** regulates blood glucose concentration. In turn, insulin secretion is turned on or off by changes in the blood glucose concentration. Thus, when blood glucose concentration is high, insulin secretion from the pancreas is turned on; insulin then acts on its target tissues (liver, muscle, and adipose) to decrease the blood glucose concentration back toward normal.

When the glucose concentration is sensed as being low enough, insulin is no longer needed and its secretion is turned off.

Positive Feedback

Positive feedback is uncommon. With positive feedback, some feature of hormone action causes *more* secretion of the hormone (see Fig. 9-3). When compared with negative feedback, which is self-limiting, positive feedback is self-augmenting. Although rare in biologic systems, when positive feedback does occur, it leads to an explosive event.

A nonhormonal example of positive feedback is the opening of nerve sodium (Na^+) channels during the **upstroke of the action potential.** Depolarization opens voltage-sensitive Na^+ channels and causes Na^+ entry into the cell, which leads to more depolarization and more Na^+ entry. This self-reinforcing process produces the rapid, explosive upstroke.

In hormonal systems, the primary example of positive feedback is the effect of **estrogen** on the secretion of follicle-stimulating hormone (**FSH**) and luteinizing hormone (**LH**) by the anterior pituitary at the midpoint of the menstrual cycle. During the follicular phase of the menstrual cycle, the ovaries secrete estrogen, which acts on the anterior pituitary to produce a rapid burst of FSH and LH secretion. FSH and LH have two effects on the ovaries: ovulation *and* stimulation of estrogen secretion. Thus, estrogen secreted from the ovaries acts on the anterior pituitary to cause secretion of FSH and LH, and these anterior pituitary hormones cause *more* estrogen secretion. In this example, the explosive event is the burst of FSH and LH that precedes ovulation.

A second example of hormonal positive feedback is **oxytocin**. Dilation of the cervix causes the posterior pituitary to secrete oxytocin. In turn, oxytocin stimulates uterine contraction, which causes further dilation of the cervix. In this example, the explosive event is parturition, the delivery of the fetus.

REGULATION OF HORMONE RECEPTORS

The previous section describes the mechanisms that regulate circulating levels of hormones, usually by negative feedback. Although circulating hormone levels are important, they are *not* the only determinant of the response of a target tissue. To respond, a target tissue must possess specific receptors that recognize the hormone. Those receptors are coupled to cellular mechanisms that produce the physiologic response. (The coupling mechanisms are discussed in the section on mechanisms of hormone action.)

The responsiveness of a target tissue to a hormone is expressed in the **dose-response relationship** in which the magnitude of response is correlated with hormone concentration. As the hormone concentration increases, the response usually increases and then levels off. **Sensitivity** is defined as the hormone concentration that produces 50% of the maximal response. If more hormone is required to produce 50% of the maximal response, then there has been a decrease in sensitivity of the target tissue. If less hormone is required, there has been an increase in sensitivity of the target tissue.

The responsiveness or sensitivity of a target tissue can be changed in one of two ways: by changing the *number* of receptors or by changing the *affinity* of the receptors for the hormone. The greater the number of receptors for a hormone, the greater the maximal response. The higher the affinity of the receptor for the hormone, the greater the likelihood of a response.

A change in the number or affinity of receptors is called down-regulation or up-regulation. **Down-regulation** means that the number of receptors or the affinity of the receptors for the hormone has decreased.

Up-regulation means that the number or the affinity of the receptors has increased. Hormones may down-regulate or up-regulate their own receptors in target tissues and even may regulate receptors for other hormones.

Down-Regulation

Down-regulation is a mechanism in which a hormone *decreases* the number or affinity of its receptors in a target tissue. Down-regulation may occur by decreasing the synthesis of new receptors, by increasing the degradation of existing receptors, or by inactivating receptors. The purpose of down-regulation is to reduce the sensitivity of the target tissue when hormone levels are high for an extended period of time. As down-regulation occurs, the response to hormone declines, although hormone levels remain high. An example of down-regulation is the effect of **progesterone** on its own receptor in the uterus (see Chapter 10).

Down-regulation can also refer to a hormone's effect on receptors for other related hormones. This type of down-regulation also is illustrated by progesterone. In the uterus, progesterone down-regulates its own receptor *and* down-regulates the receptors for estrogen. A second example of this type of down-regulation is seen in the thyroid system: Triiodothyronine, or **T₃**, decreases the sensitivity of thyrotropin-releasing hormone (TRH) receptors in the anterior pituitary. The overall effect is that chronically high levels of T_3 reduce the overall responsiveness of the hypothalamic-pituitary-thyroid axis.

Up-Regulation

Up-regulation of receptors is a mechanism in which a hormone *increases* the number or affinity of its receptors. Up-regulation may occur by increasing synthesis of new receptors, decreasing degradation of existing receptors, or activating receptors. For example, **prolactin** increases the number of its receptors in the breast, **growth hormone** increases the number of its receptors in skeletal muscle and liver, and **estrogen** increases the number of its receptors in the uterus.

A hormone also can up-regulate the receptors for other hormones. For example, estrogen not only up-regulates its own receptor in the uterus, but it also up-regulates the receptors for LH in the ovaries.

MECHANISMS OF HORMONE ACTION AND SECOND MESSENGERS

Hormone actions on target cells begin when the hormone binds to a membrane receptor, forming a hormone-receptor complex. In many hormonal systems,

Table 9-3 Mechanisms of Hormone Action

Adenylyl Cyclase Mechanism (cAMP)	Phospholipase C Mechanism (IP$_3$/Ca^{2+})	Steroid Hormone Mechanism	Tyrosine Kinase Mechanism	Guanylate Cyclase Mechanism (cGMP)
ACTH	GnRH	Glucocorticoids	Insulin	Atrial natriuretic
LH	TRH	Estrogen	IGF-1	peptide (ANP)
FSH	GHRH	Progesterone	Growth hormone	Nitric oxide (NO)
TSH	Angiotensin II	Testosterone	Prolactin	
ADH (V$_2$ receptor)	ADH (V$_1$ receptor)	Aldosterone		
HCG	Oxytocin	1,25-Dihydroxycholecalciferol		
MSH	α$_1$ Receptors	Thyroid hormones		
CRH				
Calcitonin				
PTH				
Glucagon				
β$_1$ and β$_2$ receptors				

the hormone-receptor complex is coupled to effector proteins by guanosine triphosphate (GTP)–binding proteins (G proteins). The effector proteins usually are enzymes, either adenylyl cyclase or phospholipase C. When the effector proteins are activated, a second messenger, either cAMP or IP$_3$ (inositol 1,4,5-triphosphate), is produced, which amplifies the original hormonal signal and orchestrates the physiologic actions.

The major mechanisms of hormone action on target cells are the **adenylyl cyclase** mechanism, in which cAMP is the second messenger; the **phospholipase C** mechanism, in which IP$_3$/Ca^{2+} is the second messenger; and the **steroid hormone** mechanism. In addition, insulin and insulin-like growth factors (IGFs) act on their target cells through a **tyrosine kinase** mechanism. Finally, several hormones activate **guanylate cyclase,** in which cyclic guanosine monophosphate (cyclic GMP, or cGMP) is the second messenger. The mechanisms of action of the major hormones are summarized in Table 9-3.

G Proteins

G proteins are discussed in Chapter 2 in the context of autonomic receptors. Briefly, G proteins are a family of membrane-bound proteins that couple hormone receptors to effector enzymes (e.g., adenylyl cyclase). Thus, G proteins serve as "molecular switches" that decide whether the hormone action can proceed.

At the molecular level, G proteins are heterotrimeric (i.e., they have three subunits) proteins. The three subunits are designated alpha (α), beta (β), and gamma (γ). The α subunit can bind either guanosine diphosphate (GDP) or GTP, and it contains GTPase activity. When GDP is bound to the α subunit, the G protein is inactive; when GTP is bound, the G protein is active and can perform its coupling function. Guanosine nucleotide releasing factors (GRFs) facilitate dissociation of GDP so that GTP binds more rapidly, whereas GTPase activating factors (GAPs) facilitate hydrolysis of

GTP. Thus, the relative activity of GRFs and GAPs influences the overall rate of G protein activation.

G proteins can be either stimulatory or inhibitory and are called, accordingly, **G$_s$** or **G$_i$**. Stimulatory or inhibitory activity resides in the α subunit (α$_s$ or α$_i$). Thus, when GTP is bound to the α$_s$ subunit of a G$_s$ protein, the G$_s$ protein *stimulates* the effector enzyme (e.g., adenylyl cyclase). When GTP is bound to the α$_i$ subunit of a G$_i$ protein, the G$_i$ protein *inhibits* the effector enzyme.

Adenylyl Cyclase Mechanism

The adenylyl cyclase/cAMP mechanism is utilized by many hormonal systems (see Table 9-3). This mechanism involves binding of a hormone to a receptor, coupling by a G$_s$ or G$_i$ protein, and then activation or inhibition of adenylyl cyclase, leading to increases or decreases in intracellular cAMP. cAMP, the second messenger, then amplifies the hormonal signal to produce the final physiologic actions.

The steps in the adenylyl cyclase/cAMP mechanism are shown in Figure 9-4. In this example, the hormone utilizes a G$_s$ protein (rather than a G$_i$ protein). The receptor–G$_s$–adenylyl cyclase complex is embedded in the cell membrane. When no hormone is bound to the receptor, the α$_s$ subunit of the G$_s$ protein binds GDP. In this configuration, the G$_s$ protein is **inactive.** When hormone binds to its receptor, the following steps (see Fig. 9-4) occur:

1. Hormone binds to its **receptor** in the cell membrane, producing a conformational change in the α$_s$ subunit (Step 1), which produces two changes: GDP is released from the α$_s$ subunit and is replaced by GTP, and the α$_s$ subunit detaches from the G$_s$ protein (Step 2).

2. The **α$_s$-GTP complex** migrates within the cell membrane and binds to and activates adenylyl cyclase (Step 3). Activated **adenylyl cyclase** catalyzes the

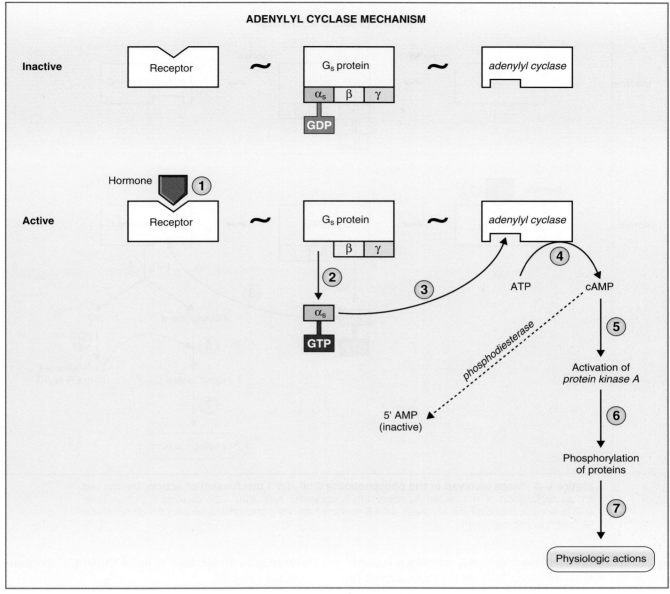

Figure 9–4 **Steps involved in the adenylyl cyclase (cAMP) mechanism of action.** See the text for an explanation of the circled numbers. AMP, Adenosine monophosphate; ATP, adenosine triphosphate; cAMP, cyclic adenosine monophosphate; GDP, guanosine diphosphate; GTP, guanosine triphosphate.

conversion of ATP to cAMP, which serves as the second messenger (Step 4). Although not shown, intrinsic GTPase activity in the G protein converts GTP back to GDP, and the α_s subunit returns to its inactive state.

3. **cAMP,** via a series of steps involving activation of **protein kinase A,** phosphorylates intracellular proteins (Steps 5 and 6). These phosphorylated proteins then execute the final physiologic actions (Step 7).

4. Intracellular cAMP is degraded to an inactive metabolite, **5′ AMP,** by the enzyme **phosphodiesterase,** thereby turning off the action of the second messenger.

Phospholipase C Mechanism

Hormones that utilize the phospholipase C (IP_3/Ca^{2+}) mechanism also are listed in Table 9-3. The mechanism involves binding of hormone to a receptor and coupling via a G_q protein to phospholipase C. Intracellular levels of IP_3 and Ca^{2+} are increased, producing the final physiologic actions. The steps in the phospholipase C (IP_3/Ca^{2+}) mechanism are shown in Figure 9-5.

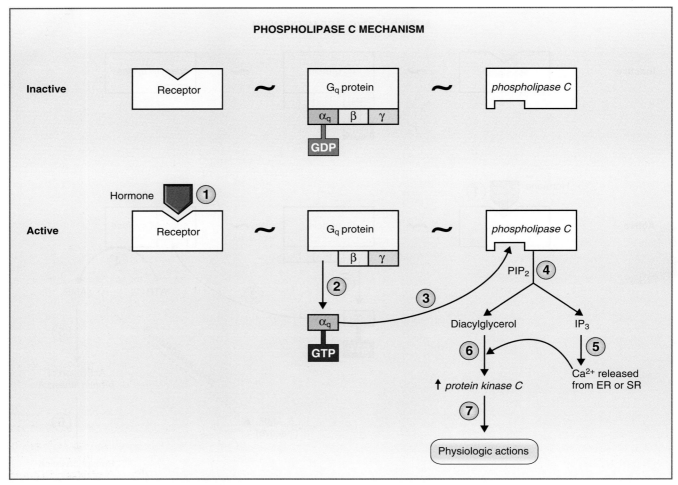

Figure 9–5 **Steps involved in the phospholipase C (IP₃/Ca²⁺) mechanism of action.** See the text for an explanation of the circled numbers. ER, Endoplasmic reticulum; GDP, guanosine diphosphate; GTP, guanosine triphosphate; IP₃, inositol 1,4,5-triphosphate; PIP₂, phosphatidylinositol 4,5-diphosphate; SR, sarcoplasmic reticulum.

The receptor–G_q–phospholipase C complex is embedded in the cell membrane. With no hormone bound to the receptor, the α_q subunit binds GDP. In this configuration, the G_q protein is **inactive.** When the hormone binds to the receptor, G_q is activated, which activates phospholipase C, in the following steps (see Fig. 9-5):

1. Hormone binds to its receptor in the cell membrane, producing a conformational change in the α_q subunit (Step 1). GDP is released from the α_q subunit, is replaced by GTP, and the α_q subunit detaches from the G_q protein (Step 2).

2. The **α_q-GTP complex** migrates within the cell membrane and binds to and activates phospholipase C (Step 3). Activated **phospholipase C** catalyzes the liberation of diacylglycerol and IP₃ from phosphatidylinositol 4,5-diphosphate (PIP₂), a membrane phospholipid (Step 4). The **IP₃** generated causes the release of **Ca²⁺** from intracellular stores in the endoplasmic or sarcoplasmic reticulum,

resulting in an increase in intracellular Ca²⁺ concentration (Step 5).

3. Together, Ca²⁺ and diacylglycerol activate **protein kinase C** (Step 6), which phosphorylates proteins and produces the final physiologic actions (Step 7).

Catalytic Receptor Mechanisms

Some hormones bind to cell surface receptors that have, or are associated with, enzymatic activity on the intracellular side of the cell membrane. These so-called **catalytic receptors** include guanylyl cyclase, serine/threonine kinases, tyrosine kinases, and tyrosine kinase-associated receptors. Guanylyl cyclase catalyzes the generation of cyclic GMP from GTP. The kinases phosphorylate serine, threonine, or tyrosine on proteins and thus add negative charge in the form of the phosphate group; phosphorylation of target proteins results in conformational changes that are responsible for the hormone's physiologic actions.

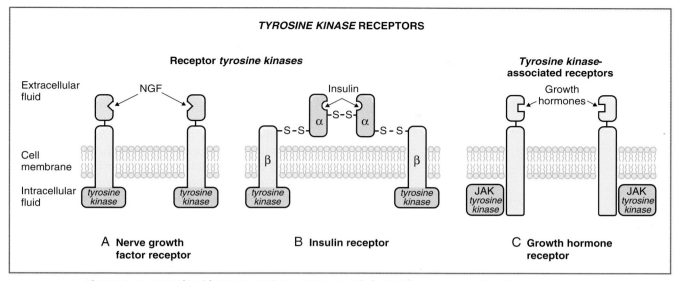

Figure 9–6 **Tyrosine kinase receptors.** Nerve growth factor **(A)** and insulin **(B)** utilize receptor tyrosine kinases that have intrinsic tyrosine kinase activity. Growth hormone **(C)** utilizes a tyrosine kinase–associated receptor. NGF, nerve growth factor; JAK, Janus family of receptor-associated tyrosine kinase.

Guanylyl Cyclase

Hormones acting through the guanylyl cyclase mechanism are also listed in Table 9-3. **Atrial natriuretic peptide (ANP)** and related natriuretic peptides act through a *receptor* guanylyl cyclase mechanism as follows (see Chapters 4 and 6). The extracellular domain of the receptor has a binding site for ANP, while the intracellular domain of the receptor has guanylyl cyclase activity. Binding of ANP causes activation of guanylyl cyclase and conversion of GTP to cyclic GMP. Cyclic GMP then activates cyclic GMP-dependent kinase, which phosphorylates the proteins responsible for ANP's physiologic actions.

Nitric oxide (NO) acts through a *cytosolic* guanylyl cyclase as follows (see Chapter 4). NO synthase in vascular endothelial cells cleaves arginine into citrulline and NO. The just-synthesized NO diffuses out of the endothelial cells into nearby vascular smooth muscle cells, where it binds to and activates soluble, or cytosolic, guanylyl cyclase. GTP is converted to cyclic GMP, which relaxes vascular smooth muscle.

Serine/Threonine Kinases

As previously discussed, numerous hormones utilize G-protein-linked receptors as part of the **adenylyl cyclase** and **phospholipase C** mechanisms (see Table 9-3). In these mechanisms, the cascade of events ultimately activates protein kinase A or protein kinase C, respectively. The activated kinases then phosphorylate serine and threonine moieties on proteins that execute the hormone's physiologic actions. In addition, **Ca^{2+}-calmodulin-dependent protein kinase (CaMK)** and **mitogen-activated protein kinases (MAPKs)** phosphorylate serine and threonine in the cascade of events leading to their biologic actions.

Tyrosine Kinases

Tyrosine kinases phosphorylate tyrosine moieties on proteins and fall in two major categories. **Receptor tyrosine kinases** have *intrinsic* tyrosine kinase activity within the receptor molecule. **Tyrosine kinase-associated receptors** do not have intrinsic tyrosine kinase activity but *associate* noncovalently with proteins that do (Fig. 9-6).

♦ **Receptor tyrosine kinases** have an extracellular binding domain that binds the hormone or ligand, a hydrophobic transmembrane domain, and an intracellular domain that contains tyrosine kinase activity. When activated by hormone or ligand, the intrinsic tyrosine kinase phosphorylates itself and other proteins.

One type of receptor tyrosine kinase is a monomer (e.g., **nerve growth factor [NGF] and epidermal growth factor receptors,** see Fig. 9-6A). In this monomeric type, binding of ligand to the extracellular domain results in dimerization of the receptor, activation of intrinsic tyrosine kinase, and phosphorylation of tyrosine moieties on itself and other proteins, leading to its physiologic actions.

Another type of receptor tyrosine kinase is already a dimer (e.g., **insulin and insulin-like growth factor [IGF] receptors,** see Fig. 9-6B). In this dimeric type, binding of the ligand (e.g., insulin) activates intrinsic tyrosine kinase and leads to phosphorylation of itself and other proteins and ultimately the hormone's physiologic actions. The mechanism of

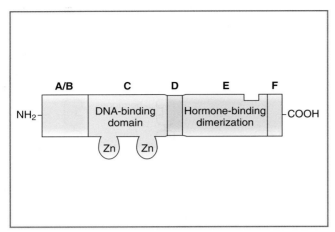

Figure 9–7 **Structure of cytosolic (or nuclear) steroid hormone receptor.** Letters A–F represent the six domains of the receptor. DNA, Deoxyribonucleic acid.

the insulin receptor is also discussed later in the chapter.

♦ **Tyrosine kinase-associated receptors** (e.g., **growth hormone receptors,** see Fig. 9-6C) also have an extracellular domain, a hydrophobic transmembrane domain, and an intracellular domain. However, unlike the receptor tyrosine kinases, the intracellular domain does not have tyrosine kinase activity but is noncovalently "associated" with tyrosine kinase such as those in the Janus kinase family (**JAK,** Janus family of receptor-associated tyrosine kinase, or "just another kinase"). Hormone binds to the extracellular domain, leading to receptor dimerization and activation of tyrosine kinase in the associated protein (e.g., JAK). The associated tyrosine kinase phosphorylates tyrosine moieties on itself, the hormone receptor, and other proteins. Downstream targets of JAK include members of the **STAT** (signal transducers and activators of transcription) family, which cause transcription of mRNAs and ultimately new proteins involved in the hormone's physiologic actions.

Steroid and Thyroid Hormone Mechanism

Steroid hormones and thyroid hormones have the same mechanism of action. In contrast to the adenylyl cyclase and phospholipase C mechanisms utilized by peptide hormones and involving cell membrane receptors and generation of intracellular second messengers, the steroid hormone mechanism involves binding to cytosolic (or nuclear) receptors (Fig. 9-7) that initiate DNA transcription and synthesis of new proteins. In further contrast to peptide hormones, which act quickly on their target cells (within minutes), steroid hormones **act slowly** (taking hours).

The steps in the steroid hormone mechanism (shown in Fig. 9-8) are described as follows:

1. The steroid hormone diffuses across the cell membrane and enters its target cell (Step 1), where it binds to a specific **receptor protein** (Step 2) that is located in either the cytosol (as shown in Fig. 9-8) or nucleus. Steroid hormone receptors are monomeric phosphoproteins that are part of a gene superfamily of intracellular receptors. Each receptor has six domains (see Fig. 9-7). The steroid hormone binds in the **E domain** located near the C-terminus. The central **C domain** is highly conserved among different steroid hormone receptors, has two zinc fingers, and is responsible for DNA-binding. With hormone bound, the receptor undergoes a conformational change and the activated hormone-receptor complex enters the nucleus of the target cell.

2. The hormone-receptor complex **dimerizes** and binds (at its C domain) to specific DNA sequences, called **steroid-responsive elements (SREs)** located in the 5′ region of target genes (Step 3).

3. The hormone-receptor complex has now become a **transcription factor** that regulates the rate of transcription of that gene (Step 4). New **messenger RNA (mRNA)** is transcribed (Step 5), leaves the nucleus (Step 6), and is translated to new proteins (Step 7) that have specific physiologic actions (Step 8). The nature of the **new proteins** is specific to the hormone and accounts for the specificity of the hormone's actions. For example, 1,25-dihydroxycholecalciferol induces the synthesis of a Ca^{2+}-binding protein that promotes Ca^{2+} absorption from the intestine; aldosterone induces synthesis of Na^+ channels (ENaC) in the renal principal cells that promote Na^+ reabsorption in the kidney; and testosterone induces synthesis of skeletal muscle proteins.

HYPOTHALAMIC-PITUITARY RELATIONSHIPS

The hypothalamus and pituitary gland function in a coordinated fashion to orchestrate many of the endocrine systems. The hypothalamic-pituitary unit regulates the functions of the thyroid, adrenal, and reproductive glands and also controls growth, milk production and ejection, and osmoregulation. It is important to visualize the anatomic relationships between the hypothalamus and the pituitary because these relationships underlie the functional connections between the glands.

The pituitary gland, which also is called the hypophysis, consists of a posterior lobe and an anterior lobe. The **posterior lobe** (or posterior pituitary) is also called the neurohypophysis. The **anterior lobe** (or anterior

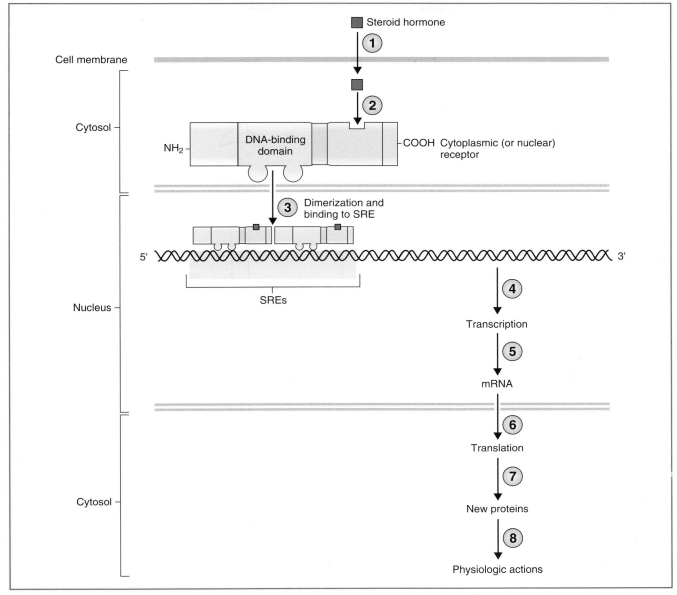

Figure 9–8 **Steps involved in the steroid hormone mechanism of action.** See the text for an explanation of the circled numbers. DNA, Deoxyribonucleic acid; mRNA, messenger ribonucleic acid; SREs, steroid-responsive elements.

pituitary) is also called the adenohypophysis. The hypothalamus is connected to the pituitary gland by a thin stalk called the **infundibulum.** Functionally, the hypothalamus controls the pituitary gland by both neural and hormonal mechanisms (Fig. 9-9).

Relationship of the Hypothalamus to the Posterior Pituitary

The posterior lobe of the pituitary gland is derived from neural tissue. It secretes two peptide hormones, antidiuretic hormone (ADH) and oxytocin, which act on their respective target tissues—the kidney, the breast, and the uterus.

The connections between the hypothalamus and the posterior lobe of the pituitary are neural. In fact, the posterior pituitary is a collection of nerve axons whose cell bodies are located in the hypothalamus. Thus, the hormones secreted by the posterior lobe (ADH and oxytocin) are actually **neuropeptides;** in other words, they are peptides released from neurons.

The cell bodies of ADH- and oxytocin-secreting neurons are located in supraoptic and paraventricular nuclei within the hypothalamus. Although both hormones are synthesized in both nuclei, **ADH** is primarily associated with **supraoptic** nuclei and **oxytocin** is primarily associated with **paraventricular** nuclei.

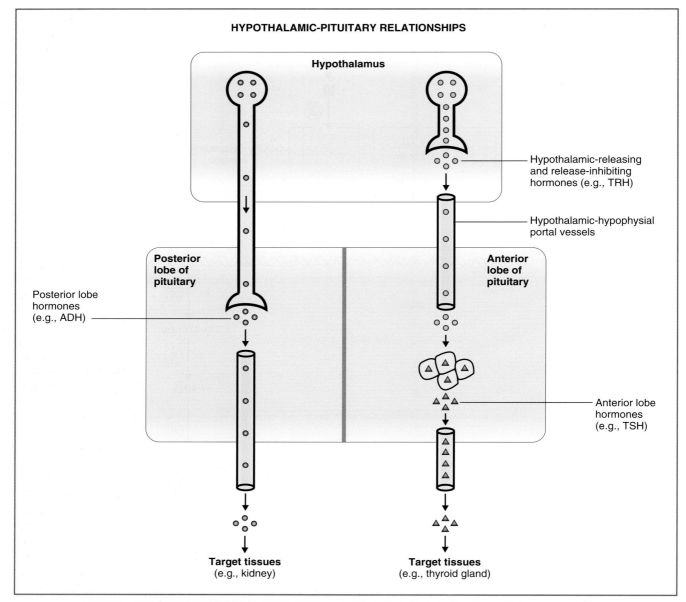

HYPOTHALAMIC-PITUITARY RELATIONSHIPS

Hypothalamus

Hypothalamic-releasing and release-inhibiting hormones (e.g., TRH)

Hypothalamic-hypophysial portal vessels

Posterior lobe of pituitary

Anterior lobe of pituitary

Posterior lobe hormones (e.g., ADH)

Anterior lobe hormones (e.g., TSH)

Target tissues (e.g., kidney)

Target tissues (e.g., thyroid gland)

Figure 9–9 **Schematic figure showing the relationship between the hypothalamus and the posterior and anterior lobes of the pituitary gland.** *Pink circles* are posterior pituitary hormones; *yellow circles* are hypothalamic hormones; *triangles* are anterior pituitary hormones. ADH, Antidiuretic hormone; TRH, thyrotropin-releasing hormone; TSH, thyroid-stimulating hormone.

Once synthesized in the cell bodies, the hormones (i.e., neuropeptides) are transported down the axons in neurosecretory vesicles and stored in bulbous nerve terminals in the posterior pituitary. When the cell body is stimulated, the neurosecretory vesicles are released from the nerve terminals by exocytosis and the secreted hormone enters nearby fenestrated capillaries. Venous blood from the posterior pituitary enters the systemic circulation, which delivers the hormones to their target tissues.

In summary, the relationship between the hypothalamus and the posterior pituitary is straightforward—a hormone-secreting neuron has its cell body in the hypothalamus and its axons in the posterior lobe of the pituitary.

Relationship of the Hypothalamus to the Anterior Pituitary

The anterior lobe of the pituitary gland is derived from primitive foregut. Unlike the posterior lobe, which is neural tissue, the anterior lobe is primarily a collection of endocrine cells. The anterior pituitary secretes six peptide hormones: thyroid-stimulating hormone (TSH), follicle-stimulating hormone (FSH), luteinizing hormone (LH), growth hormone, prolactin, and adrenocorticotropic hormone (ACTH).

The nature of the relationship between the hypothalamus and the anterior pituitary is both neural and endocrine (in contrast to the posterior lobe, which is only neural). The hypothalamus and anterior pituitary are linked directly by the **hypothalamic-hypophysial portal blood vessels,** which provide most of the blood supply to the anterior lobe.

There are both long and short hypophysial portal vessels, which are distinguished as follows: Arterial blood is delivered to the hypothalamus via the superior hypophysial arteries, which distribute the blood in a capillary network in the median eminence, called the primary capillary plexuses. These primary capillary plexuses converge to form the *long* **hypophysial portal vessels,** which travel down the infundibulum to deliver hypothalamic venous blood to the anterior lobe of the pituitary. A parallel capillary plexus forms from the inferior hypophysial arteries in the lower portion of the infundibular stem. These capillaries converge to form the *short* **hypophysial portal vessels,** which deliver blood to the anterior lobe of the pituitary. In summary, the blood supply of the anterior pituitary differs from that of other organs: Most of its blood supply is *venous* blood from the hypothalamus, supplied by the long and short hypophysial portal vessels.

There are two important implications of the portal blood supply to the anterior lobe of the pituitary: (1) The hypothalamic hormones can be delivered to the anterior pituitary directly and in high concentration, and (2) the hypothalamic hormones do not appear in the systemic circulation in high concentrations. The cells of the anterior pituitary, therefore, are the only cells in the body to receive high concentrations of the hypothalamic hormones.

The *functional* connections between the hypothalamus and the anterior lobe of the pituitary now can be understood in the context of the *anatomic* connections. Hypothalamic-releasing hormones and release-inhibiting hormones are synthesized in the cell bodies of hypothalamic neurons and travel down the axons of these neurons to the median eminence of the hypothalamus. Upon stimulation of these neurons, the hormones are secreted into the surrounding hypothalamic tissue and enter the nearby capillary plexus. The blood from these capillaries (now venous blood) drains into the hypophysial portal vessels and is delivered directly to the anterior lobe of the pituitary. There, the hypothalamic hormones act on the cells of the anterior lobe, where they stimulate or inhibit the release of the anterior pituitary hormones. The anterior pituitary hormones then enter the systemic circulation, which delivers them to their target tissues.

The hypothalamic-anterior pituitary relationship can be illustrated by considering the TRH–TSH–thyroid hormone system. **TRH** is synthesized in hypothalamic neurons and secreted in the median eminence of the hypothalamus, where it enters capillaries and then hypophysial portal vessels. It is delivered in this portal blood to the anterior lobe of the pituitary, where it stimulates TSH secretion. **TSH** enters the systemic circulation and is delivered to its target tissue, the thyroid gland, where it stimulates secretion of **thyroid hormones.**

ANTERIOR LOBE HORMONES

Six major hormones are secreted by the anterior lobe of the pituitary: TSH, FSH, LH, ACTH, growth hormone, and prolactin. Each hormone is secreted by a different cell type (except FSH and LH, which are secreted by the same cell type). The cell types are denoted by the suffix "troph," meaning nutritive. Thus, TSH is secreted by **thyrotrophs** (5%), FSH and LH by **gonadotrophs** (15%), ACTH by **corticotrophs** (15%), growth hormone by **somatotrophs** (20%), and prolactin by **lactotrophs** (15%). (The percentages give the representation of each cell type in the anterior pituitary gland.)

Each of the anterior pituitary hormones is a peptide or polypeptide. As described, the synthesis of peptide hormones includes the following steps: transcription of DNA to mRNA in the nucleus; translation of mRNA to a preprohormone on the ribosomes; and posttranslational modification of the preprohormone on the endoplasmic reticulum and the Golgi apparatus to produce the final hormone. The hormone is stored in membrane-bound secretory granules for subsequent release. When the anterior pituitary is stimulated by a hypothalamic-releasing hormone or a release-inhibiting hormone (e.g., thyrotrophs are stimulated by TRH to secrete TSH), there is exocytosis of the secretory granules; the anterior pituitary hormone (e.g., TSH) enters capillary blood and is delivered by the systemic circulation to the target tissue (e.g., thyroid gland).

The hormones of the anterior lobe are organized in "families," according to structural and functional homology. TSH, FSH, and LH are structurally related and constitute one family, ACTH is part of a second family, and growth hormone and prolactin constitute a third family.

TSH, FSH, LH, and ACTH are discussed briefly in this section and later in the chapter in the context of their actions. (TSH is discussed within the context of the thyroid gland. ACTH is discussed in the context of the adrenal cortex. FSH and LH are discussed in Chapter 10 with male and female reproductive

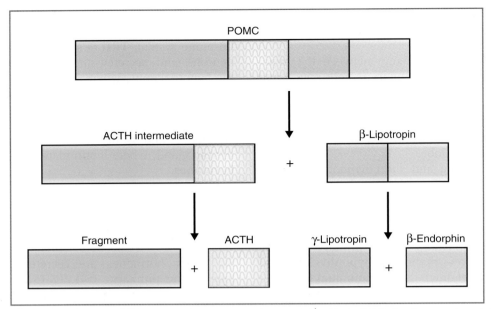

Figure 9-10 **The hormones derived from pro-opiomelanocortin (POMC).** The fragment contains γ-MSH; ACTH contains α-MSH; and γ-lipotropin contains β-MSH. ACTH, Adrenocorticotropic hormone; MSH, melanocyte-stimulating hormone.

physiology.) Growth hormone and prolactin are discussed in this section.

TSH, FSH, and LH Family

TSH, FSH, and LH are all **glycoproteins** with sugar moieties covalently linked to asparagine residues in their polypeptide chains. Each hormone consists of two subunits, α and β, which are not covalently linked; none of the subunits alone is biologically active. The **α subunits** of TSH, FSH, and LH are identical and are synthesized from the same mRNA. The **β subunits** for each hormone are different and, therefore, confer the biologic specificity (although the β subunits have a high degree of homology among the different hormones). During the biosynthetic process, pairing of the α and β subunits begins in the endoplasmic reticulum and continues in the Golgi apparatus. In the secretory granules, the paired molecules are refolded into more stable forms prior to secretion.

The placental hormone **human chorionic gonadotropin (HCG)** is structurally related to the TSH-FSH-LH family. Thus, HCG is a glycoprotein with the identical α chain and its own β chain, which confers its biologic specificity.

ACTH Family

The ACTH family is derived from a single precursor, **pro-opiomelanocortin (POMC).** The ACTH family includes ACTH, γ- and β-lipotropin, β-endorphin, and melanocyte-stimulating hormone (MSH). ACTH is the only hormone in this family with well-established physiologic actions in humans. MSH is involved in pigmentation in lower vertebrates but has little activity in humans. β-Endorphin is an endogenous opiate.

The preprohormone for this group, **preproopiomelanocortin,** is transcribed from a single gene. The signal peptide is cleaved in the endoplasmic reticulum, yielding POMC, the precursor to the ACTH family. Endopeptidases then hydrolyze peptide bonds in POMC and intermediates to produce the members of the ACTH family (Fig. 9-10). The anterior pituitary in humans produces mainly ACTH, γ-lipotropin, and β-endorphin.

It is noteworthy that MSH activity is found in POMC and in several of its products: The "fragment," which is left over from hydrolysis of the ACTH intermediate, contains γ-MSH; ACTH contains α-MSH; and γ-lipotropin contains β-MSH. These MSH-containing fragments can cause skin pigmentation in humans if their blood levels are increased. For example, in **Addison disease** (primary adrenal insufficiency), POMC and ACTH levels are increased by negative feedback. Because POMC and ACTH contain MSH activity, skin pigmentation is a symptom of this disorder.

Growth Hormone

Growth hormone is secreted throughout life. It is the single most important hormone for **normal growth** to adult stature. Considering the broad nature of this

Table 9–4 Factors Affecting Growth Hormone Secretion

Stimulatory Factors	Inhibitory Factors
Decreased glucose concentration	Increased glucose concentration
Decreased free fatty acid concentration	Increased free fatty acid concentration
Arginine	Obesity
Fasting or starvation	Senescence
Hormones of puberty (estrogen, testosterone)	Somatostatin
Exercise	Somatomedins
Stress	Growth hormone
Stage III and IV sleep	β-Adrenergic agonists
α-Adrenergic agonists	Pregnancy

task (growth), it is not surprising that growth hormone has profound effects on protein, carbohydrate, and fat metabolism.

Chemistry of Growth Hormone

Growth hormone is synthesized in the somatotrophs of the anterior lobe of the pituitary and also is called somatotropin or somatotropic hormone. Human growth hormone contains **191 amino acids** in a straight-chain polypeptide with **2 internal disulfide bridges.** The gene for growth hormone is a member of a family of genes for related peptides, prolactin and human placental lactogen. The synthesis of growth hormone is stimulated by GHRH, its hypothalamic-releasing hormone.

Human growth hormone is structurally similar to prolactin, which is synthesized by lactotrophs in the anterior lobe, and to human placental lactogen, which is synthesized in the placenta. Prolactin, a 198-amino acid straight-chain polypeptide with 3 disulfide bridges, has 75% homology with growth hormone. Human placental lactogen, a 191-amino acid straight-chain polypeptide with two disulfide bridges, has 80% homology.

Regulation of Growth Hormone Secretion

Growth hormone is secreted in a **pulsatile** pattern, with bursts of secretion occurring approximately every 2 hours. The largest secretory burst occurs within 1 hour of falling asleep (during sleep stages III and IV). The bursting pattern, in terms of both frequency and magnitude, is affected by several agents that alter the overall level of growth hormone secretion (Table 9-4).

Growth hormone secretory rates are not constant over a lifetime. The rate of secretion increases steadily from birth into early childhood. During childhood, secretion remains relatively stable. At **puberty,** there is an enormous secretory burst, induced in females by estrogen and in males by testosterone. The high pubertal levels of growth hormone are associated with both increased frequency and increased magnitude of the secretory pulses and are responsible for the **growth spurt** of puberty. After puberty, the rate of growth hormone secretion declines to a stable level. Finally, in senescence, growth hormone secretory rates and pulsatility decline to their lowest levels.

The major factors that alter growth hormone secretion are summarized in Table 9-4. **Hypoglycemia** (a decrease in blood glucose concentration) and **starvation** are potent stimuli for growth hormone secretion. Other stimuli for secretion are exercise and various forms of stress including trauma, fever, and anesthesia. The highest rates of growth hormone secretion occur during puberty, and the lowest rates occur in senescence.

Regulation of growth hormone secretion is illustrated in Figure 9-11, which shows the relationship between the hypothalamus, the anterior lobe of the pituitary, and the target tissues for growth hormone. Secretion of growth hormone by the anterior pituitary is controlled by two pathways from the hypothalamus, one stimulatory (GHRH) and the other inhibitory (somatostatin, also known as somatotropin release–inhibiting factor [SRIF]).

♦ **GHRH** acts directly on somatotrophs of the anterior pituitary to induce transcription of the growth hormone gene and, thereby, to stimulate both synthesis and secretion of growth hormone. In initiating its action on the somatotroph, GHRH binds to a membrane receptor, which is coupled through a G_s protein to *both* adenylyl cyclase and phospholipase C. Thus, GHRH stimulates growth hormone secretion by utilizing both cAMP and IP_3/Ca^{2+} as second messengers.

♦ **Somatostatin (somatotropin release–inhibiting hormone, SRIF)** is also secreted by the hypothalamus and acts on the somatotrophs to inhibit growth hormone secretion. Somatostatin inhibits growth hormone secretion by blocking the action of GHRH on the somatotroph. Somatostatin binds to its own membrane receptor, which is coupled to adenylyl cyclase by a G_i protein, inhibiting the generation of cAMP and decreasing growth hormone secretion.

Growth hormone secretion is regulated by negative feedback (see Fig. 9-11). Three feedback loops including both long and short loops are involved. (1) GHRH inhibits its own secretion from the hypothalamus via an ultrashort-loop feedback. (2) Somatomedins, which are by-products of the growth hormone action on target tissues, inhibit secretion of growth hormone by the anterior pituitary. (3) Both growth hormone and somatomedins stimulate the secretion of somatostatin by the hypothalamus. The overall effect of this third loop is *inhibitory* (i.e., negative feedback) because

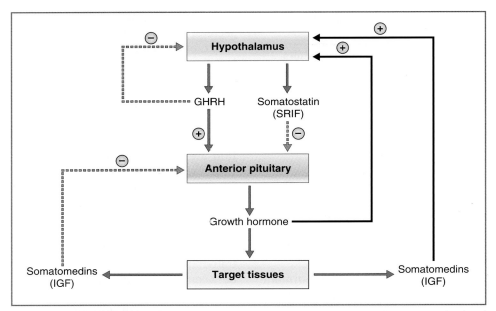

Figure 9–11 Regulation of growth hormone secretion. GHRH, Growth hormone–releasing hormone; IGF, insulin-like growth factor; SRIF, somatotropin release–inhibiting factor.

somatostatin inhibits growth hormone secretion by the anterior pituitary.

Actions of Growth Hormone

Growth hormone has multiple metabolic actions on liver, muscle, adipose tissue, and bone, as well as growth-promoting actions in virtually every other organ. The actions of growth hormone include effects on linear growth, protein synthesis and organ growth, carbohydrate metabolism, and lipid metabolism.

Some of the actions of growth hormone result from the hormone's *direct* effect on target tissues such as skeletal muscle, the liver, or adipose tissue. Other actions of growth hormone are mediated *indirectly* through the production of **somatomedins** (or insulin-like growth factors [IGFs]) in the liver. The most important of the somatomedins is somatomedin C or **IGF-1.** Somatomedins act on target tissues through IGF receptors that are similar to the insulin receptor, having **intrinsic tyrosine kinase activity** and exhibiting autophosphorylation. The growth-promoting effects of growth hormone are mediated largely through production of somatomedins.

The actions of growth hormone are described as follows:

♦ **Diabetogenic effect.** Growth hormone causes **insulin resistance** and decreases glucose uptake and utilization by target tissues such as muscle and adipose tissue. These effects are called "diabetogenic" because they produce an increase in blood glucose concentration, as occurs when insulin is lacking or when tissues are resistant to insulin (e.g., diabetes mellitus). Growth hormone also increases

lipolysis in adipose tissue. As a consequence of these metabolic effects, growth hormone causes an increase in blood insulin levels.

♦ **Increased protein synthesis and organ growth.** In virtually all organs, growth hormone increases the uptake of amino acids and stimulates the synthesis of DNA, RNA, and protein. These effects account for the hormone's growth-promoting actions: increased lean body mass and increased organ size. As noted, many of the growth effects of growth hormone are mediated by somatomedins.

♦ **Increased linear growth.** The most striking effect of growth hormone is its ability to increase linear growth. Mediated by the somatomedins, growth hormone alters every aspect of cartilage metabolism: stimulation of DNA synthesis, RNA synthesis, and protein synthesis. In growing bones, the epiphyseal plates widen and more bone is laid down at the ends of long bones. There also is increased metabolism in cartilage-forming cells and proliferation of chondrocytes.

Pathophysiology of Growth Hormone

The pathophysiology of growth hormone includes deficiency or excess of the hormone, with predictable effects on linear growth, organ growth, and carbohydrate and lipid metabolism.

Growth hormone deficiency in children results in failure to grow, short stature, mild obesity, and delayed puberty. The causes of growth hormone deficiency include defects at every step in the hypothalamic–anterior pituitary–target tissue axis:

decreased secretion of GHRH due to hypothalamic dysfunction; primary deficiencies of growth hormone secretion from the anterior pituitary; failure to generate somatomedins in the liver; and deficiency of growth hormone or somatomedin receptors in target tissues (growth hormone resistance). Growth hormone deficiency in children is treated with human growth hormone replacement.

Growth hormone excess causes **acromegaly** and is most often due to a growth hormone–secreting pituitary adenoma. The consequences of excess growth hormone differ, depending on whether the excess occurs before or after puberty. Before puberty, excessive levels of growth hormone cause **gigantism** (increased linear growth) because of intense hormonal stimulation at the epiphyseal plates. After puberty, when linear growth is complete and can no longer be influenced, excess levels of growth hormone cause increased periosteal bone growth, increased organ size, increased hand and foot size, enlargement of the tongue, coarsening of facial features, insulin resistance, and glucose intolerance. Conditions with excess secretion of growth hormone are treated with **somatostatin analogues** (e.g., **octreotide**), which, like endogenous somatostatin, inhibit growth hormone secretion by the anterior pituitary.

Prolactin

Prolactin is the major hormone responsible for **milk production** and also participates in the development of the breasts. In nonpregnant, nonlactating females and in males, blood levels of prolactin are low. However, during pregnancy and lactation, blood levels of prolactin increase, consistent with the hormone's role in breast development and lactogenesis (milk production).

Chemistry of Prolactin

Prolactin is synthesized by the lactotrophs, which represent approximately 15% of the tissue in the anterior lobe of the pituitary. The number of lactotrophs increases during pregnancy and lactation when the demand for prolactin is increased. Chemically, prolactin is related to growth hormone, having **198 amino acids** in a **single-chain polypeptide** with three internal disulfide bridges.

Stimuli that increase or decrease prolactin secretion do so by altering transcription of the prolactin gene. Thus, TRH, a stimulant of prolactin secretion, increases transcription of the prolactin gene, whereas dopamine, an inhibitor of prolactin secretion, decreases transcription of the gene.

Regulation of Prolactin Secretion

Figure 9-12 illustrates the hypothalamic control of prolactin secretion. There are two regulatory paths from the hypothalamus, one inhibitory (via dopamine, which

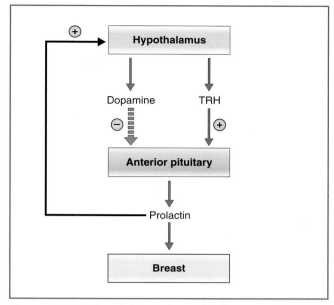

Figure 9–12 Regulation of prolactin secretion. TRH, Thyrotropin-releasing hormone.

acts by decreasing cAMP levels) and the other stimulatory (via TRH).

In persons who are not pregnant or lactating, prolactin secretion is **tonically inhibited by dopamine** (prolactin-inhibiting factor, PIF) from the hypothalamus. In other words, the inhibitory effect of dopamine dominates and overrides the stimulatory effect of TRH. In contrast to other hypothalamic-releasing or release-inhibiting hormones, which are peptides, dopamine is a catecholamine.

Two questions arise regarding this inhibitory action of dopamine: *What is the source of hypothalamic dopamine? How does dopamine reach the anterior lobe?* There are three sources and three routes: (1) The major source of dopamine is dopaminergic neurons in the hypothalamus, which synthesize and secrete dopamine into the median eminence. This dopamine enters capillaries that drain into the hypothalamic-hypophysial portal vessels and deliver dopamine directly and in high concentration to the anterior pituitary, where it inhibits prolactin secretion. (2) Dopamine also is secreted by dopaminergic neurons of the posterior lobe of the pituitary, reaching the anterior lobe by short connecting portal veins. (3) Finally, nonlactotroph cells of the anterior pituitary secrete a small amount of dopamine that diffuses a short distance to the lactotrophs and inhibits prolactin secretion by a paracrine mechanism.

The factors that alter prolactin secretion are summarized in Table 9-5. **Prolactin** inhibits its own secretion by increasing the synthesis and secretion of dopamine from the hypothalamus (see Fig. 9-12).

Table 9-5 Factors Affecting Prolactin Secretion

Stimulatory Factors	Inhibitory Factors
Pregnancy (estrogen)	Dopamine
Breast-feeding	Bromocriptine (dopamine
Sleep	agonist)
Stress	Somatostatin
TRH	Prolactin (negative feedback)
Dopamine antagonists	

TRH, Thyrotropin-releasing hormone.

This action of prolactin constitutes negative feedback because *stimulation* of dopamine secretion causes *inhibition* of prolactin secretion. **Pregnancy** and **breast-feeding** (suckling) are the most important stimuli for prolactin secretion. For example, during breast-feeding, serum prolactin levels can increase to more than tenfold the basal levels. During suckling, afferent fibers from the nipple carry information to the hypothalamus and inhibit dopamine secretion; by releasing the inhibitory effect of dopamine, prolactin secretion is increased. The effects of dopamine, dopamine agonists, and dopamine antagonists on prolactin secretion are predictable, based on feedback regulation (see Fig. 9-12). Thus, dopamine itself and dopamine agonists such as **bromocriptine** inhibit prolactin secretion, whereas dopamine antagonists stimulate prolactin secretion by "inhibiting the inhibition" by dopamine.

Actions of Prolactin

Prolactin, in a supportive role with estrogen and progesterone, stimulates development of the breasts, promotes milk secretion from the breasts during lactation, and suppresses ovulation.

♦ **Breast development.** At puberty, prolactin, with estrogen and progesterone, stimulates proliferation and branching of the mammary ducts. During pregnancy, prolactin (again with estrogen and progesterone) stimulates growth and development of the mammary alveoli, which will produce milk once parturition occurs.

♦ **Lactogenesis (milk production).** The major action of prolactin is stimulation of milk production and secretion in response to suckling. (Interestingly, pregnancy *does not* have to occur for lactation to be possible; if there is sufficient stimulation of the nipple, prolactin is secreted and milk is produced.) Prolactin stimulates milk production by inducing the synthesis of the components of milk including **lactose** (the carbohydrate of milk), **casein** (the protein of milk), and **lipids.** The mechanism of action of prolactin on the breast involves binding of prolactin to a cell membrane receptor and, via an unknown second messenger, inducing transcription of the genes for enzymes in the biosynthetic pathways for lactose, casein, and lipid.

Although prolactin levels are high during pregnancy, lactation does not occur because the high levels of estrogen and progesterone down-regulate prolactin receptors in the breast and block the action of prolactin. At parturition, estrogen and progesterone levels drop precipitously and their inhibitory actions cease. Prolactin can then stimulate lactogenesis, and lactation can occur.

♦ **Inhibition of ovulation.** In females, prolactin inhibits ovulation by inhibiting the synthesis and release of gonadotropin-releasing hormone (GnRH) (see Chapter 10). Inhibition of GnRH secretion and, secondarily, inhibition of ovulation account for the decreased fertility during breast-feeding. In males with high prolactin levels (e.g., due to a prolactinoma), there is a parallel inhibitory effect on GnRH secretion and spermatogenesis, resulting in infertility.

Pathophysiology of Prolactin

The pathophysiology of prolactin can involve either a deficiency of prolactin, which results in the inability to lactate, or an excess of prolactin, which causes galactorrhea (excessive milk production).

♦ **Prolactin deficiency** can be caused by either destruction of the entire anterior lobe of the pituitary or selective destruction of the lactotrophs. Prolactin deficiency results, predictably, in a failure to lactate.

♦ **Prolactin excess** can be caused by destruction of the hypothalamus, interruption of the hypothalamic-hypophysial tract, or prolactinomas (prolactin-secreting tumors). In cases of hypothalamic destruction or interruption of the hypothalamic-hypophysial tract, increased prolactin secretion occurs because of the *loss of tonic inhibition by dopamine.* The major symptoms of excess prolactin secretion are **galactorrhea** and **infertility** (which is caused by inhibition of GnRH secretion by the high prolactin levels). Whether the result of hypothalamic failure or a prolactinoma, prolactin excess can be treated by administration of **bromocriptine,** a dopamine agonist. Like dopamine, bromocriptine inhibits prolactin secretion by the anterior pituitary.

POSTERIOR LOBE HORMONES

The posterior lobe of the pituitary secretes antidiuretic hormone (ADH) and oxytocin. Both ADH and oxytocin are neuropeptides, synthesized in cell bodies of

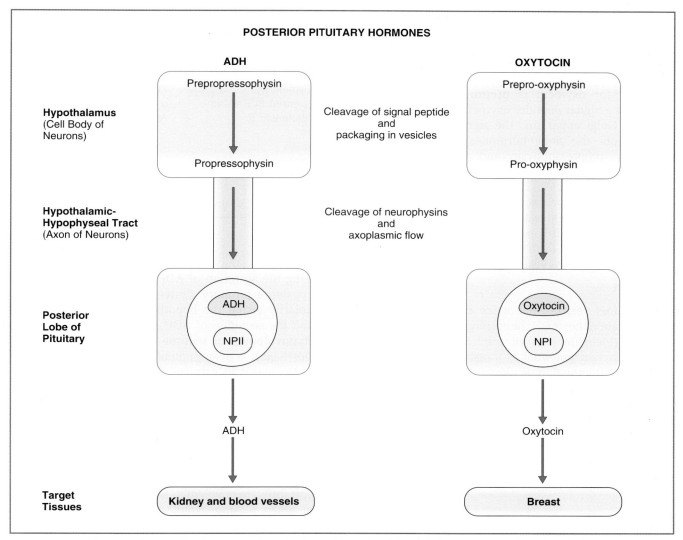

POSTERIOR PITUITARY HORMONES

Figure 9–13 Synthesis, processing, and secretion of antidiuretic hormone (ADH) and oxytocin. NPI, Neurophysin I; NPII, neurophysin II.

hypothalamic neurons and secreted from nerve terminals in the posterior pituitary.

Synthesis and Secretion of Antidiuretic Hormone and Oxytocin

Synthesis and Processing

ADH and oxytocin are homologous **nonapeptides** (containing nine amino acids) (Figs. 9-13 and 9-14) that are synthesized in the supraoptic and paraventricular nuclei of the hypothalamus. The **ADH** neurons have their cell bodies primarily in the **supraoptic nuclei** of the hypothalamus. The **oxytocin** neurons have their cell bodies primarily in **paraventricular nuclei.** While primarily dedicated to producing ADH or oxytocin, each nucleus also produces the "other" hormone.

ADH

1	2	3	4	5	6	7	8	9
Cys – Tyr	Phe	Gln – Asn – Cys – Pro	Arg	Gly	NH₂

Oxytocin

1	2	3	4	5	6	7	8	9
Cys – Tyr	Ile	Gln – Asn – Cys – Pro	Leu	Gly	NH₂

Figure 9–14 **Structures of antidiuretic hormone (ADH) and oxytocin.** Homologous amino acid sequences are shown within the *shaded boxes.*

Similar genes located in close proximity on the chromosome direct synthesis of the preprohormones for ADH and oxytocin. The peptide precursor for ADH is **prepropressophysin,** which comprises a signal peptide, ADH, neurophysin II, and a glycoprotein. The precursor for oxytocin is **prepro-oxyphysin,** which comprises a signal peptide, oxytocin, and neurophysin I. In the Golgi apparatus, the signal peptides are removed from the *prepro*hormones to form the *pro*hormones, *pro*pressophysin and *pro*-oxyphysin, and the prohormones are packaged in secretory vesicles. The secretory vesicles, containing the prohormones, then travel down the axon of the neuron, through the hypothalamic-hypophysial tract, to the posterior pituitary. En route to the posterior pituitary, the neurophysins are cleaved from their respective prohormones within the secretory vesicles.

Secretion

The secretory vesicles that arrive at the posterior pituitary contain either ADH, neurophysin II, and glycoprotein *or* oxytocin and neurophysin I. Secretion is initiated when an action potential is transmitted from the cell body in the hypothalamus, down the axon to the nerve terminal in the posterior pituitary. When the nerve terminal is depolarized by the action potential, Ca^{2+} enters the terminal, causing exocytosis of the secretory granules containing ADH or oxytocin and their neurophysins. The secreted hormones enter nearby fenestrated capillaries and are carried to the systemic circulation, which delivers the hormones to their target tissues.

Antidiuretic Hormone

ADH (or vasopressin) is the major hormone concerned with regulation of body fluid osmolarity. ADH is secreted by the posterior pituitary in response to an increase in serum osmolarity. ADH then acts on the principal cells of the late distal tubule and collecting duct to increase water reabsorption, thus decreasing body fluid osmolarity back toward normal. Osmoregulation and the actions of ADH on the kidney are discussed in Chapter 6.

Regulation of Antidiuretic Hormone Secretion

The factors that stimulate or inhibit the secretion of ADH by the posterior pituitary are summarized in Table 9-6.

Increased plasma osmolarity is the most important physiologic stimulus for increasing ADH secretion (Fig. 9-15). For example, when a person is deprived of water, serum osmolarity increases. The increase is sensed by osmoreceptors in the anterior hypothalamus. Action potentials are initiated in cell bodies of the nearby ADH neurons and propagated down the axons,

Table 9–6 Factors Affecting Antidiuretic Hormone Secretion

Stimulatory Factors	Inhibitory Factors
Increased serum osmolarity	Decreased serum osmolarity
Decreased ECF volume	Ethanol
Angiotensin II	α-Adrenergic agonists
Pain	Atrial natriuretic peptide (ANP)
Nausea	
Hypoglycemia	
Nicotine	
Opiates	
Antineoplastic drugs	

causing the secretion of ADH from nerve terminals in the posterior pituitary. Conversely, decreases in serum osmolarity signal the hypothalamic osmoreceptors to inhibit the secretion of ADH.

Hypovolemia, or volume contraction (e.g., due to hemorrhage), is also a potent stimulus for ADH secretion. Decreases in extracellular fluid (ECF) volume of 10% or more cause a decrease in arterial blood pressure that is sensed by baroreceptors in the left atrium, carotid artery, and aortic arch. This information about blood pressure is transmitted via the vagus nerve to the hypothalamus, which directs an increase in ADH secretion. ADH then stimulates water reabsorption in the collecting ducts, attempting to restore ECF volume. Importantly, hypovolemia stimulates ADH secretion, even when plasma osmolarity is lower than normal (see Fig. 9-15). Conversely, hypervolemia (volume expansion) inhibits ADH secretion, even when plasma osmolarity is higher than normal.

Pain, nausea, hypoglycemia, and various drugs (e.g., nicotine, opiates, antineoplastic agents) all stimulate the secretion of ADH. Ethanol, α-adrenergic agonists, and atrial natriuretic peptide inhibit secretion of ADH.

Actions of Antidiuretic Hormone

ADH (vasopressin) has two actions, one on the kidney and the other on vascular smooth muscle. These actions are mediated by different receptors, different intracellular mechanisms, and different second messengers.

♦ **Increase in water permeability.** The major action of ADH is to increase the water permeability of principal cells in the late distal tubule and collecting duct. The receptor for ADH on the principal cells is a **V₂ receptor,** which is coupled to adenylyl cyclase via a G_s protein. The second messenger is **cAMP,** which, via phosphorylation steps, directs the insertion of water channels, **aquaporin 2 (AQP2),** in the

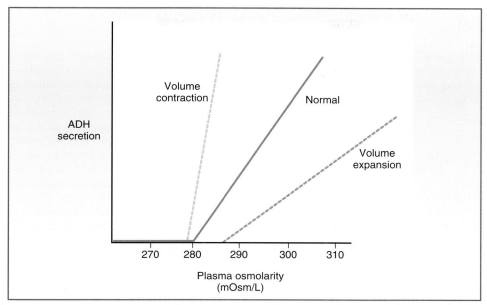

Figure 9–15 Control of antidiuretic hormone (ADH) secretion by osmolarity and extracellular fluid volume.

luminal membranes. The increased water permeability of the principal cells allows water to be reabsorbed by the collecting ducts and makes the urine concentrated, or hyperosmotic (see Chapter 6).

♦ **Contraction of vascular smooth muscle.** The second action of ADH is to cause contraction of vascular smooth muscle (as implied by its other name, vasopressin). The receptor for ADH on vascular smooth muscle is a V_1 **receptor,** which is coupled to phospholipase C via a G_q protein. The second messenger for this action is IP_3/Ca^{2+}, which produces contraction of vascular smooth muscle, constriction of arterioles, and increased total peripheral resistance.

Pathophysiology of Antidiuretic Hormone

The pathophysiology of ADH is discussed in detail in Chapter 6 and is summarized here.

Central **diabetes insipidus** is caused by failure of the posterior pituitary to secrete ADH. In this disorder, circulating levels of ADH are low, the collecting ducts are impermeable to water, and the urine cannot be concentrated. Thus, persons with central diabetes insipidus produce large volumes of dilute urine, and their body fluids become concentrated (e.g., increased serum osmolarity, increased serum Na^+ concentration). Central diabetes insipidus is treated with an ADH analogue, **dDAVP.**

In *nephrogenic* **diabetes insipidus,** the posterior pituitary is normal but the principal cells of the collecting duct are unresponsive to ADH due to a defect in the V_2 receptor, G_s protein, or adenylyl cyclase. As in central diabetes insipidus, water is not reabsorbed in the collecting ducts and the urine cannot be concentrated, resulting in excretion of large volumes of dilute urine. As a result, the body fluids become concentrated and the serum osmolarity increases. In contrast to central diabetes insipidus, however, ADH levels are elevated in nephrogenic diabetes insipidus due to stimulation of secretion by the increased serum osmolarity. Nephrogenic diabetes insipidus is treated with **thiazide diuretics.** The usefulness of thiazide diuretics in treating nephrogenic diabetes insipidus is explained as follows: (1) Thiazide diuretics inhibit Na^+ reabsorption in the early distal tubule. By preventing dilution of the urine at that site, the final, excreted urine is less dilute (than it would be without treatment). (2) Thiazide diuretics decrease glomerular filtration rate; because less water is filtered, less water is excreted. (3) Thiazide diuretics, by increasing Na^+ excretion, can cause a secondary ECF volume contraction. In response to volume contraction, proximal reabsorption of solutes and water is increased; because more water is reabsorbed, less water is excreted.

In **syndrome of inappropriate ADH (SIADH),** excess ADH is secreted from an autonomous site (e.g., oat cell carcinoma of the lung; Box 9-1). High levels of ADH cause excess water reabsorption by the collecting ducts, which dilutes the body fluids (e.g., decreases plasma osmolarity and Na^+ concentration). The urine is *inappropriately concentrated* (i.e., too concentrated for the serum osmolarity). SIADH is treated with an ADH antagonist such as **demeclocycline** or **water restriction.**

BOX 9–1   Clinical Physiology: Syndrome of Inappropriate ADH

DESCRIPTION OF CASE. A 56-year-old man with oat cell carcinoma of the lung is admitted to the hospital after having a grand mal seizure. Laboratory studies yield the following information:

Serum	Urine
[Na$^+$],110 mEq/L	Osmolarity, 650 mOsm/L
Osmolarity, 225 mOsm/L	

The man's lung tumor is diagnosed as inoperable. He is treated with an IV infusion of hypertonic NaCl and is stabilized and discharged. He is given deme-clocycline, an ADH-antagonist, and is ordered to severely limit his water intake.

EXPLANATION OF CASE. Upon his admission to the hospital, the man's serum [Na$^+$] and serum osmolarity are severely depressed (normal serum [Na$^+$], 140 mEq/L; normal serum osmolarity, 290 mOsm/L). Simultaneously, his urine is hyperosmotic, with a measured osmolarity of 650 mOsm/L. In other words, his urine is *inappropriately* concentrated, given his very dilute serum osmolarity.

Independent of the posterior pituitary, the oat cell carcinoma synthesized and secreted ADH and caused the abnormal urine and serum values. Normally, ADH is secreted by the posterior lobe of the pituitary, which is under negative-feedback regulation by serum osmolarity. When the serum osmolarity decreases below normal, ADH secretion by the posterior pituitary is inhibited. However, ADH secretion by the tumor is not under such negative feedback regulation, and ADH

secretion continues unabated (no matter how low the serum osmolarity) and causes SIADH.

The man's serum and urine values are explained as follows: The tumor is secreting large amounts of ADH (inappropriately). This ADH circulates to the kidney and acts on the principal cells of the late distal tubule and collecting duct to increase water reabsorption. The reabsorbed water is added to the total body water, diluting the solutes. Thus, serum [Na$^+$] and serum osmolarity are diluted by the excess water reabsorbed by the kidney. Although this dilution of serum osmolarity turns off ADH secretion by the posterior pituitary, it does not turn off ADH secretion by the tumor cells.

The man's grand mal seizure was caused by swelling of brain cells. The excess water reabsorbed by the kidney was distributed throughout the total body water including ICF. As water flowed into the cells, their volume increased. For brain cells, this swelling was catastrophic because the brain is encased in a fixed cavity, the skull.

TREATMENT. The man is treated promptly with an infusion of hypertonic NaCl to raise the osmolarity of his ECF. As extracellular osmolarity becomes higher than intracellular osmolarity, water flows out of the cells, driven by the osmotic gradient, and decreases ICF volume. For brain cells, the reduction in cell volume decreases the probability of another seizure.

The man's lung tumor is inoperable and will continue to secrete large quantities of ADH. His treatment includes water restriction and administration of dem-eclocycline, an ADH-antagonist that blocks the effect of ADH on water reabsorption in the principal cells.

Oxytocin

Oxytocin produces milk "letdown" or milk ejection from the lactating breast by stimulating contraction of myoepithelial cells lining the milk ducts.

Regulation of Oxytocin Secretion

Several factors cause the secretion of oxytocin from the posterior pituitary including suckling; the sight, sound, or smell of the infant; and dilation of the cervix (Table 9-7).

The major stimulus for oxytocin secretion is **suckling** of the breast. Sensory receptors in the nipple transmit impulses to the spinal cord via afferent neurons. This information then ascends in the spinothalamic tract to the brain stem and, finally, to the paraventricular nuclei of the hypothalamus. Within seconds of suckling, oxytocin is secreted from nerve terminals in the posterior pituitary. If suckling continues, new oxytocin

Table 9–7 Factors Affecting Oxytocin Secretion

Stimulatory Factors	Inhibitory Factors
Suckling	Opioids (endorphins)
Sight, sound, or smell of the infant	
Dilation of the cervix	
Orgasm	

is synthesized in the hypothalamic cell bodies, travels down the axons, and replenishes the oxytocin that was secreted.

Suckling is *not required* for oxytocin secretion; **conditioned responses** to the sight, sound, or smell of the infant also cause milk letdown. Oxytocin also is secreted in response to dilation of the cervix during labor and orgasm.

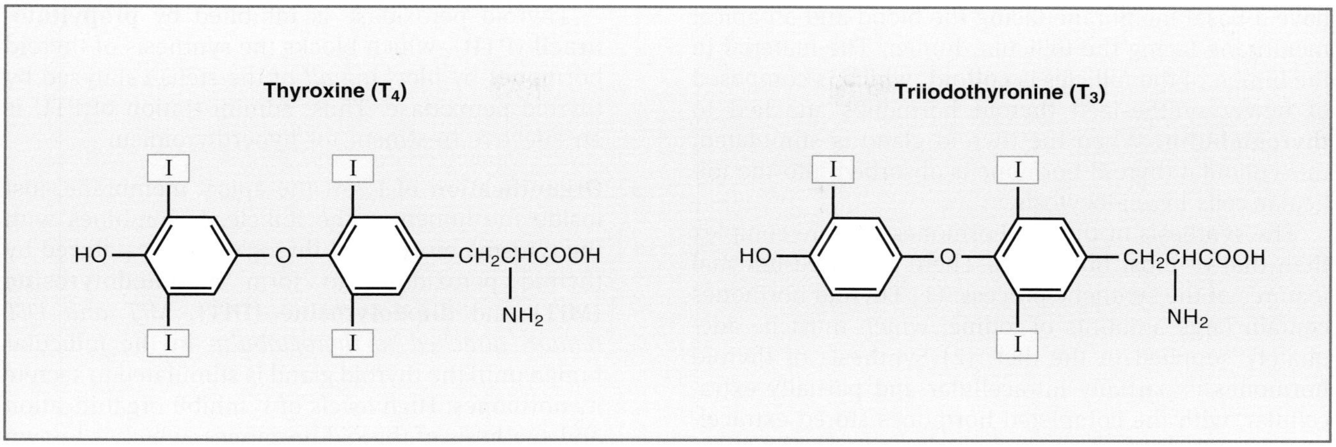

Thyroxine (T₄)

Triiodothyronine (T₃)

Figure 9-16 **Structures of the thyroid hormones thyroxine (T₄) and triiodothyronine (T₃).**

Actions of Oxytocin

♦ **Milk ejection.** Prolactin stimulates lactogenesis. The milk is stored in mammary alveoli and small milk ducts. The major action of oxytocin is to cause milk letdown. When oxytocin is secreted in response to suckling or to conditioned responses, it causes contraction of myoepithelial cells lining these small ducts, forcing the milk into large ducts. The milk collects in cisterns and then flows out through the nipple.

♦ **Uterine contraction.** At a very low concentration, oxytocin also causes powerful rhythmic contractions of uterine smooth muscle. Although it is tempting to speculate that oxytocin is the critical hormone involved in parturition, it is unclear whether oxytocin plays a physiologic role in either the initiation of or the normal course of labor. However, this action of oxytocin is the basis for its use in **inducing labor** and in **reducing postpartum bleeding.**

THYROID HORMONES

Thyroid hormones are synthesized and secreted by epithelial cells of the thyroid gland. They have effects on virtually every organ system in the body including those involved in normal growth and development. The thyroid gland was the first of the endocrine organs to be described by a deficiency disorder. In 1850, patients without thyroid glands were described as having a form of mental and growth retardation called **cretinism.** In 1891, such patients were treated by administering crude thyroid extracts (i.e., hormone replacement therapy). Disorders of thyroid deficiency and excess are among the most common of the endocrinopathies (disorders of the endocrine glands), affecting 4% to 5% of the population in the United States and an even greater

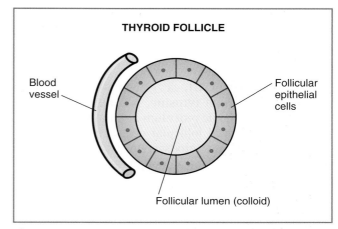

Figure 9–17 Schematic drawing of a thyroid follicle. Colloid is present in the follicular lumen.

percentage of people in regions of the world where there is iodine deficiency.

Synthesis and Transport of Thyroid Hormones

The two active thyroid hormones are triiodothyronine (T₃) and tetraiodothyronine, or thyroxine (T₄). The structures of T₃ and T₄ differ only by a single atom of iodine, as shown in Figure 9-16. Although T₃ is more active than T₄, almost all hormonal output of the thyroid gland is T₄. This "problem" of secreting the less active form is solved by the target tissues, which convert T₄ to T₃. A third compound, reverse T₃ (not shown in Fig. 9-16), has no biologic activity.

Synthesis of Thyroid Hormones

Thyroid hormones are synthesized by the **follicular epithelial cells** of the thyroid gland. The follicular epithelial cells are arranged in circular follicles 200 to 300 μm in diameter, as shown in Figure 9-17. The cells have a basal membrane facing the blood and an apical membrane facing the follicular lumen. The material in the lumen of the follicles is **colloid,** which is composed of newly synthesized thyroid hormones attached to **thyroglobulin.** When the thyroid gland is stimulated, this colloidal thyroid hormone is absorbed into the follicular cells by endocytosis.

The synthesis of thyroid hormones is more complex than that of most hormones. There are three unusual features of the synthetic process: (1) Thyroid hormones contain large amounts of iodine, which must be adequately supplied in the diet. (2) Synthesis of thyroid hormones is partially intracellular and partially extracellular, with the completed hormones stored extracellularly in the follicular lumen until the thyroid gland is stimulated to secrete. (3) As noted, although T_4 is the major secretory product of the thyroid gland, it is not the most active form of the hormone.

The steps in thyroid hormone biosynthesis in follicular epithelial cells are illustrated in Figure 9-18. The circled numbers in the figure correlate with the following steps:

1. **Thyroglobulin (TG),** a glycoprotein containing large quantities of **tyrosine,** is synthesized on the rough endoplasmic reticulum and the Golgi apparatus of the thyroid follicular cells. Thyroglobulin is then incorporated into secretory vesicles and extruded across the apical membrane into the follicular lumen. Later, the tyrosine residues of thyroglobulin will be iodinated to form the precursors of thyroid hormones.

2. **Na^+-I^- cotransport, or "I-trap."** I^- is actively transported from blood into the follicular epithelial cells against both chemical and electrical gradients. The activity of this pump is regulated by I^- levels in the body. For example, low levels of I^- stimulate the pump. When there is a dietary deficiency of I^-, the Na^+-I^- cotransport increases its activity, attempting to compensate for the deficiency. If the dietary deficiency is severe, however, even the Na^+-I^- cotransport cannot compensate and the synthesis of thyroid hormones will be decreased.

   There are several competitive inhibitors of Na^+-I^- cotransport including the anions **thiocyanate** and **perchlorate,** which block I^- uptake into follicular cells and interfere with the synthesis of thyroid hormones.

3. **Oxidation of I^- to I_2.** Once I^- is pumped into the cell, it traverses the cell to the apical membrane, where it is oxidized to I_2 by the enzyme **thyroid peroxidase.** Thyroid peroxidase catalyzes this oxidation step *and* the next two steps (i.e., organification of I_2 into thyroglobulin and the coupling reactions).

Thyroid peroxidase is inhibited by **propylthiouracil (PTU),** which blocks the synthesis of thyroid hormones by blocking *all* of the steps catalyzed by thyroid peroxidase. Thus, administration of PTU is an effective treatment for hyperthyroidism.

4. **Organification of I_2.** At the apical membrane, just inside the lumen of the follicle, I_2 combines with the tyrosine moieties of thyroglobulin, catalyzed by thyroid peroxidase, to form **monoiodotyrosine (MIT)** and **diiodotyrosine (DIT).** *MIT and DIT remain attached to thyroglobulin* in the follicular lumen until the thyroid gland is stimulated to secrete its hormones. High levels of I^- inhibit organification and synthesis of thyroid hormones, which is known as the **Wolff-Chaikoff effect.**

5. **Coupling reaction.** While still part of thyroglobulin, two separate coupling reactions occur between MIT and DIT, again catalyzed by thyroid peroxidase. In one reaction, two molecules of DIT combine to form **T_4.** In the other reaction, one molecule of DIT combines with one molecule of MIT to form **T_3.** The first reaction is faster, and as a result, approximately 10 times more T_4 is produced than T_3. A portion of MIT and DIT does not couple (is "left over") and simply remains attached to thyroglobulin. After the coupling reactions occur, thyroglobulin contains T_4, T_3, and leftover MIT and DIT. This iodinated thyroglobulin is stored in the follicular lumen as **colloid** until the thyroid gland is stimulated to secrete its hormones (e.g., by TSH).

6. **Endocytosis of thyroglobulin.** When the thyroid gland is stimulated, iodinated thyroglobulin (with its attached T_4, T_3, MIT, and DIT) is endocytosed into the follicular epithelial cells. Pseudopods are pinched off the apical cell membrane, engulf a portion of colloid, and absorb it into the cell. Once inside the cell, thyroglobulin is transported in the direction of the basal membrane by microtubular action.

7. **Hydrolysis of T_4 and T_3 from thyroglobulin by lysosomal enzymes.** Thyroglobulin droplets fuse with lysosomal membranes. Lysosomal proteases then hydrolyze peptide bonds to release T_4, T_3, MIT, and DIT from thyroglobulin. T_4 and T_3 are transported across the basal membrane into nearby capillaries to be delivered to the systemic circulation. MIT and DIT remain in the follicular cell and are recycled into the synthesis of new thyroglobulin.

8. **Deiodination of MIT and DIT.** MIT and DIT are deiodinated inside the follicular cell by the enzyme **thyroid deiodinase.** The I^- generated by this step is recycled into the intracellular pool and added to the I^- transported by the pump. The tyrosine molecules

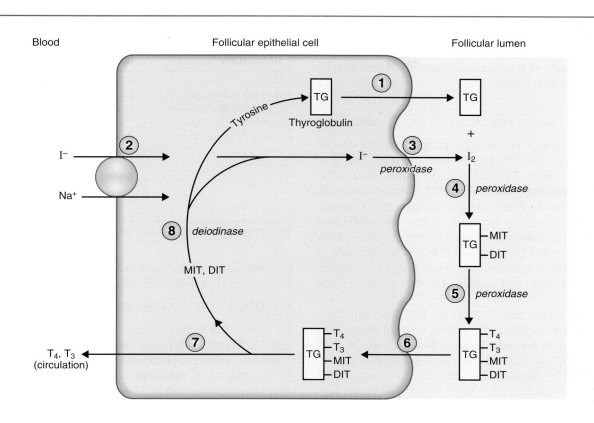

	Event	Site	Enzyme	Inhibitor
(1)	Synthesis of TG; extrusion into follicular lumen	Rough ER, Golgi apparatus		
(2)	Na^+ - I^- cotransport	Basal membrane		Perchlorate, thiocyanate
(3)	Oxidation of $I^- \rightarrow I_2$	Apical (luminal) membrane	Peroxidase	PTU
(4)	Organification of I_2 into MIT and DIT	Apical membrane	Peroxidase	PTU
(5)	Coupling reaction of MIT and DIT into T_3 and T_4	Apical membrane	Peroxidase	PTU
(6)	Endocytosis of TG	Apical membrane		
(7)	Hydrolysis of T_4 and T_3; T_4 and T_3 enter circulation	Lysosomes	Proteases	
(8)	Deiodination of residual MIT and DIT Recycling of I^- and tyrosine	Intracellular	Deiodinase	

Figure 9–18 **Steps involved in the synthesis of thyroid hormones in thyroid follicular cells.** Also see the text for an explanation of the circled numbers. DIT, Diiodotyrosine; ER, endoplasmic reticulum; MIT, monoiodotyrosine; PTU, propylthiouracil; TG, thyroglobulin; T_3, triiodothyronine; T_4, thyroxine.

are incorporated into the synthesis of new thyroglobulin to begin another cycle. Thus, both I⁻ and tyrosine are "salvaged" by the deiodinase enzyme. A deficiency of thyroid deiodinase therefore mimics dietary I⁻ deficiency.

Binding of Thyroid Hormones in the Circulation

Thyroid hormones (T_4 and T_3) circulate in the bloodstream either bound to plasma proteins or free (unbound). Most T_4 and T_3 circulates bound to **thyroxine-binding globulin (TBG).** Smaller amounts circulate bound to T_4-binding prealbumin and albumin. Still smaller amounts circulate in the free, unbound form. Because only *free* thyroid hormones are physiologically active, the role of TBG is to provide a large reservoir of circulating thyroid hormones, which can be released and added to the pool of free hormone.

Changes in the blood levels of TBG alter the fraction of free (physiologically active) thyroid hormones. For example, in **hepatic failure,** blood levels of TBG decrease because there is decreased hepatic protein synthesis. The decrease in TBG levels results in a transient increase in the level of free thyroid hormones; a consequence of increased free thyroid hormone is inhibition of synthesis of thyroid hormones (by negative feedback). In contrast, during **pregnancy,** the high level of estrogen inhibits hepatic breakdown of TBG and increases TBG levels. With a higher level of TBG, more thyroid hormone is bound to TBG and less thyroid hormone is free and unbound. The transiently decreased level of free hormone causes, by negative feedback, increased synthesis and secretion of thyroid hormones by the thyroid gland. In pregnancy, as a consequence of all these changes, levels of *total* T_4 and T_3 are increased (due to the increased level of TBG), but levels of *free,* physiologically active, thyroid hormones are normal and the person is said to be "clinically euthyroid."

Circulating levels of TBG can be indirectly assessed with the **T_3 resin uptake test,** which measures the binding of radioactive T_3 to a synthetic resin. In the test, a standard amount of radioactive T_3 is added to an assay system that contains a sample of the patient's serum and the T_3-binding resin. The rationale is that radioactive T_3 will first bind to unoccupied sites on the patient's TBG and any "leftover" radioactive T_3 will bind to the resin. Thus, T_3 resin uptake is increased when circulating levels of TBG are decreased (e.g., hepatic failure) or when endogenous T_3 levels are increased (i.e., endogenous hormone occupies more sites than usual on TBG). Conversely, T_3 resin uptake is decreased when circulating levels of TBG are increased (e.g., during pregnancy) or when endogenous T_3 levels

Table 9–8 Factors Affecting Thyroid Hormone Secretion

Stimulatory Factors	Inhibitory Factors
TSH	I⁻ deficiency
Thyroid-stimulating immunoglobulins	Deiodinase deficiency
Increased TBG levels (e.g., pregnancy)	Excessive I⁻ intake (Wolff-Chaikoff effect)
	Perchlorate; thiocyanate (inhibit Na⁺-I⁻ cotransport)
	Propylthiouracil (inhibits peroxidase enzyme)
	Decreased TBG levels (e.g., liver disease)

TBG, Thyroxine-binding globulin; TSH, thyroid-stimulating hormone.

are decreased (i.e., endogenous hormone occupies fewer sites than usual on TBG).

Activation of T_4 in Target Tissues

As noted, the major secretory product of the thyroid gland is T_4, which is not the most active form of thyroid hormone. This "problem" is solved in the target tissues by the enzyme **5′ iodinase,** which converts T_4 to T_3 by removing one atom of I_2. The target tissues also convert a portion of the T_4 to **reverse T_3** (rT_3), which is inactive. Essentially, T_4 serves as a precursor for T_3, and the relative amounts of T_4 converted to T_3 and rT_3 determine how much *active* hormone is produced in the target tissue.

In **starvation** (fasting), target tissue 5′ iodinase plays an interesting role. Starvation inhibits 5′ iodinase in tissues such as skeletal muscle, thus lowering O_2 consumption and basal metabolic rate during periods of caloric deprivation. However, brain 5′ iodinase differs from the 5′ iodinase in other tissues and is, therefore, not inhibited in starvation; in this way, brain levels of T_3 are protected even during caloric deprivation.

Regulation of Thyroid Hormone Secretion

The factors that increase or decrease the secretion of thyroid hormones are summarized in Table 9-8. Major control of the synthesis and secretion of thyroid hormones is via the hypothalamic-pituitary axis (Fig. 9-19). Thyrotropin-releasing hormone (TRH) is secreted by the hypothalamus and acts on the thyrotrophs of the anterior pituitary to cause secretion of thyroid-stimulating hormone (TSH). TSH then acts on the thyroid gland to stimulate the synthesis and secretion of thyroid hormones.

♦ **TRH,** a tripeptide, is secreted by the paraventricular nuclei of the hypothalamus. TRH then acts on the thyrotrophs of the anterior pituitary to stimulate both transcription of the TSH gene and secretion

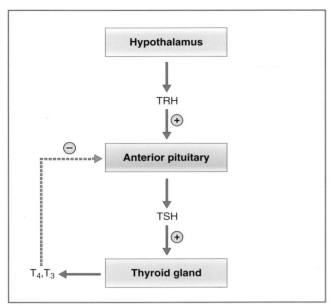

Figure 9–19 **Regulation of thyroid hormone secretion.**
TRH, Thyrotropin-releasing hormone; TSH, thyroid-stimulating
hormone; T_3, triiodothyronine; T_4, thyroxine.

of TSH. (Recall that the other action of TRH is to stimulate the secretion of prolactin by the anterior pituitary.)

♦ **TSH,** a glycoprotein, is secreted by the anterior lobe of the pituitary in response to stimulation by TRH. The role of TSH is to regulate the growth of the thyroid gland (i.e., a trophic effect) and the secretion of thyroid hormones by influencing several steps in the biosynthetic pathway. The thyrotrophs of the anterior pituitary develop and begin secreting TSH at approximately gestational week 13, the same time that the fetal thyroid gland begins secreting thyroid hormones.

TSH secretion is regulated by two reciprocal factors: (1) TRH from the hypothalamus stimulates the secretion of TSH, and (2) Thyroid hormones inhibit the secretion of TSH by down-regulating the TRH receptor on the thyrotrophs, thus decreasing their sensitivity to stimulation by TRH. This negative feedback effect of thyroid hormones is mediated by **free T_3**, which is possible because the anterior lobe contains thyroid deiodinase (converting T_4 to T_3). The reciprocal regulation of TSH secretion by TRH and negative feedback by free T_3 results in a relatively steady rate of TSH secretion, which, in turn, produces a steady rate of secretion of thyroid hormones (in contrast to growth hormone secretion, whose secretion is pulsatile).

♦ The **actions of TSH on the thyroid gland** are initiated when TSH binds to a membrane receptor, which is coupled to adenylyl cyclase via a G_s

protein. Activation of adenylyl cyclase generates **cAMP,** which serves as the second messenger for TSH. TSH has two types of actions on the thyroid gland. (1) It increases the synthesis and secretion of thyroid hormones by stimulating *each* step in the biosynthetic pathway: I^- uptake and oxidation, organification of I_2 into MIT and DIT, coupling of MIT and DIT to form T_4 and T_3, endocytosis, and proteolysis of thyroglobulin to release T_4 and T_3 for secretion. (2) TSH has a trophic effect on the thyroid gland. This trophic effect is exhibited when TSH levels are elevated for a sustained period of time and leads to hypertrophy and hyperplasia of thyroid follicular cells and increased thyroidal blood flow.

♦ The TSH receptor on the thyroid cells also is activated by **thyroid-stimulating immunoglobulins,** which are antibodies to the TSH receptor. Thyroid-stimulating immunoglobulins are components of the immunoglobulin G (IgG) fraction of plasma proteins. When these immunoglobulins bind to the TSH receptor, they produce the same response in thyroid cells as TSH: stimulation of thyroid hormone synthesis and secretion and hypertrophy and hyperplasia of the gland (i.e., hyperthyroidism). **Graves disease,** a common form of hyperthyroidism, is caused by increased circulating levels of thyroid-stimulating immunoglobulins. In this disorder, the thyroid gland is intensely stimulated by the antibodies, causing circulating levels of thyroid hormones to be increased. In Graves disease, TSH levels are actually lower than normal because the high circulating levels of thyroid hormones inhibit TSH secretion by negative feedback.

Actions of Thyroid Hormones

Thyroid hormones act on virtually every organ system in the human body (Fig. 9-20): Thyroid hormones act synergistically with growth hormone and somatomedins to promote bone formation; they increase basal metabolic rate (BMR), heat production, and oxygen consumption; and they alter the cardiovascular and respiratory systems to increase blood flow and oxygen delivery to the tissues.

The first step in the action of thyroid hormones in target tissues is **conversion of T_4 to T_3 by 5′-iodinase.** (Recall that T_4 is secreted in far greater amounts than T_3, but it also is much less active.) In an alternate pathway, T_4 can be converted to rT_3, which is physiologically inactive. Normally, the tissues produce T_3 and rT_3 in approximately equal amounts (T_3, 45% and rT_3, 55%). However, under certain conditions, the relative amounts may change. For example, pregnancy, fasting, stress, hepatic and renal failure, and β-adrenergic blocking agents all decrease the conversion of T_4 to T_3

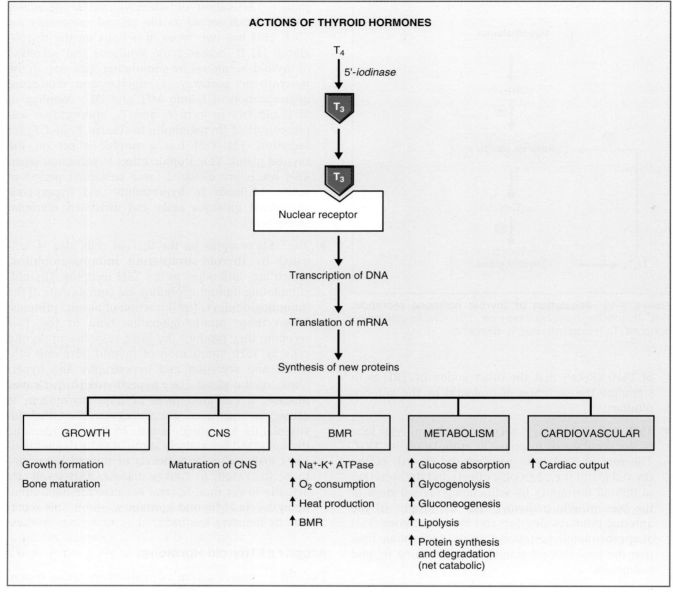

Figure 9–20 **Mechanism of action of thyroid hormones.** Thyroxine (T₄) is converted to triiodothyronine (T₃) in target tissues. The actions of T₃ on several organ systems are shown. BMR, Basal metabolic rate; CNS, central nervous system; DNA, deoxyribonucleic acid; mRNA, messenger ribonucleic acid.

(and increase conversion to rT₃), thus decreasing the amount of the active hormone. Obesity increases the conversion of T₄ to T₃, increasing the amount of the active hormone.

Once T₃ is produced inside the target cells, it enters the nucleus and binds to a **nuclear receptor.** The T₃-receptor complex then binds to a thyroid-regulatory element on DNA, where it stimulates **DNA transcription.** The newly transcribed mRNAs are translated, and new proteins are synthesized. These new proteins are responsible for the multiple actions of thyroid hormones. Other T₃ receptors located in ribosomes and

mitochondria mediate posttranscriptional and posttranslational events.

A vast array of **new proteins** are synthesized under the direction of thyroid hormones, including Na⁺-K⁺ ATPase, transport proteins, β₁-adrenergic receptors, lysosomal enzymes, proteolytic proteins, and structural proteins. The nature of the protein induced is specific to the target tissue. In most tissues, Na⁺-K⁺ ATPase synthesis is induced, which leads to increased oxygen consumption, BMR, and heat production. In myocardial cells, myosin, β₁-adrenergic receptors, and Ca²⁺ ATPase are induced, accounting for thyroid hormone–induced increases in heart rate and contractility. In liver and adipose tissue, key metabolic enzymes are induced, leading to alterations in carbohydrate, fat, and protein metabolism.

The effects of thyroid hormone (T_3) on various organ systems are as follows:

♦ **Basal metabolic rate (BMR).** One of the most significant and pronounced effects of thyroid hormone is **increased oxygen consumption** and a resulting increase in **BMR** and **body temperature.** Thyroid hormones increase oxygen consumption in all tissues *except brain, gonads, and spleen* by inducing the synthesis and increasing the activity of the **Na^+-K^+ ATPase.** The Na^+-K^+ ATPase is responsible for primary active transport of Na^+ and K^+ in all cells; this activity is highly correlated with and accounts for a large percentage of the total oxygen consumption and heat production in the body. Thus, when thyroid hormones increase Na^+-K^+ ATPase activity, they also increase oxygen consumption, BMR, and heat production.

♦ **Metabolism.** Ultimately, increased oxygen consumption depends on increased availability of substrates for oxidative metabolism. Thyroid hormones increase glucose absorption from the gastrointestinal tract and potentiate the effects of other hormones (e.g., catecholamines, glucagon, growth hormone) on gluconeogenesis, lipolysis, and proteolysis. Thyroid hormones increase both protein synthesis and degradation, but, overall, their effect is *catabolic* (i.e., net degradation), which results in decreased muscle mass. These metabolic effects occur because thyroid hormones induce the synthesis of key metabolic enzymes including cytochrome oxidase, NADPH cytochrome C reductase, α-glycerophosphate dehydrogenase, malic enzyme, and several proteolytic enzymes.

♦ **Cardiovascular and respiratory.** Because thyroid hormones increase O_2 consumption, they create a higher demand for O_2 in the tissues. Increased O_2 delivery to the tissues is possible because thyroid hormones produce an increase in cardiac output and ventilation. The **increase in cardiac output** is the result of a combination of increased heart rate and increased stroke volume (increased contractility). These cardiac effects are explained by the fact that thyroid hormones induce the synthesis of (i.e., up-regulate) cardiac β_1-adrenergic receptors. Recall that these β_1 receptors mediate the effects of the sympathetic nervous system to increase heart rate and contractility. Thus, when thyroid hormone levels are high, the myocardium has an increased number of β_1 receptors and is more sensitive to stimulation by the sympathetic nervous system. (In complementary actions, thyroid hormones also induce the synthesis of cardiac myosin and sarcoplasmic reticulum Ca^{2+} ATPase.)

♦ **Growth.** Thyroid hormone is required for growth to adult stature. Thyroid hormones act synergistically with growth hormone and somatomedins to promote bone formation. Thyroid hormones promote ossification and fusion of bone plates and bone maturation. In hypothyroidism, bone age is less than chronologic age.

♦ **Central nervous system (CNS).** Thyroid hormones have multiple effects on the CNS, and the impact of these effects is age dependent. In the **perinatal period,** thyroid hormone is *essential for normal maturation of the CNS.* Hypothyroidism in the perinatal period causes irreversible mental retardation. For this reason, screening of newborns for hypothyroidism is mandated; if it is detected in the newborn, thyroid hormone replacement can reverse the CNS effects. In **adults,** hypothyroidism causes listlessness, slowed movement, somnolence, impaired memory, and decreased mental capacity. Hyperthyroidism causes hyperexcitability, hyperreflexia, and irritability.

♦ **Autonomic nervous system.** Thyroid hormones interact with the **sympathetic nervous system** in ways that are not fully understood. Many of the effects of thyroid hormones on BMR, heat production, heart rate, and stroke volume are similar to those produced by catecholamines via **β-adrenergic receptors.** The effects of thyroid hormones and catecholamines on heat production, cardiac output, lipolysis, and gluconeogenesis appear to be synergistic. The significance of this synergism is illustrated by the effectiveness of **β-adrenergic blocking agents** (e.g., propranolol) in treating many of the symptoms of hyperthyroidism.

Pathophysiology of Thyroid Hormone

The most common endocrine abnormalities are disturbances of thyroid hormones. The constellation of signs and symptoms produced by an excess or a deficiency of thyroid hormones are predictable on the basis of the hormones' physiologic actions. Thus, disturbances of thyroid hormones will affect growth, CNS function, BMR and heat production, nutrient metabolism, and the cardiovascular system. The symptoms of hyperthyroidism and hypothyroidism, common etiologies, TSH levels, and treatments are summarized in Table 9-9.

Hyperthyroidism

The most common form of hyperthyroidism is **Graves disease,** an autoimmune disorder characterized by increased circulating levels of **thyroid-stimulating**

Table 9–9 Pathophysiology of Thyroid Hormones

	Hyperthyroidism	Hypothyroidism
Symptoms	Increased basal metabolic rate Weight loss Negative nitrogen balance Increased heat production Sweating Increased cardiac output Dyspnea (shortness of breath) Tremor, muscle weakness Exophthalmos Goiter	Decreased basal metabolic rate Weight gain Positive nitrogen balance Decreased heat production Cold sensitivity Decreased cardiac output Hypoventilation Lethargy, mental slowness Drooping eyelids Myxedema Growth retardation Mental retardation (perinatal) Goiter
Causes	Graves disease (increased thyroid-stimulating immunoglobulins) Thyroid neoplasm Excess TSH secretion Exogenous T_3 or T_4 (factitious)	Thyroiditis (autoimmune or Hashimoto thyroiditis) Surgery for hyperthyroidism I^- deficiency Congenital (cretinism) Decreased TRH or TSH
TSH Levels	Decreased (feedback inhibition of T_3 on the anterior lobe) Increased (if defect is in anterior pituitary)	Increased (by negative feedback if primary defect is in thyroid gland) Decreased (if defect is in hypothalamus or anterior pituitary)
Treatment	Propylthiouracil (inhibits peroxidase enzyme and thyroid hormone synthesis) Thyroidectomy $^{131}I^-$ (destroys thyroid) β-Adrenergic blocking agents (adjunct therapy)	Thyroid hormone replacement therapy

immunoglobulins. These immunoglobulins are antibodies to TSH receptors on thyroid follicular cells. When present, the antibodies intensely stimulate the thyroid gland, resulting in increased secretion of thyroid hormones and hypertrophy of the gland. Other causes of hyperthyroidism are thyroid neoplasm, excessive secretion of TRH or TSH, and administration of excessive amounts of exogenous thyroid hormones.

The **diagnosis of hyperthyroidism** is based on symptoms and measurement of increased levels of T_3 and T_4. TSH levels may be decreased or increased, depending on the cause of the hyperthyroidism. If the *cause* of hyperthyroidism is Graves disease, thyroid neoplasm (i.e., the disorder is in the thyroid gland), or exogenous administration of thyroid hormones (factitious hyperthyroidism), then TSH levels will be decreased by negative feedback of the high levels of T_3 on the anterior pituitary. However, if the *cause* of hyperthyroidism is increased secretion of TRH or TSH (i.e., the disorder is in the hypothalamus or anterior pituitary), then TSH levels will be increased.

The **symptoms of hyperthyroidism** are dramatic and include weight loss accompanied by increased food intake due to the increased metabolic rate; excessive heat production and sweating secondary to increased oxygen consumption; rapid heart rate due to up-regulation of β_1 receptors in the heart; breathlessness on exertion; and tremor, nervousness, and weakness due to the CNS effects of thyroid hormones. The increased activity of the thyroid gland causes it to enlarge, called **goiter.** The goiter may compress the esophagus and cause difficulty in swallowing.

Treatment of hyperthyroidism includes administration of drugs such as **propylthiouracil,** which inhibit the synthesis of thyroid hormones; surgical removal of the gland; or radioactive ablation of the thyroid gland with $^{131}I^-$.

Hypothyroidism

The most common cause of hypothyroidism is **autoimmune destruction of the thyroid gland** (thyroiditis) in which antibodies may either frankly destroy the gland or block thyroid hormone synthesis. Other causes of hypothyroidism are surgical removal of the thyroid as treatment for hyperthyroidism, hypothalamic or pituitary failure, and I⁻ deficiency. Rarely, hypothyroidism is the result of target tissue resistance caused by down-regulation of thyroid-hormone receptors.

The **diagnosis of hypothyroidism** is based on symptoms and a finding of decreased levels of T_3 and T_4. Depending on the cause of the hypothyroidism, TSH levels may be increased or decreased. If the defect is in the thyroid gland (e.g., thyroiditis), TSH levels will be increased by negative feedback; the low circulating levels of T_3 stimulate TSH secretion. If the defect is in the hypothalamus or pituitary, then TSH levels will be decreased.

The **symptoms of hypothyroidism** are opposite those seen in hyperthyroidism and include decreased metabolic rate and weight gain without increased food intake; decreased heat production and cold intolerance; decreased heart rate; slowing of movement, slurred speech, slowed mental activity, lethargy, and somnolence; periorbital puffiness; constipation; hair loss; and menstrual dysfunction. In some cases, **myxedema** develops, in which there is increased filtration of fluid out of the capillaries and edema due to accumulation of osmotically active mucopolysaccharides in interstitial fluid. When the cause of hypothyroidism is a defect in the thyroid, a **goiter** develops from the unrelenting stimulation of the thyroid gland by the high circulating levels of TSH. Finally, and of critical importance, if hypothyroidism occurs in the **perinatal period** and is untreated, it results in an irreversible form of growth and mental retardation called **cretinism.**

Treatment of hypothyroidism involves thyroid hormone replacement therapy, usually T_4. Like endogenous hormone, exogenous T_4 is converted to its active form, T_3, in the target tissues.

Goiter

Goiter (i.e., enlarged thyroid) can be associated with certain causes of hyperthyroidism and also, perhaps surprisingly, with certain causes of hypothyroidism and euthyroidism. The terms hyperthyroid, hypothyroid, and euthyroid describe, respectively, the *clinical states* of excess thyroid hormone, deficiency of thyroid hormone, and normal levels of thyroid hormone. Thus, they describe blood levels of thyroid hormone, *not* the size of the thyroid gland. The presence or absence of goiter can be understood only by analyzing the etiology of the various thyroid disorders. The central principle in understanding goiter is that high levels of TSH and substances that act like TSH (e.g., thyroid-stimulating immunoglobulins) have a trophic (growth) effect on the thyroid and cause it to enlarge.

♦ **Graves disease.** In Graves disease, the most common cause of hyperthyroidism, the high levels of thyroid-stimulating immunoglobulins drive excess secretion of T_4 and T_3 and also have a trophic effect on the thyroid gland to produce **goiter.** Although TSH levels are decreased (by negative feedback) in Graves disease, the trophic effect is due to the TSH-*like* effect of the immunoglobulins.

♦ **TSH-secreting tumor.** TSH-secreting tumors are an uncommon cause of hyperthyroidism. Increased levels of TSH drive the thyroid to secrete excess T_4 and T_3 and have a trophic effect on the thyroid gland to produce **goiter.**

♦ **Ingestion of T_4.** Ingestion of exogenous thyroid hormones, or factitious hyperthyroidism, is associated with increased levels of thyroid hormone (from the ingestion), which causes decreased levels of TSH (by negative feedback). Because TSH levels are low there is **no goiter;** in fact, with time, the thyroid gland shrinks, or involutes.

♦ **Autoimmune thyroiditis.** Autoimmune thyroiditis is a common cause of hypothyroidism, in which thyroid hormone synthesis is impaired by antibodies to peroxidase, leading to decreased T_4 and T3 secretion. TSH levels are increased (by negative feedback), and the resulting high levels of TSH have a trophic effect on the thyroid gland to produce **goiter.** That's right! The gland enlarges even though it is not effectively synthesizing thyroid hormones.

♦ **TSH deficiency (anterior pituitary failure).** TSH deficiency is an uncommon cause of hypothyroidism, where the decreased levels of TSH cause decreased thyroid hormone secretion and **no goiter.**

♦ **I⁻ deficiency.** Deficiency of I⁻ leads to transiently decreased synthesis of T_4 and T_3, which increases TSH secretion by negative feedback. Increased TSH levels then have a trophic effect on the gland, causing **goiter.** The enlarged gland (which is otherwise normal) can often maintain normal blood levels of thyroid hormone (due to the high TSH levels); in that case, the person will be clinically euthyroid and asymptomatic. If the gland cannot maintain normal blood levels of thyroid hormone, then the person will be clinically hypothyroid.

ADRENAL MEDULLA AND CORTEX

The adrenal glands are located in the retroperitoneal cavity above each kidney. The adrenal glands are actually two separate glands, the adrenal medulla and the adrenal cortex, whose secretions are essential for life. When corrected for weight, these glands receive among the highest blood flow of any organ in the body.

The **adrenal medulla,** which is in the inner zone of the gland, composes approximately 20% of the tissue. The adrenal medulla is of neuroectodermal origin and

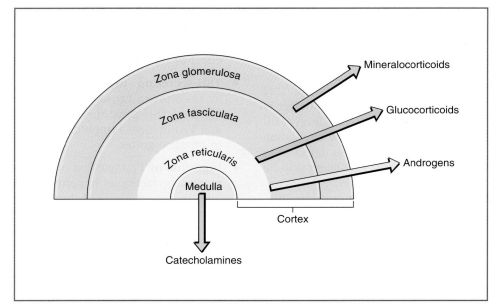

Figure 9–21 **Secretions of the adrenal medulla and adrenal cortex.** The zonae fasciculata and reticularis secrete glucocorticoids and androgens; the zona glomerulosa secretes mineralocorticoids.

secretes the catecholamines epinephrine and norepinephrine (see Chapter 2).

The **adrenal cortex,** which is in the outer zone of the gland, is of mesodermal origin and has three distinct layers. It composes 80% of the adrenal tissue and secretes adrenocortical steroid hormones. The adrenal cortex differentiates by gestational week 8 and is responsible for the production of fetal adrenal steroids throughout intrauterine life (see Chapter 10). Soon after birth, the fetal adrenal cortex begins to involute, eventually disappears, and is replaced by the three-layered adult adrenal cortex.

Synthesis of Adrenocortical Steroid Hormones

The adrenal cortex secretes three classes of steroid hormones: glucocorticoids, mineralocorticoids, and androgens. Figure 9-21 shows the three layers of the adrenal cortex in relation to the adrenal medulla. The innermost zone of the cortex, called the **zona reticularis,** and the middle (and widest) zone, called the **zona fasciculata,** synthesize and secrete glucocorticoids and adrenal androgens. The outermost zone, called the **zona glomerulosa,** secretes mineralocorticoids.

Structures of Adrenocortical Steroids

The structures of the major adrenocortical steroids are shown in Figure 9-22, which should be used as a reference throughout this section. All of the steroids of the adrenal cortex are chemical modifications of a basic steroid nucleus, which is illustrated in the structure of **cholesterol.** The basic nucleus is a carbon skeleton,

with carbons numbered from 1 through 21 and four labeled rings: A, B, C, and D. (Cholesterol is called, therefore, a 21-carbon steroid.) The **glucocorticoids,** represented by cortisol, have a ketone group at carbon 3 (C3) and hydroxyl groups at C11 and C21. The **mineralocorticoids,** represented by aldosterone, have a double-bond oxygen at C18. The **androgens,** represented in the adrenal cortex by dehydroepiandrosterone (DHEA) and androstenedione, have a double-bond oxygen at C17; androgens do not have the C20,21 side chain that is present in glucocorticoids and mineralocorticoids. Another androgen, testosterone (not shown in Fig. 9-22), is produced primarily in the testes. Estrogens (not shown), which are aromatized in the A ring and are lacking C19, are produced primarily in the ovaries.

In summary, cholesterol, progesterone, the glucocorticoids, and the mineralocorticoids are 21-carbon steroids; androgens are 19-carbon steroids; and estrogens (produced primarily in the ovaries) are 18-carbon steroids.

Biosynthetic Pathways in the Adrenal Cortex

Figure 9-23 is a schematic diagram of the biosynthetic pathways of the adrenocortical steroids. As noted earlier, the layers of the adrenal cortex are specialized to synthesize and secrete particular steroid hormones: either glucocorticoids and androgens or mineralocorticoids. The *basis for this specialization* is the presence or absence of the enzymes that catalyze various modifications of the steroid nucleus. For example, the zonae reticularis/fasciculata produce androgenic steroids because they

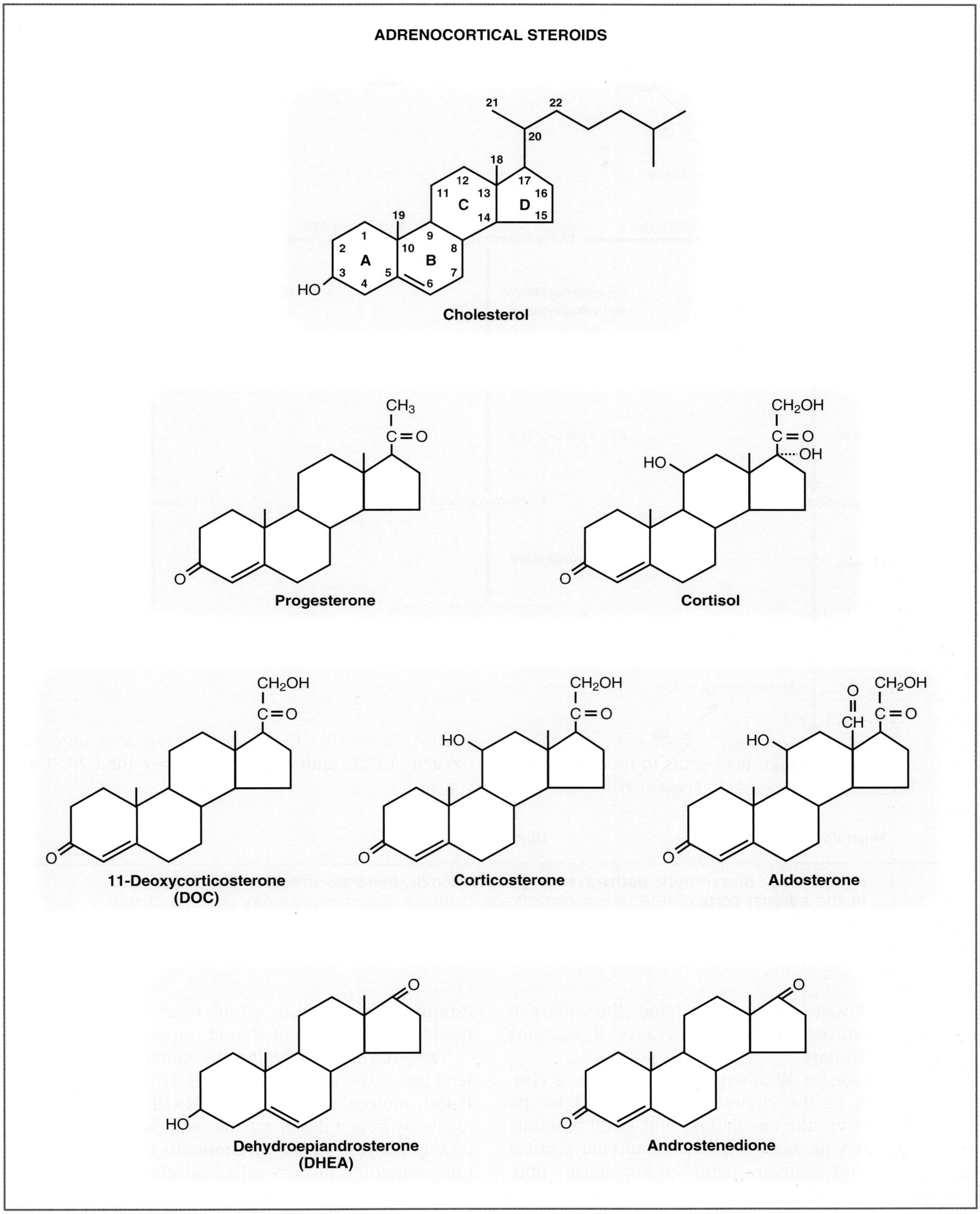

ADRENOCORTICAL STEROIDS

Figure 9–22 **Structures of adrenocortical steroids.** In the structure of cholesterol, the four rings of the steroid molecules are labeled A, B, C, and D, and the carbon atoms are numbered.

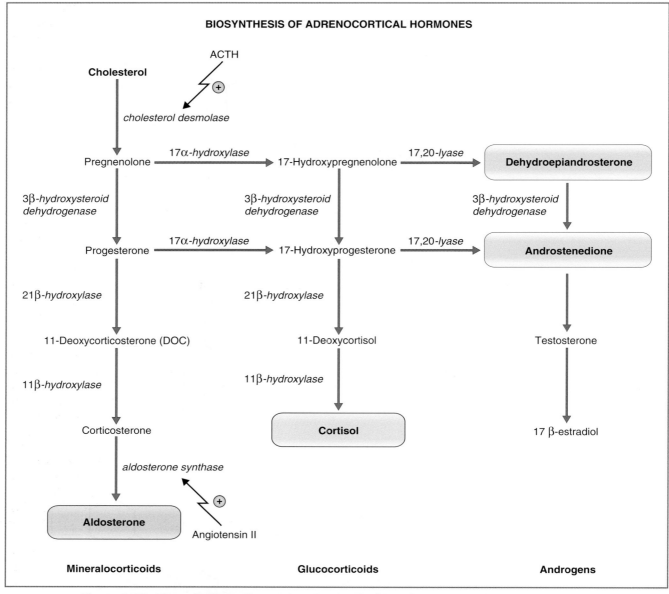

Figure 9–23 **Biosynthetic pathways for glucocorticoids, mineralocorticoids, and androgens in the adrenal cortex.** ACTH, Adrenocorticotropic hormone. The major secretory products of the adrenal cortex are shown in colored boxes.

contain 17,20-lyase; on the other hand, the zona glomerulosa produces aldosterone because it contains aldosterone synthase.

The precursor for all adrenocortical steroids is **cholesterol.** Most of the cholesterol is provided to the adrenal cortex via the circulation, and small amounts are synthesized *de novo* within the adrenal cortical cells. Cholesterol circulates bound to low-density lipoproteins. There are receptors for these lipoproteins in the membranes of adrenocortical cells; the lipoprotein-cholesterol complex binds and is transferred into the cell by endocytosis. Inside the cells, cholesterol is

esterified and stored in cytoplasmic vesicles until it is needed for synthesis of steroid hormones.

The enzymes catalyzing the conversion of cholesterol to active steroid hormones require **cytochrome P-450,** molecular oxygen, and NADPH, which serves as the hydrogen donor for the reducing steps. A flavoprotein enzyme called **adrenodoxin reductase** and an iron-containing protein called **adrenodoxin** are intermediates in the transfer of hydrogen from NADPH to the cytochrome P-450 enzymes.

For purposes of illustration, all of the biosynthetic pathways in the adrenal cortex are shown in Figure 9-23.

Remember, however, that not all layers of the cortex contain all of the steps in the pathway: Each layer has that portion of the pathway necessary to produce its primary hormones (i.e., glucocorticoids and androgens or mineralocorticoids).

The first step in each pathway is the conversion of cholesterol to pregnenolone, catalyzed by **cholesterol desmolase.** Thus, all layers of the adrenal cortex contain cholesterol desmolase. Cholesterol desmolase is the rate-limiting enzyme in the pathway, and it is stimulated by **ACTH** (see further discussion concerning regulation of cortisol secretion). Follow the pathways for the synthesis of cortisol, aldosterone, and DHEA and androstenedione:

♦ **Glucocorticoids (cortisol).** The major glucocorticoid produced in humans is **cortisol** (hydrocortisone), which is synthesized n the **zonae fasciculata/reticularis.** Thus, the zona fasciculata contains all of the enzymes required to convert cholesterol to cortisol: cholesterol desmolase, which converts cholesterol to pregnenolone; 17α-hydroxylase, which hydroxylates pregnenolone to form 17-hydroxypregnenolone; 3β-hydroxysteroid dehydrogenase, which converts 17-hydroxypregnenolone to 17-hydroxyprogesterone; and 21β-hydroxylase and 11β-hydroxylase, which hydroxylate at C11 and C21 to produce the final product, cortisol. Interestingly, some steps in the cortisol biosynthetic pathway can occur in a different order; for example, hydroxylation at C17 can occur before or after the action of 3β-hydroxysteroid dehydrogenase.

Cortisol is not the only steroid in the pathway with glucocorticoid activity; **corticosterone** is also a glucocorticoid. For example, if the 17α-hydroxylase step is blocked, the zona fasciculata still can produce corticosterone without deleterious effect. Thus, cortisol is not absolutely necessary to sustain life as long as corticosterone is being synthesized. Blocks at the cholesterol desmolase, 3β-hydroxysteroid dehydrogenase, 21β-hydroxylase, or 11β-hydroxylase steps are devastating because they prevent the production of cortisol *and* corticosterone; in these cases, death will ensue without appropriate hormone replacement therapy.

Metyrapone and ketoconazole are drugs that inhibit glucocorticoid biosynthesis. **Metyrapone** inhibits 11β-hydroxylase, the last step in cortisol synthesis. **Ketoconazole** inhibits several steps in the pathway including cholesterol desmolase, the first step.

♦ **Adrenal androgens (DHEA and androstenedione).** DHEA and androstenedione are androgenic steroids produced by the **zonae fasciculata/reticularis**. These compounds have weak androgenic activity, but in the testes, they are converted to testosterone, a more potent androgen. The precursors for the adrenal androgens are 17-hydroxypregnenolone and 17-hydroxyprogesterone, which are converted to androgens by removal of the C20,21 side chain. In males, adrenal androgens are of little significance; the testes produce their own testosterone from cholesterol and do not require the adrenal precursors (see Chapter 10). In females, however, the adrenal cortex is the major source of androgenic compounds.

Adrenal androgens have a ketone group at C17 that distinguishes them from cortisol, aldosterone, and testosterone. (Cortisol and aldosterone have side chains at C17. Testosterone has a hydroxyl group at C17.) Thus, the major adrenal androgens are called **17-ketosteroids,** which can be measured in the urine.

The zonae fasciculata/reticularis also produce small amounts of testosterone and 17β-estradiol, although the major sources for these hormones are the testes and ovaries, respectively (see Chapter 10).

♦ **Mineralocorticoids (aldosterone).** The major mineralocorticoid in the body is **aldosterone,** which is synthesized only in the **zona glomerulosa.** The steps required to convert cholesterol to corticosterone are identical to those in the zona fasciculata, and the addition of **aldosterone synthase** in the zona glomerulosa converts corticosterone to aldosterone. The zona glomerulosa *does not* produce glucocorticoids for two reasons: (1) Corticosterone, a glucocorticoid, is converted to aldosterone because this zone contains aldosterone synthase, and (2) the zona glomerulosa lacks 17α-hydroxylase and, therefore, is unable to produce cortisol from progesterone.

Aldosterone is not the only steroid with mineralocorticoid activity; **11-deoxycorticosterone** (**DOC**) and **corticosterone** also have mineralocorticoid activity. Thus, if the mineralocorticoid pathway is blocked *below the level of DOC* (e.g., absence of 11β-hydroxylase or aldosterone synthase), mineralocorticoids will continue to be produced. However, if the pathway is blocked *above the level of DOC* (e.g., absence of 21β-hydroxylase), then no mineralocorticoids will be produced.

Regulation of Secretion of Adrenocortical Steroids

As discussed previously, the synthesis and secretion of steroid hormones by the adrenal cortex depend on the stimulation of cholesterol desmolase (the first step) by **ACTH.** In the absence of ACTH, biosynthesis of adrenocortical steroid hormones ceases. Two questions arise, therefore: *What regulates the secretion of ACTH? What special regulatory factors control*

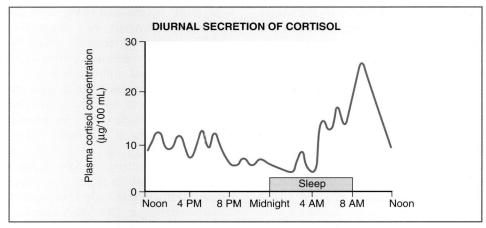

Figure 9–24 **Diurnal pattern of cortisol secretion.**

the functions of the zonae reticularis, fasciculata, and glomerulosa?

♦ The **zonae fasciculata/reticularis,** which secrete glucocorticoids and androgens, is under the exclusive control of the hypothalamic-pituitary axis. The hypothalamic hormone is corticotropin-releasing hormone (CRH), and the anterior pituitary hormone is ACTH.

♦ The **zona glomerulosa,** which secretes mineralocorticoids, depends on ACTH for the first step in steroid biosynthesis, but otherwise it is controlled separately via the renin-angiotensin-aldosterone system.

Control of the zonae fasciculata and reticularis will be discussed together, and control of the zona glomerulosa will be discussed separately.

Regulation of Glucocorticoid and Adrenal Androgen Secretion

An impressive feature of the regulation of cortisol secretion is its **pulsatile** nature and its **diurnal** (daily) pattern (Fig. 9-24). The daily profile of blood cortisol levels is characterized by an average of 10 secretory bursts during a 24-hour period. The lowest secretory rates occur during the evening hours and just after falling asleep (e.g., midnight), and the highest secretory rates occur just before awakening in the morning (e.g., 8 AM). The major burst of cortisol secretion before awakening accounts for one half of the total daily cortisol secretion. Other adrenal steroids (e.g., adrenal androgens) are secreted in similar bursting diurnal patterns. ACTH secretion also exhibits the same diurnal pattern; in fact, it is the pattern of ACTH secretion that drives the diurnal pattern of steroid hormone secretion.

The secretion of glucocorticoids by the zonae fasciculata/reticularis is regulated exclusively by the **hypothalamic-pituitary axis** (Fig. 9-25). CRH is secreted by the hypothalamus and acts on the

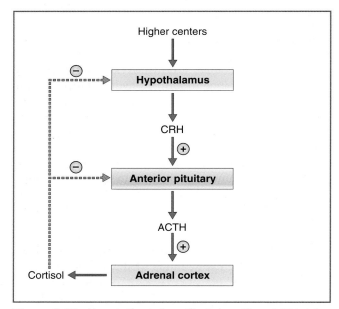

Figure 9–25 **Regulation of cortisol secretion.** ACTH, Adrenocorticotropic hormone; CRH, corticotropin-releasing hormone.

corticotrophs of the anterior pituitary to cause secretion of ACTH. In turn, ACTH acts on the cells of the adrenal cortex to stimulate the synthesis and secretion of adrenocortical hormones.

♦ **CRH** is a polypeptide containing 41 amino acids. It is secreted by cells of the paraventricular nuclei of the hypothalamus. Like other hypothalamic hormones that act on the anterior pituitary, CRH travels to the pituitary in the hypothalamic-hypophysial portal blood. In the anterior lobe, it acts on the corticotrophs by an adenylyl cyclase/cAMP mechanism to cause secretion of ACTH into the bloodstream.

♦ **ACTH,** the anterior pituitary hormone, has several effects on the adrenal cortex. The immediate effects of ACTH are to stimulate transfer of stored cholesterol to the mitochondria, to stimulate binding of cholesterol to cytochrome P-450, and to activate cholesterol desmolase. Long-term effects of ACTH include stimulation of transcription of the genes for cytochrome P-450 and adrenodoxin and up-regulation of ACTH receptors. Chronic effects of elevated ACTH levels include hypertrophy and hyperplasia of the adrenal cortical cells, mediated by local growth factors (e.g., IGF-2).

As noted, ACTH has a **pulsatile** and **diurnal** secretory pattern that drives a parallel pattern of cortisol secretion. The nocturnal peak of ACTH (i.e., preceding awakening) is driven, in turn, by a burst of CRH secretion. The "internal clock" that drives the diurnal pattern can be shifted by alternating the sleep-wake cycle (e.g., varying the time of going to sleep and awakening). The diurnal pattern is abolished by coma, blindness, or constant exposure to either light or dark.

♦ **Negative feedback** is exerted by cortisol at three points in the hypothalamic-pituitary axis. (1) Cortisol directly inhibits secretion of CRH from the hypothalamus. (2) Cortisol indirectly inhibits CRH secretion by effects on hippocampal neurons, which synapse on the hypothalamus. (3) Cortisol inhibits the action of CRH on the anterior pituitary, resulting in inhibition of ACTH secretion. Thus, chronic *deficiency* of cortisol leads to stimulation of the CRH-ACTH axis and to increased ACTH levels; chronic *excess* of cortisol leads to inhibition (suppression) of the CRH-ACTH axis and decreased ACTH levels.

♦ The **dexamethasone suppression test** is based on the negative feedback effects of cortisol on the CRH-ACTH axis. Dexamethasone is a synthetic glucocorticoid that has all of the actions of cortisol including the negative feedback effect on ACTH secretion. When a low dose of dexamethasone is given to a **healthy person,** it inhibits (or "suppresses") ACTH secretion, just as cortisol, the natural glucocorticoid, does. The decreased level of ACTH then causes decreased cortisol secretion, which is measured in the test. The major use of the dexamethasone suppression test is in persons with **hypercortisolism** (high levels of cortisol). The test is used to determine whether the hypercortisolism is due to an ACTH-secreting tumor or a cortisol-secreting tumor of the adrenal cortex. If the cause of hypercortisolism is an **ACTH-secreting tumor** of the anterior pituitary, a low dose of dexamethasone does not suppress cortisol secretion but a high dose of dexamethasone does. (The tumor's ACTH secretion is less sensitive to negative feedback by glucocorticoids than is normal anterior pituitary tissue.) If the cause of hypercortisolism is an **adrenal cortical tumor,** then neither low-dose nor high-dose dexamethasone suppresses cortisol secretion. (The

Table 9-10 Factors Affecting ACTH Secretion

Stimulatory Factors	Inhibitory Factors
Decreased blood cortisol levels	Increased blood cortisol levels
Sleep-wake transition	
Stress; hypoglycemia; surgery; trauma	Opioids
Psychiatric disturbances	Somatostatin
ADH	
α-Adrenergic agonists	
β-Adrenergic antagonists	
Serotonin	

ADH, Antidiuretic hormone.

tumor's secretion of cortisol is autonomous and is not affected by changes in the ACTH level.)

In addition to negative feedback control by the CRH-ACTH axis, other factors alter ACTH and cortisol secretion (Table 9-10). Many of these factors alter ACTH secretion via effects of higher brain centers on the hypothalamus.

Regulation of Aldosterone Secretion

The regulation of aldosterone secretion by the zona glomerulosa is different from the regulation of the secretion of cortisol and adrenal androgens. Naturally, ACTH remains essential in this process because it stimulates cholesterol desmolase, the first step in the biosynthetic pathway. (Thus, ACTH has a tonic effect on aldosterone secretion.) Like the other adrenal steroid hormones, aldosterone exhibits a diurnal pattern, with the lowest levels occurring at midnight and the highest levels occurring just before awakening. However, the primary regulation of aldosterone secretion occurs not by ACTH, but through changes in ECF volume via the renin–angiotensin II–aldosterone system and through changes in serum potassium (K^+) levels.

♦ **Renin–angiotensin II–aldosterone.** The major control of aldosterone secretion is via the renin–angiotensin II–aldosterone system. The mediator of this regulation is **angiotensin II,** which increases the synthesis and secretion of aldosterone by stimulating cholesterol desmolase and aldosterone synthase, the first and last steps in the pathway (see Fig. 9-23). In the zona glomerulosa, angiotensin II binds to AT_1 receptors that are coupled to phospholipase C via a G_q protein. Thus, the second messengers for the action of angiotensin II are IP_3/Ca^{2+}.

Regulation of the renin–angiotensin II–aldosterone axis is described in Chapter 4. Briefly, a decrease in ECF volume (e.g., due to hemorrhage or Na^+ depletion) causes a decrease in renal perfusion pressure, which increases renin secretion by the juxtaglomerular cells of the kidney. **Renin,** an enzyme, catalyzes the conversion of angiotensinogen to

Table 9-11 Actions of Adrenocortical Steroids

Actions of Glucocorticoids	Actions of Mineralocorticoids	Actions of Adrenal Androgens
Increase gluconeogenesis	Increase Na^+ reabsorption	Females: stimulate growth of pubic and axillary hair; stimulate libido
Increase proteolysis (catabolic)	Increase K^+ secretion	Males: same as testosterone
Increase lipolysis	Increase H^+ secretion	
Decrease glucose utilization		
Decrease insulin sensitivity		
Inhibit inflammatory response		
Suppress immune response		
Enhance vascular responsiveness to catecholamines		
Inhibit bone formation		
Increase GFR		
Decrease REM sleep		

GFR, Glomerular filtration rate; REM, rapid eye movement.

angiotensin I, which is inactive. **Angiotensin-converting enzyme** (**ACE**) catalyzes the conversion of angiotensin I to **angiotensin II,** which then acts on the zona glomerulosa to stimulate **aldosterone** synthesis.

In light of the role that aldosterone plays in maintaining ECF volume, the control of aldosterone secretion by the renin–angiotensin II–aldosterone system is logical. For example, decreases in ECF volume stimulate aldosterone secretion, and aldosterone stimulates Na^+ reabsorption by the kidney to help restore ECF Na^+ content and ECF volume.

♦ **Serum K^+.** The other factor that controls aldosterone secretion is the serum K^+ concentration. Increases in serum K^+ concentration increase aldosterone secretion, and decreases in serum K^+ concentration decrease aldosterone secretion. For example, an increase in serum K^+ concentration acts on adrenal cells by depolarizing them and opening voltage-sensitive Ca^{2+} channels. When Ca^{2+} channels open, intracellular Ca^{2+} concentration increases and stimulates aldosterone secretion. In light of the major role that aldosterone plays in maintaining K^+ balance, the control of aldosterone secretion by serum K^+ concentration also is logical. For example, increases in serum K^+ stimulate aldosterone secretion, and aldosterone increases K^+ secretion by the kidney, thereby decreasing serum K^+ toward normal.

Actions of Adrenocortical Steroids

Adrenocortical steroids have diverse actions, and the actions are classified as glucocorticoid (cortisol), mineralocorticoid (aldosterone), or androgenic (DHEA and androstenedione). As steroid hormones, these actions first require transcription of DNA, synthesis of specific mRNAs, and induction of new protein synthesis. These new proteins confer specificity to the steroid hormone actions in target tissues (Table 9-11).

Actions of Glucocorticoids

Glucocorticoids are essential for life. If the adrenal cortex is removed or is not functioning, exogenous glucocorticoids must be administered or death will ensue. The actions of glucocorticoids (e.g., cortisol) are essential for gluconeogenesis, vascular responsiveness to catecholamines, suppression of inflammatory and immune responses, and modulation of CNS function.

♦ **Stimulation of gluconeogenesis.** A major action of cortisol is to promote gluconeogenesis and storage of glycogen. Overall, the effects of cortisol are **catabolic** and **diabetogenic.** Cortisol affects protein, fat, and carbohydrate metabolism in a coordinated fashion to increase glucose synthesis as follows: Cortisol increases protein catabolism in muscle and decreases new protein synthesis, thereby providing additional amino acids to the liver for gluconeogenesis. Cortisol increases lipolysis, which provides additional glycerol to the liver for gluconeogenesis. Finally, cortisol decreases glucose utilization by tissues and decreases the insulin sensitivity of adipose tissue. Glucocorticoids are essential for **survival during fasting** because they stimulate these gluconeogenic routes. In hypocortisolism (e.g., primary adrenal insufficiency, Addison disease), there is hypoglycemia. In hypercortisolism (e.g., Cushing syndrome), there is hyperglycemia.

♦ **Anti-inflammatory effects.** Cortisol has three actions that interfere with the body's inflammatory response to trauma and irritants. (1) Cortisol induces the synthesis of **lipocortin,** an inhibitor of the enzyme phospholipase A_2. Phospholipase A_2 liberates arachidonic acid from membrane phospholipids and provides the precursor for the prostaglandins and leukotrienes that mediate the inflammatory response. Therefore, this component of the antiinflammatory effect of cortisol is based on inhibiting the synthesis of the precursor to prostaglandins and leukotrienes. (2) Cortisol inhibits the production of **interleukin-2 (IL-2)** and the proliferation of T lymphocytes. (3) Cortisol inhibits the release of **histamine** and **serotonin** from mast cells and platelets.

♦ **Suppression of immune response.** As previously noted, cortisol inhibits the production of IL-2 and the proliferation of T lymphocytes, which also are critical for cellular immunity. Exogenous glucocorticoids can be administered therapeutically to suppress the immune response and prevent the rejection of transplanted organs.

♦ **Maintenance of vascular responsiveness to catecholamines.** Cortisol is necessary for the maintenance of normal blood pressure and plays a permissive role in the arterioles by up-regulating α_1-adrenergic receptors. In this way, cortisol is required for the vasoconstrictive response of the arterioles to catecholamines. In hypocortisolism, there is hypotension; in hypercortisolism, there is hypertension.

♦ **Inhibition of bone formation.** Cortisol inhibits bone formation by decreasing the synthesis of type I collagen, the major component of bone matrix; by decreasing formation of new bone by osteoblasts; and by decreasing intestinal Ca^{2+} absorption.

♦ **Increases in glomerular filtration rate (GFR).** Cortisol increases GFR by causing vasodilation of afferent arterioles, thereby increasing renal blood flow and GFR.

♦ **Effects on CNS.** Glucocorticoid receptors are found in the brain, particularly in the limbic system. Cortisol decreases REM sleep, increases slow-wave sleep, and increases awake time. (Recall that the largest bursts of ACTH and cortisol occur just before awakening.)

Actions of Mineralocorticoids

The actions of mineralocorticoids (e.g., aldosterone) are described in detail in Chapter 6. Briefly, aldosterone has three actions on the late distal tubule and collecting ducts of the kidney: It increases **Na⁺ reabsorption,** it increases **K⁺ secretion,** and it increases **H⁺ secretion.** Its effects on Na⁺ reabsorption and K⁺ secretion are on the principal cells, and its effect on H⁺ secretion is on the α-intercalated cells. Thus, when aldosterone levels are increased (e.g., due to an aldosterone-secreting tumor), Na⁺ reabsorption, K⁺ secretion, and H⁺ secretion all are increased. These changes in renal transport result in ECF volume expansion and hypertension, hypokalemia, and metabolic alkalosis. Conversely, when aldosterone levels are decreased (e.g., due to adrenal insufficiency), Na⁺ reabsorption, K⁺ secretion,

and H⁺ secretion all are decreased. These changes produce ECF volume contraction and hypotension, hyperkalemia, and metabolic acidosis.

An interesting "problem" arises with respect to the actions of mineralocorticoids in their target tissues (i.e., late distal tubule and collecting ducts of the kidney). That is, the affinity of mineralocorticoid receptors for cortisol is, surprisingly, just as high as their affinity for aldosterone. Because circulating levels of cortisol are much higher than circulating levels of aldosterone, it seems that cortisol would overwhelm and dominate the mineralocorticoid receptors. How would the kidneys know that a change in aldosterone concentration had occurred and that mineralocorticoid actions are desired? The "problem" is solved by the renal cells themselves. They contain the enzyme **11β-hydroxysteroid dehydrogenase,** which converts cortisol to cortisone; in contrast to cortisol, cortisone has a low affinity for mineralocorticoid receptors. In this way, cortisol is effectively inactivated in mineralocorticoid target tissues. This unique solution allows changes in blood levels of aldosterone to be "seen" by the renal cells and not be overshadowed by the high circulating levels of cortisol. This inactivation of cortisol in mineralocorticoid target tissues also explains why, when circulating levels of cortisol are high, the cortisol has only weak mineralocorticoid activity (despite its high affinity for mineralocorticoid receptors).

Actions of Adrenal Androgens

The adrenal cortex produces the androgenic compounds, DHEA and androstenedione, which are converted to testosterone primarily in the testes. In males, adrenal androgens play only a minor role because de novo synthesis of testosterone from cholesterol in the testes is much greater than testosterone synthesis from adrenal androgenic precursors. In females, however, adrenal androgens are the *major* androgens, and they are responsible for the development of pubic and axillary hair and for libido.

In conditions such as **adrenogenital syndrome,** in which there is increased synthesis of adrenal androgens, the high levels of DHEA and androstenedione lead to masculinization in females, early development of axillary and pubic hair, and suppression of gonadal function in both males and females. Also, in the adrenogenital syndromes, due to the overproduction of adrenal androgens, there will be increased urinary levels of **17-ketosteroids.**

Pathophysiology of the Adrenal Cortex

Disorders involving the adrenal cortex are characterized by either an excess or a deficiency of adrenocortical hormones. When evaluating the pathophysiology of these disorders, it is helpful to consider the following issues:

1. *What are the symptoms and signs? Are the signs and symptoms consistent with an excess or a deficiency of one or more of the adrenocortical hormones?* The normal physiologic effects of each of the adrenocortical hormones can be used to predict the effects of hormonal excess or deficiency (see Table 9-11). A few examples are cited here.

   Cortisol promotes gluconeogenesis, and therefore, excess levels of cortisol will produce hyperglycemia; deficits of cortisol will produce hypoglycemia upon fasting. **Aldosterone** causes increased K^+ secretion by the renal principal cells; thus excess aldosterone will cause increased K^+ secretion and hypokalemia, and deficiency of aldosterone will cause decreased K^+ secretion and hyperkalemia. Aldosterone also causes increased Na^+ reabsorption by the principal cells; thus, excess aldosterone causes ECF volume expansion and hypertension, and deficiency of aldosterone causes ECF volume contraction and hypotension. Because **adrenal androgens** have testosterone-like effects, overproduction causes masculinization in females (e.g., hirsutism); deficits of adrenal androgens result in loss of pubic and axillary hair and decreased libido in females.

2. *What is the etiology of the disorder?* Disorders of the adrenal cortex can be caused by a primary defect in the adrenal cortex or by a primary defect in the hypothalamic-pituitary axis. Or, in the case of aldosterone, the defect may be in the renin-angiotensin II axis. For example, symptoms consistent with overproduction of an adrenocortical hormone (e.g., hypercortisolism) may be caused by a primary defect in the adrenal cortex. Or, the symptoms may be caused by a primary defect in the anterior pituitary or the hypothalamus, which then produces a secondary effect on the adrenal cortex. The etiology of the disorder may not be deduced until circulating levels of CRH and ACTH are measured and the feedback regulation of the CRH-ACTH axis is evaluated.

   For disorders caused by enzyme deficiencies in the steroid hormone biosynthetic pathway, the pathways can be visualized to predict the effects of a given enzyme block (see Fig. 9-23). For example, a woman with masculinization also has symptoms consistent with aldosterone deficiency (e.g., hyperkalemia) and cortisol deficiency (e.g., hypoglycemia). This constellation of symptoms suggests that there is an enzyme block preventing the synthesis of all mineralocorticoids and all glucocorticoids (e.g., deficiency of 21β-hydroxylase). Because of the block, steroid intermediates are "shunted" toward androgen production and the increased adrenal androgen levels cause masculinization. To understand the pathophysiology of the adrenal cortex, use the biosynthetic pathway shown in Figure 9-23 in combination with the actions of the steroid hormones summarized in Table 9-11. The features of each disorder are summarized in Table 9-12.

Addison Disease

Addison disease, or **primary adrenocortical insufficiency,** is commonly caused by autoimmune destruction of all zones of the adrenal cortex (Box 9-2). In this disease, there is decreased synthesis of all adrenocortical hormones, resulting in decreased circulating levels of cortisol, aldosterone, and adrenal androgens. The symptoms of Addison disease can be predicted on the basis of the known physiologic effects of these hormones. The loss of glucocorticoids (cortisol) produces hypoglycemia, anorexia, weight loss, nausea and vomiting, and weakness. The loss of mineralocorticoids (aldosterone) produces hyperkalemia, metabolic acidosis, and hypotension (due to decreased ECF volume). In women, the loss of the adrenal androgens, DHEA and androstenedione, results in decreased pubic and axillary hair and decreased libido.

Addison disease also is characterized by **hyperpigmentation** of the skin, particularly of the elbows, knees, nail beds, nipples, areolae, and on recent scars. Hyperpigmentation is a result of **increased levels of ACTH** (which contains the α-MSH fragment). Hyperpigmentation, therefore, provides an important clue about the etiology of Addison disease: ACTH levels must be high, not low, and the cause of the hypocortisolism must *not* be a primary defect in ACTH secretion from the anterior pituitary. Rather, the hypocortisolism of Addison disease must be due to a primary defect in the adrenal cortex itself (i.e., primary adrenal insufficiency), with low levels of cortisol then causing an increase in ACTH secretion by negative feedback (see Fig. 9-25).

Treatment of Addison disease includes glucocorticoid and mineralocorticoid replacement.

Secondary Adrenocortical Insufficiency

Conditions of secondary adrenocortical insufficiency occur when there is insufficient CRH (uncommon) or insufficient ACTH (resulting from failure of corticotrophs in the anterior pituitary to secrete ACTH). In either case, there is decreased ACTH, which then decreases cortisol secretion by the adrenal cortex. The cortisol deficiency then produces many of the symptoms that occur in primary adrenocortical insufficiency (e.g., hypoglycemia). There are, however, several distinctions between primary and secondary adrenocortical insufficiency. (1) In secondary adrenocortical insufficiency, ACTH levels are low, not high. (2) In secondary adrenocortical insufficiency, aldosterone levels usually are normal because aldosterone synthesis

Table 9–12 Pathophysiology of the Adrenal Cortex

Disease	Clinical Features	ACTH Levels	Treatment
Addison disease (primary adrenocortical insufficiency)	Hypoglycemia Anorexia, weight loss, nausea, vomiting Weakness Hypotension Hyperkalemia Metabolic acidosis Decreased pubic and axillary hair in females Hyperpigmentation	Increased (negative feedback effect of decreased cortisol)	Replacement of glucocorticoids and mineralocorticoids
Cushing syndrome (e.g., primary adrenal hyperplasia)	Hyperglycemia Muscle wasting Central obesity Round face, supraclavicular fat, buffalo hump Osteoporosis Striae Virilization and menstrual disorders in females Hypertension	Decreased (negative feedback effect of increased cortisol)	Ketoconazole Metyrapone
Cushing disease (excess ACTH)	Same as Cushing syndrome (see above)	Increased	Surgical removal of ACTH-secreting tumor
Conn syndrome (aldosterone-secreting tumor)	Hypertension Hypokalemia Metabolic alkalosis Decreased renin levels	—	Aldosterone antagonist (e.g., spironolactone) Surgery
21β-hydroxylase Deficiency	Virilization in females Early acceleration of linear growth Early appearance of pubic and axillary hair Symptoms of deficiency of glucocorticoids and mineralocorticoids	Increased (negative feedback effect of decreased cortisol)	Replacement of glucocorticoids and mineralocorticoids
17α-hydroxylase Deficiency	Lack of pubic and axillary hair in females Symptoms of deficiency of glucocorticoids Symptoms of excess mineralocorticoids	Increased (negative feedback effect of decreased cortisol)	Replacement of glucocorticoids Aldosterone antagonist (e.g., spironolactone)

by the zona glomerulosa requires only tonic levels of ACTH. If aldosterone levels are normal, hyperkalemia, metabolic acidosis, and ECF volume contraction are not present. (3) In secondary adrenocortical insufficiency, hyperpigmentation does not occur because levels of ACTH (containing the α-MSH fragment) are low, not high as occurs in Addison disease.

Cushing Syndrome

Cushing syndrome is the result of chronic excess of glucocorticoids. It can be caused by spontaneous overproduction of cortisol by the adrenal cortex or from the administration of pharmacologic doses of exogenous glucocorticoids. **Cushing disease** is a separate entity, also characterized by excess glucocorticoids, in which the cause is hypersecretion of ACTH from a pituitary adenoma (which then drives the adrenal cortex to secrete excess cortisol).

The symptoms of either Cushing syndrome or Cushing disease are the result of excessive glucocorticoids and adrenal androgens (Fig. 9-26). Excess cortisol causes hyperglycemia, increased proteolysis and muscle wasting, increased lipolysis and thin extremities, central obesity, round face, supraclavicular fat, buffalo hump,

BOX 9–2 Clinical Physiology: Addison Disease

DESCRIPTION OF CASE. A 45-year-old woman is admitted to the hospital with a history of progressive weakness and weight loss, occasional nausea, and darkening skin pigmentation. On physical examination, she is thin, has dark skin creases, and has diminished axillary and pubic hair. Her blood pressure is 120/80 when supine and 106/50 when standing. Her pulse rate is 100/minute when supine and 120/minute when standing. Laboratory studies yield the following values:

Serum	Urine
$[Na^+]$ 120 mEq/L	Na^+, increased
$[K^+]$, 5.8 mEq/L	K^+, decreased
$[HCO_3^-]$, 120 mEq/L	pH, increased
Osmolarity, 254 mOsm/L	Osmolarity, 450 mOsm/L

Arterial blood gases are consistent with metabolic acidosis. Blood urea nitrogen (BUN) and serum creatinine are increased. Her blood glucose concentration is low-normal, and she becomes hypoglycemic upon fasting. Serum levels of ACTH are elevated. An ACTH stimulation test shows a "flat" cortisol response (i.e., the adrenal cortex *did not* respond to ACTH).

The woman is treated with cortisol, taken twice daily, early morning and late afternoon, and fludrocortisone, a synthetic mineralocorticoid.

EXPLANATION OF CASE. The woman has primary adrenocortical insufficiency (Addison disease), in which all layers of the adrenal cortex are destroyed. None of the adrenocortical hormones, glucocorticoids, mineralocorticoids, and adrenal androgens are secreted in adequate amounts. Decreased blood levels of cortisol, via negative feedback mechanisms, then cause increased secretion of ACTH by the anterior lobe of the pituitary. The woman's abnormal serum and urine values, orthostatic hypotension, hypoglycemia, decreased body hair, and hyperpigmentation can be explained by decreased circulating levels of adrenocortical steroids as follows:

The woman has increased serum $[K^+]$ (hyperkalemia) and metabolic acidosis. Simultaneously, urinary excretion of K^+ is decreased, and urine pH is increased. These disturbances of K^+ and acid-base balance are caused by the loss of the adrenocortical hormone aldosterone. Normally, aldosterone stimulates K^+ and H^+ secretion in the renal distal tubule and collecting duct. Therefore, when there is a deficiency of aldosterone, the kidney secretes inadequate amounts of K^+ and H^+, elevating their respective blood levels and causing hyperkalemia and metabolic acidosis. (Accordingly, the excretion of K^+ and H^+ in urine is decreased.)

When the woman moves from a supine to a standing position, her blood pressure decreases and her pulse rate increases. Orthostatic hypotension, the decrease in blood pressure upon standing, is explained by a deficiency of aldosterone and a deficiency of cortisol. In addition to its effects on K^+ and H^+ secretion, aldosterone stimulates renal Na^+ reabsorption. When aldosterone is deficient, there is inadequate renal Na^+ reabsorption, which results in decreased body Na^+ content, decreased ECF volume and blood volume, and decreased arterial blood pressure (especially when standing). Lack of cortisol contributes to her hypotension by reducing vascular responsiveness to catecholamines. The increased pulse rate upon standing reflects the response of the baroreceptor reflex to this orthostatic decrease in blood pressure. A component of the baroreceptor reflex response is increased heart rate, which attempts to restore blood pressure back to normal. The woman's elevated BUN and serum creatinine reflect a decreased GFR, which is consistent with decreased ECF volume (i.e., prerenal azotemia).

The woman's decreased serum $[Na^+]$ and serum osmolarity are secondary to the ECF volume contraction. When ECF volume decreases by 10% or more, ADH secretion is stimulated. ADH then circulates to the kidney, stimulating water reabsorption, as reflected in the hyperosmotic urine. The reabsorbed water is added to the body fluids, diluting them, as reflected in the decreased $[Na^+]$ and osmolarity. ADH secreted under such hypovolemic conditions is quite appropriate for her volume status but inappropriate for her serum osmolarity.

Hypoglycemia, nausea, weight loss, and weakness are caused by a deficiency of glucocorticoids. The decreased body Na^+ content and decreased ECF volume also contribute to weight loss because a large percentage of body weight is water.

Hyperpigmentation resulted from negative feedback on the anterior pituitary by the low circulating cortisol levels. The decreased levels of cortisol stimulate secretion of ACTH, which contains the α-MSH fragment. When circulating levels of ACTH are elevated, as in Addison disease, the α-MSH component of the molecule produces darkening skin pigmentation.

The woman has decreased pubic and axillary hair from the loss of the adrenal androgens, DHEA and androstenedione. (In females, adrenal androgens are the major source of androgens.)

TREATMENT. Treatment of this patient consists of replacing the missing adrenocortical steroid hormones, which are necessary for life. She is given a synthetic mineralocorticoid (fludrocortisone) and a glucocorticoid (cortisol). Cortisol is administered twice daily, a large dose in early morning and a smaller dose in late afternoon, to simulate the normal diurnal pattern of cortisol secretion.

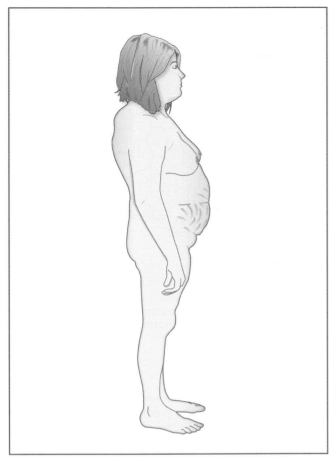

Figure 9–26 **Drawing of a woman with Cushing disease.** Note the central obesity, buffalo hump, muscle wasting, and striae.

poor wound healing, osteoporosis, and striae (caused by a loss of connective tissue). Hypertension occurs because cortisol has weak mineralocorticoid activity and because cortisol increases the responsiveness of arterioles to catecholamines (by up-regulating α_1 receptors). Excess androgens cause virilization and menstrual disorders in females.

Cushing syndrome and Cushing disease exhibit similar clinical features, but they differ in the circulating levels of ACTH. In *Cushing syndrome,* the primary defect is in the adrenal cortex, which is overproducing cortisol. Accordingly, ACTH levels are low because the high cortisol levels feed back on the anterior pituitary and inhibit ACTH secretion. In *Cushing disease,* the primary defect is in the anterior pituitary, which is overproducing ACTH; ACTH levels are elevated. As already described, the **dexamethasone suppression test,** in which a synthetic glucocorticoid is administered, can distinguish between the two disorders. In Cushing syndrome (primary adrenal defect with a normal CRH-ACTH axis), because the adrenal tumor functions autonomously, cortisol secretion is not

suppressed by either low- or high-dose dexamethasone. In Cushing disease, ACTH and cortisol secretion are suppressed by high-dose dexamethasone but not by low-dose dexamethasone.

Treatment of *Cushing syndrome* includes administration of drugs such as **ketoconazole** or **metyrapone,** which block steroid hormone biosynthesis. If drug treatment is ineffective, then bilateral adrenalectomy coupled with steroid hormone replacement may be required. Because of its different etiology, treatment of *Cushing disease* involves surgical removal of the ACTH-secreting tumor.

Conn Syndrome

Conn syndrome, or **primary hyperaldosteronism,** is caused by an aldosterone-secreting tumor. The symptoms of Conn syndrome are explainable by the known physiologic actions of aldosterone: Na^+ reabsorption, K^+ secretion, and H^+ secretion. The effects of excess aldosterone are increased ECF volume and hypertension (due to increased Na^+ reabsorption), hypokalemia (due to increased K^+ secretion), and metabolic alkalosis (due to increased H^+ secretion). In Conn syndrome, circulating renin levels are decreased because the increased ECF volume (caused by high levels of aldosterone) increases renal perfusion pressure, which inhibits renin secretion. Treatment of Conn syndrome consists of administration of an aldosterone antagonist such as **spironolactone,** followed by surgical removal of the aldosterone-secreting tumor.

21β-Hydroxylase Deficiency

Several congenital abnormalities are associated with enzyme defects in the steroid hormone biosynthetic pathways. The most common enzymatic defect is deficiency of 21β-hydroxylase, which belongs to a group of disorders called **adrenogenital syndrome.** Review Figure 9-23 to understand the consequences of this enzyme deficiency. Without 21β-hydroxylase, the adrenal cortex is unable to convert progesterone to 11-deoxycorticosterone (DOC) or to convert 17-hydroxyprogesterone to 11-deoxycortisol. In other words, the adrenal cortex does not synthesize mineralocorticoids or glucocorticoids, resulting in predictable symptoms (as previously discussed). Steroid intermediates will accumulate *above* the enzyme block and be shunted toward production of the adrenal androgens, DHEA and androstenedione, which then cause virilization in females. There will be increased urinary levels of 17-ketosteroids. If the defect is present in utero in a female fetus, the excess androgens cause masculinization of the external genitalia, with a penis-like clitoris and scrotum-like labia. If untreated in childhood, the androgen excess will cause an acceleration of linear growth, the early appearance of pubic and axillary hair, and suppression of gonadal function. ACTH levels will be elevated because of negative feedback on the anterior pituitary by the low cortisol levels, and these high ACTH levels will have a trophic effect on the adrenal cortex and cause adrenocortical hyperplasia. (Thus, the other name for this group of disorders is **congenital adrenal hyperplasia.**) Treatment of 21β-hydroxylase deficiency consists of replacement of both glucocorticoids and mineralocorticoids.

17α-Hydroxylase Deficiency

A less-common congenital abnormality of the steroid hormone biosynthetic pathway is deficiency of 17α-hydroxylase. The consequences of this defect differ from those of 21β-hydroxylase deficiency. Examination of Figure 9-23 shows that without 17α-hydroxylase, pregnenolone cannot be converted to 17-hydroxypregnenolone and progesterone cannot be converted to 17-hydroxyprogesterone. As a result, neither glucocorticoids nor adrenal androgens will be produced by the adrenal cortex. The absence of cortisol will cause predictable effects (e.g., hypoglycemia), and the absence of adrenal androgens will result in the lack of pubic and axillary hair in females. In this disorder, steroid intermediates accumulate to the *left* of the enzyme block and will be shunted toward mineralocorticoids; there will be overproduction of 11-deoxycorticosterone and corticosterone, both of which have mineralocorticoid activity. The resulting high levels of mineralocorticoids then cause hypertension, hypokalemia, and metabolic alkalosis.

Interestingly, the levels of aldosterone itself are actually *decreased* in 17α-hydroxylase deficiency. Why would this be so, if steroid intermediates are shunted toward the production of mineralocorticoids? The answer lies in the feedback regulation of the renin–angiotensin II–aldosterone system. The increased levels of 11-deoxycorticosterone and corticosterone cause symptoms of mineralocorticoid excess: hypertension, metabolic alkalosis, and hypokalemia. Hypertension inhibits renin secretion, thus leading to decreased levels of angiotensin II and aldosterone; hypokalemia also inhibits aldosterone secretion directly.

ENDOCRINE PANCREAS

The endocrine pancreas secretes two major peptide hormones, insulin and glucagon, whose coordinated functions are to regulate glucose, fatty acid, and amino acid metabolism. The endocrine pancreas also secretes somatostatin and pancreatic polypeptide, whose functions are less well established.

The endocrine cells of the pancreas are arranged in clusters called the **islets of Langerhans,** which compose 1% to 2% of the pancreatic mass. There are approximately 1 million islets of Langerhans, each containing about 2500 cells. The islets of Langerhans contain four

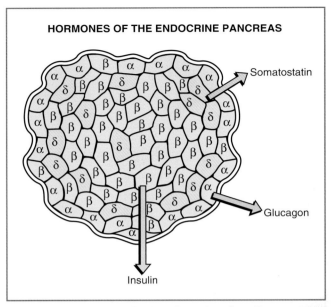

Figure 9–27 Schematic drawing showing the arrangement of cell types and the hormones they secrete in an islet of Langerhans.

cell types, and each cell secretes a different hormone or peptide (Fig. 9-27). The β cells compose 65% of the islet and secrete **insulin.** The α cells compose 20% of the islet and secrete **glucagon.** The delta (δ) **cells** compose 10% of the islet and secrete **somatostatin.** The remaining cells (not shown in Fig. 9-27) secrete **pancreatic polypeptide** or other peptides.

The central core of the islet of Langerhans contains mostly β cells, with α cells distributed around the outer rim. The δ cells are interposed between α and β cells, and their intimate contact with the other cell types suggests a paracrine function.

There are three ways in which cells of the islets of Langerhans communicate with each other and thereby alter each other's secretion (i.e., paracrine mechanisms). (1) Gap junctions connect α cells to each other, β cells to each other, and α cells to β cells. These gap junctions permit rapid cell-to-cell communication via either ionic current flow or transfer of molecules (up to 1000 molecular weight). (2) The islets receive about 10% of the total pancreatic blood flow. The **blood supply** of the endocrine pancreas is arranged so that venous blood from one cell type bathes the other cell types. Small arteries enter the core of the islet, distributing blood through a network of fenestrated capillaries and then converging into venules that carry the blood to the rim of the islet. Thus, venous blood from the β cells carries insulin to the α and δ cells. (3) The islets are innervated by adrenergic, cholinergic, and peptidergic neurons. The δ cells even have a "neuronal" appearance and send dendrite-like processes onto the β cells, suggesting intraislet neural communication.

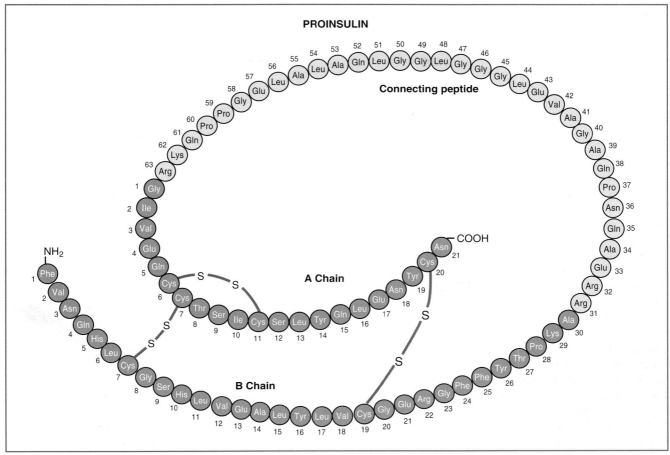

Figure 9-28 **Structure of porcine proinsulin.** The connecting peptide (C peptide) is cleaved to form insulin. (Modified from Shaw WN, Chance RR: Effect of porcine proinsulin in vitro on adipose tissue and diaphragm of the normal rat. Diabetes 17:737, 1968.)

Insulin

Insulin, which is synthesized and secreted by the β **cells,** boasts an impressive array of "firsts." It was the *first* hormone to be isolated from animal sources in a form that could be administered therapeutically to humans; the *first* hormone to have its primary and tertiary structure determined; the *first* hormone to have its mechanism of action elucidated; the *first* hormone to be measured by radioimmunoassay; the *first* hormone known to be synthesized from a larger precursor (prohormone); and the *first* hormone to be synthesized with recombinant DNA technology.

Structure and Synthesis of Insulin

Insulin is a peptide hormone consisting of two straight chains, an **A chain** (21 amino acids) and a **B chain** (30 amino acids). Two disulfide bridges link the A chain to the B chain, and a third disulfide bridge is located within the A chain.

The synthesis of insulin is directed by a gene on **chromosome 11,** a member of a superfamily of genes that encode related growth factors. The mRNA directs ribosomal synthesis of **preproinsulin,** which contains four peptides: a signal peptide, the A and B chains of insulin, and a connecting peptide (C peptide). The signal peptide is cleaved early in the biosynthetic process (while the peptide chains are still being assembled), yielding **proinsulin** (Fig. 9-28). Proinsulin is then shuttled to the endoplasmic reticulum, where, with the connecting peptide still attached, disulfide bridges form to yield a "folded" form of insulin. Proinsulin is packaged in secretory granules on the Golgi apparatus. During this packaging process, proteases cleave the connecting peptide, yielding **insulin.**

Insulin and the cleaved connecting peptide are packaged together in secretory granules, and when the β cell is stimulated, they are released in equimolar quantities into the blood. The secretion of **connecting peptide (C peptide)** is the basis of a test for β-cell function in persons with type I diabetes mellitus who are receiving injections of exogenous insulin. (In these persons, serum insulin levels do not reflect endogenous secretory rates.)

Insulin is metabolized in the liver and kidney by enzymes that break disulfide bonds. The A chains and B chains are released, now inactive, and are excreted in the urine.

Table 9-13 Factors Affecting Insulin Secretion

Stimulatory Factors	Inhibitory Factors
Increased glucose concentration	Decreased blood glucose
Increased amino acid concentration	Fasting
Increased fatty acid and ketoacid concentration	Exercise
	Somatostatin
	α-Adrenergic agonists
	Diazoxide
Glucagon	
Cortisol	
Glucose-dependent insulinotropic peptide (GIP)	
Potassium	
Vagal stimulation; acetylcholine	
Sulfonylurea drugs (e.g., tolbutamide, glyburide)	
Obesity	

Regulation of Insulin Secretion

Table 9-13 summarizes the factors that influence the secretion of insulin by β cells. Of these factors, the most important is **glucose.** Increases in blood glucose concentration rapidly stimulate the secretion of insulin. Because of the preeminence of glucose as a stimulant, it is used to describe the mechanism of insulin secretion by the β cell, as illustrated in Figure 9-29. The circled numbers in the figure correlate with the steps described as follows:

1. **Transport of glucose into the β cell.** The β-cell membrane contains **GLUT 2,** a specific transporter for glucose that moves glucose from the blood into the cell by facilitated diffusion (Step 1).

2. **Metabolism of glucose inside the β cell.** Once inside the cell, glucose is phosphorylated to glucose-6-phosphate by glucokinase (Step 2), and glucose-6-phosphate is subsequently oxidized (Step 3). ATP, one of the products of this oxidation step, appears to be the key factor that regulates insulin secretion.

3. **ATP closes ATP-sensitive K⁺ channels.** K⁺ channels in the β-cell membrane are regulated (i.e., opened or closed) by changes in ATP levels. When ATP levels inside the β cell increase, the K⁺ channels close (Step 4), which depolarizes the β-cell membrane (Step 5). (Refer to Chapter 1 for the complete discussion of why closing the K⁺ channels depolarizes the cell. Briefly, when the K⁺ channels close, K⁺ conductance decreases and the membrane potential moves away from the K⁺ equilibrium potential and is depolarized.)

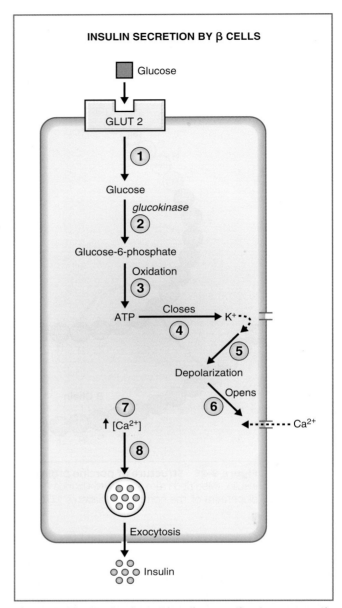

Figure 9-29 **Mechanism of insulin secretion by pancreatic β cells stimulated by glucose.** See the text for an explanation of the circled numbers. ATP, Adenosine triphosphate; GLUT 2, glucose transporter.

4. **Depolarization opens voltage-sensitive Ca²⁺ channels.** Ca²⁺ channels, also in the β-cell membrane, are regulated by changes in voltage; they are opened by depolarization and closed by hyperpolarization. The depolarization caused by ATP opens these Ca²⁺ channels (Step 6). Ca²⁺ flows into the β cell down its electrochemical gradient and the intracellular Ca²⁺ concentration increases (Step 7).

5. **Increased intracellular Ca²⁺ causes insulin secretion.** Increases in intracellular Ca²⁺ concentration cause exocytosis of the insulin-containing secretory granules (Step 8). Insulin is secreted into pancreatic

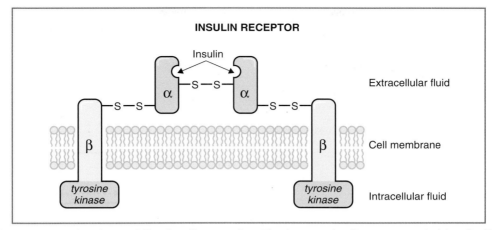

Figure 9–30 **Structure of the insulin receptor.** The two α subunits are connected by disulfide bonds; each α subunit is connected to a β subunit by a disulfide bond. The β subunits have intrinsic tyrosine kinase activity.

venous blood and then delivered to the systemic circulation. C peptide is secreted in equimolar amounts with insulin and is excreted unchanged in the urine. Therefore, the excretion rate of C peptide can be used to assess and monitor endogenous β-cell function.

Recall from Chapter 8 that oral glucose is a more powerful stimulant for insulin secretion than intravenous glucose. The reason for this difference is that oral glucose stimulates the secretion of **glucose-dependent insulinotropic peptide** (**GIP),** a gastrointestinal hormone that has an independent stimulatory effect on insulin secretion (adding to the direct effect of glucose on the β cells). Intravenous glucose does not cause the release of GIP and thus only acts directly.

Many of the other factors that affect insulin secretion do so by altering one or more steps in this basic mechanism. For example, the stimulatory effects of amino acids and fatty acids on insulin secretion utilize metabolic pathways parallel to those utilized by glucose. **Glucagon** activates a G_q protein coupled to phospholipase C, which leads to a rise in intracellular Ca^{2+} (i.e., IP_3/Ca^{2+}), causing exocytosis of insulin. **Somatostatin** inhibits the mechanism that glucagon stimulates. The **sulfonylurea drugs** (e.g., tolbutamide, glyburide) that are used to treat type II (non–insulin-dependent) diabetes mellitus stimulate insulin release from β cells by closing the ATP-dependent K^+ channels, depolarizing the cell, and mimicking the depolarization induced by glucose.

Mechanism of Action of Insulin

The action of insulin on target cells begins when the hormone binds to its receptor in the cell membrane. The **insulin receptor** is a tetramer composed of **two α subunits** and **two β subunits** (Fig. 9-30). The α subunits lie in the extracellular domain, and the β subunits span the cell membrane. A disulfide bond connects the two α subunits, and each α subunit is connected to a β subunit by a disulfide bond. The β subunits have **intrinsic tyrosine kinase activity.**

Insulin acts on its target cells, as described in the following steps:

1. **Insulin binds to the α subunits** of the tetrameric insulin receptor, producing a conformational change in the receptor. The conformational change activates tyrosine kinase in the β subunits, which phosphorylate themselves in the presence of ATP. In other words, the β subunits **autophosphorylate.**

2. Activated **tyrosine kinase** phosphorylates several other proteins or enzymes that are involved in the physiologic actions of insulin including protein kinases, phosphatases, phospholipases, and G proteins. Phosphorylation either activates or inhibits these proteins to produce the various metabolic actions of insulin.

3. The **insulin-receptor complex is internalized** (i.e., taken in) by its target cell by endocytosis. The insulin receptor is either degraded by intracellular proteases, stored, or recycled to the cell membrane to be used again. Insulin **down-regulates** its own receptor by decreasing the rate of synthesis and increasing the rate of degradation of the receptor. Down-regulation of the insulin receptor is in part responsible for the decreased insulin sensitivity of target tissues in obesity and type II diabetes mellitus.

In addition to the previously described actions, insulin also binds to elements in the nucleus, the Golgi apparatus, and the endoplasmic reticulum. Thus, insulin stimulates **gene transcription,** similar to the actions of somatomedins, IGF-1 and IGF-2.

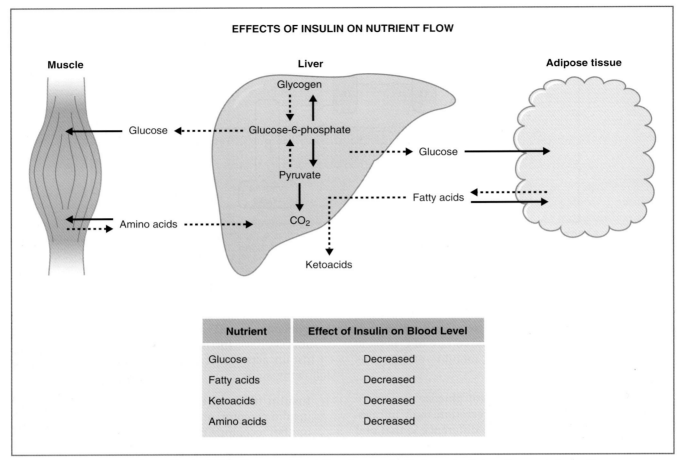

Figure 9–31 **Effects of insulin on nutrient flow in muscle, liver, and adipose tissue and result-ing effects on blood levels of nutrients.** *Solid arrows* indicate that the step is stimulated; *dashed arrows* indicate that the step is inhibited.

Actions of Insulin

Insulin is known as the hormone of **"abundance"** or plenty. When the availability of nutrients exceeds the demands of the body, insulin ensures that excess nutri-ents are stored as glycogen in the liver, as fat in adipose tissue, and as protein in muscle. These stored nutrients are then available during subsequent periods of fasting to maintain glucose delivery to the brain, muscle, and other organs. The effects of insulin on nutrient flow and the resulting changes in blood levels are summa-rized in Table 9-14 and shown in Figure 9-31. Insulin has the following actions on liver, muscle, and adipose tissue:

♦ **Decreases blood glucose concentration.** The hypo-glycemic action of insulin can be described in two ways: Insulin causes a frank decrease in blood glucose concentration, *and* insulin limits the rise in blood glucose that occurs after ingestion of carbo-hydrates. The hypoglycemic action of insulin is the result of coordinated responses that simultaneously stimulate glucose oxidation and inhibit gluconeo-genesis as follows: (1) Insulin **increases glucose**

Table 9–14 Major Actions of Insulin and the Effect on Blood Levels

Action of Insulin	Effect on Blood Level
Increases glucose uptake into cells	Decreases blood [glucose]
Increases glycogen formation	
Decreases glycogenolysis	
Decreases gluconeogenesis	
Increases protein synthesis (anabolic)	Decreases blood [amino acid]
Increases fat deposition	Decreases blood [fatty acid]
Decreases lipolysis	Decreases blood [ketoacid]
Increases K⁺ uptake into cells	Decreases blood [K⁺]

transport into target cells such as muscle and adipose by directing the insertion of glucose trans-porters **(GLUT 4)** into the cell membranes. As glucose enters the cells, the blood glucose con-centration decreases. (2) Insulin **promotes the**

formation of glycogen from glucose in the liver and in muscle and, simultaneously, inhibits glycogenolysis (glycogen breakdown). (3) Insulin **inhibits gluconeogenesis** (synthesis of glucose) by increasing the production of fructose 2,6-bisphosphate, which increases phosphofructokinase activity. In effect, substrates are directed *away from* the formation of glucose.

♦ **Decreases blood fatty acid and ketoacid concentrations.** The overall effect of insulin on fat metabolism is to inhibit the mobilization and oxidation of fatty acids and, simultaneously, to increase the storage of fatty acids. As a result, insulin decreases the circulating levels of fatty acids and ketoacids. In adipose tissue, insulin **stimulates fat deposition** and **inhibits lipolysis.** Simultaneously, insulin inhibits ketoacid (β-hydroxybutyric acid and aceto-acetic acid) formation in liver because decreased fatty acid degradation means that less acetyl coenzyme A (acetyl CoA) substrate will be available for the formation of ketoacids.

♦ **Decreases blood amino acid concentration.** The overall effect of insulin on protein metabolism is **anabolic.** Insulin increases amino acid and protein uptake by tissues, thereby decreasing blood levels of amino acids. Insulin stimulates amino acid uptake into target cells (e.g., muscle), increases protein synthesis, and inhibits protein degradation.

♦ **Other actions.** In addition to major actions on carbohydrate, fat, and protein metabolism, insulin has several additional effects. Insulin promotes **K^+ uptake into cells** (at the same time that it promotes glucose uptake) by increasing the activity of the Na^+-K^+ ATPase. This action of insulin can be viewed as "protecting" against an increase in serum K^+ concentration. When K^+ is ingested in the diet, insulin ensures that ingested K^+ will be taken into the cells with glucose and other nutrients. Insulin also appears to have a direct effect on the **hypothalamic satiety center** independent of the changes it produces in blood glucose concentration.

Pathophysiology of Insulin

The major disorder involving insulin is diabetes mellitus. In one form of diabetes mellitus (type I), there is inadequate insulin secretion; in another form (type II), there is insulin-resistance of target tissues.

♦ **Insulin-dependent diabetes mellitus,** or type I diabetes mellitus, is caused by destruction of β cells, often as a result of an autoimmune process. When pancreatic β cells do not secrete adequate amounts of insulin, there are serious metabolic consequences: Carbohydrate, fat, and protein metabolism all will be disturbed.

Type I diabetes mellitus is characterized by the following changes: **increased blood glucose concentration** from decreased uptake of glucose into cells, decreased glucose utilization, and increased gluconeogenesis; **increased blood fatty acid and ketoacid concentration** from increased lipolysis of fat, increased conversion of fatty acids to ketoacids, and decreased utilization of ketoacids by tissues; and **increased blood amino acid concentration** from increased breakdown of protein to amino acids. There also is loss of lean body mass (i.e., a catabolic state) and loss of adipose tissue.

Disturbances of fluid and electrolyte balance are present in type I diabetes mellitus. The increased levels of ketoacids cause a form of metabolic acidosis called **diabetic ketoacidosis (DKA).** The increased blood glucose concentration results in an increased filtered load of glucose, which exceeds the reabsorptive capacity of the proximal tubule. The nonreabsorbed glucose then acts as an osmotic solute in urine, producing an **osmotic diuresis,** polyuria, and thirst. The polyuria produces ECF volume contraction and hypotension. Lack of insulin also causes a shift of K^+ out of cells (recall that insulin promotes K^+ uptake), resulting in **hyperkalemia.**

Treatment of type I diabetes mellitus consists of insulin replacement therapy, which restores the ability of the body to store carbohydrates, lipids, and proteins and returns the blood values of nutrients and electrolytes to normal.

♦ **Non–insulin-dependent diabetes mellitus,** or type II diabetes mellitus, is often associated with obesity. It exhibits some, but not all, of the metabolic derangements seen in type I diabetes mellitus. Type II diabetes mellitus is caused by down-regulation of insulin receptors in target tissues and **insulin resistance.** Insulin is secreted normally by the β cells, but at normal concentrations, it cannot activate its receptors on muscle, liver, and adipose tissue; thus, insulin is unable to produce its usual metabolic effects. Typically, the blood glucose concentration is elevated in both fasting and postprandial (after eating) states. Treatment of type II diabetes mellitus includes caloric restriction and weight reduction; treatment with **sulfonylurea drugs** (e.g., tolbutamide or glyburide), which stimulate pancreatic insulin secretion; and treatment with biguanide drugs (e.g., **metformin**), which up-regulate insulin receptors on target tissues.

Glucagon

Glucagon is synthesized and secreted by the **α cells** of the islets of Langerhans. In most respects (i.e., regulation of secretion, actions, and effect on blood levels), glucagon is the "mirror image" of insulin. Thus, while insulin is the hormone of "abundance," glucagon is the

Table 9–15 Factors Affecting Glucagon Secretion

Stimulatory Factors	Inhibitory Factors
Fasting	Insulin
Decreased glucose concentration	Somatostatin
	Increased fatty acid and ketoacid concentration
Increased amino acid concentration (especially arginine)	
Cholecystokinin (CCK)	
β-Adrenergic agonists	
Acetylcholine	

hormone of "starvation." In contrast to insulin, which promotes storage of metabolic fuels, glucagon promotes their mobilization and utilization.

Structure and Synthesis of Glucagon

Glucagon is a single straight-chain polypeptide with 29 amino acids. It is a member of a family of peptides that includes the gastrointestinal hormones secretin and gastric inhibitory peptide (GIP). All of the peptides in the family share structural features and overlap in their physiologic actions (see Chapter 8, Fig. 8-6).

As with other peptide hormones, glucagon is synthesized as preproglucagon. The signal peptide and other peptide sequences are removed to produce glucagon, which then is stored in dense granules until it is secreted by the α cells. Both glucose and insulin inhibit the synthesis of glucagon; insulin-sensitive and cAMP-sensitive elements are present on the gene for preproglucagon.

Regulation of Glucagon Secretion

The actions of glucagon are coordinated to increase and maintain the blood glucose concentration. Thus, the factors that cause stimulation of glucagon secretion are those that inform the α cells that a decrease in blood glucose has occurred (Table 9-15).

The major factor stimulating the secretion of glucagon is **decreased blood glucose concentration.** Coordinating with this stimulatory effect of low blood glucose is a separate inhibitory action of insulin. Thus, the presence of insulin reduces or *modulates* the effect of low blood glucose concentration to stimulate glucagon secretion. In the absence of insulin (i.e., type I diabetes mellitus), however, the glucagon response to hypoglycemia is exaggerated and may lead to severe, perpetuated hyperglycemia.

Glucagon secretion also is stimulated by the ingestion of protein, specifically by the amino acids **arginine** and **alanine.** The response of the α cells to amino acids is blunted if glucose is administered simultaneously (partially mediated by the inhibitory effect of insulin on glucagon secretion). Thus, glucose and amino acids have offsetting or opposite effects on glucagon secretion (in contrast to their effects on insulin secretion, which are complementary).

Other factors stimulating glucagon secretion are **cholecystokinin** (CCK), which is secreted from the gastrointestinal tract when protein or fat is ingested, and **fasting** and **intense exercise.** Some of the stimulatory effects on glucagon secretion are mediated by activation of sympathetic α-adrenergic receptors.

Actions of Glucagon

The **mechanism of action** of glucagon on its target cells begins with hormone binding to a cell membrane receptor, which is coupled to **adenylyl cyclase** via a G_s protein. The second messenger is **cAMP,** which activates protein kinases that phosphorylate various enzymes; the phosphorylated enzymes then mediate the physiologic actions of glucagon.

As the hormone of starvation, glucagon promotes mobilization and utilization of stored nutrients to maintain the blood glucose concentration in the fasting state. The major actions of glucagon are on the liver (in contrast to insulin, which acts on liver, adipose, and muscle tissue). The effects of glucagon on the flow of nutrients are illustrated in Figure 9-32. Glucagon has the following effects on blood levels, which are summarized in Table 9-16 and described as follows:

♦ **Increases blood glucose concentration.** Glucagon increases the blood glucose concentration by the following coordinated actions: (1) Glucagon stimulates glycogenolysis and simultaneously inhibits glycogen formation from glucose, and (2) Glucagon increases gluconeogenesis by decreasing the production of fructose 2,6-bisphosphate, which decreases phosphofructokinase activity. Thus, substrate is directed *toward* the formation of glucose. Amino acids are utilized for gluconeogenesis, and the resulting amino groups are incorporated into urea.

♦ **Increases blood fatty acid and ketoacid concentration.** Glucagon increases lipolysis and inhibits fatty acid synthesis, which also shunts substrates toward gluconeogenesis. The ketoacids β-hydroxybutyric acid and acetoacetic acid are produced from fatty acids.

Somatostatin

Pancreatic somatostatin, a polypeptide with 14 amino acids, is secreted by the **δ cells** of the islets of Langerhans. (The gastrointestinal counterpart of somatostatin has 28 amino acids and shares many of the physiologic actions of the pancreatic hormone.) Secretion of somatostatin is stimulated by the ingestion of *all* forms of

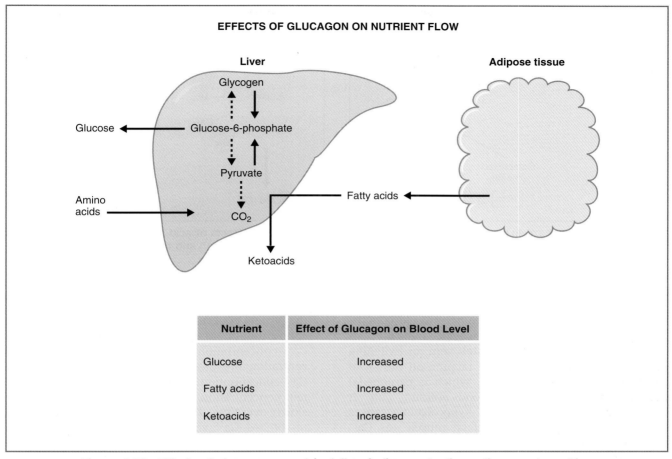

EFFECTS OF GLUCAGON ON NUTRIENT FLOW

Nutrient	Effect of Glucagon on Blood Level
Glucose	Increased
Fatty acids	Increased
Ketoacids	Increased

Figure 9–32 **Effects of glucagon on nutrient flow in liver and adipose tissue and resulting effects on blood levels of nutrients.** *Solid arrows* indicate that the step is stimulated; *dashed arrows* indicate that the step is inhibited.

Table 9–16 Major Actions of Glucagon and Effect on Blood Levels

Action of Glucagon	Effect on Blood Level
Increases glycogenolysis	Increases blood [glucose]
Increases gluconeogenesis	
Increases lipolysis	Increases blood [fatty acid]
Increases ketoacid formation	Increases blood [ketoacid]

nutrients (i.e., glucose, amino acids, and fatty acids), by several gastrointestinal hormones, by glucagon, and by β-adrenergic agonists. Secretion of somatostatin is inhibited by insulin via an intraislet paracrine mechanism.

Pancreatic somatostatin **inhibits secretion of insulin and glucagon** via paracrine actions on the α and β cells. Thus, somatostatin is secreted by the δ cells in response to a meal, diffuses to the nearby α and β cells, and inhibits secretion of their respective hormones. Apparently, the function of somatostatin is to modulate or limit the responses of insulin and glucagon to ingestion of food.

REGULATION OF CALCIUM AND PHOSPHATE METABOLISM

Forms of Ca^{2+} in Blood

The total Ca^{2+} concentration in blood is normally 10 mg/dL (Fig. 9-33). Of the total Ca^{2+}, 40% is bound to plasma proteins, mainly albumin. The remaining 60%, which is not protein-bound, is ultrafilterable. The ultrafilterable component includes a small portion that is complexed to anions (e.g., phosphate, sulfate, citrate) and free, ionized Ca^{2+}. Free, **ionized Ca^{2+}** amounts to 50% of the total (i.e., 5 mg/dL), and it is the *only form of Ca^{2+} that is biologically active.*

Hypocalcemia is a decrease in the plasma Ca^{2+} concentration. The symptoms of hypocalcemia are

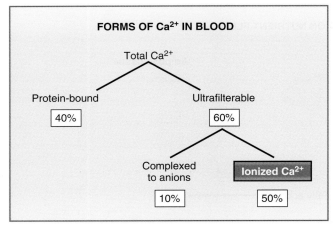

Figure 9-33 **Forms of Ca²⁺ in blood.** Percentages give percent of total Ca²⁺ concentration in each form. Only free, ionized Ca²⁺ is physiologically active.

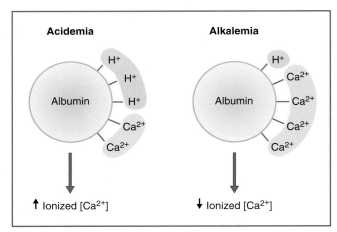

Figure 9-34 **Effects of acid-base disturbances on plasma protein-binding of Ca²⁺ and the ionized Ca²⁺ concentration in blood.**

hyperreflexia, spontaneous twitching, muscle cramps, and tingling and numbness. Specific indicators of hypocalcemia include the **Chvostek sign,** or twitching of the facial muscles elicited by tapping on the facial nerve, and the **Trousseau sign,** which is carpopedal spasm upon inflation of a blood pressure cuff. It may be surprising to learn that hypocalcemia causes twitching and cramping of skeletal muscle (as Ca²⁺ is required for cross-bridge cycling in muscle contraction). However, the Ca²⁺ that initiates the cross-bridge cycle in skeletal muscle contraction is *intracellular* Ca²⁺. This discussion of the effects of hypocalcemia refers to low *extracellular* Ca²⁺. Decreased extracellular Ca²⁺ causes increased excitability of excitable cells including sensory and motor nerves and muscle. Decreased extracellular Ca²⁺ lowers (makes more negative) the threshold potential; by lowering threshold potential, less inward current is required to depolarize to threshold and to fire action potentials. Thus, hypocalcemia produces tingling and numbness (effects on sensory nerves) and spontaneous muscle twitches (effects on motoneurons and the muscle itself).

Hypercalcemia is an increase in the plasma Ca²⁺ concentration. Manifestations of hypercalcemia include constipation, polyuria, polydipsia, and neurologic signs of hyporeflexia, lethargy, coma, and death.

Changes in plasma protein concentration, changes in complexing anion concentration, and acid-base disturbances may alter the forms of Ca²⁺ in plasma. Such changes will be physiologically significant, however, only if they alter the ionized Ca²⁺ concentration because that is the form with biologic activity.

♦ **Changes in plasma protein concentration** alter the *total* Ca²⁺ concentration in the same direction as the protein concentration; thus, increases in protein concentration are associated with increases in total Ca²⁺ concentration, and decreases in protein concentration are associated with decreases in total Ca²⁺ concentration. Because changes in plasma protein concentration usually are chronic and develop slowly over time, they do not cause a parallel change in *ionized* Ca²⁺ concentration. Regulatory mechanisms such as those involving parathyroid hormone (see later) sense any transient change in ionized Ca²⁺ concentration and have time to make the appropriate correction.

♦ **Changes in anion concentration** alter the ionized Ca²⁺ concentration by changing the fraction of Ca²⁺ complexed with anions. For example, if the plasma phosphate concentration increases, the fraction of Ca²⁺ that is complexed increases, thereby decreasing the ionized Ca²⁺ concentration. If the plasma phosphate concentration decreases, the complexed Ca²⁺ decreases and the ionized Ca²⁺ increases.

♦ **Acid-base abnormalities** alter the ionized Ca²⁺ concentration by changing the fraction of Ca²⁺ bound to plasma albumin, as illustrated in Figure 9-34. Albumin has negatively charged sites, which can bind either H⁺ ions or Ca²⁺ ions. In **acidemia,** there is an excess of H⁺ in blood; thus, more H⁺ binds to albumin, leaving fewer sites for Ca²⁺ to bind. In acidemia, the free ionized Ca²⁺ concentration increases because less Ca²⁺ is bound to albumin. In **alkalemia,** there is a deficit of H⁺ in blood, and less H⁺ will be bound to albumin, leaving more sites for Ca²⁺ to bind. Thus, in alkalemia (e.g., **acute respiratory alkalosis**) the free, ionized Ca²⁺ concentration decreases, often accompanied by symptoms of hypocalcemia.

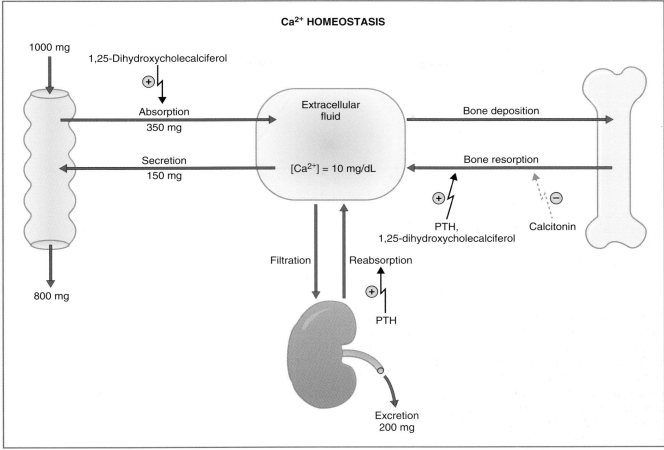

Ca²⁺ HOMEOSTASIS

Figure 9-35 **Ca²⁺ homeostasis in an adult eating 1000 mg/day of elemental Ca²⁺.** Hormonal effects on Ca²⁺ absorption from the gastrointestinal tract, bone remodeling, and Ca²⁺ reabsorption in the kidney are shown. PTH, Parathyroid hormone.

Overall Calcium Homeostasis

Ca²⁺ homeostasis involves the coordinated interaction of three organ systems (bone, kidney, and intestine) and three hormones (parathyroid hormone, calcitonin, and vitamin D). The relationship between the organ systems and the hormones in maintaining Ca²⁺ balance is depicted in Figure 9-35.

To illustrate, the "person" shown in Figure 9-35 is said to be in Ca²⁺ balance. In this person, net excretion of Ca²⁺ by the kidney is equal to net absorption of Ca²⁺ from the gastrointestinal tract.

If the person ingests 1000 mg of elemental Ca²⁺ daily, approximately 350 mg is absorbed from the gastrointestinal tract, a process that is stimulated by the active form of vitamin D, 1,25-dihydroxycholecalciferol. However, about 150 mg/day is secreted into the gastrointestinal tract in salivary, pancreatic, and intestinal fluids. Thus, *net absorption of Ca²⁺* is 200 mg/day (350 mg-150 mg), and the remaining 800 mg/day (of the 1000 mg ingested) is excreted in feces. The absorbed Ca²⁺ enters the Ca²⁺ pool in ECF.

The person depicted in Figure 9-35 is presumed to have no net gain or loss of Ca²⁺ from bone. Nevertheless, there is continuous **bone remodeling,** in which new bone is formed (deposited) and old bone is resorbed. Bone resorption is stimulated by parathyroid hormone and 1,25-dihydroxycholecalciferol and is inhibited by calcitonin.

Ultimately, to maintain Ca²⁺ balance, the kidneys must excrete the same amount of Ca²⁺ that is absorbed from the gastrointestinal tract, or, in this case, 200 mg/day. The renal mechanisms (which are discussed in Chapter 6) include filtration of Ca²⁺, followed by extensive reabsorption.

Parathyroid Hormone

The role of parathyroid hormone (PTH) is to regulate the concentration of Ca²⁺ in ECF (i.e., plasma or serum). When the plasma Ca²⁺ concentration decreases, PTH is secreted by the parathyroid glands. In turn, PTH has physiologic actions on bone, kidney, and intestine that

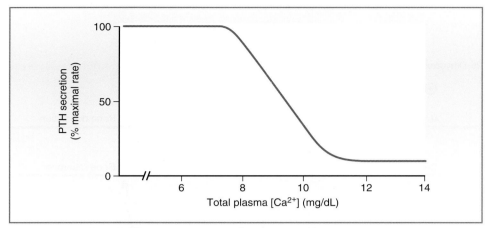

Figure 9–36 **Relationship between plasma Ca²⁺ concentration and parathyroid hormone (PTH) secretion.**

are coordinated to increase the plasma Ca^{2+} concentration back to normal.

Structure of Parathyroid Hormone

There are four parathyroid glands in humans, located in the neck under the thyroid gland. The **chief cells** of the parathyroid glands synthesize and secrete PTH, a single-chain polypeptide with 84 amino acids. The molecule's biologic activity resides entirely in the N-terminal 34 amino acids. PTH is synthesized on the ribosomes as **preproPTH,** which has 115 amino acids. A 25-amino acid signal peptide sequence is cleaved while synthesis of the molecule is being completed on the ribosomes. The 90-amino acid **proPTH** then is transported to the Golgi apparatus, where 6 more amino acids are cleaved, yielding the final 84-amino acid form of the hormone. PTH is packaged in secretory granules for subsequent release.

Regulation of Parathyroid Hormone Secretion

PTH secretion is regulated by the **plasma Ca²⁺ concentration.** As shown in Figure 9-36, when the total Ca^{2+} concentration is in the normal range (i.e., 10 mg/dL) or higher, PTH is secreted at a low (basal) level. However, when the plasma Ca^{2+} concentration decreases to less than 10 mg/dL, PTH secretion is stimulated, reaching maximal rates when the Ca^{2+} concentration is 7.5 mg/dL. The relationship between *total* Ca^{2+} concentration and PTH secretion is shown in Figure 9-36, although it is actually the *ionized* Ca^{2+} concentration that regulates secretion by the parathyroid glands. The response of the parathyroid glands to a decrease in ionized Ca^{2+} concentration is remarkably prompt, occurring within seconds. Furthermore, the faster the ionized Ca^{2+} falls, the greater the PTH secretory response.

It may seem paradoxical that the chief cells would secrete PTH in response to a *decrease* in Ca^{2+} concentration because many endocrine glands secrete their hormones in response to an *increase* in intracellular Ca^{2+} concentration. Actually, this is no paradox because what is sensed by the chief cells is a decrease in *extracellular* Ca^{2+} concentration, not a decrease in *intracellular* Ca^{2+}. The mechanism of PTH secretion is explained as follows: The parathyroid cell membrane contains **Ca²⁺ sensing receptors** that are linked, via a G protein (G_q), to phospholipase C. When the extracellular Ca^{2+} concentration is increased, Ca^{2+} binds to the receptor and activates phospholipase C. Activation of phospholipase C leads to increased levels of IP_3/Ca^{2+}, which *inhibits* PTH secretion. When extracellular Ca^{2+} is decreased, there is decreased Ca^{2+} binding to the receptor, which *stimulates* PTH secretion.

In addition to these acute (rapid) changes in PTH secretion, chronic (long-term) changes in plasma Ca^{2+} concentration alter transcription of the gene for prepro-PTH, synthesis and storage of PTH, and growth of the parathyroid glands. Thus, **chronic hypocalcemia** (decreased plasma Ca^{2+} concentration) causes **secondary hyperparathyroidism,** which is characterized by increased synthesis and storage of PTH and hyperplasia of the parathyroid glands. On the other hand, **chronic hypercalcemia** (increased plasma Ca^{2+} concentration) causes decreased synthesis and storage of PTH, increased breakdown of stored PTH, and release of inactive PTH fragments into the circulation.

Magnesium (**Mg²⁺**) has parallel, although less important, effects on PTH secretion. Thus, like hypocalcemia, hypomagnesemia stimulates PTH secretion and hypermagnesemia inhibits PTH secretion. An exception is the case of severe hypomagnesemia associated with chronic Mg^{2+} depletion (e.g., alcoholism);

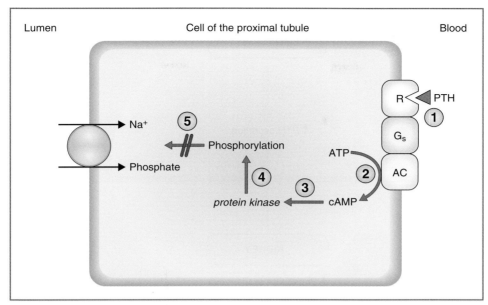

Figure 9–37 **Mechanism of action of PTH on the renal proximal tubule.** See the text for an explanation of the circled numbers. AC, Adenylyl cyclase; ATP, adenosine triphosphate; cAMP, cyclic adenosine monophosphate; G_s, stimulatory G protein; PTH, parathyroid hormone; R, receptor for PTH.

severe hypomagnesemia *inhibits* PTH synthesis, storage, and secretion by the parathyroid glands.

Actions of Parathyroid Hormone

PTH has actions on bone, kidney, and intestine, all of which are coordinated to produce an increase in plasma Ca^{2+} concentration. The actions on bone and kidney are direct and are mediated by cAMP; the action on intestine is indirect, via activation of vitamin D.

The **mechanism of action** of PTH on bone and kidney is initiated when PTH binds to its receptor on the cell membrane of the target tissue. The receptor for PTH is coupled, via a G_s protein, to **adenylyl cyclase,** as illustrated for one of its actions, inhibition of renal phosphate reabsorption, in Figure 9-37. The circled numbers in the figure correlate with the steps described as follows: The action of PTH on the renal proximal tubule begins at the basolateral membrane, where the hormone binds to its receptor. The receptor is coupled, via a G_s protein, to adenylyl cyclase (Step 1). When activated, adenylyl cyclase catalyzes the conversion of ATP to cAMP (Step 2), which activates a series of protein kinases (Step 3). Activated protein kinases phosphorylate intracellular proteins (Step 4), leading to the final physiologic action at the luminal membrane, inhibition of Na^+-phosphate cotransport (Step 5). Inhibition of Na^+-phosphate cotransport results in decreased phosphate reabsorption and phosphaturia (increased phosphate excretion).

The actions of PTH on bone, kidney, and intestine are summarized in Figure 9-38 and are described as follows:

♦ **Bone.** PTH has several actions on bone, some direct and some indirect. In bone, **PTH receptors** are located on **osteoblasts** but not on osteoclasts. Initially and transiently, PTH causes an increase in **bone formation** by a direct action on osteoblasts. (This brief action is the basis for the usefulness of intermittent synthetic PTH administration in the **treatment of osteoporosis.**) In a second, long-lasting action on osteoclasts, PTH causes an increase in **bone resorption.** This second action on osteoclasts is indirect and mediated by cytokines released from osteoblasts; these cytokines then increase the number and activity of the bone-resorbing osteoclasts. Thus, the bone-forming cells, osteoblasts, are required for the bone-resorbing action of PTH on osteoclasts. When PTH levels are chronically elevated, as in hyperparathyroidism, the rate of bone resorption is persistently elevated, which increases the serum Ca^{2+} concentration.

The *overall* effect of PTH on bone is to promote bone resorption, delivering *both* Ca^{2+} and phosphate to ECF. Hydroxyproline that is released from bone matrix is excreted in urine.

Alone, the effects of PTH on bone cannot account for its overall action to increase the plasma-ionized Ca^{2+} concentration. The phosphate released from bone will complex with Ca^{2+} in ECF and limit the rise in ionized Ca^{2+} concentration. Thus, an additional mechanism must coordinate with the PTH effect on bone to cause the plasma ionized Ca^{2+} concentration to increase. (That additional mechanism is the phosphaturic action of PTH.)

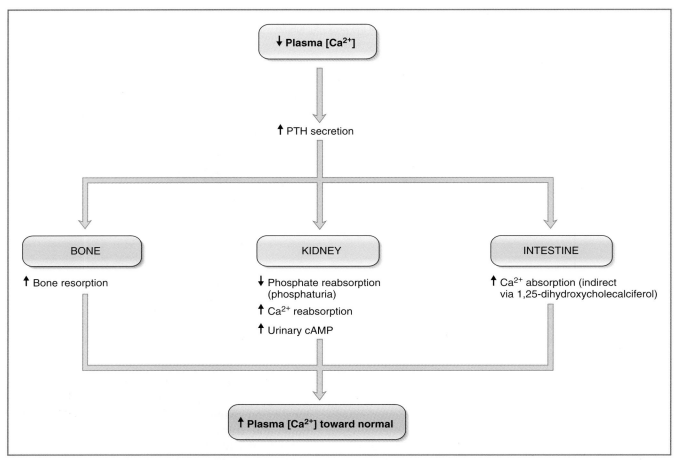

Figure 9–38 **Regulation of PTH secretion and PTH actions on bone, kidney, and intestine.** cAMP, Cyclic adenosine monophosphate; PTH, parathyroid hormone.

◆ **Kidney.** PTH has two actions on the kidney. (1) PTH **inhibits phosphate reabsorption** by inhibiting Na^+-phosphate cotransport in the proximal convoluted tubule. As a result of this action, PTH causes **phosphaturia,** an increased excretion of phosphate in urine. The cAMP generated in cells of the proximal tubule is excreted in urine and is called nephrogenous or **urinary cAMP.** The phosphaturic action of PTH is critical because the phosphate that was resorbed from bone is excreted in the urine; this phosphate would have otherwise complexed Ca^{2+} in ECF. Excreting phosphate in urine "allows" the plasma ionized Ca^{2+} concentration to increase! (2) PTH **stimulates Ca^{2+} reabsorption.** This second renal action of PTH is on the distal convoluted tubule and complements the increase in plasma Ca^{2+} concentration that resulted from the combination of bone resorption and phosphaturia.

◆ **Small intestine.** PTH does not have direct actions on the small intestine, although indirectly it stimulates intestinal Ca^{2+} absorption via activation of vitamin D. PTH stimulates renal 1α-hydroxylase, the enzyme that converts 25-hydroxycholecalciferol to the active form, 1,25-dihydroxycholecalciferol. In turn, 1,25-dihydroxycholecalciferol stimulates intestinal Ca^{2+} absorption.

Pathophysiology of Parathyroid Hormone

The pathophysiology of the PTH system can involve an excess of PTH, a deficiency of PTH, or target tissue resistance to PTH. Disorders associated with PTH are summarized in Table 9-17.

◆ **Primary hyperparathyroidism.** Primary hyperparathyroidism is most commonly caused by parathyroid adenomas (tumors), which secrete excessive amounts of PTH (Box 9-3). The consequences of primary hyperparathyroidism are predictable from the known physiologic actions of PTH on bone, kidney, and intestine: increased circulating levels of PTH, hypercalcemia, and hypophosphatemia. **Hypercalcemia** results from increased bone resorption, increased renal Ca^{2+} reabsorption, and increased intestinal Ca^{2+} absorption. **Hypophosphatemia** results

Table 9–17 Pathophysiology of Parathyroid Hormone

Disorder	PTH	1,25-Dihydroxy-cholecalciferol	Bone	Urine	Serum [Calcium]	Serum [Phosphate]
Primary Hyper-parathyroidism	↑*	↑ (PTH effect on 1α-hydroxylase)	↑ Resorption	↑ Urine phosphate (phosphaturia) ↑ Urine Ca^{2+} (due to high filtered load) ↑ Urine cAMP	↑	↓
Surgical Hypo-parathyroidism	↓*	↓ (PTH effect on 1α-hydroxylase)	↓ Resorption	↓ Urine phosphate ↓ Urine cAMP	↓	↑
Pseudohypo-parathyroidism	↑	↓	↓ Resorption (defective G_s)*	↓ Urine phosphate ↓ Urine cAMP (defective G_s)*	↓	↑
Humoral Hyper-calcemia of Malignancy (↑ PTH-rp*)	↓	↑	↑ Resorption	↑ Urine phosphate (phosphaturia) ↑ Urine Ca^{2+} (due to high filtered load) ↑ Urine cAMP	↑	↓
Chronic Renal Failure	↑ (secondary)	↓*	Osteomalacia (due to ↓ 1,25-dihydroxy-cholecalciferol) ↑ Resorption (due to ↑ PTH)	↓ Urine phosphate (due to ↓ GFR)*	↓ (due to ↓ 1,25-dihydroxy-cholecalciferol)	↑ (due to ↓ urine phosphate)

*Primary events or disturbances.

BOX 9–3 Clinical Physiology: Primary Hyperparathyroidism

DESCRIPTION OF CASE. A 52-year-old woman reports that she suffers from symptoms of generalized weakness, easy fatigability, loss of appetite, and occasional vomiting. Also, she reports that her urine output is higher than normal and that she is unusually thirsty. Laboratory tests show hypercalcemia (increased serum [Ca^{2+}]), hypophosphatemia (decreased serum phosphate concentration), and phosphaturia (increased urinary phosphate excretion). Suspecting that the woman may have a disorder of the parathyroid glands, her physician orders a PTH level, which is found to be significantly elevated.

The woman undergoes surgery, and a single parathyroid adenoma is located and removed. The woman's blood and urine values return to normal. She regains her strength and reports feeling well.

EXPLANATION OF CASE. The woman has primary hyperparathyroidism caused by a single parathyroid adenoma, a benign lesion. The tumor secretes large

amounts of PTH chemically identical to the hormone secreted by the normal parathyroid glands. This excess PTH acts directly on bone and kidney and indirectly on the intestine to cause hypercalcemia and hypophosphatemia. Her hypercalcemia results from the effects of PTH to increase bone resorption, renal Ca^{2+} reabsorption, and intestinal Ca^{2+} absorption via activation of vitamin D to 1,25-dihydroxycholecalciferol. Her hypophosphatemia is caused by the effect of PTH to decrease renal phosphate reabsorption and produce phosphaturia.

Most of the woman's symptoms including hyporeflexia, weakness, loss of appetite, and vomiting are caused by hypercalcemia. Her polyuria and polydipsia result from deposition of Ca^{2+} in the inner medulla of the kidney, where ADH acts on the collecting ducts. High Ca^{2+} in the inner medulla inhibits the action of ADH on the collecting ducts, causing a form of nephrogenic diabetes insipidus.

TREATMENT. Surgery was curative for this patient.

from decreased renal phosphate reabsorption and phosphaturia.

Persons with primary hyperparathyroidism excrete excessive amounts of phosphate, cAMP, and Ca^{2+} in their urine. The increased urinary Ca^{2+} (hypercalciuria) can precipitate in the urine as Ca^{2+}-phosphate or Ca^{2+}-oxalate stones. The presence of hypercalciuria may seem surprising because the direct effect of PTH on the renal tubule is to *increase* Ca^{2+} reabsorption, thus decrease Ca^{2+} excretion. The presence of hypercalciuria is explained, however, because the high plasma Ca^{2+} concentration in primary hyperparathyroidism results in a high filtered load of Ca^{2+}, which overwhelms the reabsorptive capacity of the nephron—the Ca^{2+} that is not reabsorbed is spilled into the urine. Persons with primary hyperparathyroidism are said to have **"stones," "bones,"** and **"groans"**—stones from hypercalciuria, bones from increased bone resorption, and groans from constipation. Treatment of primary hyperparathyroidism usually is parathyroidectomy (surgical removal of the parathyroid glands).

♦ **Secondary hyperparathyroidism.** The causes of secondary hyperparathyroidism are different from the causes of primary hyperparathyroidism. In primary hyperparathyroidism, the disorder is *in* the parathyroid gland, which is secreting excessive PTH. In secondary hyperparathyroidism, the parathyroid glands are normal but are stimulated to secrete excessive PTH *secondary* to **hypocalcemia,** which can be caused by vitamin D deficiency or chronic renal failure. In secondary hyperparathyroidism, circulating levels of PTH are elevated and blood levels of Ca^{2+} are low or normal but never high.

♦ **Hypoparathyroidism.** Hypoparathyroidism is a relatively common, inadvertent consequence of thyroid surgery (for treatment of thyroid cancer or Graves disease) or parathyroid surgery (for treatment of hyperparathyroidism). Autoimmune and congenital hypoparathyroidism are less common. The characteristics of hypoparathyroidism are predictable: low circulating levels of PTH, hypocalcemia, and hyperphosphatemia. **Hypocalcemia** results from decreased bone resorption, decreased renal Ca^{2+} reabsorption, and decreased intestinal Ca^{2+} absorption. **Hyperphosphatemia** results from increased phosphate reabsorption. This disorder usually is treated with the combination of an oral Ca^{2+} supplement and the active form of vitamin D, 1,25-dihydroxycholecalciferol.

♦ **Pseudohypoparathyroidism.** Patients with pseudo-hypoparathyroidism type Ia were described in the early 1940s by the endocrinologist Fuller Albright as follows: They had hypocalcemia, hyperphosphatemia, and a characteristic phenotype consisting of short stature, short neck, obesity, subcutaneous calcification, and shortened fourth metatarsals and metacarpals. Thereafter, this phenotype was called **Albright hereditary osteodystrophy.**

As in hypoparathyroidism, patients with pseudohypoparathyroidism have hypocalcemia and hyperphosphatemia. However, in pseudohypoparathyroidism, circulating levels of PTH are increased rather than decreased, and administration of exogenous PTH produces no phosphaturic response and no increase in urinary cAMP. It is now known that pseudohypoparathyroidism is an inherited autosomal dominant disorder in which the **G_s protein** for PTH in kidney and bone is defective. When PTH binds to its receptor in these tissues, it does not activate adenylyl cyclase or produce its usual physiologic actions. As a result, hypocalcemia and hyperphosphatemia develop.

♦ **Humoral hypercalcemia of malignancy.** Some malignant tumors (e.g., lung, breast) secrete PTH-related peptide **(PTH-rp),** which is structurally homologous with the PTH secreted by the parathyroid glands. PTH-rp is not only structurally similar but has all the physiologic actions of PTH including increased bone resorption, inhibition of renal phosphate reabsorption, and increased renal Ca^{2+} reabsorption. Together, the effects of PTH-rp on bone and kidney cause hypercalcemia and hypophosphatemia, a blood profile similar to that seen in primary hyperparathyroidism. However, in humoral hypercalcemia of malignancy, circulating levels of PTH are low, not high (as would occur in primary hyperparathyroidism); PTH secretion by the parathyroid glands, which are normal, is suppressed by the hypercalcemia. Humoral hypercalcemia of malignancy is treated with **furosemide,** which inhibits renal Ca^{2+} reabsorption and increases Ca^{2+} excretion, and inhibitors of bone resorption such as **etidronate.**

♦ **Familial hypocalciuric hypercalcemia (FHH).** This autosomal dominant disorder is characterized by decreased urinary Ca^{2+} excretion and increased serum Ca^{2+} concentration. It is caused by inactivating mutations of the **Ca^{2+} sensing receptors** in the parathyroid glands (that regulate PTH secretion) and parallel Ca^{2+} receptors in the thick, ascending limb of the kidney (that mediate Ca^{2+} reabsorption). When the renal receptors are defective, a high serum Ca^{2+} concentration is incorrectly sensed as "normal" and Ca^{2+} reabsorption is increased (leading to decreased urinary Ca^{2+} [hypocalciuria] and increased serum Ca^{2+} concentration). Because the Ca^{2+} receptors in the parathyroid glands are also defective, they incorrectly sense the increased serum Ca^{2+} as normal

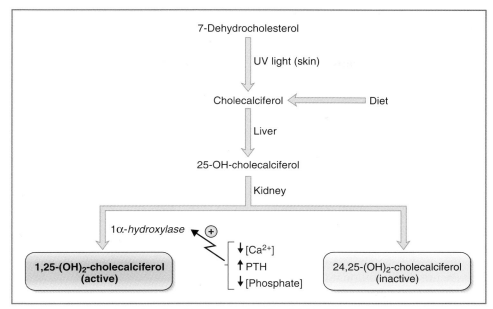

Figure 9–39 **Steps involved in the synthesis of 1,25-dihydroxycholecalciferol.**
PTH, Parathyroid hormone; UV, ultraviolet.

and PTH secretion is not inhibited as it would be in normal persons.

Calcitonin

Calcitonin is a straight-chain peptide with 32 amino acids. It is synthesized and secreted by the **parafollicular** or C ("C" for calcitonin) cells of the thyroid gland. The calcitonin gene directs the synthesis of preprocalcitonin and a signal peptide is cleaved to yield procalcitonin; other peptide sequences are then removed, and the final hormone, calcitonin, is stored in secretory granules for subsequent release.

The major stimulus for calcitonin secretion is increased plasma Ca^{2+} concentration (contrast this with the stimulus for PTH secretion, decreased plasma Ca^{2+} concentration). The major action of calcitonin is to inhibit osteoclastic bone resorption, which decreases the plasma Ca^{2+} concentration.

In contrast to PTH, calcitonin *does not* participate in the minute-to-minute regulation of the plasma Ca^{2+} concentration in humans. In fact, a physiologic role for calcitonin in humans is uncertain because neither thyroidectomy (with decreased calcitonin levels) nor thyroid tumors (with increased calcitonin levels) cause a derangement of Ca^{2+} metabolism, as would be expected if calcitonin had important regulatory functions.

Vitamin D

Vitamin D, in conjunction with PTH, is the second major regulatory hormone for Ca^{2+} and phosphate metabolism. The roles of PTH and vitamin D can be distinguished as follows: The role of *PTH* is to maintain the plasma Ca^{2+} concentration, and its actions are coordinated to increase the ionized Ca^{2+} concentration toward normal. The role of *vitamin D* is to promote mineralization of new bone, and its actions are coordinated to increase *both* Ca^{2+} and phosphate concentrations in plasma so that these elements can be deposited in new bone mineral.

Synthesis of Vitamin D

Vitamin D (**cholecalciferol**) is provided in the diet and is produced in the skin from cholesterol. Vitamin D has formal "hormone" status because cholecalciferol itself is inactive and must be successively hydroxylated to an active metabolite. Hydroxylation of cholecalciferol is regulated by negative feedback mechanisms. The pathways for vitamin D metabolism are shown in Figure 9-39.

There are two sources of cholecalciferol in the body: It is either ingested in the diet or synthesized in the skin from 7-dehydrocholesterol in the presence of ultraviolet light. As noted, cholecalciferol itself is physiologically inactive. It is hydroxylated in the liver to form **25-hydroxycholecalciferol,** which also is inactive. This hydroxylation step occurs in the endoplasmic reticulum and requires NADPH, O_2, and Mg^{2+}, but not cytochrome P-450. 25-Hydroxycholecalciferol is bound to an α-globulin in plasma and is the principal circulating form of vitamin D.

In the **kidney,** 25-hydroxycholecalciferol undergoes one of two routes of hydroxylation: It can be hydroxylated at the C1 position to produce **1,25-dihydroxycholecalciferol,** which is the physiologically *active* form, or it can be hydroxylated at C24 to produce **24,25-dihydroxycholecalciferol,** which is *inactive.*

C1 hydroxylation is catalyzed by the enzyme **1α-hydroxylase,** which is regulated by several factors including the plasma Ca^{2+} concentration and PTH. C1 hydroxylation occurs in the renal mitochondria and requires NADPH, O_2, Mg^{2+}, and cytochrome **P-450.**

Regulation of Vitamin D Synthesis

Whether the renal cells produce 1,25-dihydroxycholecalciferol (the active metabolite) or 24,25-dihydroxycholecalciferol (the inactive metabolite) depends on the "status" of Ca^{2+} in the body. When Ca^{2+} is sufficient, with an adequate dietary intake of Ca^{2+} and normal or increased plasma Ca^{2+} concentration, the inactive metabolite is preferentially synthesized because there is no need for more Ca^{2+}. When Ca^{2+} is insufficient, with a low dietary intake of Ca^{2+} and decreased plasma Ca^{2+} concentration, the active metabolite is preferentially synthesized to ensure that additional Ca^{2+} will be absorbed from the gastrointestinal tract.

The production of the active metabolite, 1,25-dihydroxycholecalciferol, is regulated by changing the activity of the **1α-hydroxylase enzyme** (see Fig. 9-39). 1α-Hydroxylase activity is increased by each of the following three factors: decreased plasma Ca^{2+} concentration, increased circulating levels of PTH, and decreased plasma phosphate concentration.

Actions of Vitamin D

The overall role of vitamin D (1,25-dihydroxycholecalciferol) is to increase the plasma concentrations of *both* Ca^{2+} and phosphate and to increase the $Ca^{2+} \times$ phosphate product to promote mineralization of new bone. To increase plasma Ca^{2+} and phosphate concentrations, vitamin D has coordinated actions on intestine, kidney, and bone. Because 1,25-dihydroxycholecalciferol is a steroid hormone, its mechanism of action involves stimulation of gene transcription and synthesis of new proteins, which have the following physiologic actions:

♦ **Intestine.** The major actions of 1,25-dihydroxycholecalciferol are on the intestine. There, 1,25-dihydroxycholecalciferol increases both Ca^{2+} and phosphate absorption, although far more is known about its effect on Ca^{2+} absorption. In the intestine, 1,25-dihydroxycholecalciferol induces the synthesis of a vitamin D–dependent Ca^{2+}-binding protein called **calbindin D-28 K,** a cytosolic protein that can bind four Ca^{2+} ions.

The mechanism of Ca^{2+} absorption in intestinal epithelial cells is illustrated in Figure 9-40. Ca^{2+} diffuses from the lumen into the cell, down its electrochemical gradient (Step 1). It is bound inside the cell to calbindin D-28K (Step 2) and subsequently is pumped across the basolateral membrane by a Ca^{2+} ATPase (Step 3). The exact role of calbindin

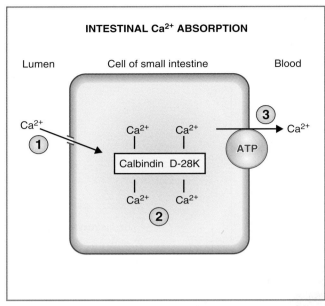

Figure 9–40 Role of calbindin D-28K in intestinal Ca^{2+} absorption. 1,25-Dihydroxycholecalciferol induces the synthesis of calbindin D-28K. See the text for an explanation of the circled numbers. ATP, Adenosine triphosphate.

D-28K in promoting absorption in intestinal epithelial cells is uncertain. It may act as a shuttle, moving Ca^{2+} across the cell from lumen to blood, or it may act as a Ca^{2+} buffer to keep intracellular free Ca^{2+} low, thus maintaining the concentration gradient for Ca^{2+} diffusion across the luminal membrane.

♦ **Kidney.** The actions of 1,25-dihydroxycholecalciferol on the kidney are parallel to its actions on the intestine—it stimulates both Ca^{2+} and phosphate reabsorption. In the kidney, the actions of 1,25-dihydroxycholecalciferol are clearly distinguishable from those of PTH. PTH stimulates Ca^{2+} reabsorption and inhibits phosphate reabsorption, and 1,25-dihydroxycholecalciferol stimulates the reabsorption of *both* ions.

♦ **Bone.** In bone, 1,25-dihydroxycholecalciferol acts synergistically with PTH to stimulate osteoclast activity and bone resorption. This action may seem paradoxical because the overall action of 1,25-dihydroxycholecalciferol is to promote bone mineralization. However, mineralized "old" bone is resorbed to provide more Ca^{2+} and phosphate to ECF so that "new" bone can be mineralized (bone remodeling).

Pathophysiology of Vitamin D

In children, vitamin D deficiency causes **rickets,** a condition in which insufficient amounts of Ca^{2+} and phosphate are available to mineralize the growing bones. Rickets is characterized by growth failure and skeletal deformities. This condition is rare in areas of the world where vitamin D is supplemented and when there is adequate exposure to sunlight. In adults, vitamin D deficiency results in **osteomalacia,** in which new bone fails to mineralize, resulting in bending and softening of the weight-bearing bones.

Vitamin D resistance occurs when the kidney is unable to produce the active metabolite, 1,25-dihydroxycholecalciferol. This condition is called "resistant" because no matter how much vitamin D is supplemented in the diet, it will be inactive because the C1 hydroxylation step in the kidney is absent or is inhibited. Vitamin D resistance can be caused by the congenital absence of 1α-hydroxylase or, more commonly, by **chronic renal failure.** Chronic renal failure is associated with a constellation of bone abnormalities including osteomalacia, a consequence of the inability of the diseased renal tissue to produce 1,25-dihydroxycholecalciferol, the active form of vitamin D.

SUMMARY

■ The endocrine glands synthesize and secrete hormones, which circulate to their target tissues. Chemically, hormones may be classified as peptides, steroids, or amines. Hormone levels are measured by radioimmunoassay.

■ Peptide hormones are synthesized by transcription of genes to mRNAs and translation of mRNAs to preprohormones. Signal peptides and other peptide sequences are cleaved from preprohormones to form the peptide hormones, which are packaged in secretory granules. Steroid hormones are synthesized from cholesterol in the adrenal cortex, testes, ovaries, and placenta. Amine hormones are derivatives of tyrosine.

■ Hormone synthesis and secretion is regulated by negative and positive feedback mechanisms. Negative feedback is self-limiting; positive feedback is self-augmenting. Hormone receptors are also regulated by increasing (up-regulation) or decreasing (down-regulation) their number or activity.

■ Mechanisms of hormone action (and their second messengers) include adenylyl cyclase (cAMP), phospholipase C (IP_3/Ca^{2+}), steroid hormone mechanism, and the tyrosine kinase mechanism.

■ The connection between the hypothalamus and the posterior lobe of the pituitary is neuronal. The cell bodies are in the hypothalamus, and the hormones are secreted from nerve terminals in the posterior lobe of the pituitary. The hypothalamus is connected to the anterior lobe of the pituitary by hypothalamic-hypophysial portal blood vessels.

■ Hormones of the anterior lobe are TSH, FSH, LH, ACTH, growth hormone, and prolactin. Hormones of the posterior lobe are ADH and oxytocin.

■ Growth hormone is required for growth to normal stature and has actions on carbohydrate metabolism, protein synthesis, organ growth, and bone growth. Many of the actions of growth hormone are mediated by somatomedins. In children, a deficiency of growth hormone causes growth retardation. Excess growth hormone causes acromegaly.

■ Prolactin is responsible for breast development and lactogenesis. Prolactin secretion is under tonic inhibition, mediated by dopamine from the hypothalamus. Excess prolactin secretion (e.g., prolactinoma) causes galactorrhea, which can be treated with dopamine agonists (e.g., bromocriptine).

■ ADH is responsible for osmoregulation by increasing water reabsorption in the principal cells of the kidney. ADH secretion is stimulated by increases in serum osmolarity and by decreases in ECF volume. Deficiency of ADH causes diabetes insipidus; excess ADH causes SIADH.

■ Oxytocin secretion is stimulated by suckling and is responsible for milk ejection from the lactating breast.

■ Thyroid hormones are synthesized by thyroid follicular cells. Tyrosines of thyroglobulin are iodinated, yielding MIT and DIT. Coupling of MIT and DIT produces T_3 and T_4. T_4 is activated to T_3 in target tissues. The actions of thyroid hormones include increased Na^+-K^+ ATPase, increased oxygen consumption and BMR, and increased cardiac output. Hyperthyroidism is commonly caused by thyroid-stimulating immunoglobulins (Graves disease) and exhibits weight loss, increased BMR, excess heat production, rapid heart rate, and nervousness. Hypothyroidism exhibits weight gain, decreased BMR, cold intolerance, slowed movements, and lethargy.

■ Adrenocortical steroid hormones are glucocorticoids, mineralocorticoids, and adrenal androgens, all of which are synthesized from cholesterol. Glucocorticoids stimulate gluconeogenesis and have antiinflammatory and immunosuppressive actions. Mineralocorticoids stimulate Na^+ reabsorption and K^+ and H^+ secretion by the kidney. Addison disease is primary adrenocortical insufficiency. Cushing syndrome is overproduction of glucocorticoids. Conn syndrome is overproduction of mineralocorticoids.

■ The islets of Langerhans have three cell types: α, which secrete glucagon; β, which secrete insulin; and δ, which secrete somatostatin. Insulin is the hormone of "abundance" and promotes storage of glucose as glycogen, storage of fatty acids in adipose, and storage of amino acids as protein. Deficiency of insulin is type I diabetes mellitus; insulin resistance of target tissues is type II diabetes mellitus. Glucagon is the hormone of "starvation" and promotes utilization of stored nutrients.

■ Ca^{2+} homeostasis is controlled by the interplay of bone, kidney, and intestine, and the actions of the hormones PTH, calcitonin, and vitamin D. The function of PTH is to increase serum ionized Ca^{2+} concentration by increasing bone resorption, increasing intestinal Ca^{2+} absorption, increasing renal Ca^{2+} reabsorption, and decreasing renal phosphate reabsorption. Hyperparathyroidism is associated with hypercalcemia and hypophosphatemia. Hypoparathyroidism is associated with hypocalcemia and hyperphosphatemia. Vitamin D is converted to its active form, 1,25-dihydroxycholecalciferol, in the kidney. The function of vitamin D is to promote bone mineralization by increasing the Ca^{2+} and phosphate concentrations in ECF. Its actions are to increase intestinal and renal Ca^{2+} and phosphate absorption and to increase bone resorption. Deficiency of vitamin D causes rickets in children and osteomalacia in adults.

Challenge Yourself

Each numbered question begins with an endocrine disorder or a disturbance to an endocrine system. The disorder or disturbance is followed by a list of parameters (e.g., blood level of various substances). For each parameter, predict whether it is increased, decreased, or unchanged.

1 **Addison Disease**
Cortisol
ACTH
Blood glucose

2 **Nephrogenic Diabetes Insipidus**
ADH
Urine osmolarity

3 **Conn Syndrome**
Serum K^+
Blood pressure
Renin

4 **Cushing Disease**
ACTH
Cortisol
Blood glucose

5 **Surgical Hypoparathyroidism**
Serum Ca^{2+}
Serum phosphate
Urinary cyclic AMP

6 **Car Accident That Severs the Hypothalamic-Pituitary Stalk**
Prolactin
ADH
Serum osmolarity
PTH

7 **Autoimmune Destruction of the Thyroid**
T_4
TSH
Basal metabolic rate
T_3 resin uptake

8 **21β-Hydroxylase Deficiency**
ACTH
Cortisol
Deoxycorticosterone (DOC)
Aldosterone
Dehydroepiandrosterone (DHEA)
Urinary 17-ketosteroids

9 **Administration of Synthetic Glucocorticoid (Dexamethasone) to a Normal Person**
ACTH
Cortisol

10 **Lung Cancer Producing Parathyroid Hormone-Related Peptide (PTH-rp)**
Serum Ca^{2+}
PTH

11 **17α-Hydroxylase Deficiency**
Blood pressure
Blood glucose
DHEA
Aldosterone

SELECTED READINGS

Bell GI, Pictet RL, Rutter WJ, et al: Sequence of human insulin gene. Nature 284:26, 1980.

DeGroot LJ: Endocrinology, 3rd ed. Philadelphia, WB Saunders, 1994.

Gharib SD, Wierman ME, Shupnik MA, et al: Molecular biology of the pituitary gonadotropins. Endocr Rev 11:177, 1990.

Gilman AG: Guanine nucleotide-binding regulatory proteins and dual control of adenylate cyclase. J Clin Invest 73:1, 1984.

Norman A, Roth J, Orci L: The vitamin D endocrine system: Steroid metabolism, hormone receptors, and biological response (calcium-binding proteins). Endocr Rev 3:331, 1982.

Olefsky JM: The insulin receptor: A multifunctional protein. Diabetes 39:1009, 1991.

Tepperman J, Tepperman HM: Metabolic and Endocrine Physiology, 5th ed. Chicago, Year Book, 1987.

Ullrich A, Bell JR, Chen EY, et al: Human insulin receptor and its relation to the tyrosine kinase family of oncogenes. Nature 313:756, 1985.

Unger RH, Dobbs RE, Orci L: Insulin, glucagon, and somatostatin secretion in the regulation of metabolism. Ann Rev Physiol 40:307, 1978.

Reproductive Physiology

The gonads are endocrine glands whose functions are to support development and maturation of the male and female germ cells. The male gonads, the testes, are responsible for development and maturation of sperm and synthesis and secretion of the male sex steroid hormone, testosterone. The female gonads, the ovaries, are responsible for development and maturation of ova and synthesis and secretion of the female sex steroid hormones, estrogen and progesterone.

SEXUAL DIFFERENTIATION

Sexual differentiation includes the development of the gonads, internal genital tract, and external genitalia. "Maleness" or "femaleness" can be characterized in three ways: (1) genetic sex, whether the sex chromosomes are XY or XX; (2) gonadal sex, whether the gonads are testes or ovaries; and (3) phenotypic or genital sex, whether the person looks like a male or a female (Fig. 10-1).

Genetic Sex

Genetic sex is determined by the sex chromosomes—XY in males and XX in females. During the first 5 weeks of gestational life, the gonads are indifferent or bipotential—they are neither male nor female. At gestational weeks 6 to 7 in genetic males, the testes begin to develop; at gestational week 9 in genetic females, the ovaries begin to develop. Therefore, genetic sex normally determines gonadal sex, and the gonads appear in males slightly before they appear in females.

Gonadal Sex

Gonadal sex is defined by the presence of either male gonads or female gonads, namely, the testes or the ovaries. The gonads comprise germ cells and steroid hormone–secreting cells.

The testes, the male gonads, consist of three cell types: germ cells, Sertoli cells, and Leydig cells. The **germ cells** produce spermatogonia, the **Sertoli cells** synthesize a glycoprotein hormone called antimüllerian hormone, and the **Leydig cells** synthesize testosterone.

The ovaries, the female gonads, also have three cell types: germ cells, granulosa cells, and theca cells. The **germ cells** produce oogonia. The meiotic oogonia are surrounded by granulosa cells and stroma, and in this configuration, they are called oocytes. They remain in the prophase of meiosis until ovulation occurs. The **theca cells** synthesize

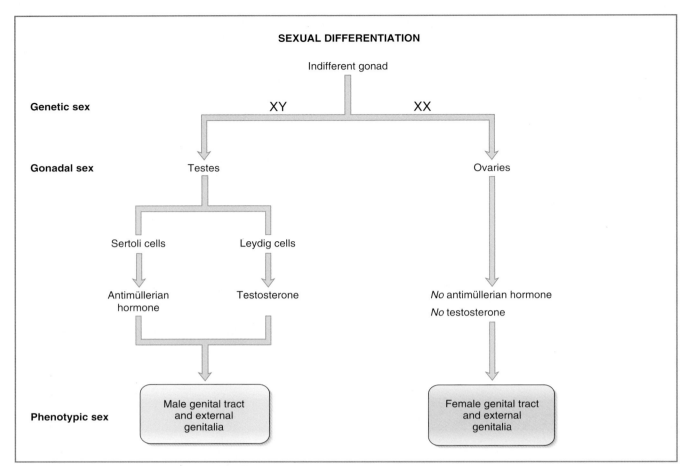

SEXUAL DIFFERENTIATION

Figure 10–1 **Determination of genetic sex, gonadal sex, and phenotypic sex.**

progesterone and, together with the **granulosa cells,** synthesize estradiol.

There are two key differences between the male and female gonads that influence phenotypic sex: (1) The testes synthesize antimüllerian hormone, and the ovaries do not; and (2) the testes synthesize testosterone, and the ovaries do not. Antimüllerian hormone and testosterone are decisive in determining that the fetus will be a phenotypic male. If there are no testes and, therefore, no antimüllerian hormone or testosterone, the fetus will become a phenotypic female by "default."

Phenotypic Sex

Phenotypic sex is defined by the physical characteristics of the internal genital tract and the external genitalia. In **males,** the internal genital tract includes the prostate, seminal vesicles, vas deferens, and epididymis. The external genitalia in males are the scrotum and the penis. In **females,** the internal genitalia are the fallopian tubes, uterus, and upper one third of the vagina. The external genitalia in females are the clitoris, labia majora, labia minora, and lower two thirds of the vagina. As previously noted, phenotypic sex is determined by the hormonal output of the gonads as follows:

♦ **Male phenotype.** Gonadal males have testes that synthesize and secrete **antimüllerian hormone** and **testosterone,** both of which are required for the development of the male phenotype. Embryologically, the wolffian ducts give rise to the epididymis, vas deferens, seminal vesicles, and ejaculatory ducts. Testosterone, which is present in gonadal males, stimulates the growth and differentiation of the wolffian ducts. Testosterone from each testis acts ipsilaterally (same side) on its own wolffian duct. In this action on the wolffian ducts, testosterone does *not* have to be converted to dihydrotestosterone (discussed later in chapter). At the same time, antimüllerian hormone produced by testicular Sertoli cells causes atrophy of a second set of ducts, the müllerian ducts. (The müllerian ducts *would have become* the female genital tract if they had not been suppressed by antimüllerian hormone.) The external male genitalia, the penis and scrotum, differentiate at gestational weeks 9 to 10. Growth and

BOX 10–1 Clinical Physiology: Androgen Insensitivity Syndrome

DESCRIPTION OF CASE. A girl who is apparently normal begins to develop breasts at age 11, and at age 13, she is considered to have larger-than-average breasts among her peers. However, by age 16, she has not begun to menstruate and has scant pubic and axillary hair. Upon pelvic examination, a gynecologist notes the presence of testes and a short vagina, but no cervix, ovaries, or uterus. Chromosomal evaluation reveals that the girl has an XY genotype. Suspecting a form of androgen insensitivity syndrome (a testicular feminization), the physician orders androgen-binding studies in genital skin fibroblasts. The studies show no binding of testosterone or dihydrotestosterone, suggesting that androgen receptors in the tissue are absent or defective. She has mildly elevated levels of plasma testosterone and elevated levels of luteinizing hormone (LH). The young woman's testes are removed, and she is treated with intermittent estrogen replacement therapy. She is advised, however, that she will never have menstrual cycles or be able to bear children.

EXPLANATION OF CASE. This girl has a female phenotype with female external genitalia (lower vagina, clitoris, and labia). At puberty, she develops breasts. However, she has a male genotype (XY) and male gonads (testes).

The basis for her disorder, a form of androgen insensitivity syndrome, is lack of androgen receptors in target tissues, which results in resistance to androgens.

Her testes, which are normal, secreted both antimüllerian hormone and testosterone in utero. As in normal males, antimüllerian hormone suppressed development of the müllerian ducts in utero; therefore, the girl has no fallopian tubes, uterus, or upper vagina. The testes also secreted testosterone in utero, which *should have* stimulated growth and differentiation of the wolffian ducts into the male genital tract and development of the male external genitalia. The male genital tract and external genitalia *did not* develop, however, because the target tissues lack androgen receptors. Thus, although the testes secreted normal amounts of testosterone, testosterone could not act on the tissues of the male genital tract. (Lack of androgen receptors also explains the girl's scant body hair at puberty.) The female phenotype (short vagina, labia, and clitoris) is present because, in the absence of testosterone receptors, the fetus became a phenotypic female by "default."

The girl's breasts developed at puberty because her testes are producing estradiol from testosterone, stimulated by the high circulating levels of LH. The estradiol then promotes breast development.

TREATMENT. In androgen insensitivity syndrome, because the testes can develop a neoplasm, they are removed. Following removal of the testes (and, therefore, removal of the testicular source of estradiol), the girl is treated with estrogen therapy to maintain her breasts. She will not be able to bear children, however, because she lacks ovaries and a uterus.

---

development of the external male genitalia depend on conversion of testosterone to dihydrotestosterone and the presence of androgen receptors on the target tissues (Box 10-1).

♦ **Female phenotype.** Gonadal females have ovaries that secrete **estrogen,** but they do not secrete antimüllerian hormone or testosterone. Thus, in females, *no testosterone* is available to stimulate growth and differentiation of the wolffian ducts into the internal male genital tract, and *no antimüllerian hormone* is available to suppress differentiation of the müllerian ducts. Consequently, the müllerian ducts develop into the internal female tract (fallopian tubes, uterus, and upper one third of the vagina). Like the internal genital tract, the development of the external female genitalia (clitoris, labia majora, labia minora, and lower two thirds of the vagina) does not require any hormones, although growth of these structures to normal size depends on the presence of estrogen.

If a gonadal female is exposed to high levels of androgens in utero (e.g., from excessive production by the adrenal cortex) when the external genitalia are differentiating, then a male phenotype results. If such exposure occurs after differentiation of the external genitalia, the female phenotype is retained, but perhaps with enlargement of the clitoris (Box 10-2).

PUBERTY

Gonadotropin Secretion Over the Lifetime

In both males and females, gonadal function is driven by the hypothalamic-pituitary axis, whose activity varies over the life span, as shown in Figure 10-2.

Secretion of gonadotropin-releasing hormone (GnRH), the hypothalamic hormone, begins at gestational week 4, but its levels remain low until puberty. Secretion of follicle-stimulating hormone (FSH) and luteinizing hormone (LH), the anterior pituitary hormones, begins between gestational weeks 10 and 12. Like GnRH, the levels of FSH and LH remain low until puberty. During childhood, FSH levels are relatively higher than LH levels.

At puberty and throughout the reproductive years, the secretory pattern changes: Secretion of GnRH, FSH,

BOX 10–2 Clinical Physiology: Congenital Adrenal Hyperplasia

DESCRIPTION OF CASE. At birth, a baby is found to have ambiguous external genitalia. There is no penis, and a clitoris is significantly enlarged. Chromosomal evaluation reveals that the baby has an XX genotype. She is found to have ovaries but no testes. Tests confirm that the baby has a form of adrenal hyperplasia in which there is congenital lack of the adrenal cortical enzyme 21β-hydroxylase. Treatment involves surgical reconstruction of the external genitalia to conform to the female phenotype and the administration of glucocorticoids and mineralocorticoids. The child will be raised as a female.

EXPLANATION OF CASE. The baby has a congenital absence of 21β-hydroxylase, the adrenal enzyme that normally converts steroid precursors to mineralocorticoids and cortisol (see Chapter 9, Fig. 9-23). As a result of this defect, steroid precursors accumulate behind the enzyme block and are directed toward the production of the adrenal androgens, dehydroepiandrosterone and androstenedione. The high levels of androgens caused masculinization of the external genitalia (enlargement of the clitoris) in utero. The

genotype is XX (female), and the internal organs are female including ovaries, fallopian tubes, uterus, and upper vagina. The fallopian tubes, uterus, and upper vagina developed because, without testes, there was no source of antimüllerian hormone to suppress differentiation of müllerian ducts into the female genital tract. There is hyperplasia of the adrenal cortex because the absence of cortisol increases secretion of adrenocorticotropic hormone (ACTH), which then has a trophic effect on the adrenal cortex.

TREATMENT. Surgical correction of the ambiguous external genitalia involves reconstruction to conform to a phenotypic female. Because the baby has normal ovaries, fallopian tubes, and uterus, she should begin normal menstrual cycles at puberty and have a normal reproductive capacity. Hormone replacement therapy has two goals: (1) to replace the missing adrenal glucocorticoids and mineralocorticoids and (2) to suppress ACTH secretion (by the negative feedback of glucocorticoids on the anterior pituitary) to reduce the adrenal output of androgens and prevent further masculinization.

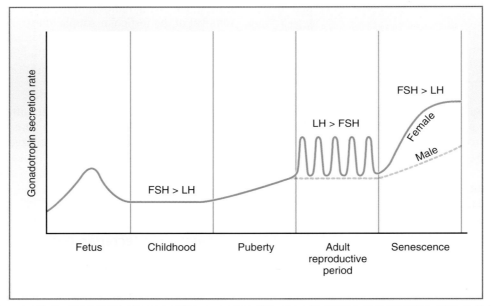

Figure 10–2 Gonadotropin secretion over the life span in males and females. FSH, Follicle-stimulating hormone; LH, luteinizing hormone.

and LH increases and becomes pulsatile. The relative levels of FSH and LH reverse, with LH levels becoming higher than FSH levels. In addition, in females, there is a 28-day cycle of gonadotropin secretion called the menstrual cycle.

Finally, in senescence, gonadotropin secretion rates increase further, with FSH levels becoming higher than LH levels, as they were in childhood.

Pulsatile Secretion of GnRH, FSH, and LH

The primary event at puberty is the initiation of **pulsatile secretion of GnRH.** This new pattern of GnRH secretion drives a parallel **pulsatile secretion of FSH and LH** by the anterior lobe of the pituitary. One of the earliest events of puberty is the appearance of large nocturnal pulses of LH during REM sleep. Another significant event early in puberty is an increased sensitivity of the GnRH receptor in the anterior pituitary. Thus, at puberty, GnRH up-regulates its own receptor in the anterior pituitary, and a given concentration of GnRH produces a greater stimulation of FSH and LH secretion. In addition, there is a shift in the relative secretion rates of the two anterior pituitary hormones; at puberty and throughout the reproductive period, LH levels are greater than FSH levels (compared with childhood and senescence, when FSH is greater than LH).

Pulsatile secretion of FSH and LH stimulates secretion of the gonadal steroid hormones, testosterone and estradiol. Increased circulating levels of the sex steroid hormones are then responsible for the appearance of the secondary sex characteristics at puberty.

The onset of the maturational process at puberty is genetically programmed, and familial patterns are evident. For example, the age at menarche (the onset of menses) is similar between mothers and daughters. The mechanisms underlying the onset of pulsatile GnRH secretion, however, remain a mystery. There may be gradual maturation of the hypothalamic neurons that synthesize and secrete GnRH. The central nervous system and nutritional status may alter the process; for example, extreme stress or caloric deprivation in girls delays the onset of puberty. It has been suggested that melatonin plays a role in the onset of puberty. Melatonin, secreted by the pineal gland, *may be* a natural inhibitor of GnRH release. Melatonin levels are highest during childhood and decline in adulthood, and this decline may release an inhibition of GnRH secretion. In support of a role for melatonin is the observation that removal of the pineal gland precipitates early puberty.

Characteristics of Puberty

As noted, the biologic events at puberty are set in motion by the onset of pulsatile activity in the hypothalamic–anterior pituitary axis. In turn, this pulsatile, or bursting, activity causes the testes and ovaries to secrete their respective sex hormones, testosterone and estrogen, that are responsible for the development of the secondary sex characteristics. Pulsatility of the hypothalamic-pituitary axis is *required* for normal reproductive function, as illustrated by the treatment of persons with delayed puberty caused by GnRH deficiency. If a GnRH analogue is administered in intermittent pulses to replicate the normal pulsatile secretory pattern, puberty is initiated and reproductive function is established. However, if a long-acting GnRH analogue is administered, puberty is not initiated. The events of puberty and their timing are illustrated in Figure 10-3.

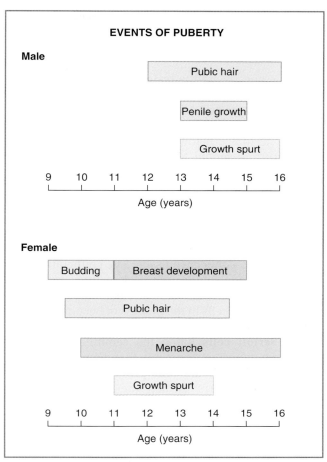

Figure 10–3 **Major events of puberty in males and females.**

In **boys,** puberty is associated with activation of the hypothalamic-pituitary axis, Leydig cell proliferation in the testes, and increased synthesis and secretion of testosterone by the Leydig cells. There is growth of the testes, largely because of an increased number of seminiferous tubules. There is growth of the sex accessory organs such as the prostate. There is a pronounced linear growth spurt, and the epiphyses close when adult height is attained. As plasma levels of testosterone increase, facial, pubic, and axillary hair appears and there is growth of the penis, lowering of the voice, and initiation of spermatogenesis **(spermarche).**

In **girls,** puberty also is associated with the activation of the hypothalamic-pituitary axis, which drives the synthesis of estradiol by the ovaries. The first observable sign of puberty in girls is budding of the breasts, which is followed in approximately 2 years by **menarche,** the onset of menstrual cycles. The growth spurt and closure of the epiphyses typically begin and end earlier in girls than in boys. The appearance of pubic and axillary hair precedes menarche and is dependent on increased secretion of adrenal androgens, called **adrenarche.**

MALE REPRODUCTIVE PHYSIOLOGY

Structure of the Testes

The male gonads are the **testes,** which have two functions: spermatogenesis and secretion of testosterone. Normally, the testes occupy the scrotum, which lies outside the body cavity and is maintained at 35° to 36°C, or 1° to 2°C below body temperature. This lower temperature, essential for normal spermatogenesis, is maintained by a countercurrent arrangement of testicular arteries and veins, which facilitates heat exchange.

Eighty percent of the adult testis is composed of **seminiferous tubules,** which produce the sperm. The seminiferous tubules are convoluted loops, 120 to 300 μm in diameter, which are arranged in lobules and surrounded by connective tissue. The epithelium lining the seminiferous tubules consists of three cell types: spermatogonia, which are the stem cells; spermatocytes, which are cells in the process of becoming sperm; and Sertoli cells, which support the developing sperm.

The **Sertoli cells** lining the seminiferous tubules have three important functions that support spermatogenesis. (1) The Sertoli cells provide nutrients to the differentiating sperm (which are isolated from the bloodstream). (2) Sertoli cells form tight junctions with each other, creating a barrier between the testes and the bloodstream called the **blood-testes barrier.** The blood-testes barrier imparts a selective permeability, admitting "allowable" substances such as testosterone to cross but prohibiting noxious substances that might damage the developing sperm. (3) Sertoli cells secrete an aqueous fluid into the lumen of the seminiferous tubules, which helps to transport sperm through the tubules into the epididymis.

The remaining 20% of the adult testis is connective tissue interspersed with **Leydig cells.** The function of the Leydig cells is synthesis and secretion of testosterone, the male sex steroid hormone. Testosterone has both local (paracrine) effects that support spermatogenesis in the testicular Sertoli cells and endocrine effects on other target organs (e.g., skeletal muscle and the prostate).

Spermatogenesis

Spermatogenesis occurs continuously throughout the reproductive life of the male, from puberty until senescence. Spermatogenesis occurs along the length of the seminiferous tubules, and the process can be divided into three phases: (1) **Mitotic divisions** of spermatogonia generate the spermatocytes, which are destined to become mature sperm; (2) **meiotic divisions** of the spermatocytes, which decrease the chromosome number and produce haploid spermatids; and (3) spermiogenesis, in which spermatids are transformed into mature sperm through the loss of cytoplasm and the development of flagella (Fig. 10-4). One full cycle of spermatogenesis requires about **64 days.** There is a temporal organization to the spermatogenic cycle, called the **spermatogenic wave,** which ensures that mature spermatozoa are produced continuously. Two million spermatogonia begin this process daily, and because each spermatogonium gives rise to 64 spermatozoa, 128 million sperm are produced daily.

Storage of Sperm, Ejaculation, and Function of Sex Accessory Glands

Sperm leave the testes through ducts that carry them to the **epididymis,** the primary location for the maturation and storage of sperm. They remain viable in the epididymis for several months.

During **sexual arousal,** contractions of the smooth muscle around the ducts advance sperm through the epididymis. At **ejaculation,** sperm are expelled into the **vas deferens** and then into the urethra. The ampulla of the vas deferens provides another storage area for sperm and secretes a fluid rich in **citrate** and **fructose,** which nourishes the ejaculated sperm.

The **seminal vesicles** secrete a fluid rich in fructose, citrate, prostaglandins, and fibrinogen. As the vas deferens empties its sperm into the ejaculatory duct, each seminal vesicle contributes its secretions, which also will be nutritive for the ejaculated sperm. The prostaglandins present in seminal fluid may assist in fertilization in two ways: (1) Prostaglandins react with cervical mucus to make it more penetrable by sperm; and (2) prostaglandins induce peristaltic contractions in the female reproductive tract (i.e., the uterus and fallopian tubes) to propel the sperm up the tract.

The **prostate gland** adds its own secretion to the ejaculate, a milky aqueous solution rich in citrate, calcium, and enzymes. The prostatic secretion is slightly alkaline, which increases sperm motility and aids in fertilization by neutralizing acidic secretions from the vas deferens and the vagina. Collectively, the combined secretions of the male sex accessory glands compose 90% of the volume of semen, and sperm compose the remaining 10%.

Ejaculated sperm cannot immediately fertilize an ovum: They must reside in the female reproductive tract for 4 to 6 hours for **capacitation** to occur. Capacitation is a process in which inhibitory factors in the seminal fluid are washed free, cholesterol is withdrawn from the sperm membrane, and surface proteins are redistributed. Calcium influx into the sperm increases their motility, and the motion of the sperm becomes "whiplike." Capacitation also results in the **acrosomal reaction** in which the acrosomal membrane fuses with the outer sperm membrane. This fusion creates pores

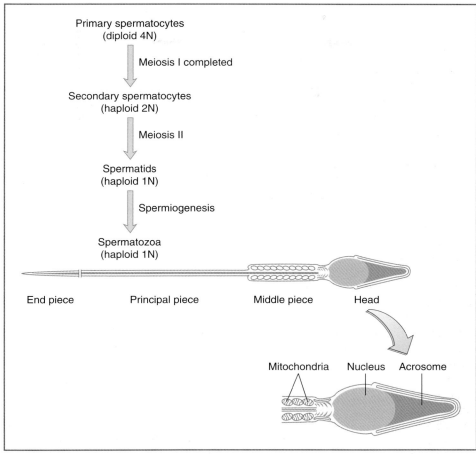

Primary spermatocytes
(diploid 4N)

Meiosis I completed

Secondary spermatocytes
(haploid 2N)

Meiosis II

Spermatids
(haploid 1N)

Spermiogenesis

Spermatozoa
(haploid 1N)

End piece   Principal piece   Middle piece   Head

Mitochondria   Nucleus   Acrosome

Figure 10–4   Development and structure of the spermatozoon.

through which hydrolytic and proteolytic enzymes can escape from the acrosome, creating a path for sperm to penetrate the protective coverings of the ovum.

Synthesis and Secretion of Testosterone

Testosterone, the major androgenic hormone, is synthesized and secreted by the Leydig cells of the testes. The steroidogenic pathways in the testes, shown in Figure 10-5, are similar to those previously described for the adrenal cortex (see Chapter 9, Fig. 9-23), with two important differences: (1) The testes *lack* the enzymes 21β-hydroxylase and 11β-hydroxylase and therefore cannot synthesize glucocorticoids or mineralocorticoids; and (2) the testes have an additional enzyme, **17β-hydroxysteroid dehydrogenase,** which converts androstenedione to testosterone. Thus, the androgenic end product of the testes is testosterone rather than dehydroepiandrosterone (DHEA) and androstenedione (the androgenic end products of the adrenal cortex).

Testosterone is not active in *all* androgenic target tissues. In *some* tissues, **dihydrotestosterone** is the active androgen. In those tissues, testosterone is converted to dihydrotestosterone by the enzyme **5α-reductase.**

Ninety-eight percent of the circulating testosterone is bound to plasma proteins, such as **sex steroid–binding globulin** and albumin. Because only free (unbound) testosterone is biologically active, sex steroid–binding globulin essentially functions as a reservoir for the circulating hormone. The synthesis of sex steroid–binding globulin is stimulated by estrogens and inhibited by androgens.

Regulation of the Testes

Both functions of the testes, spermatogenesis and secretion of testosterone, are controlled by the hypothalamic-pituitary axis (Fig. 10-6). The hypothalamic hormone is gonadotropin-releasing hormone (GnRH), and the anterior pituitary hormones are follicle-stimulating hormone (FSH) and luteinizing hormone (LH).

GnRH

GnRH is a decapeptide that is secreted by hypothalamic neurons in the **arcuate nuclei.** GnRH is secreted into

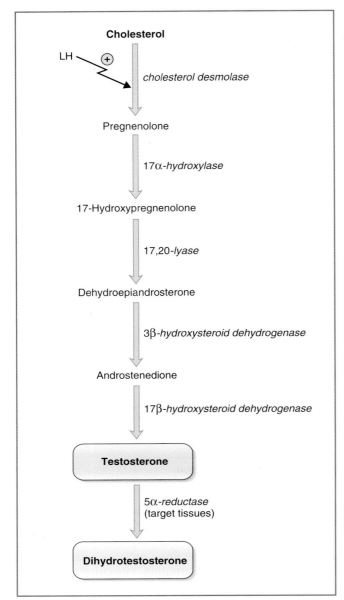

Figure 10–5 Biosynthetic pathway for testosterone synthesis in the testes. Dihydrotestosterone is synthesized from testosterone in target tissues that contain 5α-reductase. LH, Luteinizing hormone.

hypothalamic-hypophysial portal blood and then delivered in high concentration directly to the anterior lobe of the pituitary. Recall that throughout the reproductive period GnRH secretion is **pulsatile** and drives a parallel pulsatile secretory pattern of FSH and LH from the anterior lobe. (Note that if GnRH is administered continuously, it inhibits FSH and LH secretion.)

FSH and LH

FSH and LH are the anterior pituitary hormones (gonadotropins) that stimulate the testes to perform their spermatogenic and endocrine functions. FSH and LH are members of the glycoprotein hormone family that includes TSH and HCG; all members of the family have identical α subunits but unique β subunits that confer biologic activity. **FSH** stimulates spermatogenesis and Sertoli cell function. **LH** stimulates the Leydig cells to synthesize testosterone by increasing the activity of cholesterol desmolase. Thus, the function of LH in the testes parallels the function of ACTH in the adrenal cortex: It stimulates the first step in the steroidogenic pathway.

Testosterone, secreted by the Leydig cells, has functions both locally within the testes (paracrine effects) and on other target tissues (endocrine effects). Intratesticularly, testosterone diffuses from the Leydig cells to the nearby Sertoli cells, where it reinforces the spermatogenic action of FSH. Extratesticularly, testosterone is secreted into the general circulation and delivered to its target tissues.

Negative Feedback

The hypothalamic-pituitary axis in the male is controlled by **negative feedback,** which has two paths. In the first path, **testosterone** itself feeds back on both the hypothalamus and the anterior lobe, where it inhibits the secretion of GnRH and LH. At the hypothalamic level, testosterone decreases both the frequency and amplitude of the GnRH pulses. In the second path, the Sertoli cells secrete a substance called **inhibin.** Inhibin is a glycoprotein that is a feedback inhibitor of FSH secretion by the anterior pituitary. Thus, the Sertoli cells, which produce sperm, synthesize their own feedback inhibitor that serves as an "indicator" of the spermatogenic activity of the testes.

Negative feedback control of the hypothalamic-pituitary axis is illustrated when circulating levels of testosterone are decreased (e.g., testes are removed). Under such conditions, the frequency and amplitude of GnRH, FSH, and LH pulses are *increased* because of decreased feedback inhibition by testosterone on the hypothalamus and anterior pituitary.

Actions of Androgens

In some target tissues, testosterone is the active androgenic hormone. In other target tissues, testosterone must be activated to dihydrotestosterone by the action of **5α-reductase** (Box 10-3). Table 10-1 is a summary of the target tissues for testosterone and dihydrotestosterone and their respective actions.

♦ **Testosterone** is responsible for the fetal differentiation of the internal male genital tract: the epididymis, vas deferens, and seminal vesicles. At puberty, testosterone is responsible for increased muscle mass, the pubertal growth spurt, closure of the epiphyseal plates, growth of the penis and seminal

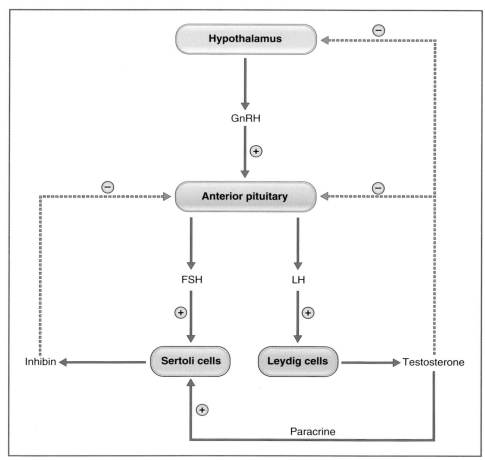

Figure 10–6 **Control of gonadotropin-releasing hormone (GnRH), follicle-stimulating hormone (FSH), and luteinizing hormone (LH) secretion in males.**

vesicles, deepening of the voice, spermatogenesis, and libido. Finally, as mentioned previously, testosterone mediates negative feedback effects on the anterior pituitary and the hypothalamus.

♦ **Dihydrotestosterone** is responsible for fetal differentiation of the external male genitalia (i.e., the penis, scrotum, and prostate); for male hair distribution and male pattern baldness; for sebaceous gland activity; and for growth of the prostate.

    5α-Reductase inhibitors such as **finasteride** block the conversion of testosterone to dihydrotestosterone and, therefore, block the production of active androgens in some target tissues. Because the growth of the prostate gland and male pattern baldness depend on dihydrotestosterone rather than testosterone, 5α-reductase inhibitors can be used as a treatment for **benign prostatic hypertrophy** and hair loss in males.

The **mechanism of action** of androgens begins with binding of testosterone or dihydrotestosterone to an androgen-receptor protein in the cells of target tissues.

The androgen-receptor complex moves into the nucleus, where it initiates gene transcription. New messenger ribonucleotides (mRNAs) are generated and translated into new proteins that are responsible for the various physiologic actions of androgens.

FEMALE REPRODUCTIVE PHYSIOLOGY

The female gonads are the **ovaries,** which, together with the uterus and the fallopian tubes, constitute the female reproductive tract. The ovaries, analogous to the testes in the male, have two functions: oogenesis and secretion of the female sex steroid hormones, progesterone and estrogen. Each adult ovary is attached to the uterus by ligaments, and running through these ligaments are the ovarian arteries, veins, lymphatic vessels, and nerves.

    The ovary has three zones. The **cortex** is the outer and largest zone. It is lined by germinal epithelium and contains all of the oocytes, each of which is enclosed in a follicle. The ovarian follicles are also responsible

BOX 10–3   Clinical Physiology: 5α-Reductase Deficiency

DESCRIPTION OF CASE. Jenny was born with what appeared to be an enlarged clitoris, although neither her parents nor the doctor questioned the abnormality. Now, at 13 years old, Jenny's girlfriends are developing breasts and having menstrual periods, but she is experiencing none of these changes. In fact, her voice is deepening, she is becoming muscular like the boys, and her enlarged clitoris is growing larger. Jenny is diagnosed with a form of male pseudohermaphroditism that is caused by a deficiency of 5α-reductase. On physical examination, she had no ovaries, no uterus, a blind vaginal pouch, a small prostate, a penis, descended testes, and hypospadias (urethral opening low on the underside of the penis). She had a male musculature but no body hair, facial hair, or acne. Her genotype was confirmed as 46, XY, and blood work showed a high-normal level of testosterone and a low level of dihydrotestosterone. Fibroblasts from genital skin had no 5α-reductase activity.

EXPLANATION OF CASE. Jenny is a genotypic male with testes and no ovaries. Her testes secrete testosterone, but she lacks the enzyme 5α-reductase. In normal males, some androgenic target tissues contain 5α-reductase, which converts testosterone to dihydrotestosterone; in those tissues, dihydrotestosterone is the active androgen. Androgenic actions that utilize dihydrotestosterone include differentiation of the external male genitalia, stimulation of hair follicles, male pattern baldness, activity of sebaceous glands, and growth of the prostate. Other androgenic target tissues in normal males do not contain 5α-reductase and do not synthesize dihydrotestosterone; in those tissues, testosterone is active. Androgenic actions that respond directly to testosterone include differentiation of internal male genital tract (epididymis, vas deferens, seminal vesicles), development of muscle mass, pubertal growth spurt, growth of the penis, deepening of the voice, spermatogenesis, and libido.

As a genetic male (46, XY), the presence of the Y chromosome determined that Jenny would have testes. Prenatally, the testes synthesized antimüllerian hormone and testosterone. Antimüllerian hormone suppressed development of the müllerian ducts into the internal female genital tract, so Jenny has no fallopian tubes, uterus, or upper one third of the vagina. Testosterone caused differentiation of the wolffian ducts into the internal male genital tract (epididymis, vas deferens, seminal vesicles), a process that does not require dihydrotestosterone and thus occurred even though she is lacking 5α-reductase. However, differentiation of the external male genitalia (e.g., penis, scrotum) requires dihydrotestosterone. Thus, deficiency of 5α-reductase meant that Jenny's external genitalia were not normally developed. At puberty, the clitoris grew and became more like a penis because of the high-normal circulating level of testosterone; apparently, with high enough levels, the androgen receptors that mediate growth of the external genitalia can be activated. Her voice deepened and she acquired skeletal muscle mass, actions that are mediated by testosterone and do not require conversion to dihydrotestosterone. Despite acquiring many masculine characteristics, Jenny did not develop body and facial hair because the hair follicles require dihydrotestosterone. Jenny did not develop breasts because she did not have ovaries, which in normal females are the source of the estrogen required for breast development.

TREATMENT. If Jenny chooses to continue life as a woman, it will be necessary to remove her testes, which are producing the testosterone that is causing her to be selectively masculinized (e.g., growth of penis, deepening of voice, muscle mass). In addition, because she lacks ovaries, Jenny has no endogenous source for the estrogen needed for breast development and female fat distribution; thus, she would require treatment with supplemental estrogen. She may elect to have surgical correction of the introitus; however, even with the surgery, she will not be able to bear children because she lacks ovaries and an internal female genital tract. If Jenny chooses to live the rest of her life as a man, she will be treated with androgenic compounds that do not require 5α-reduction for activity. The supplemental androgens will complete the masculinization process including development of male body and facial hair, sebaceous gland activity, growth of the prostate and, in later life, male pattern baldness.

Table 10–1   Actions of Androgens on Target Tissues

Mediated by Testosterone	Mediated by Dihydrotestosterone
Differentiation of epididymis, vas deferens, and seminal vesicles	Differentiation of penis, scrotum, and prostate
Increased muscle mass	Male hair pattern
Pubertal growth spurt	Male pattern baldness
Cessation of pubertal growth spurt (epiphyseal closure)	Sebaceous gland activity
Growth of penis and seminal vesicles	Growth of prostate
Deepening of voice	
Spermatogenesis	
Negative feedback on anterior pituitary	
Libido	

for steroid hormone synthesis. The **medulla** is the middle zone and is a mixture of cell types. The **hilum** is the inner zone, through which blood vessels and lymphatics pass.

The ovarian steroid hormones have both paracrine and endocrine functions. Locally, within the ovaries, the ovarian steroid hormones act to support the development of the ova. Systemically, the ovarian steroid hormones act on a variety of target tissues including uterus, breast, and bone.

The functional unit of the ovaries is the **single ovarian follicle,** which comprises one germ cell surrounded by endocrine cells. When fully developed, the ovarian follicle serves several critical roles: It will provide nutrients for the developing oocyte; release the oocyte at the proper time (ovulation); prepare the vagina and fallopian tubes to aid in fertilization of the egg by a sperm; prepare the lining of the uterus for implantation of the fertilized egg; and, in the event of fertilization, maintain steroid hormone production for the fetus until the placenta can assume this role.

Oogenesis

In the developing ovaries, primordial germ cells produce oogonia by mitotic divisions until gestational weeks 20 to 24. At that time, there are approximately 7 million oogonia. Beginning at gestational weeks 8 to 9, some of these oogonia enter the prophase of meiosis and become primary oocytes. The meiotic process continues until approximately 6 months after birth, at which point all oogonia have become oocytes. The oocytes remain in a state of suspended prophase; the first meiotic division will not be completed until ovulation occurs many years later. Simultaneously, there is attrition of oocytes. At birth, only 2 million oocytes remain; by puberty, only 400,000 oocytes remain; by menopause (which marks the end of the reproductive period), few, if any, oocytes remain. Whereas males continuously produce spermatogonia and spermatocytes, females do not produce new oogonia and function from a declining pool of oocytes.

The **development of ovarian follicles** occurs in the following stages, which are illustrated in Figure 10-7:

1. **First stage.** The first stage of follicular development parallels prophase of the oocyte. Thus, the first stage of the ovarian follicle lasts many years. The shortest duration for the first stage is approximately 13 years (the approximate age at first ovulation); the longest duration is 50 years (the approximate age at menopause). As the primary oocyte grows, the granulosa cells proliferate and nurture the oocyte with nutrients and steroid hormones. During this stage, the primordial follicle develops into a **primary follicle,** theca interna cells develop, and granulosa cells begin to secrete fluid. No follicle progresses beyond this first stage in prepubertal ovaries.

2. **Second stage.** The second stage of follicular development occurs much more rapidly than the first stage. This stage takes place over a period of 70 to 85 days and is present only during the reproductive period. During each menstrual cycle, a few follicles enter this sequence. A fluid containing steroid hormones, mucopolysaccharides, proteins, and FSH accumulates in a central area of the follicle called the antrum. The steroid hormones reach the antrum by direct secretion from granulosa cells. The granulosa and theca cells continue to grow. At the end of the second stage, the follicle is called a **graafian follicle** and has an average diameter of 2 to 5 mm.

3. **Third stage.** The third and final stage of follicular development is the most rapid, occurring 5 to 7 days after menses (menses marks the end of the previous cycle). A single graafian follicle achieves dominance over its cohorts, and the cohorts regress. Within 48 hours, the **dominant follicle** grows to 20 mm in diameter. On day 14 of a 28-day menstrual cycle, **ovulation** occurs and the dominant follicle ruptures and releases its oocyte into the peritoneal cavity. At this time, the first meiotic division is completed and the resulting secondary oocyte enters the nearby fallopian tube, where it begins the second meiotic division. In the fallopian tube, if fertilization by a sperm occurs, the second meiotic division is completed, producing the haploid ovum with 23 chromosomes.

The residual elements of the ruptured primary follicle form the **corpus luteum.** The corpus luteum is composed primarily of granulosa cells but also of theca cells, capillaries, and fibroblasts. The corpus luteum synthesizes and secretes steroid hormones, which are necessary for implantation and maintenance of the zygote should fertilization occur. If fertilization *does* occur, the corpus luteum will secrete steroid hormones until the placenta assumes this role, later in pregnancy. If fertilization *does not occur,* the corpus luteum regresses during the next 14 days (the second half of the menstrual cycle) and is replaced by a scar called the **corpus albicans.**

Synthesis and Secretion of Estrogen and Progesterone

The ovarian steroid hormones, progesterone and 17β-estradiol, are synthesized by the ovarian follicles through the combined functions of the **granulosa cells** and the **theca cells** (Fig. 10-8). Virtually all steps in the biosynthetic pathway are the same as those discussed

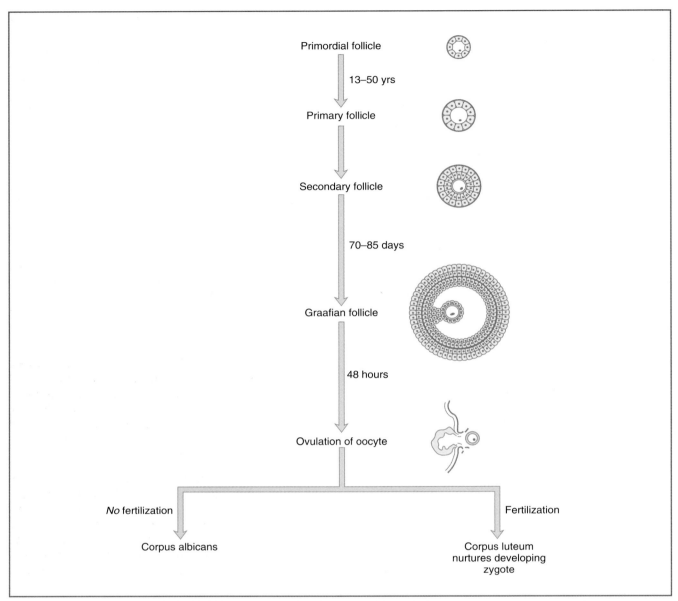

Primordial follicle

13–50 yrs

Primary follicle

Secondary follicle

70–85 days

Graafian follicle

48 hours

Ovulation of oocyte

No fertilization

Fertilization

Corpus albicans

Corpus luteum
nurtures developing
zygote

Figure 10–7 **Development of the oocyte from a primordial follicle.** If fertilization occurs, the corpus luteum secretes steroid hormones and supports the developing zygote. If no fertilization occurs, the corpus luteum regresses and becomes the corpus albicans.

previously for the adrenal cortex and the testes. Recall that the adrenal cortex produces all intermediates up to the level of androstenedione, but because it lacks the enzyme 17β-hydroxysteroid dehydrogenase, it does not produce testosterone. Recall also that the testes, having 17β-hydroxysteroid dehydrogenase, produce testosterone as their major hormonal product. In the ovaries, *all* steps in the biosynthetic pathway are present *including* **aromatase,** which converts testosterone to 17β-estradiol, the major ovarian estrogen.

Progesterone and 17β-estradiol are synthesized as follows: **Theca cells** synthesize and secrete progesterone.

Theca cells also synthesize androstenedione; this androstenedione diffuses from the theca cells to the nearby granulosa cells, which contain 17β-hydroxysteroid dehydrogenase and aromatase. In the **granulosa cells,** androstenedione is converted to testosterone and testosterone is then converted to 17β-estradiol. FSH and LH each have roles in the biosynthetic process. **LH** stimulates cholesterol desmolase in the theca cells, the first step in the biosynthetic pathway (parallel to its role in the testes). **FSH** stimulates aromatase in the granulosa cells, the last step in the synthesis of 17β-estradiol.

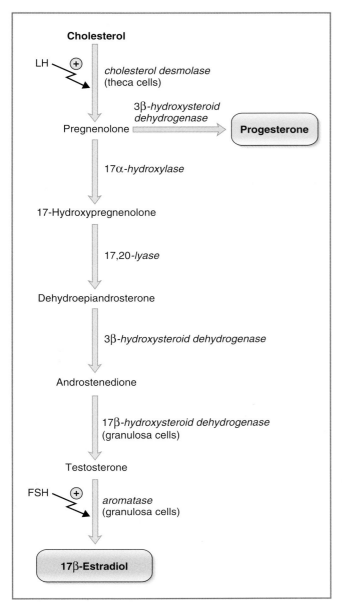

Figure 10–8 **Biosynthetic pathway for progesterone and 17β-estradiol in the ovaries.** Luteinizing hormone (LH) stimulates cholesterol desmolase in theca cells. Follicle-stimulating hormone (FSH) stimulates aromatase in granulosa cells.

Regulation of the Ovaries

As noted, the ovaries have two functions: oogenesis and secretion of the female sex steroid hormones. Both functions are controlled by the hypothalamic-pituitary axis. As in the testes, the hypothalamic hormone is GnRH and the anterior pituitary hormones are FSH and LH.

GnRH

Like testicular function in the male, ovarian function in the female is driven by **pulsatile** activity of the hypothalamic-pituitary axis. GnRH is delivered directly to the anterior lobe of the pituitary in high concentration, where it stimulates pulsatile secretion of FSH and LH. FSH and LH then act on the ovaries to stimulate follicular development and ovulation and to stimulate the synthesis of the female sex steroid hormones.

FSH and LH

To understand the hypothalamic-pituitary control of the ovaries, it is necessary to appreciate its cyclic behavior. Every 28 days a sequence of follicular development, ovulation, and formation and degeneration of a corpus luteum is repeated in the **menstrual cycle.** The first 14 days of the menstrual cycle involve follicular development and are called the **follicular phase.** The last 14 days of the menstrual cycle are dominated by the corpus luteum and are called the **luteal phase.** At the midpoint of the cycle, between the follicular and luteal phases, **ovulation** occurs.

The actions of FSH and LH on follicular development and on ovulation are explained as follows:

◆ **FSH.** The granulosa cells are the only ovarian cells with FSH receptors. Initial actions of FSH stimulate the growth of granulosa cells in primary follicles and stimulate estradiol synthesis. The locally produced estradiol then supports the trophic effect of FSH on follicular cells. Thus, the two effects of FSH on the granulosa cells are mutually reinforcing: more cells, more estradiol, more cells.

◆ **LH.** Ovulation is initiated by LH. Just prior to ovulation, the concentration of LH in blood rises sharply and induces rupture of the dominant follicle, releasing the oocyte. LH also stimulates formation of the corpus luteum, a process called luteinization, and maintains steroid hormone production by the corpus luteum during the luteal phase of the menstrual cycle.

Negative and Positive Feedback

In females, the hypothalamic-pituitary axis is controlled by *both* **negative and positive feedback,** depending on the phase of the menstrual cycle (Fig. 10-9).

◆ In the **follicular phase** of the menstrual cycle, FSH and LH stimulate synthesis and secretion of estradiol by follicular cells. One of the actions of estradiol is *negative* feedback on the anterior pituitary cells to inhibit further secretion of FSH and LH. Thus, the follicular phase is dominated by negative feedback effects of estradiol.

◆ At **midcycle,** the pattern changes. Estradiol levels rise sharply as a result of the proliferation of follicular cells and the stimulation of estradiol synthesis that occurred during the follicular phase. When a

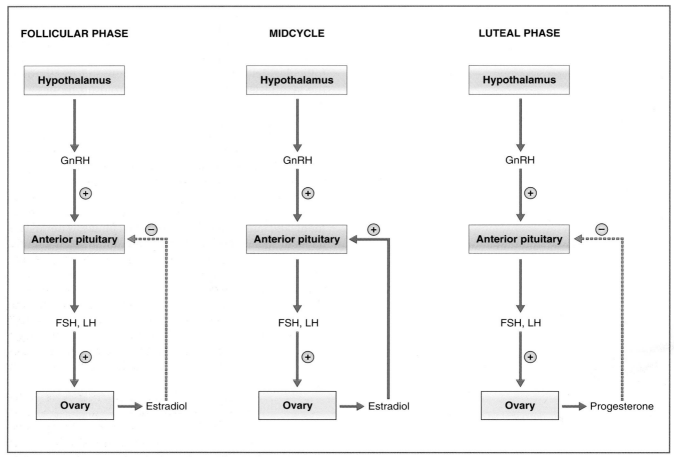

Figure 10–9 **Control of follicle-stimulating hormone (FSH) and luteinizing hormone (LH) secretion in females during the menstrual cycle.** The follicular and luteal phases are characterized by negative feedback of estradiol and progesterone, respectively, on the anterior pituitary. Midcycle is characterized by positive feedback of estradiol on the anterior pituitary. GnRH, Gonadotropin-releasing hormone.

critical level of estradiol is reached (of at least 200 picograms per milliliter of plasma), estradiol has a *positive* feedback effect on the anterior pituitary, by upregulating GnRH receptors in the anterior pituitary, thus causing *further secretion* of FSH and LH. This burst of hormone secretion by the anterior pituitary, called the **ovulatory surge of FSH and LH,** then triggers ovulation of the mature oocyte.

♦ In the **luteal phase** of the menstrual cycle, the major hormonal secretion of the ovaries is progesterone. One of the actions of progesterone is *negative* feedback on the anterior pituitary to inhibit secretion of FSH and LH. Thus, the luteal phase is dominated by negative feedback effects of progesterone.

♦ **Inhibin** is produced by ovarian granulosa cells. As in the testes, it inhibits FSH secretion from the anterior pituitary.

♦ **Activin** is also produced by ovarian granulosa cells and stimulates FSH secretion.

Actions of Estrogen and Progesterone

The physiologic actions of estrogen and progesterone are summarized in Tables 10-2 and 10-3. In general, the two ovarian steroid hormones function in a coordinated fashion to support reproductive activity of the female including development of the ovum, development and maintenance of the corpus luteum to sustain a fertilized ovum, maintenance of pregnancy, and preparation of the breasts for lactation.

Usually, estrogen and progesterone complement or enhance each other's actions in the female reproductive tract. Occasionally, they antagonize or modulate each other's actions. Over the course of the menstrual cycle, estrogen secretion by the ovaries precedes progesterone secretion, preparing the target tissues to respond to progesterone. An example of this "preparation" is seen in the up-regulation of progesterone receptors by estrogen in several target tissues. Without estrogen and its up-regulatory action, progesterone has little biologic activity. Conversely, progesterone

Table 10–2 Actions of Estrogens on Target Tissues

Maturation and maintenance of uterus, fallopian tubes, cervix, and vagina
Responsible at puberty for the development of female secondary sex characteristics
Requisite for development of the breasts
Responsible for proliferation and development of ovarian granulosa cells
Up-regulation of estrogen, progesterone, and LH receptors
Negative *and* positive feedback effects on FSH and LH secretion
Maintenance of pregnancy
Lowering of uterine threshold to contractile stimuli
Stimulation of prolactin secretion
Blocking the action of prolactin on the breast
Decreasing LDL cholesterol
Anti-osteoporosis

FSH, Follicle-stimulating hormone; LDL, low-density lipoproteins; LH, luteinizing hormone.

Table 10–3 Actions of Progesterone on Target Tissues

Maintenance of secretory activity of uterus during luteal phase
Development of the breasts
Negative feedback effects on FSH and LH secretion
Maintenance of pregnancy
Raising uterine threshold to contractile stimuli during pregnancy

FSH, Follicle-stimulating hormone; LH, luteinizing hormone.

down-regulates estrogen receptors in some target tissues, decreasing their responsiveness to estrogen.

Development of the Female Reproductive Tract

At puberty, the ovaries, driven by pulsatile secretion of FSH and LH, begin to secrete estrogen. In turn, estrogen promotes the growth and development of the female reproductive tract: the uterus, fallopian tubes, cervix, and vagina. Progesterone is also active in these tissues, usually increasing their secretory activity. Thus, in the **uterus,** estrogen causes cell proliferation, cell growth, and increased contractility; progesterone increases secretory activity and decreases contractility. In the **fallopian tubes,** estrogen stimulates ciliary activity and contractility, aiding in the movement of sperm toward the uterus; progesterone increases secretory activity and decreases contractility. In the **vagina,** estrogen stimulates proliferation of epithelial cells; progesterone stimulates differentiation but inhibits proliferation of epithelial cells.

Menstrual Cycle

Over the course of the menstrual cycle, estrogen and progesterone are responsible for the changes that occur in the endometrium, cervix, and vagina and are responsible for feedback regulation of FSH and LH secretion by the anterior pituitary.

Based on a "typical" 28-day cycle, the **follicular phase** of the menstrual cycle is the 14-day period preceding ovulation. This phase, which is also called the **proliferative phase,** is dominated by estrogen. 17β-Estradiol, whose secretion increases markedly during this phase, has significant effects on the endometrial lining of the uterus, preparing it for the *possibility* of accepting a fertilized ovum: Estradiol stimulates growth of the endometrium, growth of glands and stroma, and elongation of the spiral arteries, which supply the endometrium. Estradiol also causes the cervical mucus to become copious, watery, and elastic. When spread on a glass slide, cervical mucus from the follicular phase produces a pattern known as "ferning." This characteristic of cervical mucus has physiologic significance: Channels form in the watery mucus, creating openings in the cervix through which sperm can be propelled.

The **luteal phase** of a 28-day menstrual cycle is the 14-day period following ovulation. This phase also is called the **secretory phase** and is dominated by progesterone. Proliferation of the endometrium slows, and its thickness decreases. The uterine glands become more tortuous, accumulate glycogen in vacuoles, and increase their mucus secretions. The stroma of the endometrium becomes edematous. The spiral arteries elongate more and become coiled. Progesterone secretion decreases the quantity of cervical mucus, which then becomes thick and nonelastic and does not "fern" on a slide. (Because the opportunity for fertilization has passed, the cervical mucus need not be penetrable by sperm.)

Breasts

Development of adult breasts is absolutely dependent on estrogen. The breasts, or mammary glands, are composed of lobular ducts lined by a milk-secreting epithelium. Small ducts converge and empty into larger ducts that converge at the nipple. These glandular structures are embedded in adipose tissue. At puberty, with the onset of estrogen secretion, the lobular ducts grow and the area around the nipple, the areola, enlarges. Estrogen also increases the amount of adipose tissue, giving the breasts their characteristic female shape. Progesterone collaborates with estrogen by stimulating secretory activity in the mammary ducts.

Pregnancy

The highest levels of estrogen and progesterone occur during pregnancy, synthesized in early pregnancy by the corpus luteum and in mid-to-late pregnancy by the placenta. Both estrogen and progesterone have multiple roles in pregnancy. Estrogen stimulates growth of the myometrium, growth of the ductal system of the breasts, prolactin secretion, and enlargement of the external genitalia. Progesterone maintains the endometrial lining of the uterus and increases the uterine threshold to contractile stimuli, thus preserving the pregnancy until the fetus is ready to be delivered.

Other Actions of Estrogen and Progesterone

In addition to those actions previously discussed, estrogen contributes to the pubertal growth spurt, closure of the epiphyses at the end of the growth spurt, and the deposition of subcutaneous fat (i.e., female fat distribution). Progesterone has a mild thermogenic action, which increases basal body temperature during the luteal phase of the menstrual cycle. This increase in basal body temperature during the luteal phase is the basis for the "rhythm" method of contraception, in which the increase in temperature can be used retrospectively to determine the time of ovulation.

Events of the Menstrual Cycle

The menstrual cycle recurs approximately every 28 days over the reproductive period of the female: from puberty until menopause. The events of the cycle include development of an ovarian follicle and its oocyte, ovulation, preparation of the reproductive tract to receive the fertilized ovum, and shedding of the endometrial lining if fertilization does not occur. The cycle length can vary from 21 to 35 days, but the average length is 28 days. The variability in cycle length is attributable to variability in the duration of the follicular phase; the luteal phase is constant. The hormonal changes and events of a 28-day menstrual cycle are illustrated in Figure 10-10 and described in the following steps. *By convention, day 0 marks the onset of menses from the previous cycle.*

1. **Follicular or proliferative phase.** The follicular phase occurs from day 0 until day 14. During this period, a primordial follicle develops into a graafian follicle and neighboring follicles become atretic (degenerate or regress). After the neighboring follicles degenerate, the remaining follicle is called the **dominant follicle.** Early in the follicular phase, receptors for FSH and LH are up-regulated in ovarian theca and granulosa cells and the gonadotropins stimulate the synthesis of estradiol. The follicular phase is dominated by **17β-estradiol,** whose levels steadily increase. The high levels of estradiol cause proliferation of the endometrial lining of the uterus and inhibit FSH and LH secretion by the anterior pituitary by negative feedback (see Fig. 10-9).

2. **Ovulation.** Ovulation occurs on day 14 of a 28-day menstrual cycle. Regardless of cycle length, ovulation typically occurs *14 days prior to menses.* For example, in a 35-day cycle, ovulation occurs on day 21, or 14 days before menses; in a 24-day cycle, ovulation occurs on day 10. Ovulation follows a burst of estradiol secretion at the end of the follicular phase: The burst of estradiol has a positive feedback effect on FSH and LH secretion by the anterior pituitary (called the FSH and LH surge). The **FSH and LH surge** then causes ovulation of the mature ovum. At ovulation, cervical mucus increases in quantity and becomes watery and more penetrable by sperm. Estradiol levels decrease just after ovulation, but they will increase again during the luteal phase.

3. **Luteal or secretory phase.** The luteal phase occurs from days 14 to 28, ending with the onset of menses. During the luteal phase, the corpus luteum develops and begins synthesizing estradiol and progesterone. The high levels of **progesterone** during this phase stimulate secretory activity of the endometrium and increase its vascularity. Thus, in the follicular phase, estradiol causes the endometrial lining to proliferate; in the luteal phase, progesterone is preparing the endometrium to receive a fertilized ovum. Basal body temperature increases during the luteal phase because progesterone increases the hypothalamic temperature set-point. The cervical mucus becomes less abundant and thicker, and it is now "too late" for sperm to fertilize the ovum. Late in the luteal phase, if fertilization has not occurred, the corpus luteum regresses. With this regression, the luteal source of estradiol and progesterone is lost, and blood levels of the hormones decrease abruptly.

4. **Menses.** Regression of the corpus luteum and the abrupt loss of estradiol and progesterone cause the endometrial lining and blood to be sloughed (menses or menstrual bleeding). Typically, menses lasts 4 to 5 days, corresponding to days 0 to 4 or 5 of the next menstrual cycle. During this time, primordial follicles for the *next* cycle are being recruited and are beginning to develop.

Pregnancy

If the ovum is fertilized by a sperm, the fertilized ovum begins to divide and will become the fetus. The period of development of the fetus is called **pregnancy** or **gestation,** which, in humans, lasts approximately 40 weeks.

During pregnancy, the levels of estrogen and progesterone increase steadily. Their functions include maintenance of the endometrium, development of the breasts for lactation after delivery, and suppression of the development of new ovarian follicles. In early

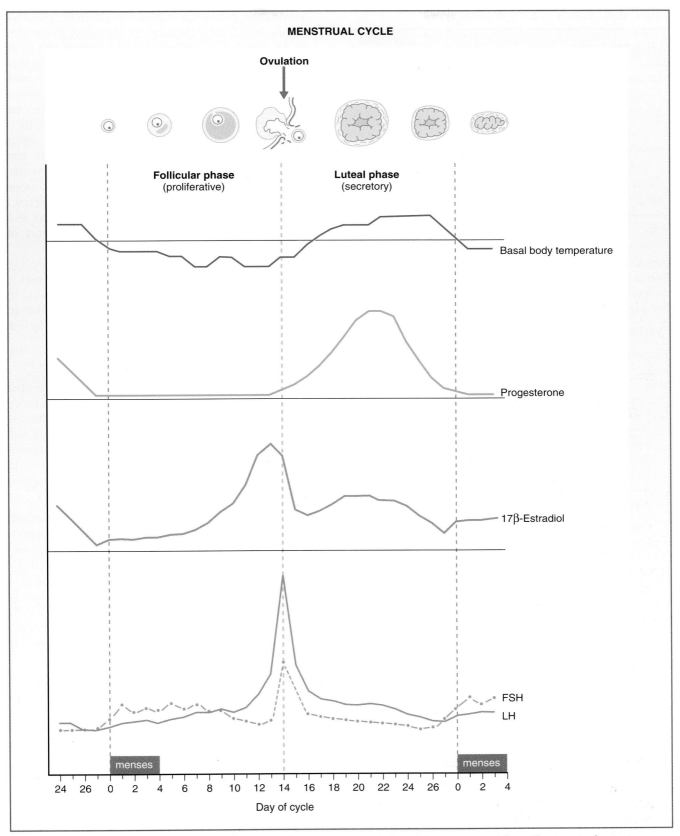

Figure 10–10 Events of the menstrual cycle. Days of the cycle are counted from the onset of menses from the previous cycle. Ovulation occurs on day 14 of a 28-day cycle. FSH, Follicle-stimulating hormone; LH, luteinizing hormone.

Table 10–4 Events of Early Pregnancy

Event	Days after Ovulation
Ovulation	0 day
Fertilization	1 day
Entrance of blastocyst into uterine cavity	4 days
Implantation	5 days
Formation of trophoblast and attachment to endometrium	6 days
Onset of trophoblast secretion of HCG	8 days
HCG "rescue" of corpus luteum	10 days

HCG, Human chorionic gonadotropin.

pregnancy (the first trimester), the source of steroid hormones is the corpus luteum; in mid-to-late pregnancy (the second and third trimesters), the source is the placenta.

Events of Early Pregnancy

The events of early pregnancy are summarized in Table 10-4. The timetable is based on the number of days after ovulation and includes the following steps:

1. **Fertilization** of the ovum takes place within 24 hours of ovulation, in a distal portion of the oviduct called the **ampulla.** Once a sperm penetrates the ovum, the second polar body is extruded and the fertilized ovum begins to divide. Four days after ovulation the fertilized ovum, the **blastocyst,** with approximately 100 cells, arrives in the uterine cavity.

2. **Implantation.** The blastocyst floats freely in the uterine cavity for 1 day and then implants in the endometrium 5 days after ovulation. The receptivity of the endometrium to the fertilized ovum is critically dependent on a **low estrogen/progesterone ratio** and corresponds to the period of highest progesterone output by the corpus luteum. At the time of implantation, the blastocyst consists of an inner mass of cells, which will become the fetus, and an outer rim of cells called the **trophoblast.** The trophoblast invades the endometrium and forms an attachment to the maternal membranes. Thus, the trophoblast contributes the *fetal* portion of the placenta. At the point of implantation, under stimulation by progesterone, the endometrium differentiates into a specialized layer of **decidual cells.** Eventually, the decidua will envelop the entire conceptus. Trophoblastic cells proliferate and form the **syncytiotrophoblast,** whose function is to allow the blastocyst to penetrate deep into the endometrium.

3. **Secretion of HCG and "rescue" of the corpus luteum.** The trophoblast, which will become the placenta, begins secreting human chorionic gonadotropin (HCG) approximately 8 days after ovulation. HCG, which has biologic activity similar to LH, is critical because it "informs" the corpus luteum that fertilization has occurred. The corpus luteum, now under the direction of HCG, continues to synthesize progesterone and estrogen, which maintain the endometrium for implantation. In other words, HCG from the trophoblast (placenta) "rescues" the corpus luteum from regression. (Without fertilization and the stimulation by HCG, the corpus luteum regresses 12 days after ovulation, at which point it stops producing steroid hormones, and menses occurs.) The high levels of estrogen and progesterone also suppress the development of the next cohort of ovarian follicles.

Production of HCG increases dramatically during the first weeks of pregnancy. The **pregnancy test** is based on the excretion of large amounts of HCG in urine, which are measurable. HCG is detectable in maternal urine 9 days after ovulation, even before the next expected menses.

Hormones of Pregnancy

The duration of pregnancy is, by convention, counted from the date of the last menstrual period. Pregnancy lasts approximately 40 weeks from the onset of the last menstrual period, or 38 weeks from the date of the last ovulation. Pregnancy is divided into three trimesters, each of which corresponds to approximately 13 weeks. Hormone levels during pregnancy are depicted in Figure 10-11.

◆ **First trimester.** HCG is produced by the trophoblast, beginning about 8 days after fertilization. As previously described, HCG "rescues" the corpus luteum from regression and, with an LH-like action, stimulates corpus luteal production of progesterone and estrogen. HCG levels are maximal at approximately gestational week 9 and then decline. Although HCG continues to be produced for the duration of pregnancy, its function beyond the first trimester is unclear.

◆ **Second and third trimesters.** During the second and third trimesters, the placenta, in concert with the mother and the fetus, assumes responsibility for production of steroid hormones. The pathways for the synthesis of progesterone and estrogen are shown in Figure 10-12.

Progesterone is produced by the placenta as follows: Cholesterol enters the placenta from the maternal circulation. In the placenta, cholesterol is converted to pregnenolone, which then is converted to progesterone.

Estriol, the major form of estrogen during pregnancy, is produced through a coordinated interplay

HORMONES OF PREGNANCY

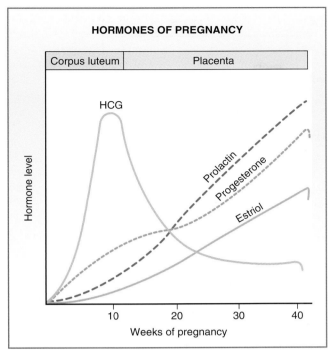

Figure 10–11 **Hormones of pregnancy.** Number of weeks of pregnancy are counted from the onset of the last menses. HCG, Human chorionic gonadotropin.

of the mother and the placenta, and, importantly, requires the fetus. Again, cholesterol is supplied to the placenta from the maternal circulation and is converted to pregnenolone in the placenta. Pregnenolone then enters the fetal circulation and is converted to dehydroepiandrosterone-sulfate (DHEA-sulfate) in the **fetal adrenal cortex.** DHEA-sulfate is hydroxylated to 16-OH DHEA-sulfate in the **fetal liver.** 16-OH DHEA-sulfate then crosses back to the placenta, where a sulfatase enzyme removes sulfate and aromatase converts it to estriol.

Parturition

Parturition, the delivery of the fetus, occurs approximately 40 weeks after the onset of the last menstrual period. The mechanism of parturition is unclear, although roles for estrogen, progesterone, cortisol, oxytocin, prostaglandins, relaxin, and catecholamines have been proposed. The following events occur near term and may contribute to parturition:

♦ Once the fetus reaches a critical size, **distention** of the uterus increases its contractility. Uncoordinated contractions, known as Braxton Hicks contractions, begin approximately 1 month before parturition.

♦ Near term, the fetal hypothalamic-pituitary-adrenal axis is activated and the fetal adrenal cortex produces significant amounts of **cortisol.** Cortisol increases the **estrogen/progesterone ratio,** which

increases the sensitivity of the uterus to contractile stimuli. Recall that estrogen and progesterone have opposite effects on uterine contractility: Estrogen increases contractility, and progesterone decreases it.

♦ Estrogen stimulates (and progesterone inhibits) local production of the **prostaglandins** PGE_2 and PGF_2-α. Thus, the increasing estrogen/progesterone ratio stimulates local prostaglandin production. Prostaglandins increase the intracellular calcium concentration of uterine smooth muscle, thereby increasing its contractility.

♦ The role that **oxytocin** plays in normal parturition is puzzling. Oxytocin is a powerful stimulant of uterine contractions (indeed, it is used to induce labor). Evidence indicates that the uterine oxytocin receptors are up-regulated toward the end of gestation. It is also known that dilation of the cervix, as occurs during the progression of labor, stimulates oxytocin secretion. Yet maternal blood levels of oxytocin *do not* increase near term, leaving the physiologic role of oxytocin uncertain.

There are three stages of **normal labor.** In the **first stage,** uterine contractions originating at the fundus and sweeping downward move the head of the fetus toward the cervix and progressively widen and thin the cervix. In the **second stage,** the fetus is forced through the cervix and delivered through the vagina. In the **third stage,** the placenta separates from the uterine decidual tissue and is delivered. During this last stage, powerful contractions of the uterus also serve to constrict uterine blood vessels and limit postpartum bleeding. After delivery of the placenta, hormone concentrations return to their prepregnant levels, except for prolactin, whose levels remain high if the mother breast-feeds the infant (see Fig. 10-11).

Lactation

Throughout pregnancy, estrogen and progesterone stimulate the growth and development of the breasts, preparing them for lactation. Estrogen also stimulates prolactin secretion by the anterior pituitary, and prolactin levels steadily increase over the course of pregnancy (see Fig. 10-11). However, although prolactin levels are high during pregnancy, lactation *does not* occur because estrogen and progesterone block the action of prolactin on the breast. After parturition, when estrogen and progesterone levels fall precipitously, their inhibitory effects on the breast are removed and lactation can proceed. As described in Chapter 9, lactation is maintained by suckling, which stimulates the secretion of both oxytocin and prolactin.

As long as lactation continues, there is **suppression of ovulation** because prolactin inhibits GnRH secretion

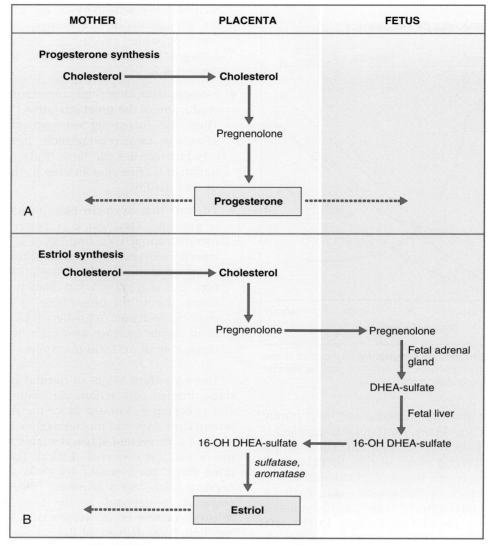

Figure 10–12 **Synthesis of progesterone (A) and estriol (B) during pregnancy.** Progesterone is synthesized entirely by the placenta. Estriol synthesis requires the placenta, the fetal adrenal gland, and the fetal liver. DHEA, Dehydroepiandrosterone.

by the hypothalamus and FSH and LH secretion by the anterior pituitary. Although not 100% effective, breast-feeding is a de facto method of contraception and family spacing in some regions of the world.

Hormonal Contraception

Oral contraceptives contain combinations of estrogen and progesterone or progesterone alone. The combination preparations exert contraceptive effects primarily through negative feedback effects on the anterior pituitary (i.e., by inhibiting FSH and LH secretion, they prevent ovulation). The combination preparations also reduce fertility by changing the character of the cervical mucus so that it is hostile to penetration by sperm and by decreasing the motility of the fallopian tubes. The contraceptive effect of progesterone alone is based

primarily on its effects on cervical mucus and tubal motility.

Higher-dose preparations of estrogen and progesterone inhibit ovulation and may interfere with implantation; these preparations can be used as **postcoital contraceptives,** or "morning after" pills.

Menopause

Menopause is the cessation of menstrual cycles in women, and it occurs at approximately 50 years of age. For several years preceding menopause, anovulatory cycles (menstrual cycles in which ovulation does not occur) become more common and the number of functioning ovarian follicles decreases. Accordingly, estrogen secretion gradually declines and eventually ceases.

Because of the decreased level of estrogen, there is reduced negative feedback on the anterior pituitary and, accordingly, increased secretion and pulsatility of FSH and LH at menopause.

The symptoms of menopause are caused by the loss of the ovarian source of estrogen and include thinning of the vaginal epithelium, decreased vaginal secretions, decreased breast mass, accelerated bone loss, vascular instability ("hot flashes"), and emotional lability. (Because estrogen can be produced from androgenic precursors in adipose tissue, obese women tend to be less symptomatic than nonobese women.) **Estrogen replacement therapy** is aimed at replacing the ovarian source of estrogen, thus minimizing or preventing the symptoms of menopause.

SUMMARY

■ Genetic sex is determined by the sex chromosomes, either XX or XY. Gonadal sex is defined by the presence of testes or ovaries. Phenotypic sex is determined by the hormonal output of the gonads.

■ Puberty in males and females is initiated by the pulsatile secretion of GnRH, which drives the pulsatile secretion of FSH and LH. Pulsatile secretion of FSH and LH drives the testes and ovaries to secrete their respective sex steroid hormones (testosterone, and progesterone and estrogen).

■ In males, the testes are responsible for spermatogenesis and secretion of testosterone. Testosterone is synthesized from cholesterol by the Leydig cells. In some target tissues, testosterone must be converted to dihydrotestosterone by the action of 5α-reductase. Testosterone acts locally to support spermatogenesis, as well as on extratesticular target tissues such as skeletal muscle.

■ Regulation of the testes is via negative feedback effects of testosterone and inhibin on the hypothalamus and anterior pituitary.

■ In females, the ovaries are responsible for oogenesis and secretion of progesterone and estrogen. Progesterone and 17β-estradiol are synthesized from cholesterol by theca and granulosa cells, respectively. Theca cells synthesize progesterone and testosterone, and granulosa cells convert testosterone to 17β-estradiol by the action of aromatase.

■ The menstrual cycle has a follicular (proliferative) phase and a luteal (secretory) phase. The follicular phase is dominated by estrogen, and the luteal phase is dominated by progesterone. Ovulation occurs on day 15 of a 28-day menstrual cycle. If fertilization occurs, the corpus luteum synthesizes steroid hormones to support the developing zygote. If fertilization does not occur, the corpus luteum regresses and menses occurs.

■ Early pregnancy is supported by steroid hormones produced by the corpus luteum, as directed by HCG from the trophoblast. The second and third trimesters of pregnancy are supported by steroid hormones from the placenta. Progesterone, estriol, and prolactin levels increase steadily during pregnancy.

■ Menopause is the cessation of menstrual cycles. During this period, the number of functioning ovarian follicles decreases, estrogen secretion declines, and the circulating levels and pulsatility of FSH and LH secretion increase.

Challenge Yourself

Answer each question with a word, phrase, sentence, or numerical solution. When a list of possible answers is supplied with the question, one, more than one, or none of the choices may be correct. Correct answers are supplied at the end of the book.

1 *In which of the following causes of delayed puberty would pulsatile administration of gonadotropin-releasing hormone (GnRH) be effective: hypothalamic dysfunction; Leydig cell dysfunction; androgen insensitivity syndrome?*

2 *Which step in testosterone synthesis is activated by luteinizing hormone (LH): androstenedione to testosterone; cholesterol to pregnenolone; testosterone to dihydrotestosterone?*

3 *Which steroidogenic enzyme is not present in the gonads: 17α-hydroxylase; 21β-hydroxylase; cholesterol desmolase?*

4 *Which hormone maintains the corpus luteum of pregnancy: LH; human chorionic gonadotropin (HCG); estradiol; progesterone?*

5 *Which of the following organs are needed to synthesize estrogen during the third trimester of pregnancy: corpus luteum; maternal ovaries; placenta; fetal liver; maternal adrenal cortex; maternal liver; fetal adrenal cortex?*

6 *During which period of the menstrual cycle does the dominant follicle produce most of its estrogen: days 1–4; days 5–14; days 15–20; days 21–25; days 26–28?*

7 *During which period of the menstrual cycle does the corpus luteum regress (if fertilization does not occur): days 1–4; days 5–14; days 15–20; days 21–25; days 26–28?*

8 *In a genetic male with deficiency of 5α-reductase, which of the following masculine features is/are present: testes; muscle mass; male hair distribution; epididymis; deepening of the voice?*

9 *Which of the following is present in androgen insensitivity disorder? Male phenotype, testes, increased levels of androgen receptors, vagina.*

10 *Which step in ovarian estradiol synthesis is stimulated by FSH? Cholesterol → pregnenolone, androstenedione → testosterone, testosterone → 17β-estradiol.*

SELECTED READINGS

Pohl CR, Knobil E: The role of the central nervous system in the control of ovarian function in higher primates. Ann Rev Physiol 44:583, 1982.

Veldhuis JD: The hypothalamic-pituitary axis. In Yen SSC, Jaffe RB (eds): Reproductive Endocrinology. Philadelphia, WB Saunders, 1991.

White PC, New MI, Dupont B: Congenital adrenal hyperplasia. N Engl J Med 316:1519, 1987.

Yen SSC: The human menstrual cycle: Neuroendocrine regulation. In Yen SSC, Jaffe RB (eds): Reproductive Endocrinology. Philadelphia, WB Saunders, 1991.

Appendix I
Common Abbreviations and Symbols

ACE	angiotensin converting enzyme		**ERP**	effective refractive period
ACh	acetylcholine		**ERV**	expiratory reserve volume
AchE	acetylcholinesterase		**FRC**	functional residual capacity
ACTH	adrenocorticotropic hormone		**FSH**	follicle-stimulating hormone
ADH	antidiuretic hormone		**GABA**	γ-aminobutyric acid
ADP	adenosine diphosphate		**GDP**	guanosine diphosphate
ANP	atrial natriuretic peptide, or atriopeptin		**GFR**	glomerular filtration rate
ANS	autonomic nervous system		**GHRH**	growth hormone–releasing hormone
ATP	adenosine triphosphate		G_i	inhibitory G protein
ATPase	adenosine triphosphatase		**GIP**	glucose-dependent insulinotropic peptide
AV node	atrioventricular node		**GMP**	guanosine monophosphate
BMR	basal metabolic rate		**GnRH**	gonadotropin-releasing hormone
BTPS	body temperature, pressure, saturated		**GRP**	gastrin-releasing peptide
BUN	blood urea nitrogen		G_s	stimulatory G protein
C	compliance or clearance		**GTP**	guanosine triphosphate
cAMP	cyclic adenosine monophosphate		**HCG**	human chorionic gonadotropin
CCK	cholecystokinin		**HGH**	human growth hormone
cGMP	cyclic guanosine monophosphate		**IC**	inspiratory capacity
CN	cranial nerve		**ICF**	intracellular fluid
CNS	central nervous system		**IGF**	insulin-like growth factor
COMT	catechol-*O*-methyltransferase		IP_3	inositol 1,4,5-triphosphate
COPD	chronic obstructive pulmonary disease		**IPSP**	inhibitory postsynaptic potential
CRH	corticotropin-releasing hormone		λ	length constant
CSF	cerebrospinal fluid		**LH**	luteinizing hormone
DHEA	dehydroepiandrosterone		**MAO**	monoamine oxidase
DIT	diiodotyrosine		**MEPP**	miniature end plate potential
DNA	deoxyribonucleic acid		**MIT**	monoiodotyrosine
DOC	11-deoxycorticosterone		**mRNA**	messenger ribonucleic acid
2,3-DPG	2,3-diphosphoglycerate		**MSH**	melanocyte-stimulating hormone
DPPC	dipalmitoyl phosphatidylcholine		**NE**	norepinephrine
ECF	extracellular fluid		**NO**	nitric oxide
ECG	electrocardiogram		**P**	pressure
EPP	end plate potential		**Pa**	mean arterial pressure
EPSP	excitatory postsynaptic potential		**PAH**	*para*-aminohippuric acid
ER	endoplasmic reticulum		P_B	barometric pressure

PIF	prolactin-inhibiting factor
PIP$_2$	phosphatidylinositol 4,5-diphosphate
PLC	phospholipase C
PNS	peripheral nervous system
POMC	pro-opiomelanocortin
PTH	parathyroid hormone
PTH-rp	parathyroid hormone-related peptide
PTU	propylthiouracil
Q	blood flow or airflow
σ	reflection coefficient
R	resistance
RBF	renal blood flow
RNA	ribonucleic acid
RPF	renal plasma flow
RRP	relative refractory period
RV	residual volume
SA node	sinoatrial node
SERCA	sarcoplasmic and endoplasmic reticulum Ca^{2+} ATPase
SIADH	syndrome of inappropriate antidiuretic hormone

SNP	supranormal period
SR	sarcoplasmic reticulum
SRIF	somatotropin-release inhibiting factor
STPD	standard temperature, pressure, dry
τ	time constant
T$_3$	triiodothyronine
T$_4$	thyroxine
TBG	thyroxine-binding globulin
TBW	total body water
TLC	total lung capacity
T$_m$	transport maximum
TPR	total peripheral resistance
TRH	thyrotropin-releasing hormone
TSH	thyroid-stimulating hormone
TV or V$_T$	tidal volume
V	volume
V̇	urine or gas flow rate
V̇$_A$	alveolar ventilation
VC	vital capacity
VIP	vasoactive inhibitory peptide
VMA	3-methoxy-4-hydroxymandelic acid

Appendix II
Normal Values and Constants

Plasma, Serum, or Blood Concentrations

Substance	Average Normal Value	Range	Comments
Bicarbonate (HCO_3^-)	24 mEq/L	22–26 mEq/L	Venous blood; measured as total CO_2
Calcium (Ca^{2+}), ionized	5 mg/dL		
Calcium (Ca^{2+}), total	10 mg/dL		
Chloride (Cl^-)	100 mEq/L	98–106 mEq/L	
Creatinine	1.2 mg/dL	0.5–1.5 mg/dL	
Glucose	80 mg/dL	70–100 mg/dL	Fasting
Hematocrit	0.45	0.4–0.5	Men, 0.47; women, 0.41
Hemoglobin	15 g/dL		
Hydrogen ion (H^+)	40 nEq/L		Arterial blood
Magnesium (Mg^{2+})	0.9 mmol/L		
Osmolarity	287 mOsm/L	280–298 mOsm/L	Osmolality is mOsm/kg H_2O
O_2 saturation	98%	96%–100%	Arterial blood
P_{CO_2}, arterial	40 mm Hg		
P_{CO_2}, venous	46 mm Hg		
P_{O_2}, arterial	100 mm Hg		
P_{O_2}, venous	40 mm Hg		
pH, arterial	7.4	7.37–7.42	
pH, venous	7.37		
Phosphate	1.2 mmol/L		
Potassium (K^+)	4.5 mEq/L		
Protein, albumin	4.5 g/dL		
Protein, total	7 g/dL	6–8 g/dL	
Sodium (Na^+)	140 mEq/L		
Urea nitrogen (BUN)	12 mg/dL	9–18 mg/dL	Varies with dietary protein
Uric acid	5 mg/dL		

Other Parameters and Values

System	Parameter	Average Normal Value	Comments
Cardiovascular	Cardiac output, rest	5 L/min	
	Cardiac output, exercise	15 L/min	Maximum value
	Stroke volume	80 mL	
	Heart rate, rest	60/min	
	Heart rate, exercise	180/min	Maximum value
	Ejection fraction	0.55	Stroke volume/end diastolic volume
	Systemic arterial pressure (Pa)	100 mm Hg	Systolic, 120 mm Hg
			Diastolic, 80 mm Hg
	Pulmonary arterial pressure	15 mm Hg	Systolic, 25 mm Hg
			Diastolic, 8 mm Hg
	Right atrial pressure	2 mm Hg	
	Left atrial pressure	5 mm Hg	Pulmonary wedge pressure
Respiratory	Barometric pressure (P_B)	760 mm Hg	Sea level
	Water vapor pressure (P_{H_2O})	47 mm Hg	At 37°C
	Total lung capacity	6.0 L	
	Functional residual capacity	2.4 L	
	Vital capacity	4.7 L	
	Tidal volume	0.5 L	
	STPD	273 K, 760 mm Hg	Standard conditions, dry
	BTPS	310 K, 760 mm Hg, 47 mm Hg	Body conditions, saturated
	Solubility of O_2 in blood	0.003 mL O_2/100 mL blood/mm Hg	
	Solubility of CO_2 in blood	0.07 mL CO_2/100 mL blood/mm Hg	
	CO_2 production	200 mL/min	
	O_2 consumption	250 mL/min	
	Respiratory exchange quotient	0.8	CO_2 production/O_2 consumption
	Hematocrit	0.45	
	Hemoglobin concentration	15 g/dL	
	O_2-binding capacity of hemoglobin	1.34 mL O_2/g Hb	At 100% saturation
Renal	Body water, total	60% of body weight	
	Body water, ICF	40% of body weight	
	Body water, ECF	20% of body weight	Interstitial fluid and plasma
	Glomerular filtration rate (GFR)	120 mL/min	Males, 120 mL/min
			Females, 95 mL/min
	Renal plasma flow (RPF)	650 mL/min	Clearance of PAH
	Renal blood flow	1200 mL/min	
	Filtration fraction	0.2	GFR/RPF
	Serum anion gap	10–16 mEq/L	$[Na^+] - ([Cl^-] + [HCO_3^-])$

Weak Acids and Bases	pK	Other Values	
Acetoacetic acid	3.8	Body surface area (for 70-kg man)	1.73 m^2
Ammonia (NH_3/NH_4^+)	9.2	Body weight	70 kg
β-hydroxybutyric acid	4.8	Faraday constant	96,500 coulombs/equivalent
Carbonic acid (HCO_3^-/CO_2)	6.1	Gas constant (R)	0.082 L-atm/mol-K
Creatinine	5.0	2.3 RT/F	60 mV at 37°C
Hemoglobin, deoxygenated	7.9		
Hemoglobin, oxygenated	6.7		
Lactic acid	3.9		
Phosphoric acid ($HPO_4^{-2}/H_2PO_4^-$)	6.8		

Challenge Yourself Answers

CHAPTER 1

1. Solution B, negative; or Solution A, positive
2. 150 mmol/L urea
3. Increases
4. Upstroke of the action potential
5. 25 quanta
6. Botulinus toxin
7. Action potential in nerve fiber; opening Ca^{2+} channels in presynaptic terminal; ACh release from presynaptic terminal; binding of ACh to nicotinic receptors; opening ligand-gated ion channels; MEPP; EPP; action potential in muscle fiber
8. Approximately equal to (Hint: Passive tension is negligible in this range.)
9. Substance P, vasopressin
10. Double (Hint: $\Delta C = 10 - 1 = 9$. If both sides doubled, $\Delta C = 20 - 2 = 18$.)
11. L-Dopa, dopamine, norepinephrine
12. Increasing nerve diameter: increases; increasing internal resistance (R_i): decreases; increasing membrane resistance (R_m): increases; decreasing membrane capacitance (C_m): increases; increasing length constant: increases; increasing time constant: decreases.
13. Depolarizes; causes muscle weakness by closing inactivation gates on Na^+ channels so that they are unavailable to carry Na^+ current for upstroke of muscle action potential
14. Conformational change in myosin that reduces its affinity for actin
15. Nicotinic receptor antagonist; inhibitor of choline reuptake; inhibitor of ACh release
16. Water flows from A to B. (Hint: Calculated π_{eff} of Solution B is higher than that of Solution A, and water flows from low to high π_{eff}.)

CHAPTER 2

1. Dilation of airways; relaxation of bladder wall
2. Muscarinic; sphincter
3. Ganglia in or near target tissues (Hints: All postganglionic neurons have nicotinic receptors; sweat glands have sympathetic cholinergic innervation; all preganglionic neurons are cholinergic.)
4. Inhibits (or blocks); β_1 receptors
5. Effect of epinephrine to increase cardiac contractility; effect of epinephrine to increase heart rate
6. Phenylethanolamine-N-methyltransferase
7. α_1-adrenergic agonist (would constrict vascular smooth muscle, further elevating blood pressure); β_1-adrenergic agonist (would increase heart rate and contractility, further elevating blood pressure)
8. Muscarinic, contraction, muscarinic, relaxation
9. α_q binds to GDP, α_q binds to GTP, activation of phospholipase C, generation of IP_3, release of Ca^{2+} from intracellular stores, activation of protein kinase
10. Slowing of conduction velocity in AV node; gastric acid secretion; erection; sweating on a hot day

CHAPTER 3

1. Right optic nerve
2. To the left (Hint: Postrotatory nystagmus is in the opposite direction of the original rotation.)
3. One
4. Knee-jerk reflex; stretch reflex (Hint: Knee-jerk is an example of stretch reflex.)
5. Phasic

6 Light; conversion of 11-*cis* rhodopsin to all-*trans* rhodopsin; transducin; decreased cyclic GMP; closure of Na^+ channels; hyperpolarization; release of neurotransmitter

7 *More* negative; *decreases* likelihood of action potentials

8 Golgi tendon organs: activated
Ia afferent fibers: unchanged (Hint: Ia afferents are involved in the stretch reflex.)
Ib afferent fibers: activated
Inhibitory interneurons: activated
α motoneurons: inhibited

9 Protein; glucose; K^+

10 Initial rotation to the right—right canal is activated; head stops rotating—left canal is activated.

11 Wider; more compliant; lower

CHAPTER 4

1 mm Hg/mL/min or mm Hg/L/min

2 800 milliseconds (Hint: 60 seconds in a minute)

3 Ventricular action potential; Ca^{2+} release from sarcoplasmic reticulum; Ca^{2+} binding to troponin C; tension; Ca^{2+} accumulation by sarcoplasmic reticulum

4 0.50 (Hint: Heart rate is not needed for the calculation.)

5 Isovolumetric relaxation (Hint: Ventricle is filling during atrial systole.)

6 Increased; increased

7 77 mL (Hint: First, calculate stroke volume from cardiac output and heart rate; then use calculated stroke volume and stated end-diastolic volume to calculate end-systolic volume.)

8 Net filtration; driving force is 9 mm Hg

9 All will decrease.

10 End-diastolic volume (or preload)

11 Increased phosphorylation of phospholamban; increased action potential duration

12 Phase 0

13 Excitability

14 Increased heart rate (Hint: Each change, by itself, leads to increased heart rate.)

15 Heart rate; resistance of cutaneous vascular beds; angiotensin II levels (Hint: Unstressed volume decreases due to venoconstriction.)

16 Decreased radius (Hint: $T = P \times r$. Thus, if P increases, r must decrease to maintain a constant wall tension.)

17 Pulmonary (Hint: Pulmonary blood flow is 100% of cardiac output.)

18 Increased contractility (Hints: End-diastolic volume is preload, and aortic pressure is afterload.)

19 Rapid ventricular ejection

20 Decreased; decreased

21 Decreased cardiac output caused by increased aortic pressure (Hint: Pressure work is more costly than volume work.)

22 Total resistance decreases from 3.33 to 2.5.

23 Blood vessel A (Hint: Velocity = flow/area.)

24 Dicrotic notch: arterial pressure trace
β_1 receptors: sinoatrial node and ventricular muscle
L_{max}: Length-tension curve
Radius to the fourth power: resistance of blood vessels or resistance equation
Phospholamban: sarcoplasmic reticulum
Negative dromotropic effect: AV node
Pulse pressure: arteries or arterial pressure
Normal automaticity: SA node
Ejection fraction: ventricle

25 Rapid ventricular ejection, isovolumetric ventricular relaxation

26 Diameter of splanchnic arterioles, TPR

27 End-systolic volume

28 Sympathetic effect to increase contractility

CHAPTER 5

1 1500 mL

2 Milliliters or liters (Hint: FEV_1 is the volume expired in the first second of forced expiration, not a fractional volume.)

3 547.5 mm Hg (Hint: $[740 - 47] \times 0.79$.)

4 39.3 mL/min/mm Hg (Hint 1: $V_{CO} = D_L \times \Delta P$. Hint 2: P_{CO} in room air = $[P_B - 47 \text{ mm Hg}] \times 0.001$, and P_{CO} in blood is initially zero.)

5 Increased H^+ concentration, increased P_{CO_2}, increased 2,3-diphosphoglycerate (DPG) concentration (Hint: Increased P_{50} = right shift.)

6 None of changes listed causes a change in O_2-binding capacity of hemoglobin. (Hint: O_2-binding capacity is the milliliter of O_2 bound to 1 g of hemoglobin at 100% saturation. Right- and left-shifts change the percent saturation but do not alter the amount of O_2 that can be bound at 100% saturation.)

7 P_{O_2} is decreased and P_{CO_2} is increased.

8 $P_{A_{O_2}}$

9 Blood flow, ventilation, P_{CO_2}

10 $\dot{V}/\dot{Q}$ defects, fibrosis, right-to-left shunt

11 Inspiratory capacity

12 Vital capacity, FEV_1 (Hint: FEV_1/FVC is decreased in obstructive but increased in restrictive.)

13 3.5 L/minute (Hints: Calculate V_D first as 200 mL. Several of the given values are not needed for the calculation.)

14 FRC increases.

15 Airway pressure = +15 cm H_2O and intrapleural pressure = +20 cm H_2O.

16 High altitude

17 Decreased $P_{I_{O_2}}$, decreased $P_{A_{O_2}}$, decreased $P_{a_{O_2}}$, hyperventilation, decreased $P_{a_{CO_2}}$, increased pH

18 FEV_1: forced vital capacity curve or measurement
$\dot{V}/\dot{Q}$ = 0: lung region where there is airway obstruction, or shunt
$P_A > P_a$: apex of lung
Afterload of right ventricle: pulmonary artery or pulmonary arterial pressure
γ chains: fetal hemoglobin
P_{50}: O_2-hemoglobin dissociation curve
Slope of pressure-volume curve: compliance
Normal pressure lower than P_B: intrapleural space
D_L: alveolar/pulmonary capillary barrier
$P_{O_2} < 60$ mm Hg stimulates breathing: peripheral chemoreceptors, or carotid bodies

19 Equal to systemic arterial P_{O_2}

20 Decrease

CHAPTER 6

1 Efferent arteriole

2 At all plasma glucose concentrations below threshold

3 Oncotic pressure is increased. (Hint: More fluid filtered out of glomerular capillaries leads to increased plasma protein concentration.)

4 Below T_m (Hint: Below T_m, the assumption that renal vein PAH ≈ 0 is correct.)

5 306.7 mOsm/L (Hints: New total body water = 45 L; NaCl dissociates into two particles; new total body osmoles = 13,800 mOsm.)

6 Unchanged (Hint: If GFR is constant and urine flow rate increases, urine inulin concentration decreases.)

7 Increased

8 Bowman's space or early proximal convoluted tubule (Hint: $[TF/P]_{inulin}$ is lowest before any water reabsorption has occurred.)

9 Bowman's space or early proximal convoluted tubule

10 Decreased (Hint: Na^+-K^+-$2Cl^-$ cotransporter is required for countercurrent multiplication, which establishes corticopapillary gradient.)

11 Central diabetes insipidus

12 Decreased

13 mg/min (or amount/time)

14 Decreased

15 Lack of insulin, spironolactone, hyperosmolarity

16 Inhibition of Na^+-phosphate cotransport, decreased urinary Ca^{2+} excretion

17 Net reabsorption, 1100 mg/min

18 Midpoint of distal convoluted tubule or early distal tubule

19 Clearance of PAH below T_m (Hints: Clearance of glucose below threshold is zero; clearance of inulin is GFR; clearance of PAH below T_m is RPF.)

20 K^+ on a very high-potassium diet, inulin, Na^+, HCO_3^-, glucose (below threshold)

CHAPTER 7

1 Weak acid "A"

2 7.9 mEq/L

3 Increased (Hint: compensatory hyperventilation for metabolic acidosis.)

4 Diarrhea, salicylate overdose, chronic renal failure

5 Loop diuretics, thiazide diuretics (Hint: Carbonic anhydrase inhibitors and K^+-sparing diuretics produce metabolic acidosis.)

6 Metabolic acidosis; anion gap is 29 mEq/L.

7 mOsm/L

8 Vomiting, morphine overdose, obstructive lung disease, hyperaldosteronism

9 Filtration of HCO_3^- across glomerular capillaries; Na^+-H^+ exchange; conversion of HCO_3^- to H_2CO_3; conversion of H_2CO_3 to CO_2 and H_2O; conversion of H_2CO_3 to H^+ and HCO_3^-; facilitated diffusion of HCO_3^-

10 70 mEq/day

11 The patient with chronic respiratory acidosis will have the higher HCO_3^- and the higher pH (closer to normal).

12 No; metabolic acidosis and respiratory acidosis

13 Decreases (toward normal)

14 Filtered load of HPO_4^{-2} (Hints: Amount of H^+ in the urine is determined by urinary buffers; urine pH is free H^+ concentration, not amount of H^+. Most NH_3 in urine is synthesized in proximal tubule cells, not filtered.)

15 Diabetic ketoacidosis

CHAPTER 8

1 Contraction of the gallbladder, stimulation of HCO_3^- secretion, stimulation of pancreatic enzyme secretion

2 Decreased intracellular cyclic AMP levels

3 Less negative (Hint: Membrane potentials are expressed as intracellular potential with respect to extracellular potential.)

4 Absorption of more solute than water

5 Increases cyclic AMP levels, activates α_s subunit of GTP-binding protein

6 Sucrose

7 Emulsification of lipids in the intestinal lumen, action of pancreatic lipase, micelles, formation of cholesterol ester, chylomicrons

8 HCO_3^-

9 Trypsinogen to trypsin, procarboxypeptidase to carboxypeptidase

10 Duodenum

11 Gastrin secretion: G cells or gastric antrum
Na$^+$–bile salt cotransport: ileum
H$^+$-K$^+$ ATPase: gastric parietal cells
Intrinsic factor secretion: gastric parietal cells
Omeprazole action: H$^+$-K$^+$ ATPase in gastric parietal cells
Na$^+$-glucose cotransporter: apical (luminal) membrane of intestinal epithelial cells
Secondary bile acids (or bile salts): intestinal lumen

12 Inhibition of H$^+$-K$^+$ ATPase

13 Increased body fat, increased insulin levels

14 Contraction of circular muscle, action of acetylcholine on circular muscle

CHAPTER 9

1 Cortisol: Decreased
ACTH: Increased
Blood glucose: Decreased

2 ADH: Increased
Urine osmolarity: Decreased, or dilute or hyposmotic

3 Serum K$^+$: Decreased
Blood pressure: Increased
Renin: Decreased (Hint: Increased blood pressure inhibits renin secretion.)

4 ACTH: Increased
Cortisol: Increased
Blood glucose: Increased

5 Serum Ca^{2+}: Decreased
Serum phosphate: Increased
Urinary cyclic AMP: Decreased

6 Prolactin: Increased
ADH: Decreased
Serum osmolarity: Increased (Hint: due to decreased ADH)
PTH: No change

7 T$_4$: Decreased
TSH: Increased
Basal metabolic rate: Decreased
T$_3$ resin uptake: Decreased (Hint: due to decreased T$_3$ levels)

8 ACTH: Increased
Cortisol: Decreased
Deoxycorticosterone (DOC): Decreased
Aldosterone: Decreased
Dehydroepiandrosterone (DHEA): Increased (Hint: shunting of intermediates toward adrenal androgens)
Urinary 17-ketosteroids: Increased

9 ACTH: Decreased
Cortisol: Decreased (Hint: decreased secretion of *endogenous* cortisol)

10 Serum Ca^{2+}: Increased
PTH: Decreased (Hint: Increased serum Ca^{2+} inhibits endogenous PTH secretion.)

11 Blood pressure: Increased (Hint: Mineralocorticoids accumulate to left of block.)
Blood glucose: Decreased
DHEA: Decreased
Aldosterone: Decreased (Hint: Excess deoxycorticosterone and corticosterone cause increased blood pressure, which inhibits renin secretion.)

CHAPTER 10

1 Hypothalamic dysfunction

2 Cholesterol to pregnenolone

3 21β-hydroxylase

4 HCG

5 Placenta; fetal liver; fetal adrenal cortex

6 Days 5–14

7 Days 26–28

8 Testes; muscle mass; epididymis; deepening of the voice

9 Male phenotype, testes, vagina

10 Testosterone → 17β-estradiol

Index

Page numbers followed by *f* indicate figures; *t*, tables; *b*, boxes.